THE COMPLETE CARB COUNTER FOR DIABETES

YOUR ESSENTIAL COMPANION TO
CARBOHYDRATES GRAMS COUNTING FOR A
BETTER DIABETES MEAL PLANNING

DR. H. MAHER

Medical Disclaimer: Because each individual is different and has particular dietary needs or restrictions, the dieting and nutritional information provided in this book does not constitute professional advice and is not a substitute for expert medical advice. Individuals should always check with a doctor before undertaking "a dieting, weight loss, or exercise regimen and should continue only under a doctor's supervision. While we provide the advice and information in this book in the hopes of helping individuals improve their overall health, multiple factors influence a person's results, and individual results may vary. When a doctor's advice to a particular individual conflicts with advice provided in this book, that individual should always follow the doctor's advice. Patients should not stop taking any of their medications without the consultation of their physician.

CONTENTS

Introduction   vii

PART I
CARB COUNTING AND HEALTHY DIET FOR DIABETES

1. Diabetes Overview   3
2. Adhering to a diabetes healthy lifestyle   10
3. Food, Weight Loss and Diabetes   14
4. The Glycemic Index Diet Explained   21
5. Carb Counting and Glycemic Index   28
6. Eating Low Glycemic and Anti-Inflammatory Foods   32
7. Avoiding High Glycemic and Inflammatory Foods   38
8. Eating Whole and minimally Processed foods   42
9. Food Processing Classification: Overview   56
10. Understanding the Food Nutrition Labels   66

PART II
THE CARBS AND CALORIES COUNTER FOR OVER 12000 FOODS

11. Baked Foods   73
12. Beans and Lentils   159
13. Beverages   204
14. Breakfast Cereals   255
15. Dairy and Egg Products   294
16. Fast Foods   332
17. Fats and Oils   406
18. Fish and Seafood   430
19. Fruits & Fruits Products   467
20. Grains and Pasta   508
21. Meats and Poultry   523
22. Nuts and Seeds   547
23. Prepared Meals   563
24. Restaurant Foods   641
25. Snacks   653

26. Soups and Sauces   682

27. Spices and Herbs   734

28. Vegetables & vegetables products   740

Health and Nutrition Websites   779

INTRODUCTION

Diabetes is a chronic metabolic illness marked by unsuitable hyperglycemia due to a lack of insulin or insulin resistance. Its adverse health effects can significantly reduce life expectancy. Several lifestyle factors and dietary habits affect the incidence of type 1 and type 2 diabetes, such as types and amounts of food ingested, weight gain, obesity, physical activity, watching TV or sedentary time, sleep quality.

Carb, or carbohydrates counting, means that you keep track of the carbohydrates in all your meals, snacks, and drinks. Carb counting is an essential tool for people with diabetes that help them match their activity level and medicines to the food they eat. For many people with diabetes, carbs counting is used as the primary tool to manage their blood sugar efficiently, which can also help them:

- avoid high spikes in blood sugar levels
- stay healthy longer, and/or reduce the severity of some diabetes complications
- improve their quality of life.

- prevent diabetes complications such as eye disorders, kidney disease, foot ulcers, heart disease, and stroke

The carb counting diet for diabetes is a targeted balanced diet with sufficient and right nutritional elements to battle diabetes, prevent diabetes complications, lower inflammation, improve mental health, and help you lose weight. Both nutritional deficiency and excess are tied with diseases and poor health conditions. Nutritional excess, particularly in highly-processed foods, refined carbohydrates, saturated fats, trans-fatty acids, sugar-sweetened foods, and sodium, can result in severe diabetes complications, poor glycemic control, cardiovascular disease, bone disorders, as well as obesity. In contrast, nutritional deficiencies can lead to impairments of body function, weight loss, fatigue, and conditions associated with vitamin and mineral deficiencies.

How many carbs should I eat?

Eating to lower the levels of blood sugar is not a one-size-fits-all approach. Different people, even twins, may respond to the same foods very differently because everyone's body is different. The amount of carbohydrates you can eat and stay in your target blood glucose range depends closely on several factors including your age, weight, and activity level.

On average, people with diabetes should target to get nearly half of their calories from carbohydrates. Thus, if you normally consume about 1,900 calories a day to maintain a healthy weight, then you have to aim to eat about 900-1000 calories from carbs. Considering that carbs provide 4 calories per gram, fat provides 9 calories per gram, and protein provides 4 calories per gram, you have to eat 225-250 grams of carb a day.

In order to keep your blood sugar levels stable throughout the day, you should eat nearly the same amount of carbs at each meal.

This book is based on the USDA (U.S. Department of Agriculture) National Nutrient Database for Standard Reference SR11-SR28, Release 28, which is the primary source of food composition data in the United States. It is designed to help you count carbohydrates and calories accurately and easily. Alphabetical listings make locating your foods easy and quick. Foods are divided into 19 categories:

- Beverages
- Baby Foods
- Baked Foods
- Beans and Lentils
- Breakfast Cereals
- Dairy and Egg Products
- Fast Foods
- Fats and Oils
- Fish & Seafood
- Fruits & Fruits Products
- Grains and Pasta
- Meats and Poultry
- Nuts and Seeds
- Prepared Meals
- Restaurant Foods
- Snacks
- Soups and Sauces
- Spices and Herbs
- Vegetables & vegetable products

PART I

CARB COUNTING AND HEALTHY DIET FOR DIABETES

1

DIABETES OVERVIEW

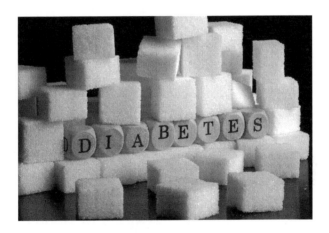

Diabetes is a chronic metabolic illness marked by unsuitable hyperglycemia due to a lack of insulin or insulin resistance. Its adverse health effects can seriously reduce life expectancy significantly by ten years. Several lifestyle factors and dietary habits affect the incidence of type 1 and type 2 diabetes, such as types and amounts of food ingested, weight gain, obesity, physical activity, watching TV or sedentary time, sleep quality.

Diabetes mellitus refers to a chronic disease that influences how the body utilizes food for energy and is marked by abnormally high blood glucose levels. Insulin — the hormone made by the pancreas — allows glucose to get into body cells to provide energy. When blood sugar levels rise after eating, your pancreas releases a sufficient amount of insulin into the blood. Insulin then reduces blood sugar to keep it in the normal range. In people who have diabetes, the pancreas cannot perform this fundamental function, or the body's cells do not respond adequately to the produced insulin. The blood sugar level then increases, and sugar accumulates in the body and becomes toxic to the vital organs. Having a high glucose level in the blood can cause severe health problems. It can cause severe damages to the eyes, kidneys, heart, and nerves irreversibly.

Diabetes Mellitus is the most common chronic endocrine disorder caused mainly by inflammation according to recent high-quality research. There are three main types of diabetes:

- 1. Type 1 diabetes

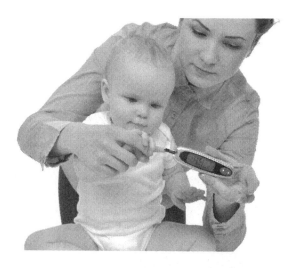

Type 1 diabetes is a chronic autoimmune disease characterized by the immune system's destruction of insulin-producing pancreatic *beta* cells. The body will no longer make insulin due to irreversible damages to the insulin-producing cells. Without insulin hormones, glucose can not get into the body's cells and the blood glucose increases above normal. People with type 1 must then inject daily insulin doses and follow a strict diet to stay alive and prevent the severe adverse effect. Type 1 diabetes generally appears in children and young adults but may occur at any age.

In 2016, the U.S. Food and Drug Administration (FDA) approved artificial pancreas to replace the manual blood glucose checking and the injection of insulin shots. These automated devices act like your real pancreas in controlling blood sugar and releasing insulin when the patient's blood sugar becomes too high. The artificial pancreas also releases a small flow of insulin continuously.

Symptoms of type 1 diabetes are serious and usually happen quickly, over a few days to weeks. Symptoms can include

- frequent thirst and urination
- increased hunger
- unexplained weight loss
- blurred vision
- frequent infections
- fatigue and tiredness

Unfortunately, type 1 diabetes is chronic immune-mediated and remains incurable. However, as you'll see in the chapter, "Vitamin D Optimal Doses", you will be able to improve the management of the disease significantly and prevent the development of diabetes-related chronic diseases.

- 2. Type 2 diabetes

Prediabetes. Even if a person is not sick, he may suffer from prediabetes without knowing it. This term refers to an intermediate stage characterized by an abnormally higher blood glucose level than usual. That represents a warning signal that informs people with prediabetes diagnosis that they are at increased risk of type 2 diabetes mellitus if they don't take appropriate and urgent action, especially if they have other risk factors, including:

- overweight,
- obesity,
- sedentary lifestyle,
- high blood pressure.

In Type 2 diabetes, the mechanism is different from type 1 diabetes: insulin is normally secreted by the pancreas but with lower efficiency. Therefore, without sufficient insulin, the glucose stays in the blood. Type 2 diabetes is induced by several factors, including lifestyle factors, strict diets, overweight, obesity, Hyperthyroidism, and genes.

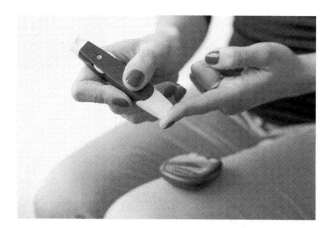

Type 2 diabetes can also develop at any age. However, it's more common after the age of forty.

- **3. Gestational diabetes**

Gestational diabetes is the high blood sugar that develops during pregnancy in women who did not have diabetes before becoming pregnant. Gestational diabetes is more frequent in the second or third trimester but can occur at any time of pregnancy and usually disappears after giving birth.

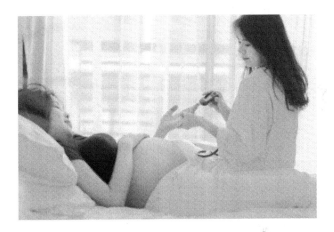

Women diagnosed with it are at higher risk of developing type 2 diabetes later in life, particularly for women with favoring factors (obesity, imbalanced diet, sedentary lifestyle, metabolic syndrome...).

Symptoms

Diabetes symptoms may vary depending on the level of blood sugar. Some people with prediabetes or type 2 diabetes may not experience frank symptoms at first. Conversely, with type 1 diabetes, symptoms come on quickly and severely.

Bellow a list of common symptoms and signs of type 1 and type 2 diabetes, and gestational diabetes:

- increased craving
- frequent urination
- excessive hunger
- weight loss
- ketones in urine
- fatigue and tiredness
- increased irritability
- blurred vision
- slow-healing wounds and cuts
- frequent infections

- ## 4. The A1C Test and Diabetes

The A1C test (also called hemoglobin A1C or HbA1c test) is a blood test that measures the average levels of your blood sugar over the past two to three months. The A1C test is one of the commonly used tests to diagnose the risk of prediabetes or type 2 diabetes. The A1C test is the main tool for diabetes management, as patients use it to achieve their individual A1C goals.

How does the test work?

The A1C (HbA1c) test measures the amount of sugar in your blood that is attached to hemoglobin, a protein inside your red blood cells that carries oxygen. When sugar enters your bloodstream, it binds with hemoglobin. The A1C (HbA1c) test measures the percentage of your red blood cells that are coated with glucose. Thus, a higher A1C (HbA1c) level indicates poor blood glucose control and warns of an elevated risk of developing severe diabetes complications.

If you have a diabetes condition, you should get an A1C (HbA1c) test at least twice a year to make sure diabetes is under close control and your blood glucose is in your target range.

Interpreting the A1C results

A normal A1C (HbA1c) level is under 5.7%. In healthy people, the normal range for the A1c (HbA1c) level is in the range of 4% to 5.6%

A level of A1C (HbA1c) in the range of 5.7% to 6.4% indicates prediabetes and a higher chance of developing diabetes.

A level of A1C (HbA1c) equal to or high than 6.5% indicates diabetes.

2

ADHERING TO A DIABETES HEALTHY LIFESTYLE

Over time, having an excess of sugar in your blood can cause complications ranging from mild to severe. Diabetes complications are often interrelated, share the same contributing causes, and combine in a dangerous way that may alter the overall health condition. For example, nearly 50% of all patients diagnosed with type 2 diabetes have high blood pressure (hypertension), which may constrict and narrow the blood vessels throughout the body, including the nerves, the eyes, and the kidney. On the other side, having high levels of glucose in your blood for a prolonged time can harm blood vessels that supply oxygen throughout your body, including the eyes, heart, kidneys, and brain. Damages that occur can lead to severe and long-term complications.

Diabetes also induces significant quantitative changes in the amount of circulating lipids characterized by an increase in triglycerides (a type of lipid in the blood), a reduction in HDL cholesterol (good), and an increase in LDL cholesterol (bad). These changes are associated with an increased risk of heart disease and stroke.

The main complications of diabetes

Diabetes complications are long-term problems that develop gradually. Diabetes complications can lead to severe damage if untreated.

- diabetic retinopathy. People with diabetes are at risk of developing an eye disorder called retinopathy due to elevated high blood pressure. Retinopathy can affect patients' eyesight and cause partial vision loss and blindness.
- diabetic foot ulcers. Foot problems are severe diabetes complications that result from concomitant actions, including damages to the nerve and impaired blood circulation. Nerve damages known as diabetic neuropathy combined with reduced blood flow affect the feeling in your feet and make it difficult for sores and cuts to heal. In some serious cases, gangrenes develop and can lead to amputation.
- diabetic nephropathy. This severe diabetes complication is common among type 1 and types 2 diabetes patients who poorly control their blood glucose. Over time, uncontrolled diabetes can lead to irreversible damages to blood vessel clusters that filter waste and extra water out of your blood. This severe condition can lead to kidney damage and kidney failure. Your kidneys are also involved in the control of blood pressure, and such damages may cause hypertension which in turn worsen kidney diseases.
- heart disease and stroke. Over time, high blood glucose can harm blood vessels and nerves that control your heart and supply oxygen to the brain and heart. Individuals with diabetes are at higher risk of developing heart disease and strokes.
- erectile dysfunction. Poor and prolonged blood glucose control may damage nerves and small blood vessels that control the erection.
- chronic inflammatory diseases. Poorly controlled diabetes

may cause damage to the whole body, trigger and worsen inflammation. In turn, inflammation causes and aggravates insulin resistance leading to much-elevated blood glucose levels.

A healthy lifestyle

Adhering to the carb counting diet for diabetes is more than selecting foods you eat, restricting your carbohydrates intake, and avoiding high glycemic index foods; it's also about sticking to the proper lifestyle that promotes better diabetes management, healthier life, and well-being. Thus, you have to focus simultaneously on your diet and lifestyle to reap all benefits of the carb counting diet for diabetes and improve your blood sugar control.

You can only focus on diet and keep your habits, but you'll not experience optimum health and win your battle against diabetes. The two significant areas in which change is highly advised are physical activity and sleeping habits. Practicing regular physical activity will drive many beneficial effects in improving blood sugar control and insulin sensitivity. It will also help you prevent, delay, and reduce morbidities and complications associated with diabetes Mellitus. Sleeping well helps your body and brain function correctly, boost your immune system, improve your mental health, and can improve your diabetes management and prevent, or delay, diabetes complications. By committing to these easy and positive changes, you will expect to achieve better blood glucose control, positive health outcomes, and prevent diabetes complications.

Based on the best and latest science of how and what to eat, the diabetes glycemic index lifestyle is meant to be your global road map for managing diabetes, which is the key to preventing, reducing, or delaying complications. You are advised to use "ABCDEs of diabetes" as a way to manage your new diabetes glycemic index lifestyle:

- A- A stands for A1C, or HbA1c test, which assesses your blood glucose control over the past two to three months. So, get a regular A1C (HbA1c) test to measure your average blood glucose and target to stay under 7% as much as possible.
- B- B refers to blood pressure. Nearly half of people with type 2 diabetes suffer from hypertension. Try to keep your blood pressure below 130/80 mm Hg (or 140/90 mm Hg in some cases).
- C- C refers to cholesterol. Total blood cholesterol, HDL cholesterol (good), LDL cholesterol (bad), and triglycerides levels should be monitored. Your doctor will use the information and, if needed, develop a strategy to reduce your risks.
- D- D refers to diet. It refers to adhering to the carb counting diet for diabetes and, if indicated, drug therapy. Your doctor may prescribe medicines that may help you lower your blood glucose, blood pressure (if applicable), cholesterol, and triglyceride levels (if applicable).
- E- E refers to exercice. You should practice regular physical activities for at least 150 minutes per week (e.g., 30 minutes, 6 days a week).

3

FOOD, WEIGHT LOSS AND DIABETES

Eating to lower the levels of blood sugar is not a one-size-fits-all approach. Different people, even twins, may respond to the same foods very differently. However, following the diabetic carb counting dietary pattern will ensure you get the most of its beneficial effects. People who adhere to this diet more closely have consistently lower levels of blood sugar levels, lower blood pressure, increased LDL cholesterol, reduced HDL cholesterol, and reduced triglycerides than those following other diets. It is considered healthier than modern fad diets (e.g., keto diet, low-carb, high-fat diets) because it is centered around controlling carbohydrates intakes, eating whole, unprocessed, or minimally processed foods, and avoiding high glycemic foods and pro-inflammatory agents.

- **Diet, Weight Loss, and Diabetes**

For years, hundreds of diets have been created with a lot of promises in terms of weight loss, inflammation reduction, diabetes reversal. Low-fat diets, low carb high fats diets were thought to be the best approaches to lose weight, control diabetes, and achieve a healthy weight. However, a growing body of evidence shows that these diets often don't work:

- low-fat diets have the tendency to replace fat with easily digested carbohydrates.
- low-carb high-fat diets overlook the importance of carbohydrates and often replace carbohydrates with highly processed fat-containing foods.
- fad diets often overlook the body's fundamental need for a balanced diet

The best diets, those that work, restrict calories to some extent, supply sufficient and high-quality nutrients, banish bad foods, and balance hormones that help lower your blood sugar, improve your glycemic control, and regulate your weight. Diets do this in three main ways:

1. getting you to eat sufficient good foods and/or banish bad ones
2. getting you aware of foods and nutrients you should include in your diet to achieve weight loss, better diabetes control, and prevent complications.
3. changing some of your bad eating habits and the ways you consider highly processed foods and refined carbohydrates

The best diet for losing weight and/or diabetes control is one that is good for all body parts, from your brain to your heart to your pancreas. It is also a diet you can embrace and live with for a long time. In other words, a powerful diet rooted in nature that offers a flexible eating pattern, provides healthy choices, banishes unhealthy foods, and doesn't require an extensive (and probably expensive) shopping list or supplements.

A diabetic balanced diet with sufficient and right nutritional elements is critical for battling diabetes, weight gain, and obesity. Both nutritional deficiency and excess are tied with diseases and poor health conditions. Nutritional excess, particularly in highly-processed foods, refined carbohydrates, saturated fats, trans-fatty acids, sugar-sweetened foods, and sodium, can result in severe chronic inflammatory illnesses such as autoimmune disease, cardiovascular disease, bone disorders, diabetes as well as obesity. In contrast, nutritional deficiencies can lead to impairments of body function, weight loss, fatigue, and conditions associated with vitamin and mineral deficiencies.

One diet that allows that is a Low glycemic type diet. Such a diet—and its many variations—usually include:

- several servings of plant foods (e.g., vegetables, fruits) a day
- whole and minimally processed foods
- daily serving of seeds and nuts
- healthy fats and oils high in omega-3 fatty acids (canola, cod liver oil, fatty fish, flaxseed oil, Walnut oil, sunflower oil, etc.)
- lean protein mainly from fish, poultry, and nuts
- limited amounts of red meat
- limited amounts of sodium
- very limited quantities of refined carbohydrates (e.g., white flour, white, rice, white sugar, brown sugar, honey, corn syrup)
- limited alcoholic drinks
- NO high glycemic index foods
- NO trans fats
- NO highly processed foods

- **Dietary carbohydrates and diabetes**

Increased intake of carbohydrates-containing foods with a higher glycemic index is found to cause a high spike in blood sugar and insulin release, making it harder to control diabetes, increasing the risk of developing diabetes for healthy people, increasing the risk of severe complications, and worsening inflammation. Conversely, eating carbohydrates-containing foods with a low glycemic index is associated with positive health outcomes, including modulating inflammation, regulating immune system responses, and will help you gain close control over your blood sugar.

In addition, many studies have established that the quality of carbohydrates has a significant impact on inflammation, and the occurrence of diabetes complications. Low-quality carbohydrates such as highly processed foods and refined carbs are associated with increased inflammation, both acute and chronic, impaired immune system responses, poor blood glucose control, and increased risk of diabetes complications. Conversely, high-quality foods such as whole foods or minimally processed food with low glycemic index food are linked with better health outcomes, including better control of blood glucose, and reduced acute and chronic inflammation.

- **Dietary fats and diabetes**

Another important nutrient you should consider as part of a carb counting diet for diabetes is fat. Eating the right amount of the right type of fat is essential whether you are managing diabetes or aiming to achieve a healthy weight.

In addition, fats are higher in calories per gram compared to proteins or carbohydrates. A gram of dietary fat has nearly 9 calories, while a gram of carbohydrate has roughly 4 calories or protein has about 4 calories. Thus, you should be aware of serving sizes when eating fats.

Eating the right types of fat is also critical for managing type 1 and type 2 diabetes and lowering the risk of developing some chronic diseases such as heart illnesses, strokes, kidneys diseases, and chronic inflammatory diseases.

Several studies have established that replacing trans fats and saturated fats with unsaturated fats (monounsaturated and polyunsaturated) reduces the risk of cardiovascular diseases in high-risk populations, including individuals with diabetes.

In addition, studies also found that replacing trans fats and saturated fat intake with low glycemic carbohydrates (e.g., wholegrain, fiber-rich fruits, fiber-rich vegetables, beans) results in cardiovascular benefits without altering the blood glucose control.

On the other side, a growing body of evidence has revealed how dietary fat intake affects the inflammatory status and focused on the gut microbiome as an important factor explaining the increase of inflammation biomarkers and fat intake. Trans fats are tied with various adverse health effects, worsen inflammation, and trigger some diabetes complications. The consumption of high amounts of saturated fats increases the LDL cholesterol (bad form) promotes and aggravates inflammation.

The American Diabetes Association recommends swapping saturated and trans fats in your diet by healthiest choices such as monounsaturated and polyunsaturated fats.

Healthy fats such as omega-3 fatty acids are associated with decreased inflammation and reduced risk of developing some chronic conditions. Several studies have investigated the role of omega-3 fatty acids in association with metformin to reduce triglyceride levels in diabetic patients with hypertriglyceridemia. Omega-3 fatty acids were found effective in reducing the triglyceride level significantly by 20-65%. Omega-3 fatty acids were also found to improve the effectiveness of statins and thus decrease the risk of cardiovascular diseases among diabetic patients with hypertriglyceridemia.

• **The Essential Role of Vitamin D**

It is established that Vitamin D is essential for normal glucose metabolism and improvement of insulin sensitivity. Therefore, vitamin D supplementation appears to promote glucose-mediated insulin secretion allowing vitamin D to play a beneficial role in glucose metabolism by:

1. regulating insulin secretion and promoting the survival of beta-cells, which results in releasing insulin in a tightly regulated manner to maintain blood glucose levels in the adequate range.
2. regulating the calcium flux within beta-cells, which results in improving insulin secretion directly because insulin secretion is a calcium-dependent process. Vitamin D stimulates insulin secretion and benefits beta-cell secretory function when calcium levels are adequate.
3. modulating the adaptive and innate immune responses which results in a preventative effect on autoimmune such as type 1 diabetes. Vitamin D modulates the immune system's response and prevents the destruction of insulin-secreting pancreatic beta-cells, which causes the development of type 1 diabetes.
4. reducing substantially systemic inflammation involved in insulin resistance and the development of type 2 diabetes. Recent studies have established that vitamin D plays an essential role in modulating the inflammation system by inhibiting the proliferation of pro-inflammatory cells and regulating the production of inflammatory cytokines.

5. improving insulin sensitivity and enhancing pancreatic beta-cell function.

4

THE GLYCEMIC INDEX DIET EXPLAINED

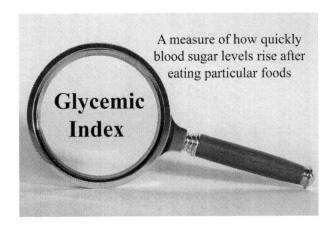

The primary foundation of the glycemic index diet for diabetes relies on the studies that established the strong relationship between what people eat and how it impacts their blood glucose level. In the past, carbohydrates were only classified according to their chemical structure as being either simple or complex. However, this division does not take into account the effects of carbohydrates on blood sugar, inflammation, and chronic diseases. The glycemic index (GI) system was developed to better categorize carbohydrate-containing foods. The GI system assigns values to foods based on how quickly and how high those foods cause spikes in blood glucose levels. Foods low on the glycemic index scale tend to release glucose in the blood slowly and steadily. In contrast, foods high on the glycemic index scale are quickly digested and absorbed and cause significant fluctuations in blood glucose.

The reasoning behind the Glycemic index Diet for Diabetes is logical, strong and aims to select the foods that are considered low glycemic and avoid foods causing high fluctuations in blood sugar. Thus eating adequate portion sizes of low glycemic whole foods will result in better glycemic control, decreased inflammation, and reduced risk of diabetes complications.

* **The Glycemic Index Diet**

The glycemic index (GI) was initially developed in the early 1980s to scientifically determine how different foods containing carbohydrates — vegetables, legumes, fruits, processed foods, and dairy products — affect blood sugar levels. Since that initial research led by Dr. Jenkins took place more than 35 years ago, many scientists identified the opportunity that the glycemic index could be a powerful tool for maintaining weight, improving effective weight-loss diets, and managing diabetes.

The glycemic index isn't formally a diet in the sense that you have to conform to strict rules, follow particular meal plans or eliminate some foods from your daily meals. Instead, it's a scientific method of identifying how carbohydrates in foods affect blood sugar levels and measuring how slowly or quickly the carbohydrates in foods raise blood sugar. Thus, the Glycemic Index referential is particularly important to know if you want to maintain weight, lose weight or if you're going to take more control of diabetes and specific health issues.

The "glycemic index (GI) diet" refers to a targeted diet plan that uses the glycemic index as the primary and only guides for meal planning. Unlike other diet plans that provide strict recommendations, the glycemic index diet doesn't specify the daily amount of calories, carbohydrates, protein, or fats for weight maintenance or weight loss. Still, it provides an effective eating plan with more flexibility and sustainable results in terms of weight loss, weight management, diabetes control, and inflammation-healing and prevention.

- **Understanding GI values**

The glycemic index ranks carbohydrates on a scale from 0 to 100:

- low glycemic foods comprise foods that have a rating of 55 or less
- medium glycemic foods comprise foods that have a rating in the range of 56 to 69
- high glycemic foods comprise foods that cause high spikes in blood sugar. Their glycemic index values are equal to or higher to 70

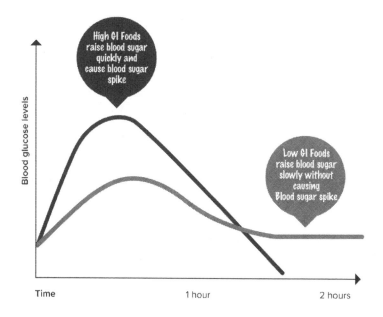

Comparing the GI values may help guide your food choices. For example, muesli has a GI value of 86 ± 4. A Smoothie drink, a banana has a GI value of 30 ± 4.

* **How does Glycemic Index (GI) Diet work?**

Eating according to the Glycemic Index Diet looks simple, because all you need to know is where different foods fall on the 0 to 100 glycemic index (GI).

* You fill up on low GI foods (GI value: 55 and under)
* Eat smaller amounts of medium GI foods (GI value:56 to 69)
* And mostly avoid high GI foods (GI value: 70 and up)

Lists of foods in the 14 categories are available in this book:

- Beef, Lamb, Veal, Pork & Poultry
- Beverages
- Bread & Bakery Products
- Breakfast Cereals
- Dairy Products & Alternatives
- Soups, Pasta, and Noodles
- Fish & Fish Products
- Fruit and Fruit Products
- Legumes and Nuts
- Meat Sandwiches and Ham
- Mixed Meals and Convenience Foods
- Recipe
- Snack Foods and Confectionery
- Vegetables

Besides referring to these lists as needed, there is no difficult weighing or measuring and no need to track your calories intake. However, you will have to concoct your eating plan and menus yourself.

- **How Is Glycemic Index Measured?**

Glycemic Index values of foods are measured using valid and proven scientific methods and cannot be guessed just by looking at the composition of specific food or the nutrition facts on food packaging.

Thus, the GI calculation follows the international standard method and provides values that are commonly accepted. The Glycemic Index value of food is calculated by feeding over ten healthy people a portion of the food object of the study and containing fifty grams of digestible carbohydrate and then measuring the effect for each participant on his blood glucose levels (blood glucose response) over the next two hours.

The second part of the process consists of giving the same participants an equal carbohydrate portion of the glucose (used as the reference food) and measuring their blood glucose response over the next two hours.

The Glycemic Index value for the food is then calculated for each participant by using a simple formula (dividing the blood glucose response for the food by their blood glucose response for the glucose (reference food)). The final value of the Glycemic Index for the food is the average Glycemic Index value for the participants (over 10).

Carbohydrates with a low GI value (55 or less) are more slowly digested, absorbed, and metabolized and cause a smaller and slower rise in blood glucose and, therefore, usually, insulin levels.

A low glycemic diet or foods are associated with reduced risks of chronic disease. Foods that have a low glycemic index are known for their property to release glucose in the blood slowly and regularly. Conversely, Foods that have a high glycemic index are known for their property to release glucose rapidly. Researches suggest that foods with a low glycemic index (LGI foods) are ideal for weight loss diets and foster lasting weight loss, in addition to their positive effect on the pancreas (insulin release), eyes, and kidney.

- **The Glycemic Load Concept**

Basing your food choices only on the GI means that you're focusing on only one aspect of the food and ignoring other important aspects, such as the quality and quantity of the carbohydrates in the foods. Here comes the importance of the glycemic load, which combines the two criteria and provides, when available, an additional tool for better weight loss control and effective diabetes management.

Glycemic Load was introduced later to fill the gap and represents another critical tool to track carbohydrates quality and quantity. Glycemic Load (GL) combines both the quality and amount of carbohydrates following a simple formula:

Glycemic Load (GL) = GI x Carbohydrate (grams) content per portion ÷ 100

For example, an apple that has a GI of 32 and contains 13 grams of carbohydrates is considered as more healthier than Sweet potato that has a GL of 11 using the glycemic load tool.

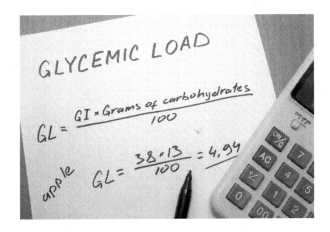

Like the glycemic index, the glycemic load (GL) of a food can be classified as:

- **Low:** 10 or less
- **Medium:** 11 – 19
- **High:** 20 or more

5

CARB COUNTING AND GLYCEMIC INDEX

It is well established now that both the amount and the type of carbohydrate in food affect blood sugar levels. The total amount of carbohydrates in food was believed to provide a good prediction of the blood glucose response. Thus, eating fifty grams of pure sugar would cause the same blood glucose response as any fifty-gram carbohydrates-containing food. Which is completely wrong!!!

Because the quality of carbohydrates matters and does have a significant effect on blood glucose, using the glycemic index (GI) may be very helpful in tightly managing blood glucose. In other words, carbohydrate counting is essential but maybe not sufficient in some cases, especially if you are not rigorous about tracking all carbs you eat or drink. In this special case, the glycemic index system provides an additional tool to allow you'll gain more control of diabetes management using this powerful tool (GI) and make smarter food choices.

In fact, carbohydrates in the food you ingest will raise your blood glucose levels. How fast they raise your blood glucose depends on the quality of the carbs and what you eat with them. For example, sugar levels in fruit or vegetable juice induce a notable spike in blood sugar levels, while sugar in the whole fruits or vegetables is digested more slowly. Carbohydrates-containing foods will be slowly digested if consumed with fat, fiber, or protein, thus inducing smoother increases in blood sugar levels.

Carb, or carbohydrates counting, means that you keep track of the carbohydrates in all your meals, snacks, and drinks. Carb counting is an essential tool for people with diabetes that help them match their activity level and medicines to the food they eat. For many people with diabetes, carbs counting is used as the primary tool to manage their blood sugar efficiently, which can also help them:

- avoid high spikes in blood sugar levels
- stay healthy longer, and/or reduce the severity of some diabetes complications
- improve their quality of life.
- prevent diabetes complications such as eye disorders, kidney disease, foot ulcers, heart disease, and stroke

If you take mealtime insulin, also known as fast-acting insulins, you'll have to count carbohydrates to match your insulin dose to your intake of carbs.

Types of Carbohydrates in Your Diet

When you eat carbohydrates, your body breaks them down into glucose (blood sugar), which are absorbed into the bloodstream. As the glucose level rises in your body, the pancreas releases insulin, a peptide hormone responsible for maintaining normal blood glucose levels. Insulin moves glucose from the blood into the cells, where it can be used as an energy source. Dietary carbohydrates can be divided into three major categories:

- Sugars: Short-chain carbs found in foods such as fructose, glucose, sucrose, and galactose.
- Starches: Long-chain of glucose molecules, which get transformed into glucose during digestion.
- Fibers: are divided into soluble and insoluble.

Carbohydrates can also be divided according to their chemical composition into simple and complex carbs:

- Complex carbohydrates are formed by sugar molecules that are linked together in complex and long chains. Complex carbs are found in vegetables, fruits, peas, beans, and whole grains and contain natural fiber. These types of food are healthy.
- Simple carbohydrates are transformed quickly by the body and induce an increased sugar blood level. They are found in high amounts in processed foods and refined sugars. The consumption of this type of carbs is associated with health problems like type 2 diabetes, obesity, metabolism problem. Simple carbs foods are also deprived of essential nutrients and vitamins.

Choosing the best carbohydrate-containing foods

The quality of the carbohydrates you eat is crucial in adjusting the level of some hormones that influences diabetes, inflammation or controls weight gain, including insulin, cortisol, leptin, peptide YY. For instance, frequently eating low-quality carbs (high glycemic foods) will lead to frequent blood sugar spikes, which will:

- let controlling your blood sugar levels hard,
- promote or worsen inflammation,

- cause weight gain, obesity,
- cause insulin resistance for healthy individuals
- dysregulate cortisol levels.

Conversely, the soluble and insoluble fibers in whole foods (low glycemic foods) are known to offset glucose conversion, prevent higher insulin supplies, and avoid irregular blood sugar variations that induce an excess of cortisol and insulin release.

How many carbs should I eat?

Eating to lower the levels of blood sugar is not a one-size-fits-all approach. Different people, even twins, may respond to the same foods very differently because everyone's body is different. The amount of carbohydrates you can eat and stay in your target blood glucose range depends closely on several factors including your age, weight, and activity level.

On average, people with diabetes should target to get nearly half of their calories from carbohydrates. Thus, if you normally consume about 1,900 calories a day to maintain a healthy weight, then you have to aim to eat about 900-1000 calories from carbs. Considering that carbs provide 4 calories per gram, fat provides 9 calories per gram, and protein provides 4 calories per gram, you have to eat 225-250 grams of carb a day.

In order to keep your blood sugar levels stable throughout the day, you should eat nearly the same amount of carbs at each meal.

6

EATING LOW GLYCEMIC AND ANTI-INFLAMMATORY FOODS

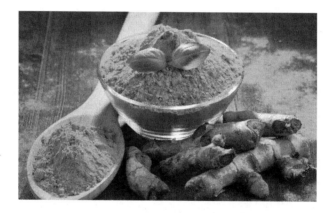

Growing lines of evidence indicate that various dietary polyphenols and flavonoids positively influence blood sugar at different levels, help control and prevent diabetes complications. Antioxidants also play a beneficial and protective role of the pancreatic beta-cells against glucose toxicity in diabetic patients. Thus, consuming polyphenols-rich foods, flavonoids-rich foods, and antioxidants will help you closely control your blood sugar levels, reduce the risk of developing chronic inflammatory diseases and prevent diabetes complications.

- I. Eating low glycemic index vegetables and fruits

In the glycemic index diet for diabetes, you have to eat low glycemic index fruits and vegetables to keep close control of your blood sugar level. In addition, non-starchy vegetables and fruits are good sources of anti-inflammatory nutrients such as polyphenols, antioxidants, and flavonoids which contribute to lowering inflammation and, in turn, reducing the risk of diabetes complications.

The serving sizes for low glycemic index vegetables and fruits are equivalent to:

- 1 cup raw or salad vegetables
- 1/2 cup cooked vegetables
- 3/4 cup (6oz) vegetable juice homemade and unsweetened
- ½ cup of cooked beans, lentils, and peas
- 1 medium piece of fruit
- 1 cup (6 oz) of sliced fruits
- ½ cup (4 oz) of fruit juice

The total vegetable intake (per day) is equivalent to 8-10 servings. You have to vary your meals using the maximal recommended amount as follows:

- "Dark-Green Vegetables" group up to 2 servings
- "Red & Orange Vegetables" group up to 3 servings
- "Beans, Peas, Lentils" group up to 2 servings
- "Starchy Vegetables" group up to 1 serving
- "Other Vegetables" group up to 3 servings

The total fruit intake is equivalent to 2-4 servings per day.

- 2. Increasing your Omega-3 Fatty Acids intake

Omega-3 fatty acids are a healthy type of polyunsaturated fats associated with beneficial health effects such as

- decreasing inflammation
- improving heart health
- supporting mental health
- decreasing liver fat
- helping in the prevention of many chronic conditions
- promoting bone health

Strategies to increase your weekly intake of omega-3 fatty acids include regularly eating omega-3-rich nuts and seeds—such as chia seed, flaxseed, Hemp seed—, eating fatty fish—such as salmon, sardines, anchovies, mackerel, and herring. The weekly fish intake is equivalent to 10 servings (a serving is equal to 3 to 4 ounces). So target eating 6-8 servings of fatty fish per week.

- 3. Choosing healthy fats

The carb counting diet for diabetes is rich in omega-3 and lower in omega-6 than most diets. High levels of omega-3 combined with a low (omega-6/omega-3) are associated with many health benefits, including a significant reduction of unnecessary inflammation and diabetes complications. For example, a ratio (omega-6/omega-3) of 4/1 was correlated to a 70% reduction in mortality. So, based on recent studies, you have to keep the ratio (omega-6/omega-3) in the range of 1/1 and 4/1, which is associated with positive health outcomes.

Strategies to achieve an adequate ratio (omega-6/omega-3) include

- consuming fatty fish (e.g., sardines, mackerels, salmon, herring, anchovies) twice a week,
- consuming nuts and seeds (e.g., flax seeds, chia seeds, walnuts) twice a week.

- **4. Increasing olive oil consumption**

Recent studies have established that an extra virgin olive oil-rich diet reduces glucose levels, LDL cholesterol (bad), and triglycerides. And thus, prevents a series of illnesses that are very common among diabetic patients.

The anti-diabetes benefits of Extra Virgin Olive Oil (EVOO) increase with the daily ingested amount. A minimum of extra virgin olive oil of four tablespoons per day is necessary to provide beneficial anti-diabetes and antioxidant effects. When cooking, EVOO is an excellent choice as it has been well established that it helps reduce blood sugar levels, reduce blood pressure, lower bad cholesterol (LDL), and decrease inflammation. The nutritional composition of virgin olive is comprised of mainly

- monounsaturated fatty acids (69.2% for extra virgin olive oil), mainly Oleic acid (omega-9)
- saturated fats (15.4% for extra virgin olive oil) mainly Stearic acid and Palmitic Acid
- polyunsaturated (9.07% for extra virgin olive oil), mainly Linoleic acid (omega-3)
- Polyphenols
- Vitamin E, Carotenoids, and Squalene

Strategies to increase your daily intake of olive oil include

- replacing butter with EVOO,

- using olive oil as finishing oil for your meals,
- replacing the oil you use for cooking,
- roasting, and frying with EVOO.

- **5. Including anti-inflammatory spices in your eating plan**

Over the several last decades, extensive research has revealed that some spices and their active components exhibit tremendous anti-inflammatory benefits. Thus, spices have been found to prevent or decrease the severity of diabetes complications as well as a number of chronic conditions such as arthritis, asthma, multiple sclerosis, cardiovascular diseases, lupus, cancer, and neurodegenerative diseases. The most common spices used for their anti-inflammatory activities are

- turmeric,
- green tea,
- garlic,
- ginger,
- cayenne pepper,
- black pepper,
- black cumin,
- clove,
- cumin,
- ginseng,
- cardamom,
- parsley
- cinnamon,
- rosemary,
- chives,
- basil,
- cilantro

In addition, spices have a unique property to add flavor to any meal without adding fats or salt. Therefore, you should consider integrating herbs as part of your daily diet when cooking.

Some strategies for getting more herbs and spices in your diet include

- using some fresh herbs as the main ingredient (e.g., herb salad, tabbouleh salad),
- replacing some green vegetables in salads with herbs,
- substituting (or reducing) salt in a recipe with spices,
- replacing mayonnaise with basil-olive oil preparation,
- drinking 3–4 cups of green tea daily.

- **6. Drinking more water**

Water is critical for life. Without water, there is no life. All of the organs of our body, such as the heart, brain, lungs, and muscles, contain a significant quantity of water and need water to stay healthy.

Every day we lose water, and we need to replace it through a regular water supply. Otherwise, we can suffer from dehydration, which may alter the normal body's functions.

The recommended water intake for men aged 19+ is 3 liters (13 cups), and for women aged 19+ is 2.2 liters (9 cups) each day.

7

AVOIDING HIGH GLYCEMIC AND INFLAMMATORY FOODS

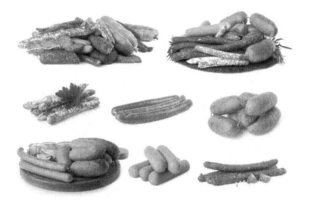

- 1. Limiting moderate glycemic index foods and avoiding high glycemic foods

Eating according to the carb counting diet looks simple because all you need to do is counting the grams of carbohydrates in all foods you eat and keeping the amount of carbohydrates ingested at each meal under close control to prevent fluctuations in blood sugar.

Avoiding high glycemic index foods will let you take more control of your glycemic level. You may follow these simple and complementary guidelines:

- Eat smaller amounts of moderate glycemic index foods (GI value:56 to 69)
- And mostly avoid high glycemic index foods (GI value: 70 and up)

- ## 2. Excluding Trans-Fats containing Foods

Trans-fatty acids are mostly industrially manufactured fats produced during the hydrogenation process that adds hydrogen to liquid vegetable oils to transform the liquid to a solid form at room temperature. Trans fats give foods a desirable taste and texture. However, unlike other dietary fats, consuming trans-fatty acids raises the level of your bad cholesterol (LDL), lowers your good cholesterol (HDL) levels, increases your risk of developing severe cardiovascular conditions certain cancers, and aggravates inflammation. Trans fats may be present in several food products, including:

- fried fast foods, including french fries, fried chicken, battered fish, mozzarella sticks, and doughnuts
- margarine
- peanut butter
- baked goods, such as cakes, pies, and cookies made with margarine or vegetable shortening
- vegetable shortening

Strategies to reduce drastically trans fats intake include

- avoiding or reducing intakes of fried fast foods—including

french fries, fried chicken, battered fish, mozzarella sticks, and doughnuts—margarine, peanut butter, frozen pizza, baked goods made with margarine or vegetable shortening
- eating smaller portion sizes
- consuming trans-fat-containing foods less frequently.

- **3. Eating a little less red meat but enough proteins**

There is little evidence that red meat may contribute to inflammation and alter glycemic control, while some recent studies revealed that unprocessed red meat might be associated with less inflammation and is safe for people with diabetes. However, there is a consensus about the danger of consuming processed red meat such as sausage, bacon, salami, and hot dogs. A 2012 study funded and supported by some health and nutrition government agencies has established the link between processed red meal consumption and increased total mortality. It also revealed that daily unprocessed red meat consumption raised the risk of total mortality by 13%. The study revealed that replacing one serving of red meat per day with other proteins sources such as fish, poultry, and nuts could decrease the risk of mortality by 7-19%.

These findings suggest that you should restrict your red meat intake to reduce inflammation, prevent and delay diabetes complications.

Eating an adequate amount of protein is extremely important for your health because proteins play a crucial role in your body's vital processes and metabolisms, such as building and repairing tissues, building muscles, blood, hair, and skin, regulating some inflammatory response, and producing hormones, enzymes, and other body chemicals. The weekly recommended proteins intake is equivalent to

- 30 servings of animal proteins (mainly lean white meat, and eggs)
- 10 servings of seafood
- 5 servings of nuts and seeds

By restricting red meat intake in the range of 1/5 to 1/4 of animal proteins (e.g., 6 to 7.5 servings of red meat per week), you may experience improvement in your overall health and reduction of some symptoms caused by inflammation.

8

EATING WHOLE AND MINIMALLY PROCESSED FOODS

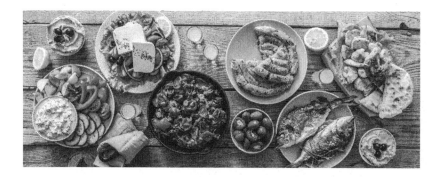

Most Americans don't eat whole foods anymore. They eat processed and highly-processed foods that are generally inferior to unprocessed or minimally processed foods. In fact, highly-processed foods are generally industrially-made and contain many ingredients, including high-fructose corn syrup, trans fats, monosodium glutamate, artificial sweeteners, flavors, colors, and other chemical additives. Highly-processed foods are believed to be a significant contributor to the obesity epidemic in the world, promoting diabetes, chronic inflammation, and the prevalence of autoimmune diseases. Therefore, we must distinguish between healthy processed foods to include in the carb counting diet for diabetes and those to exclude because they are considered unhealthy and pro-inflammatory. For this reason, the next chapter (chapter 10) is fundamental because it contains foods groups based on the NOVA classification system. To adhere to the carb counting diet for diabetes, you must get familiar with the four NOVA foods groups.

Whole food refers to unprocessed or minimally processed food— a nature-made food without added sugars, fat, sodium, flavorings, or other artificial ingredients. It has not been broken down by the man intervention into its components and refined into a new form. Whole Foods are generally close to their natural state, unprocessed and unrefined. Whole foods have little to no additives or preservatives.

A carb counting diet for diabetes is not a specific diet. Instead, it refers to an eating plan that primarily counts carbohydrates and selects whole and minimally processed foods that result in many health benefits, including better glycemic control, diabetes complication prevention, inflammation reduction, and hypertension prevention and treatment.

- **The carb counting diet for diabetes main principles**

The carb counting diet for diabetes is a balanced, easy, long-term, and sustainable diet that counts carbohydrates, selects whole, minimally processed foods, and limits animal products. It mainly focuses on plants, including vegetables, fruits, whole grains, legumes, seeds, and nuts, which should make up most of what you eat. You then have to design your eating plan around **unprocessed and minimally processed foods (NOVA group 1 of foods)** and, as much as you can, **avoid those that are processed (NOVA group 2 of** foods) and **absolutely exclude highly-processed (NOVA group 3 of foods).**

The carb counting diet for diabetes supplies your body with low glycemic unprocessed or minimally processed foods **(NOVA group 1 of foods)**, with little to no unhealthy added constituents.

Carbohydrates, Proteins, and Fats: How do macronutrients fit into the carb counting diet for diabetes?

1. Carbohydrates

The choice of high-quality macronutrients is crucial for the success of the carb counting diet for diabetes.

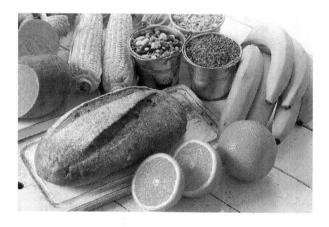

- **Knowing how carbohydrates can work for you or against you**

Eating a carb counting diet for diabetes isn't just about counting carbohydrates and eating unprocessed and minimally processed foods; a large part of controlling your blood glucose is strongly impacted by the type of carbohydrates you eat.

Types of Carbohydrates in Your Diet

When you eat carbohydrates, your body breaks them down into glucose, which is absorbed into the bloodstream. As the glucose level rises in your body, the pancreas releases insulin, a peptide hormone responsible for maintaining normal blood glucose levels. Insulin moves glucose from the blood into the cells, where it can be used as an energy source. Dietary carbohydrates can be divided into three major categories:

- sugars: Short-chain carbs found in foods such as fructose, glucose, sucrose, and galactose.
- starches: Long-chain of glucose molecules, which get transformed into glucose during digestion.
- fibers: are divided into soluble and insoluble.

Carbohydrates can also be divided according to their chemical composition into simple and complex carbs:

- complex carbohydrates are formed by sugar molecules that are linked together in complex and long chains. Complex carbs are found in vegetables, fruits, peas, beans, and whole grains and contain natural fiber. These types of food are considered healthy.
- simple carbohydrates are transformed quickly by the body and induce blood sugar spikes. They are found in high amounts in processed foods and refined sugars. The consumption of this type of carbs is associated with medical conditions such as type 2 diabetes, obesity, metabolism problem. Simple carbs foods are also deprived of essential nutrients and vitamins.

Choosing the best carbohydrate-containing foods

The quality of the carbohydrates you eat is crucial in adjusting the level of some hormones that influences inflammation or controls weight gain, including insulin, cortisol, leptin, peptide YY. For instance, low-quality carbs (high glycemic foods) are quickly digested and lead to blood glucose spikes, which may aggravate diabetes, worsen inflammation, cause weight gain, obesity, insulin resistance, and increased cortisol levels. Conversely, the soluble and insoluble fibers in whole foods (low glycemic foods) are known to offset glucose conversion, prevent higher insulin supplies, and avoid irregular blood sugar variations that induce an excess of cortisol and insulin release.

2. Protein

Eating an adequate amount of protein is extremely important for your health because it plays a crucial role in your body's vital processes and metabolisms, such as building and repairing tissues, building muscles, blood, hair, and skin, and producing hormones, enzymes, and other body chemicals.

Unlike carbohydrates and fat, your body does not store protein, and you need to eat the necessary amount to keep the right hormonal balance and a healthy body.

Plus, eating protein reduces levels of ghrelin (the hunger hormone) and stimulates the production of the satiety hormones (PYY and GLP-1)

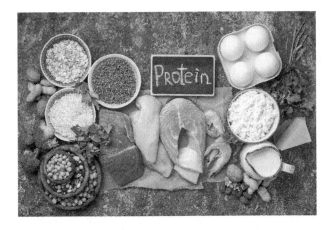

When you eat protein, it's transformed into amino acids, which help your body with various processes such as building muscle and regulating immune function.

However, many studies have established that red meat, processed meats, and highly processed meats promote and aggravate inflammation.

On the adapted whole foods diet, animal protein is consumed very moderately following the degree of food processing. You have to select animal sources of protein from the NOVA food group 1 (unprocessed or minimally processed), which include:

- poultry meat (fresh, chilled, or frozen), whole, steaks, fillets, and other cuts
- fish (fresh, chilled, or frozen), whole, steaks, fillets, and other cuts

You have also to choose vegetable sources of protein from the NOVA food group 1 (unprocessed or minimally processed), which include:

- lentils

- chickpeas
- green peas
- nuts
- seeds
- quinoa
- wild rice
- broccoli
- spinach
- asparagus
- artichokes
- sweet potatoes
- Brussels sprouts

Guidelines for individualized protein intake

The RDA (international Recommended Dietary Allowance) for protein is 0.8 g per kg of body weight, regardless of age. This recommendation is derived as the minimum amount to maintain nitrogen balance; however, it is not optimized for women's needs or physical activity levels.

Based on a recent body of evidence, the protein recommended intake from all sources can be adjusted to 1.4-1.8 grams per kg of your body weight.

The Protein Quality

The optimal source of protein is based on the calculation of the PDCAA (Protein Digestibility Corrected Amino Acid) Score or the DIAA (Digestibility Indispensable Amino Acid) Score. Thus, animal-based foods were identified as a superior source of protein because they offer a complete composition of essential amino acids, with higher bioavailability and digestibility (>90%). Thus, you have to eat a combination of animal proteins and plant proteins, mainly in the NOVA group 1 of foods (unprocessed and minimally processed).

Collagen, an essential ingredient

The most abundant type of protein in your body is collagen. Ligaments, tendons, skin, hair, nails, discs, and bones are collagen. Collagen is rich in amino acids that play an essential role in the building of joint cartilage. It also plays an important role in strengthening and rebuilding the lining of our digestive tract, thus healing gut inflammation and subsequently improving the immune system and helping modulate inflammation.

During the normal aging process, your body begins to experience a decline in the synthesis of collagen proteins. According to studies, this decline in collagen production starts around 30, at a rate of 1% per year. At the age of fifty, the rate jump to up to 3%, causing health issues::

- Muscle stiffness
- Aging joint
- Wrinkles and fine lines
- Lack of tone
- Aging skin
- Healing of wounds slower
- Frequent fatigue.

Consuming more collagen will boost your body's collagen protection. So it is recommended that your daily intake of collagen represent up to 25% of protein.

The beneficial effects include:

- Decreased gut inflammation.

- Improved intestinal health.

- Less articular pain.

- Less hair loss.

- Better skin.

• Increased muscle mass.

Foods rich in collagen

Here are some of the best collagen-rich foods you can add to your diet:

Bone broth

Made by simmering bones, tendons, ligaments, and skin of beef, bone broth is an excellent source of collagen and several essential amino acids. Bone broth is also available in powder, bar, or even capsules, so you can add it to your diet as a supplement.

Spirulina

This seaweed is an excellent source of plant-based amino acids, which are a key component of collagen. Spirulina can be found in dried form at most health food stores.

Codfish

Codfish, like most other types of white fish, is a good source of collagen in addition to selenium, vitamin B6 and phosphorus.

Eggs

Eggs are a good source of collagen, including glycine and proline.

---

3. Fats

After carbohydrates and proteins, it is essential to optimize the choice of your dietary fat.

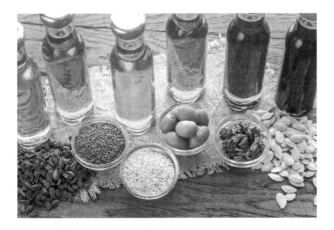

What is fat, and why it is essential for your health?

Dietary fats are found in both animals and vegetables and are essential for your living since they provide your body energy and support cell growth.

Fats also provide some valuable benefits and play essential roles, including:

- helping your body absorb some nutrients such as vitamins A, D, E, and K.
- helping your body produce the necessary hormones.
- regulating inflammation and immunity issues.
- maintaining the health of your cells (skin, hair cells)

How many different fats are there?

There are four major fats in food, based on their chemical structures and physical properties:

- Saturated fat (bad fat; reduce your intake of saturated fat): is a kind of fat in which the fatty acid chain of carbon atoms holds as many hydrogen atoms as possible (saturated with hydrogens). This form of saturated fat is associated with various adverse health effects, including aggravation of inflammation.

- Trans fat (very bad fat; to exclude completely): (trans-unsaturated fatty acids or trans fatty acids) are a form of unsaturated fat associated with various adverse health effects and known to worsen inflammation.
- Monounsaturated fats (healthy fat): are a type of unsaturated fat but have only one double bond. These fats are associated with positive health effects and may replace bad fats. Monounsaturated fats are found in olive oil, avocados, and some nuts
- Polyunsaturated fat (healthy fat): The two major classes of polyunsaturated fats are omega-3 and omega-6 fatty acids. However, many studies have shown that omega-3 and omega-6 have different inflammatory properties. Omega-3 fatty acids have powerful anti-inflammatory effects, while omega-6 tend to promote inflammation.

What is cholesterol?

Cholesterol is a waxy, fat-like substance found in all the cells in your body. Plus, your body needs some cholesterol to produce steroid hormones, vitamin D, and bile acid that helps you digest fats. Contrary to popular belief, your body makes all the cholesterol it needs in the liver. Cholesterol is supplied in small quantities (less than 15%) by plant and animals foods.

More than 85% of the cholesterol in your bloodstream comes from your liver rather than from the food you eat. Dietary cholesterol has little impact on raising blood cholesterol levels, which is valuable information from a diet perspective.

A recent and growing body of evidence has pointed to inflammation as the most important cause of cardiovascular diseases rather than cholesterol. While a high cholesterol level in the blood can be dangerous, maintaining the right balance of cholesterol is essential for your health.

What types of fat should you eat?

Eating an adapted whole foods diet implies selecting fats found naturally in food and not being processed. You have then to choose fat-rich foods belonging to the NOVA group 1 of foods (unprocessed and minimally processed foods).

Examples of healthy sources of fat include:

- butter and ghee (clarified butter)
- cheese
- avocado (the fruit or avocado oil)
- cacao butter and powder
- sardines, anchovies
- salmon
- olives and olive oil
- macadamias and macadamia oil
- almonds and almonds oil
- Brazil nuts and Brazil nuts oil
- hazelnuts and hazelnuts oil
- pecan and pecan oil

What Are Fatty Acids?

Fatty acids are a form of hydrocarbon chains with carboxyl at one end and methyl at the other. The bioloGical activity of fatty acids is determined by the length of their carbon chain and their double bonds' number and position.

While saturated fatty acids do not contain double bonds within the acyl chain, unsaturated fatty acids include at least one double bond.

When two or more double bonds are present in their chain, unsaturated fatty acids are referred to as Dietary polyunsaturated fatty acids (PUFAs) and have been associated with cholesterol-lowering properties. The two families of PUFA are omega-3 and omega-6.

What Are Omega-3 Fatty Acids?

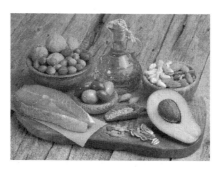

Omega-3 fatty acids are a type of polyunsaturated fats that the body can't produce. Omega-3 fatty acids are essential fats, so you have to get them from your diet.

There are various types of omega-3 fats, which differ by their chemical structure. The three most common types of omega-3 are:

- Eicosapentaenoic acid (EPA)
- Docosahexaenoic acid (DHA)
- Alpha-linolenic acid (ALA)

What Are Omega-6 Fatty Acids?

Like omega-3, omega-6 fatty acids are polyunsaturated fatty acids. omega-6 fatty acids are abundant and account for most polyunsaturated fatty acids in the food supply.

Following different recommendations and guidelines, we recommend a ratio of 4/1 omega-6 to omega-3 or less, which means that for 400 milligrams of omega-6, you have to consume 100 milligrams of omega-3. However, the Western diet has a very high ratio between 10/1 and 50/1.

Why and how is the excess of omega-6 harmful?

A high amount of omega-6 polyunsaturated fatty acids associated with a very high ratio of omega-6/omega-3 is a constant in most Western diets, including the keto diet. That increases the pathogenesis of several diseases, such as cancer, cardiovascular disease, autoimmune and inflammatory diseases. Conversely, high levels of omega-3 associated with a low ratio of omega-6/omega-3 induce health benefits. For example, a ratio omega-6/omega-3 of 4/1 was correlated to a 70% reduction in mortality.

This explains why the notion of the omega-6 / omega-3 ratio is essential in weight loss and health management.

Consuming fatty fish twice a week, eating whole foods, choosing dairy products and meat from grass-fed animals can help you improve your omega-6:omega-3 ratio.

9

FOOD PROCESSING CLASSIFICATION: OVERVIEW

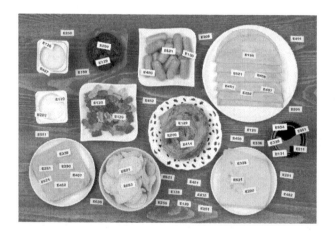

Food processing has been practiced for centuries in form of cooking, dehydrating, fermenting, ultraviolet radiation, and salt preservation. However, modern food processing methods are more sophisticated and complex, and alter considerably foods, by adding many ingredients including trans fats, high-fructose corn syrup, salts, artificial sweeteners, flavors, colors, and other chemical additives. The U.S. Department of Agriculture (USDA) defines processed food as one that has undergone any procedure that alters it from its natural state. Thus, the current definition of processed food is broad, making a diet—like the whole foods diet— that excludes all processed food very hard and challenging to follow.

Therefore, we have to distinguish between healthy processed foods to include in the whole foods diet and those to exclude because considered unhealthy and pro-inflammatory.

Because of the huge heterogeneity among industrially processed foods, researchers have developed frameworks to classify foods based on the category or complexity of processing operations, ranging from minimally to highly processed. The NOVA classification system groups all foods based on the nature, complexity, and outcomes of the industrial processes they undergo. The NOVA classification system is recognized as a legitimate system to classify foods according to their degree of processing by the World Health Organisation (WHO), and the Food and Agriculture Organization (FAO).

NOVA classifies foods and food products into four distinct groups.

- group 1 of the NOVA classification: Unprocessed, natural, or minimally processed foods
- group 2 of the NOVA classification: Processed culinary ingredients
- group 3 of the NOVA classification: Processed foods
- group 4 of the NOVA classification: Ultra-processed foods

However, it can be sometimes challenging to distinguish food that has been minimally processed, processed or highly processed. For example:

1. Plain yogurt belongs to group 1 (minimally processed), but adding food additives such as artificial sweeteners, stabilizers, or preservatives made it ultra-processed (group 4).

2. Freshly made pizzas made from wheat flour, water, salt and yeast, garlic clove, onions, green peppers, black olives, organic mozzarella cheese, raw parmesan cheese, red pepper, belongs to group 3 (processed), but adding food additives such as artificial sweeteners, stabilizers, or changing mozzarella cheese with a non-dairy cheese analog for pizza made it ultra-processed (group 4).

Group 1: Unprocessed or minimally processed foods

Unprocessed foods are obtained directly from plants or animals and include the natural edible food parts of plants and animals.

Minimally processed foods are obtained from unprocessed or natural foods after minimal industrial processing that aims to enhance the edibility and digestibility of food or to increase its shelf life and storability without changing its nutritional content. Food undergoes minor transformations such as removal of non-edible or unwanted parts, crushing, drying, fractioning, grinding, roasting, refrigeration, freezing, vacuum packaging, boiling, pasteurization, non-alcoholic fermentation. The most commonly eaten unprocessed or minimally processed foods are:

- Natural, packaged, cut, chilled, or frozen vegetables
- Natural, packaged, cut, chilled, or frozen fruits
- Natural, packaged, cut, chilled, or frozen salads
- nuts, and other seeds without sugar or salt
- bulk or packaged grains such as wholegrain, brown, parboiled rice, or corn kernel
- fresh and dried herbs and spices (e.g., basil, dill, oregano, pepper, rosemary, thyme, cinnamon, mint, parsley)
- garlic powder

- fresh or pasteurized fruit juices with no added sugar or other ingredients
- fresh or pasteurized vegetable juices with no added sugar or other ingredients
- fresh and dried mushrooms
- cereal grains (e.g. wheat, barley, rye, oats, and sorghum)
- chickpeas, lentils, beans, black beans, peas, chicken beans, and other legumes
- flours made from maize, wheat, corn, or oats, including flours fortified with iron, folic acid, vitamin B (thiamin and niacin)
- flakes, and grits made from maize, wheat, corn, or oats, including flours fortified with iron, folic acid, vitamin B (thiamin and niacin)
- meat (fresh, chilled, or frozen), whole, steaks, fillets, and other cuts
- poultry meat (fresh, chilled, or frozen), whole, steaks, fillets, and other cuts
- fish (fresh, chilled, or frozen), whole, steaks, fillets, and other cuts
- dried or fresh pasta, couscous, and polenta made from water and the grits/flakes/flours described above
- fresh or pasteurized milk
- yogurt unsweetened without added sugar, flavor, or additives
- eggs
- tea
- herbal infusions
- coffee
- dried fruits
- water (tap, spring, and mineral)

Group 2: Processed Culinary Ingredients

The next category of processed foods includes products extracted from unprocessed, minimally processed foods, or directly from nature by pressing, grinding, crushing, milling, drying, or refining.

This group of food referred to as processed culinary ingredients is rather considered as ingredients for cooking various, delicious, and nutritious meals or dishes at home and elsewhere. They are rarely consumed by themselves but used in combination with foods.

The most commonly used processed culinary ingredients foods are:

- oils made from seeds, including sunflower oil, soybean oil, corn oil, cottonseed oil, rapeseed oil, canola oil, grapeseed oil, safflower oil
- oils made from nuts, including almond oil, hazelnut oil, Brazil nut oil, Walnut oil, Macadamia nut oil, and pecan oil.
- oils made from fruits, including olive oil, avocado oil, peach oil, apricot oil, coconut oil
- vegetable oils with added anti-oxidants
- butter
- salted butter
- sugar (white, brown, and other types) obtained from cane or beet
- molasses obtained from cane or beet
- honey (natural)
- lard
- coconut fat
- maple syrup
- cane syrup
- Agave syrup
- salt (refined or raw, mined or from seawater)
- table salt with added drying agents
- potato starch

- corn starch
- starches extracted from other plants
- balsamic vinegar
- Cane vinegar
- Coconut vinegar
- Malt vinegar
- any combination of two items of the NOVA group 2 "processed culinary ingredients"
- any item of the NOVA group 2 "processed culinary ingredients" with added vitamins or minerals, such as iodized salt

Group 3: Processed Foods

Processed foods are made by adding salt, oil, fat, sugar, or other ingredients from group 2 to group 1 food. The transformation processes include preservation, cooking, fermentation. These foods usually are made from at least two or three ingredients and can be eaten without further preparation. This group of food includes cheeses, smoked and cured meats, freshly-made bread, salted and sugared nuts, bacon, tinned fruit in syrup, cider, beer, and wine.

Processed foods usually keep an equivalent nutritional value and most nutrients and constituents of the original food. However, when excessive sugar, salt, or saturated oil are added, foods of group 3 become nutritionally unbalanced and may aggravate inflammation.

The most commonly eaten processed foods are::

- legumes canned or bottled preserved in salt (brine) or vinegar, or by pickling
- vegetables canned or bottled preserved in salt (brine) or vinegar, or by pickling

- fruit canned or bottled, packed in syrup
- fruits in sugar syrup (with or without added antioxidants)
- canned fish, such as sardine and tuna, with or without added preservatives
- fish (salted, dried, smoked)
- cured meat (salted, dried, smoked)
- tomato extract concentrates, or pastes, (with salt and/or sugar)
- beef jerky
- freshly-made cheeses
- freshly-made bread made of wheat flour, salt, yeast, and water
- bacon
- nuts (salted or sugared)
- seeds (salted or sugared)
- fermented alcoholic beverages such as alcoholic cider, beer, and wine
- fermented non-alcoholic beverages such as cider

Group 4: Ultra-processed foods

Also commonly referred to as highly processed foods, Ultra-processed foods usually contain substances that you would never add when cooking homemade food. These are foods from group 3 that undergo "heavily" transformation to maintain or improve their taste, texture, safety, freshness, or appearance by the incorporation of substances:

- derived from foods—such as sugar, oils, fats, carbohydrates, and proteins,—or
- derived from food constituents—such as hydrogenated fats and modified starch—, or
- synthesized in laboratories—such as flavor enhancers,

preservatives, antioxidants, colors, and other food additives—

Ultra-processed foods are defined as "formulations of several ingredients mostly of exclusive industrial use which, besides sugar, salt, oils, and fats, include food ingredients not used in culinary preparations, in particular, flavor enhancers, preservatives, colors, antioxidants, sweeteners, emulsifiers, and other additives used to provide sensory attributes of natural or minimally processed foods and their culinary preparations or to disguise undesirable sensory attributes of the final product such as odor, appearance, texture, flavor, and taste of foods"

The most commonly eaten ultra-processed foods are:

- Industrialized breads
- packaged breads
- Pre-prepared meals (packaged)
- Pre-prepared fish (packaged)
- Pre-prepared vegetables (packaged)
- pre-prepared pizza and pasta dishes
- pre-prepared pasta dishes
- pre-prepared poultry 'nuggets' and 'sticks'
- pre-prepared fish 'nuggets' and 'sticks'
- Breakfast cereals
- Sausages and other reconstituted meat products
- fatty packaged snacks
- sweet savory or salty packaged snacks
- savory or salty packaged snacks
- biscuits (cookies)
- chocolates
- candies
- gum and jelly products
- sweet fillings
- confectionery products in general

- pasties
- buns and cakes
- industrially-made chips (e.g. potato chips, banana chips, lentil chips)
- soft drinks
- fruit drinks
- fruit juices
- fast foods
- tortilla Chips
- chip Dips
- microwave Popcorn
- pretzels
- salty snacks in general
- ice creams
- frozen desserts
- pre-prepared burgers
- hot dogs
- sausages
- cola, soda, and other carbonated soft drinks
- animal products made from remnants
- energy and sports drinks
- packaged hamburger and hot dog buns
- instant soups
- instant noodles
- canned, packaged sauces
- canned, packaged, or powdered desserts
- canned, packaged, or powdered drink mixes
- canned, packaged, or powdered seasonings
- canned, packaged, powdered desserts, drink mixes, and seasonings
- flavored cheese crackers
- baked products made with ingredients other than those in group 2 (processed culinary ingredients) such as hydrogenated vegetable fat, emulsifiers, flavors, and other food additives.

- breakfast cereals and bars
- dairy drinks, including chocolate milk
- sweetened and/or flavored yogurts, including fruit yogurts
- infant formulas and drinks
- meal replacement shakes or powders
- sweetened juices made from concentrate
- pastries
- cakes and cake mixes
- margarine and spreads
- distilled beverages such as whisky, vodka, gin, rum, tequila.

10

UNDERSTANDING THE FOOD NUTRITION LABELS

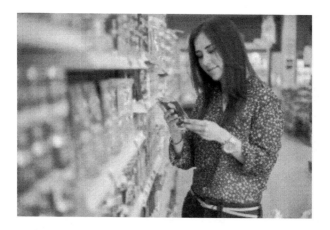

Food labeling regulation is complex, and food labels are filled with a multitude of numbers, percentages, and unusual ingredients making them difficult for consumers to understand. Products nutrition labels are often localized on the front, back, or side of the packaging. Food manufacturers must list on the product label all ingredients in the food to inform consumers what the food contains and to provide support in making healthier choices of processed foods.

Nutrition Facts label

A Nutrition Facts label breaks down the nutritional content of the food to help consumers to make healthier choices and compare between similar products. It includes

- the serving size,
- total fat,
- total carbohydrates,
- dietary fiber,
- protein,
- and vitamins per serving of the food

Example of using nutrition facts label:

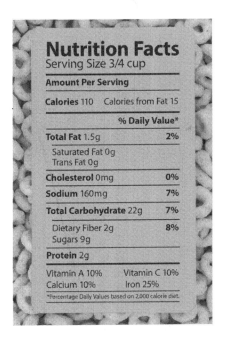

1. The first step is to check the **serving size**. All the values on this label are for a 3/4-cup serving.
2. **calorie** is an important value to many consumers. The label lists the calorie amount for one serving of food (110 calories for 3/4-cup in this example). So if you eat 1.5 cups, the total calorie is 220 calories.
3. **total fat** shows you types of fats in the food, including saturated fat, and trans fat. Avoid foods with trans fat. The total fat per 3/4-cup is 1.5 g
4. **total Carbohydrate** shows you types of carbohydrates in the food, including dietary fiber and sugar.
5. protein shows you the amount of protein in the food,
6. choose foods with lower calories, and that contain little amount of sugar, little amount of sodium, a high amount of fiber, more vitamins, and minerals.

Ingredients list

In addition to the nutrition label, food manufacturers are required to display ingredients label in their products. This is where consumers find all information about the constituents of the food, and can find if this product is suitable for them or not.

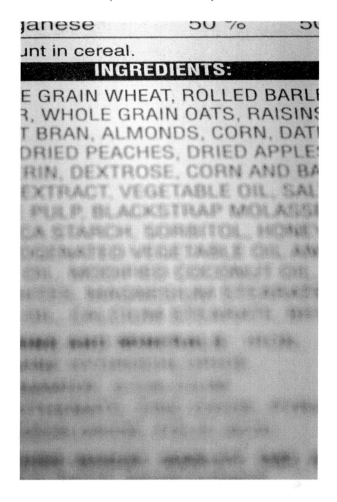

janese   5U %   5(

int in cereal.

INGREDIENTS:

E GRAIN WHEAT, ROLLED BARLI
R, WHOLE GRAIN OATS, RAISIN?
T BRAN, ALMONDS, CORN, DAT
DRIED PEACHES, DRIED APPLE?
RIN, DEXTROSE, CORN AND BA

Ingredients are listed in descending order of predominance—ingredients used in the greatest amount are listed first—. Food manufacturers are required to list food additives by their class name (e.g. acidity regulator, antioxidant, color, emulsifier, flavor enhancer, gelling agent, stabilizer, sweetener, thickener), followed by the name of the food additive or the food additive number.

PART II

THE CARBS AND CALORIES COUNTER FOR OVER 12000 FOODS

11

BAKED FOODS

🍙 Air Filled Fritter Or Fried Puff Without Syrup Puerto Rican Style ☞ serving size: 1 turnover = 57 g; Calories = 248.5; Total Carb (g) = 28.7; Net Carb (g) = 28.4; Fat (g) = 13.5; Protein = 3.7

🍙 Andreas Gluten Free Soft Dinner Roll ☞ serving size: 1 roll = 69 g; Calories = 177.3; Total Carb (g) = 27.8; Net Carb (g) = 25.8; Fat (g) = 5.7; Protein = 3.9

🍙 Apple Strudel ☞ serving size: 1 oz = 28.4 g; Calories = 77.8; Total Carb (g) = 11.7; Net Carb (g) = 11; Fat (g) = 3.2; Protein = 0.9

🍙 Archway Home Style Cookies Chocolate Chip Ice Box ☞ serving size: 1 serving = 24 g; Calories = 119.3; Total Carb (g) = 15.6; Net Carb (g) = 15.1; Fat (g) = 5.9; Protein = 1

🍙 Archway Home Style Cookies Coconut Macaroon ☞ serving size: 1 serving = 22 g; Calories = 101.2; Total Carb (g) = 13.5; Net Carb (g) = 12.3; Fat (g) = 5; Protein = 0.7

🍙 Archway Home Style Cookies Date Filled Oatmeal ☞ serving size: 1 serving = 25 g; Calories = 100; Total Carb (g) = 17; Net Carb (g) = 16.5; Fat (g) = 3; Protein = 1.2

Archway Home Style Cookies Dutch Cocoa ☞ serving size: 1 serving = 24 g; Calories = 103.4; Total Carb (g) = 16.7; Net Carb (g) = 16; Fat (g) = 3.6; Protein = 1.1

Archway Home Style Cookies Frosty Lemon ☞ serving size: 1 serving = 26 g; Calories = 111.8; Total Carb (g) = 16.8; Net Carb (g) = 16.7; Fat (g) = 4.4; Protein = 1.1

Archway Home Style Cookies Iced Molasses ☞ serving size: 1 serving = 28 g; Calories = 117.6; Total Carb (g) = 19.4; Net Carb (g) = 19.1; Fat (g) = 4; Protein = 1

Archway Home Style Cookies Iced Oatmeal ☞ serving size: 1 serving = 28 g; Calories = 121.8; Total Carb (g) = 18.7; Net Carb (g) = 18.1; Fat (g) = 4.6; Protein = 1.4

Archway Home Style Cookies Molasses ☞ serving size: 1 serving = 26 g; Calories = 104.8; Total Carb (g) = 18; Net Carb (g) = 17.7; Fat (g) = 3.1; Protein = 1.1

Archway Home Style Cookies Oatmeal ☞ serving size: 1 serving = 25 g; Calories = 105.3; Total Carb (g) = 17; Net Carb (g) = 16.3; Fat (g) = 3.5; Protein = 1.4

Archway Home Style Cookies Oatmeal Raisin ☞ serving size: 1 serving = 26 g; Calories = 105.6; Total Carb (g) = 18; Net Carb (g) = 17.3; Fat (g) = 3.1; Protein = 1.3

Archway Home Style Cookies Old Fashioned Molasses ☞ serving size: 1 serving = 26 g; Calories = 105.6; Total Carb (g) = 18.3; Net Carb (g) = 18.1; Fat (g) = 3.1; Protein = 1.1

Archway Home Style Cookies Old Fashioned Windmill Cookies ☞ serving size: 1 serving = 20 g; Calories = 93.6; Total Carb (g) = 14.4; Net Carb (g) = 14.1; Fat (g) = 3.5; Protein = 1

Archway Home Style Cookies Peanut Butter ☞ serving size: 1 serving = 21 g; Calories = 100.8; Total Carb (g) = 12.3; Net Carb (g) = 11.7; Fat (g) = 5.1; Protein = 1.9

Archway Home Style Cookies Raspberry Filled ☞ serving size: 1 serving = 25 g; Calories = 100; Total Carb (g) = 16.5; Net Carb (g) = 15.9; Fat (g) = 3.3; Protein = 1.1

Archway Home Style Cookies Reduced Fat Ginger Snaps ☞ serving size: 1 serving = 32 g; Calories = 135.7; Total Carb (g) = 24.4; Net Carb (g) = 24; Fat (g) = 3.6; Protein = 1.5

Archway Home Style Cookies Strawberry Filled ☞ serving size: 1 serving = 25 g; Calories = 100; Total Carb (g) = 16.5; Net Carb (g) = 15.9; Fat (g) = 3.3; Protein = 1.1

Archway Home Style Cookies Sugar Free Oatmeal ☞ serving size: 1 serving = 24 g; Calories = 106.1; Total Carb (g) = 16.1; Net Carb (g) = 15.7; Fat (g) = 5; Protein = 1.3

Arepa Dominicana ☞ serving size: 1 piece (4" x 2" x 1-3/4") = 115 g; Calories = 307.1; Total Carb (g) = 35.1; Net Carb (g) = 32.3; Fat (g) = 16.1; Protein = 6.5

Artificial Blueberry Muffin Mix Dry ☞ serving size: 1 muffin = 31 g; Calories = 126.2; Total Carb (g) = 24; Net Carb (g) = 24; Fat (g) = 2.7; Protein = 1.5

Bagel (Oat Bran) ☞ serving size: 1 mini bagel (2-1/2 inch dia) = 26 g; Calories = 66.3; Total Carb (g) = 13.9; Net Carb (g) = 12.9; Fat (g) = 0.3; Protein = 2.8

Bagel Multigrain ☞ serving size: 1 miniature = 26 g; Calories = 65; Total Carb (g) = 12.7; Net Carb (g) = 11.6; Fat (g) = 0.4; Protein = 2.7

Bagel Multigrain With Raisins ☞ serving size: 1 miniature = 26 g; Calories = 66.3; Total Carb (g) = 13.5; Net Carb (g) = 12.4; Fat (g) = 0.4; Protein = 2.5

Bagel Oat Bran ☞ serving size: 1 miniature = 26 g; Calories = 65; Total Carb (g) = 12.7; Net Carb (g) = 11.6; Fat (g) = 0.4; Protein = 2.7

Bagel Pumpernickel ☞ serving size: 1 miniature = 26 g; Calories

= 65; Total Carb (g) = 12.7; Net Carb (g) = 11.6; Fat (g) = 0.4; Protein = 2.7

🍞 Bagel Wheat Bran ☞ serving size: 1 miniature = 26 g; Calories = 65; Total Carb (g) = 12.7; Net Carb (g) = 11.6; Fat (g) = 0.4; Protein = 2.7

🍞 Bagel Wheat With Raisins ☞ serving size: 1 miniature = 26 g; Calories = 66.3; Total Carb (g) = 13.5; Net Carb (g) = 12.4; Fat (g) = 0.4; Protein = 2.5

🍞 Bagel Whole Grain White ☞ serving size: 1 miniature = 26 g; Calories = 65; Total Carb (g) = 12.7; Net Carb (g) = 11.6; Fat (g) = 0.4; Protein = 2.7

🍞 Bagel Whole Wheat ☞ serving size: 1 miniature = 26 g; Calories = 65; Total Carb (g) = 12.7; Net Carb (g) = 11.6; Fat (g) = 0.4; Protein = 2.7

🍞 Bagel Whole Wheat With Raisins ☞ serving size: 1 miniature = 26 g; Calories = 66.3; Total Carb (g) = 13.5; Net Carb (g) = 12.4; Fat (g) = 0.4; Protein = 2.5

🍞 Bagels ☞ serving size: 1 bagel = 99 g; Calories = 261.4; Total Carb (g) = 51.9; Net Carb (g) = 50.3; Fat (g) = 1.3; Protein = 10.5

🍞 Bagels Multigrain ☞ serving size: 1 piece bagel = 81 g; Calories = 195.2; Total Carb (g) = 38.5; Net Carb (g) = 33.4; Fat (g) = 1; Protein = 8

🍞 Bagels Plain Enriched Without Calcium Propionate (Includes Onion Poppy Sesame) ☞ serving size: 1 oz = 28.4 g; Calories = 78.1; Total Carb (g) = 15.2; Net Carb (g) = 14.5; Fat (g) = 0.5; Protein = 3

🍞 Bagels Plain Unenriched With Calcium Propionate (Includes Onion Poppy Sesame) ☞ serving size: 1 oz = 28.4 g; Calories = 78.1; Total Carb (g) = 15.2; Net Carb (g) = 14.5; Fat (g) = 0.5; Protein = 3

🍞 Bagels Plain Unenriched Without Calcium Propionate(Includes Onion Poppy Sesame) ☞ serving size: 1 oz = 28.4 g; Calories = 78.1; Total Carb (g) = 15.2; Net Carb (g) = 14.5; Fat (g) = 0.5; Protein = 3

Bagels Wheat ☞ serving size: 1 bagel = 98 g; Calories = 245; Total Carb (g) = 47.9; Net Carb (g) = 43.9; Fat (g) = 1.5; Protein = 10

Bagels Whole Grain White ☞ serving size: 1/2 piece bagel 1 serving = 43 g; Calories = 109.7; Total Carb (g) = 23.4; Net Carb (g) = 21.4; Fat (g) = 0; Protein = 4

Baklava ☞ serving size: 1 piece (2" x 2" x 1-1/2") = 78 g; Calories = 333.8; Total Carb (g) = 29.3; Net Carb (g) = 27.2; Fat (g) = 22.7; Protein = 5.2

Basbousa ☞ serving size: 1 piece (about 3 x 2-1/2") = 82 g; Calories = 252.6; Total Carb (g) = 41.1; Net Carb (g) = 40.5; Fat (g) = 8.5; Protein = 4.1

Biscuit Baking Powder Or Buttermilk Type Made From Home Recipe ☞ serving size: 1 small (1-1/2" dia) = 14 g; Calories = 49.6; Total Carb (g) = 6.2; Net Carb (g) = 6; Fat (g) = 2.3; Protein = 1

Biscuit Baking Powder Or Buttermilk Type Made From Mix ☞ serving size: 1 small (1-1/2" dia) = 14 g; Calories = 45.4; Total Carb (g) = 6.5; Net Carb (g) = 6.3; Fat (g) = 1.6; Protein = 1

Biscuit Cheese ☞ serving size: 1 biscuit (2" dia) = 30 g; Calories = 103.8; Total Carb (g) = 14.4; Net Carb (g) = 14; Fat (g) = 4.1; Protein = 2.4

Biscuit Cinnamon-Raisin ☞ serving size: 1 biscuit (3" dia) = 64 g; Calories = 220.8; Total Carb (g) = 34.2; Net Carb (g) = 33; Fat (g) = 8; Protein = 3.7

Biscuit Dough Fried ☞ serving size: 1 piece = 43 g; Calories = 150.5; Total Carb (g) = 18.4; Net Carb (g) = 17.5; Fat (g) = 7.5; Protein = 2.8

Biscuit Whole Wheat ☞ serving size: 1 small (1-1/2" dia) = 14 g; Calories = 43.7; Total Carb (g) = 6.4; Net Carb (g) = 5.5; Fat (g) = 1.7; Protein = 1.3

Biscuits Mixed Grain Refrigerated Dough ☞ serving size: 1 oz =

28.4 g; Calories = 74.7; Total Carb (g) = 13.5; Net Carb (g) = 13.5; Fat (g) = 1.6; Protein = 1.7

🎲 Biscuits Plain Or Buttermilk Dry Mix ☞ serving size: 1 cup, purchased = 120 g; Calories = 513.6; Total Carb (g) = 76.1; Net Carb (g) = 73.6; Fat (g) = 18.5; Protein = 9.6

🎲 Biscuits Plain Or Buttermilk Frozen Baked ☞ serving size: 1 oz = 28.4 g; Calories = 96; Total Carb (g) = 15.3; Net Carb (g) = 14.9; Fat (g) = 3.1; Protein = 1.8

🎲 Biscuits Plain Or Buttermilk Prepared From Recipe ☞ serving size: 1 oz = 28.4 g; Calories = 100.3; Total Carb (g) = 12.7; Net Carb (g) = 12.2; Fat (g) = 4.6; Protein = 2

🎲 Biscuits Plain Or Buttermilk Refrigerated Dough Higher Fat ☞ serving size: 1 biscuit = 58 g; Calories = 178.1; Total Carb (g) = 26.9; Net Carb (g) = 26.5; Fat (g) = 6.1; Protein = 3.9

🎲 Biscuits Plain Or Buttermilk Refrigerated Dough Higher Fat Baked ☞ serving size: 1 biscuit = 51 g; Calories = 165.2; Total Carb (g) = 25; Net Carb (g) = 23.6; Fat (g) = 5.7; Protein = 3.5

🎲 Biscuits Plain Or Buttermilk Refrigerated Dough Lower Fat ☞ serving size: 1 serving 1 biscuit = 58 g; Calories = 156.6; Total Carb (g) = 25.3; Net Carb (g) = 24.2; Fat (g) = 4.5; Protein = 3.9

🎲 Biscuits Plain Or Buttermilk Refrigerated Dough Lower Fat Baked ☞ serving size: 1 oz = 28.4 g; Calories = 90.6; Total Carb (g) = 14.7; Net Carb (g) = 14; Fat (g) = 2.6; Protein = 2.2

🎲 Blueberry Pie ☞ serving size: 1 oz = 28.4 g; Calories = 65.9; Total Carb (g) = 9.9; Net Carb (g) = 9.6; Fat (g) = 2.8; Protein = 0.5

🎲 Bread Banana Prepared From Recipe Made With Margarine ☞ serving size: 1 oz = 28.4 g; Calories = 92.6; Total Carb (g) = 15.5; Net Carb (g) = 15.2; Fat (g) = 3; Protein = 1.2

🎲 Bread Barley Toasted ☞ serving size: 1 small or thin/very thin slice = 22 g; Calories = 66.2; Total Carb (g) = 11.5; Net Carb (g) = 10.5; Fat (g) = 1.1; Protein = 2.6

Bread Boston Brown Canned ☞ serving size: 1 oz = 28.4 g; Calories = 55.4; Total Carb (g) = 12.3; Net Carb (g) = 11; Fat (g) = 0.4; Protein = 1.5

Bread Caressed Puerto Rican Style ☞ serving size: 1 slice = 25 g; Calories = 68.3; Total Carb (g) = 12.3; Net Carb (g) = 11.9; Fat (g) = 1.1; Protein = 1.9

Bread Caressed Toasted Puerto Rican Style ☞ serving size: 1 slice = 23 g; Calories = 69; Total Carb (g) = 12.5; Net Carb (g) = 12; Fat (g) = 1.2; Protein = 2

Bread Chapati Or Roti Plain Commercially Prepared ☞ serving size: 1 piece = 68 g; Calories = 202; Total Carb (g) = 31.5; Net Carb (g) = 28.2; Fat (g) = 5.1; Protein = 7.7

Bread Chapati Or Roti Whole Wheat Commercially Prepared Frozen ☞ serving size: 1 piece = 43 g; Calories = 128.6; Total Carb (g) = 19.8; Net Carb (g) = 15.7; Fat (g) = 4; Protein = 3.4

Bread Cheese ☞ serving size: 1 slice = 48 g; Calories = 195.8; Total Carb (g) = 21.5; Net Carb (g) = 20.5; Fat (g) = 10; Protein = 5

Bread Cheese Toasted ☞ serving size: 1 small or thin/very thin slice = 22 g; Calories = 98.6; Total Carb (g) = 10.8; Net Carb (g) = 10.3; Fat (g) = 5; Protein = 2.5

Bread Cinnamon ☞ serving size: 1 slice 1 serving = 28 g; Calories = 70.8; Total Carb (g) = 12.4; Net Carb (g) = 11.4; Fat (g) = 1.5; Protein = 2

Bread Cornbread Dry Mix Enriched (Includes Corn Muffin Mix) ☞ serving size: 1 oz = 28.4 g; Calories = 118.7; Total Carb (g) = 19.7; Net Carb (g) = 17.9; Fat (g) = 3.5; Protein = 2

Bread Cornbread Dry Mix Prepared With 2% Milk 80%

Margarine And Eggs ☞ serving size: 1 muffin = 51 g; Calories = 168.3; Total Carb (g) = 27.8; Net Carb (g) = 26.6; Fat (g) = 4.9; Protein = 3.4

🍞 Bread Cornbread Dry Mix Unenriched (Includes Corn Muffin Mix) ☞ serving size: 1 oz = 28.4 g; Calories = 118.7; Total Carb (g) = 19.7; Net Carb (g) = 17.9; Fat (g) = 3.5; Protein = 2

🍞 Bread Cornbread Prepared From Recipe Made With Low Fat (2%) Milk ☞ serving size: 1 oz = 28.4 g; Calories = 75.5; Total Carb (g) = 12.4; Net Carb (g) = 12.4; Fat (g) = 2; Protein = 1.9

🍞 Bread Cracked-Wheat ☞ serving size: 1 oz = 28.4 g; Calories = 73.8; Total Carb (g) = 14.1; Net Carb (g) = 12.5; Fat (g) = 1.1; Protein = 2.5

🍞 Bread Crumbs Dry Grated Plain ☞ serving size: 1 oz = 28.4 g; Calories = 112.2; Total Carb (g) = 20.4; Net Carb (g) = 19.2; Fat (g) = 1.5; Protein = 3.8

🍞 Bread Crumbs Dry Grated Seasoned ☞ serving size: 1 oz = 28.4 g; Calories = 108.8; Total Carb (g) = 19.5; Net Carb (g) = 18.1; Fat (g) = 1.6; Protein = 4

🍞 Bread Cuban Toasted ☞ serving size: 1 small or thin/very thin slice = 9 g; Calories = 26.9; Total Carb (g) = 5.1; Net Carb (g) = 4.9; Fat (g) = 0.2; Protein = 1.1

🍞 Bread Dough Fried ☞ serving size: 1 slice or roll = 26 g; Calories = 99.3; Total Carb (g) = 11.7; Net Carb (g) = 11.3; Fat (g) = 4.9; Protein = 2.1

🍞 Bread Egg ☞ serving size: 1 oz = 28.4 g; Calories = 81.5; Total Carb (g) = 13.6; Net Carb (g) = 12.9; Fat (g) = 1.7; Protein = 2.7

🍞 Bread Egg Challah Toasted ☞ serving size: 1 small or thin/very thin slice = 18 g; Calories = 56.7; Total Carb (g) = 9.5; Net Carb (g) = 9; Fat (g) = 1.2; Protein = 1.9

🍞 Bread Egg Toasted ☞ serving size: 1 oz = 28.4 g; Calories = 89.5; Total Carb (g) = 14.9; Net Carb (g) = 14.2; Fat (g) = 1.9; Protein = 3

Bread French Or Vienna Toasted (Includes Sourdough) ☞ serving size: 1 oz = 28.4 g; Calories = 90.6; Total Carb (g) = 17.6; Net Carb (g) = 16.7; Fat (g) = 0.6; Protein = 3.7

Bread French Or Vienna Whole Wheat ☞ serving size: 1 slice 1 serving = 48 g; Calories = 114.7; Total Carb (g) = 23.6; Net Carb (g) = 21.6; Fat (g) = 0.5; Protein = 4

Bread Fruit ☞ serving size: 1 slice = 41 g; Calories = 148.4; Total Carb (g) = 19.4; Net Carb (g) = 18.8; Fat (g) = 7.1; Protein = 2.4

Bread Gluten Free Toasted ☞ serving size: 1 small or thin/very thin slice = 22 g; Calories = 60.1; Total Carb (g) = 11.1; Net Carb (g) = 10; Fat (g) = 1.3; Protein = 1

Bread Gluten-Free White Made With Potato Extract Rice Starch And Rice Flour ☞ serving size: 1 slice = 34 g; Calories = 108.8; Total Carb (g) = 18; Net Carb (g) = 16.8; Fat (g) = 3.6; Protein = 1.1

Bread Gluten-Free White Made With Rice Flour Corn Starch And/or Tapioca ☞ serving size: 1 slice = 35 g; Calories = 86.8; Total Carb (g) = 16; Net Carb (g) = 14.5; Fat (g) = 1.8; Protein = 1.5

Bread Gluten-Free White Made With Tapioca Starch And Brown Rice Flour ☞ serving size: 1 slice = 28 g; Calories = 83.4; Total Carb (g) = 14.3; Net Carb (g) = 12.8; Fat (g) = 2.2; Protein = 1.5

Bread Gluten-Free Whole Grain Made With Tapioca Starch And Brown Rice Flour ☞ serving size: 1 slice = 25 g; Calories = 77.3; Total Carb (g) = 12.3; Net Carb (g) = 11; Fat (g) = 2.3; Protein = 1.8

Bread Irish Soda Prepared From Recipe ☞ serving size: 1 oz = 28.4 g; Calories = 82.4; Total Carb (g) = 15.9; Net Carb (g) = 15.2; Fat (g) = 1.4; Protein = 1.9

Bread Italian ☞ serving size: 1 oz = 28.4 g; Calories = 73.6; Total Carb (g) = 13.7; Net Carb (g) = 13.1; Fat (g) = 0.8; Protein = 2.7

Bread Italian Grecian Armenian ☞ serving size: 1 small or

thin/very thin slice = 24 g; Calories = 65; Total Carb (g) = 12; Net Carb (g) = 11.3; Fat (g) = 0.8; Protein = 2.1

🍞 Bread Italian Grecian Armenian Toasted ☞ serving size: 1 small or thin/very thin slice = 22 g; Calories = 65.6; Total Carb (g) = 12.1; Net Carb (g) = 11.3; Fat (g) = 0.8; Protein = 2.1

🍞 Bread Lard Puerto Rican Style ☞ serving size: 1 slice = 25 g; Calories = 70; Total Carb (g) = 13.9; Net Carb (g) = 13.4; Fat (g) = 0.7; Protein = 1.7

🍞 Bread Lard Toasted Puerto Rican Style ☞ serving size: 1 slice = 23 g; Calories = 71.5; Total Carb (g) = 14.2; Net Carb (g) = 13.7; Fat (g) = 0.7; Protein = 1.8

🍞 Bread Made From Home Recipe Or Purchased At A Bakery Ns As To Major Flour ☞ serving size: 1 small or thin/very thin slice = 33 g; Calories = 89.1; Total Carb (g) = 16.5; Net Carb (g) = 16; Fat (g) = 1.1; Protein = 2.8

🍞 Bread Made From Home Recipe Or Purchased At A Bakery Toasted Ns As To Major Flour ☞ serving size: 1 small or thin/very thin slice = 30 g; Calories = 89.1; Total Carb (g) = 16.5; Net Carb (g) = 15.9; Fat (g) = 1.1; Protein = 2.8

🍞 Bread Multi-Grain (Includes Whole-Grain) ☞ serving size: 1 oz = 28.4 g; Calories = 75.3; Total Carb (g) = 12.3; Net Carb (g) = 10.2; Fat (g) = 1.2; Protein = 3.8

🍞 Bread Naan Plain Commercially Prepared Refrigerated ☞ serving size: 1 piece = 90 g; Calories = 261.9; Total Carb (g) = 45.4; Net Carb (g) = 43.4; Fat (g) = 5.1; Protein = 8.7

🍞 Bread Naan Whole Wheat Commercially Prepared Refrigerated ☞ serving size: 1 piece = 106 g; Calories = 303.2; Total Carb (g) = 49; Net Carb (g) = 43.9; Fat (g) = 7.1; Protein = 10.8

🍞 Bread Native Water Puerto Rican Style ☞ serving size: 1 slice =

25 g; Calories = 69.3; Total Carb (g) = 13; Net Carb (g) = 12.5; Fat (g) = 0.8; Protein = 2.2

🍞 Bread Native Water Toasted Puerto Rican Style ☞ serving size: 1 slice = 23 g; Calories = 70.2; Total Carb (g) = 13.1; Net Carb (g) = 12.7; Fat (g) = 0.8; Protein = 2.2

🍞 Bread Nut ☞ serving size: 1 slice = 49 g; Calories = 192.1; Total Carb (g) = 24.4; Net Carb (g) = 23.7; Fat (g) = 9.4; Protein = 3.2

🍞 Bread Oat Bran ☞ serving size: 1 oz = 28.4 g; Calories = 67; Total Carb (g) = 11.3; Net Carb (g) = 10; Fat (g) = 1.2; Protein = 3

🍞 Bread Oat Bran Toasted ☞ serving size: 1 oz = 28.4 g; Calories = 73.6; Total Carb (g) = 12.4; Net Carb (g) = 11; Fat (g) = 1.4; Protein = 3.2

🍞 Bread Oatmeal ☞ serving size: 1 oz = 28.4 g; Calories = 76.4; Total Carb (g) = 13.8; Net Carb (g) = 12.6; Fat (g) = 1.2; Protein = 2.4

🍞 Bread Oatmeal Toasted ☞ serving size: 1 oz = 28.4 g; Calories = 82.9; Total Carb (g) = 15; Net Carb (g) = 13.7; Fat (g) = 1.4; Protein = 2.6

🍞 Bread Onion ☞ serving size: 1 small or thin/very thin slice = 24 g; Calories = 56.6; Total Carb (g) = 10.6; Net Carb (g) = 10.2; Fat (g) = 0.7; Protein = 1.8

🍞 Bread Onion Toasted ☞ serving size: 1 small or thin/very thin slice = 18 g; Calories = 46.8; Total Carb (g) = 8.7; Net Carb (g) = 8.4; Fat (g) = 0.6; Protein = 1.5

🍞 Bread Pan Dulce Sweet Yeast Bread ☞ serving size: 1 slice (average weight of 1 slice) = 63 g; Calories = 231.2; Total Carb (g) = 35.5; Net Carb (g) = 34.1; Fat (g) = 7.3; Protein = 5.9

🍞 Bread Paratha Whole Wheat Commercially Prepared Frozen ☞ serving size: 1 piece = 79 g; Calories = 257.5; Total Carb (g) = 35.8; Net Carb (g) = 28.2; Fat (g) = 10.4; Protein = 5

🍞 Bread Pita White Unenriched ☞ serving size: 1 oz = 28.4 g; Calo-

ries = 78.1; Total Carb (g) = 15.8; Net Carb (g) = 15.2; Fat (g) = 0.3; Protein = 2.6

Bread Potato ☞ serving size: 1 slice = 32 g; Calories = 85.1; Total Carb (g) = 15.1; Net Carb (g) = 13; Fat (g) = 1; Protein = 4

Bread Potato Toasted ☞ serving size: 1 small or thin/very thin slice = 24 g; Calories = 70.1; Total Carb (g) = 12.4; Net Carb (g) = 10.8; Fat (g) = 0.8; Protein = 3.3

Bread Pound Cake Type Pan De Torta Salvadoran ☞ serving size: 1 serving = 55 g; Calories = 214.5; Total Carb (g) = 28.2; Net Carb (g) = 27.3; Fat (g) = 9.6; Protein = 3.9

Bread Protein (Includes Gluten) ☞ serving size: 1 oz = 28.4 g; Calories = 69.6; Total Carb (g) = 12.4; Net Carb (g) = 11.6; Fat (g) = 0.6; Protein = 3.4

Bread Protein (Includes Gluten) Toasted ☞ serving size: 1 oz = 28.4 g; Calories = 76.7; Total Carb (g) = 13.7; Net Carb (g) = 12.7; Fat (g) = 0.7; Protein = 3.7

Bread Pumpernickel ☞ serving size: 1 oz = 28.4 g; Calories = 71; Total Carb (g) = 13.5; Net Carb (g) = 11.6; Fat (g) = 0.9; Protein = 2.5

Bread Pumpkin ☞ serving size: 1 slice = 60 g; Calories = 180; Total Carb (g) = 25.8; Net Carb (g) = 25; Fat (g) = 7.5; Protein = 2.9

Bread Puri Wheat ☞ serving size: 1 puri (approx 4-4/5" dia) = 36 g; Calories = 142.6; Total Carb (g) = 14.1; Net Carb (g) = 12.9; Fat (g) = 8.8; Protein = 2.2

Bread Raisin Enriched ☞ serving size: 1 oz = 28.4 g; Calories = 77.8; Total Carb (g) = 14.9; Net Carb (g) = 13.6; Fat (g) = 1.2; Protein = 2.2

Bread Raisin Enriched Toasted ☞ serving size: 1 oz = 28.4 g; Calories = 84.3; Total Carb (g) = 16.2; Net Carb (g) = 14.8; Fat (g) = 1.4; Protein = 2.4

▧ Bread Raisin Unenriched ☞ serving size: 1 oz = 28.4 g; Calories = 77.8; Total Carb (g) = 14.9; Net Carb (g) = 13.6; Fat (g) = 1.2; Protein = 2.2

▧ Bread Reduced-Calorie Oat Bran ☞ serving size: 1 oz = 28.4 g; Calories = 57.1; Total Carb (g) = 11.7; Net Carb (g) = 8.3; Fat (g) = 0.9; Protein = 2.3

▧ Bread Reduced-Calorie Oat Bran Toasted ☞ serving size: 1 oz = 28.4 g; Calories = 67.9; Total Carb (g) = 14; Net Carb (g) = 9.9; Fat (g) = 1.1; Protein = 2.7

▧ Bread Reduced-Calorie Oatmeal ☞ serving size: 1 oz = 28.4 g; Calories = 59.6; Total Carb (g) = 12.3; Net Carb (g) = 12.3; Fat (g) = 1; Protein = 2.2

▧ Bread Reduced-Calorie Rye ☞ serving size: 1 oz = 28.4 g; Calories = 57.7; Total Carb (g) = 11.5; Net Carb (g) = 8.1; Fat (g) = 0.8; Protein = 2.6

▧ Bread Reduced-Calorie Wheat ☞ serving size: 1 oz = 28.4 g; Calories = 61.6; Total Carb (g) = 12.1; Net Carb (g) = 8.9; Fat (g) = 0.8; Protein = 3.8

▧ Bread Reduced-Calorie White ☞ serving size: 1 oz = 28.4 g; Calories = 58.8; Total Carb (g) = 12.6; Net Carb (g) = 9.8; Fat (g) = 0.7; Protein = 2.5

▧ Bread Rice Bran ☞ serving size: 1 oz = 28.4 g; Calories = 69; Total Carb (g) = 12.4; Net Carb (g) = 11; Fat (g) = 1.3; Protein = 2.5

▧ Bread Rice Bran Toasted ☞ serving size: 1 oz = 28.4 g; Calories = 75; Total Carb (g) = 13.4; Net Carb (g) = 11.9; Fat (g) = 1.4; Protein = 2.8

▧ Bread Roll Mexican Bollilo ☞ serving size: 1 piece = 98 g; Calories = 311.6; Total Carb (g) = 54.7; Net Carb (g) = 52.5; Fat (g) = 5.7; Protein = 10.4

▧ Bread Rye Toasted ☞ serving size: 1 oz = 28.4 g; Calories = 80.7; Total Carb (g) = 15.1; Net Carb (g) = 13.3; Fat (g) = 1; Protein = 2.7

🍞 Bread Salvadoran Sweet Cheese (Quesadilla Salvadorena) ☞ serving size: 1 serving (approximate serving size) = 55 g; Calories = 205.7; Total Carb (g) = 26.3; Net Carb (g) = 25.9; Fat (g) = 9.4; Protein = 3.9

🍞 Bread Spanish Coffee ☞ serving size: 1 piece = 85 g; Calories = 292.4; Total Carb (g) = 49.5; Net Carb (g) = 47.9; Fat (g) = 7.4; Protein = 6.5

🍞 Bread Sprouted Wheat Toasted ☞ serving size: 1 slice = 24 g; Calories = 49.7; Total Carb (g) = 8.9; Net Carb (g) = 7.5; Fat (g) = 0; Protein = 3.5

🍞 Bread Sticks Plain ☞ serving size: 1 cup, small pieces = 46 g; Calories = 189.5; Total Carb (g) = 31.5; Net Carb (g) = 30.1; Fat (g) = 4.4; Protein = 5.5

🍞 Bread Stuffing Bread Dry Mix ☞ serving size: 1 oz = 28.4 g; Calories = 109.6; Total Carb (g) = 21.6; Net Carb (g) = 20.7; Fat (g) = 1; Protein = 3.1

🍞 Bread Stuffing Bread Dry Mix Prepared ☞ serving size: 1 oz = 28.4 g; Calories = 55.4; Total Carb (g) = 5.4; Net Carb (g) = 5.1; Fat (g) = 3.4; Protein = 0.8

🍞 Bread Stuffing Cornbread Dry Mix ☞ serving size: 1 oz = 28.4 g; Calories = 110.5; Total Carb (g) = 21.8; Net Carb (g) = 17.7; Fat (g) = 1.2; Protein = 2.8

🍞 Bread Stuffing Cornbread Dry Mix Prepared ☞ serving size: 1 oz = 28.4 g; Calories = 50.8; Total Carb (g) = 6.2; Net Carb (g) = 5.4; Fat (g) = 2.5; Protein = 0.8

🍞 Bread Sweet Potato Toasted ☞ serving size: 1 small or thin/very thin slice = 22 g; Calories = 57.9; Total Carb (g) = 10.9; Net Carb (g) = 10.5; Fat (g) = 0.7; Protein = 1.8

🍞 Bread Vegetable ☞ serving size: 1 slice = 44 g; Calories = 114; Total Carb (g) = 21.4; Net Carb (g) = 20.5; Fat (g) = 1.4; Protein = 3.6

🍞 Bread Vegetable Toasted ☞ serving size: 1 slice = 40 g; Calories = 114; Total Carb (g) = 21.4; Net Carb (g) = 20.5; Fat (g) = 1.4; Protein = 3.6

🍞 Bread Wheat Sprouted ☞ serving size: 1 slice 1 serving = 38 g; Calories = 71.4; Total Carb (g) = 12.9; Net Carb (g) = 10.9; Fat (g) = 0; Protein = 5

🍞 Bread Wheat Sprouted Toasted ☞ serving size: 1 slice 1 serving = 38 g; Calories = 77.9; Total Carb (g) = 14; Net Carb (g) = 11.8; Fat (g) = 0; Protein = 5.4

🍞 Bread Wheat Toasted ☞ serving size: 1 oz = 28.4 g; Calories = 88.9; Total Carb (g) = 15.8; Net Carb (g) = 14.5; Fat (g) = 1.2; Protein = 3.7

🍞 Bread White Commercially Prepared Low Sodium No Salt ☞ serving size: 1 oz = 28.4 g; Calories = 75.8; Total Carb (g) = 14.1; Net Carb (g) = 13.4; Fat (g) = 1; Protein = 2.3

🍞 Bread White Commercially Prepared Toasted Low Sodium No Salt ☞ serving size: 1 oz = 28.4 g; Calories = 83.2; Total Carb (g) = 15.4; Net Carb (g) = 15.4; Fat (g) = 1.1; Protein = 2.6

🍞 Bread White Made From Home Recipe Or Purchased At A Bakery ☞ serving size: 1 small or thin/very thin slice = 33 g; Calories = 89.1; Total Carb (g) = 16.5; Net Carb (g) = 16; Fat (g) = 1.1; Protein = 2.8

🍞 Bread White Made From Home Recipe Or Purchased At A Bakery Toasted ☞ serving size: 1 small or thin/very thin slice = 30 g; Calories = 89.1; Total Carb (g) = 16.5; Net Carb (g) = 15.9; Fat (g) = 1.1; Protein = 2.8

🍞 Bread White Prepared From Recipe Made With Low Fat (2%) Milk ☞ serving size: 1 oz = 28.4 g; Calories = 80.9; Total Carb (g) = 14.1; Net Carb (g) = 13.5; Fat (g) = 1.6; Protein = 2.2

🍞 Bread White Prepared From Recipe Made With Nonfat Dry

Milk ☞ serving size: 1 oz = 28.4 g; Calories = 77.8; Total Carb (g) = 15.2; Net Carb (g) = 14.7; Fat (g) = 0.7; Protein = 2.2

Bread White Wheat ☞ serving size: 1 slice = 28 g; Calories = 66.6; Total Carb (g) = 12.3; Net Carb (g) = 9.7; Fat (g) = 0.6; Protein = 3

Bread White With Whole Wheat Swirl ☞ serving size: 1 small or thin/very thin slice = 24 g; Calories = 62.2; Total Carb (g) = 11.1; Net Carb (g) = 10; Fat (g) = 0.8; Protein = 2.6

Bread White With Whole Wheat Swirl Toasted ☞ serving size: 1 small or thin/very thin slice = 22 g; Calories = 65.6; Total Carb (g) = 11.8; Net Carb (g) = 10.7; Fat (g) = 0.9; Protein = 2.6

Bread Whole Wheat Made From Home Recipe Or Purchased At Bakery ☞ serving size: 1 small or thin/very thin slice = 33 g; Calories = 81.8; Total Carb (g) = 15.7; Net Carb (g) = 13.4; Fat (g) = 1.3; Protein = 3

Bread Whole Wheat Made From Home Recipe Or Purchased At Bakery Toasted ☞ serving size: 1 small or thin/very thin slice = 30 g; Calories = 81.6; Total Carb (g) = 15.6; Net Carb (g) = 13.4; Fat (g) = 1.4; Protein = 3

Bread Whole Wheat Toasted ☞ serving size: 1 small or thin/very thin slice = 22 g; Calories = 60.9; Total Carb (g) = 10.3; Net Carb (g) = 8.9; Fat (g) = 0.8; Protein = 3

Bread Whole-Wheat Prepared From Recipe ☞ serving size: 1 oz = 28.4 g; Calories = 79; Total Carb (g) = 14.6; Net Carb (g) = 12.9; Fat (g) = 1.5; Protein = 2.4

Bread Whole-Wheat Prepared From Recipe Toasted ☞ serving size: 1 oz = 28.4 g; Calories = 86.6; Total Carb (g) = 16; Net Carb (g) = 14.1; Fat (g) = 1.7; Protein = 2.6

Bread Zucchini ☞ serving size: 1 slice = 40 g; Calories = 120; Total Carb (g) = 17; Net Carb (g) = 16.6; Fat (g) = 5.1; Protein = 2

Breadsticks Nfs ☞ serving size: 1 small stick = 28 g; Calories =

95.8; Total Carb (g) = 12.4; Net Carb (g) = 11.8; Fat (g) = 3.6; Protein = 3.4

🍴 Breadsticks Soft From Fast Food / Restaurant ☞ serving size: 1 small stick = 26 g; Calories = 88.9; Total Carb (g) = 11.5; Net Carb (g) = 10.9; Fat (g) = 3.3; Protein = 3.2

🍴 Breadsticks Soft From Frozen ☞ serving size: 1 small stick = 26 g; Calories = 81.1; Total Carb (g) = 12.1; Net Carb (g) = 11.4; Fat (g) = 2.4; Protein = 2.8

🍴 Breadsticks Soft Nfs ☞ serving size: 1 small stick = 28 g; Calories = 95.8; Total Carb (g) = 12.4; Net Carb (g) = 11.8; Fat (g) = 3.6; Protein = 3.4

🍴 Breadsticks Soft With Parmesan Cheese From Fast Food / Restaurant ☞ serving size: 1 small stick = 28 g; Calories = 96.3; Total Carb (g) = 12.3; Net Carb (g) = 11.6; Fat (g) = 3.7; Protein = 3.5

🍴 Breakfast Tart Low Fat ☞ serving size: 1 tart = 52 g; Calories = 193.4; Total Carb (g) = 39.9; Net Carb (g) = 39.2; Fat (g) = 3.1; Protein = 2.1

🍴 Brioche ☞ serving size: 1 piece = 77 g; Calories = 322.6; Total Carb (g) = 27.6; Net Carb (g) = 26.5; Fat (g) = 20.7; Protein = 6.7

🍴 Butter Croissants ☞ serving size: 1 oz = 28.4 g; Calories = 115.3; Total Carb (g) = 13; Net Carb (g) = 12.3; Fat (g) = 6; Protein = 2.3

🍴 Cake Angelfood Commercially Prepared ☞ serving size: 1 piece (1/12 of 12 oz cake) = 28 g; Calories = 72.2; Total Carb (g) = 16.2; Net Carb (g) = 15.8; Fat (g) = 0.2; Protein = 1.7

🍴 Cake Angelfood Dry Mix Prepared ☞ serving size: 1 piece (1/12 of 10 inch dia) = 50 g; Calories = 128.5; Total Carb (g) = 29.4; Net Carb (g) = 29.3; Fat (g) = 0.2; Protein = 3.1

🍴 Cake Batter Raw Chocolate ☞ serving size: 1 tablespoon = 14 g; Calories = 40.6; Total Carb (g) = 5.7; Net Carb (g) = 5.5; Fat (g) = 1.9; Protein = 0.6

Cake Batter Raw Not Chocolate ☞ serving size: 1 tablespoon = 15 g; Calories = 42.2; Total Carb (g) = 6.2; Net Carb (g) = 6.1; Fat (g) = 1.7; Protein = 0.6

Cake Boston Cream Pie Commercially Prepared ☞ serving size: 1 oz = 28.4 g; Calories = 71.6; Total Carb (g) = 12.2; Net Carb (g) = 11.8; Fat (g) = 2.4; Protein = 0.7

Cake Cherry Fudge With Chocolate Frosting ☞ serving size: 1 oz = 28.4 g; Calories = 75; Total Carb (g) = 10.8; Net Carb (g) = 10.7; Fat (g) = 3.6; Protein = 0.7

Cake Cream Without Icing Or Topping ☞ serving size: 1 cake (8" dia) = 510 g; Calories = 1887; Total Carb (g) = 234.3; Net Carb (g) = 232.3; Fat (g) = 95.5; Protein = 24.8

Cake Dobos Torte ☞ serving size: 1 cake (8-1/2" dia) = 1472 g; Calories = 5740.8; Total Carb (g) = 818.1; Net Carb (g) = 809.3; Fat (g) = 263; Protein = 52.8

Cake Fruitcake Commercially Prepared ☞ serving size: 1 oz = 28.4 g; Calories = 92; Total Carb (g) = 17.5; Net Carb (g) = 16.4; Fat (g) = 2.6; Protein = 0.8

Cake Gingerbread Dry Mix ☞ serving size: 1 oz = 28.4 g; Calories = 124.1; Total Carb (g) = 21.2; Net Carb (g) = 20.7; Fat (g) = 3.9; Protein = 1.2

Cake Ice Cream And Cake Roll Chocolate ☞ serving size: 1 ice cream roll (12 oz) = 340 g; Calories = 1064.2; Total Carb (g) = 138.3; Net Carb (g) = 132.8; Fat (g) = 55.4; Protein = 11.9

Cake Ice Cream And Cake Roll Not Chocolate ☞ serving size: 1 ice cream roll (12 oz) = 340 g; Calories = 1067.6; Total Carb (g) = 144.9; Net Carb (g) = 143.2; Fat (g) = 51.1; Protein = 10.9

Cake Jelly Roll ☞ serving size: 1 jelly roll = 506 g; Calories = 1852; Total Carb (g) = 284.9; Net Carb (g) = 281.8; Fat (g) = 70.4; Protein = 20.3

🍰 Cake Or Cupcake Applesauce With Icing Or Filling ☞ serving size: 1 regular cupcake = 75 g; Calories = 318; Total Carb (g) = 34.9; Net Carb (g) = 34.1; Fat (g) = 19.4; Protein = 2.9

🍰 Cake Or Cupcake Banana With Icing Or Filling ☞ serving size: 1 regular cupcake = 75 g; Calories = 326.3; Total Carb (g) = 36; Net Carb (g) = 35; Fat (g) = 19.8; Protein = 3.1

🍰 Cake Or Cupcake Banana Without Icing Or Filling ☞ serving size: 1 regular cupcake = 50 g; Calories = 212; Total Carb (g) = 23.5; Net Carb (g) = 22.5; Fat (g) = 12.5; Protein = 2.7

🍰 Cake Or Cupcake Carrot With Icing Or Filling ☞ serving size: 1 regular cupcake = 75 g; Calories = 321; Total Carb (g) = 34.4; Net Carb (g) = 33.4; Fat (g) = 19.9; Protein = 3.1

🍰 Cake Or Cupcake Carrot Without Icing Or Filling ☞ serving size: 1 regular cupcake = 50 g; Calories = 206.5; Total Carb (g) = 21.8; Net Carb (g) = 20.8; Fat (g) = 12.6; Protein = 2.7

🍰 Cake Or Cupcake Chocolate Devil's Food Or Fudge Without Icing Or Filling ☞ serving size: 1 regular cupcake = 50 g; Calories = 163; Total Carb (g) = 22.8; Net Carb (g) = 22.1; Fat (g) = 7.6; Protein = 2.4

🍰 Cake Or Cupcake German Chocolate With Icing Or Filling ☞ serving size: 1 regular cupcake = 75 g; Calories = 300.8; Total Carb (g) = 38.6; Net Carb (g) = 36.6; Fat (g) = 16.4; Protein = 2.9

🍰 Cake Or Cupcake Gingerbread ☞ serving size: 1 regular cupcake = 50 g; Calories = 154; Total Carb (g) = 25.3; Net Carb (g) = 24.7; Fat (g) = 5.1; Protein = 2

🍰 Cake Or Cupcake Lemon With Icing Or Filling ☞ serving size: 1 regular cupcake = 75 g; Calories = 289.5; Total Carb (g) = 41.3; Net Carb (g) = 41; Fat (g) = 13; Protein = 2.6

🍰 Cake Or Cupcake Lemon Without Icing Or Filling ☞ serving

size: 1 regular cupcake = 50 g; Calories = 172; Total Carb (g) = 22.7; Net Carb (g) = 22.5; Fat (g) = 8; Protein = 2.3

🍰 Cake Or Cupcake Marble With Icing Or Filling ☞ serving size: 1 regular cupcake = 75 g; Calories = 292.5; Total Carb (g) = 40.9; Net Carb (g) = 40; Fat (g) = 14.2; Protein = 2.4

🍰 Cake Or Cupcake Marble Without Icing Or Filling ☞ serving size: 1 regular cupcake = 50 g; Calories = 167.5; Total Carb (g) = 22.8; Net Carb (g) = 22.4; Fat (g) = 7.8; Protein = 2.4

🍰 Cake Or Cupcake Nut With Icing Or Filling ☞ serving size: 1 regular cupcake = 75 g; Calories = 303; Total Carb (g) = 40.3; Net Carb (g) = 39.7; Fat (g) = 15.1; Protein = 3.1

🍰 Cake Or Cupcake Nut Without Icing Or Filling ☞ serving size: 1 regular cupcake = 50 g; Calories = 212.5; Total Carb (g) = 23.1; Net Carb (g) = 22.4; Fat (g) = 12.4; Protein = 3.3

🍰 Cake Or Cupcake Oatmeal ☞ serving size: 1 regular cupcake = 50 g; Calories = 185; Total Carb (g) = 31.6; Net Carb (g) = 30.9; Fat (g) = 6.3; Protein = 1.6

🍰 Cake Or Cupcake Peanut Butter ☞ serving size: 1 regular cupcake = 50 g; Calories = 206.5; Total Carb (g) = 26.9; Net Carb (g) = 26.4; Fat (g) = 10.5; Protein = 2.6

🍰 Cake Or Cupcake Pumpkin With Icing Or Filling ☞ serving size: 1 regular cupcake = 75 g; Calories = 308.3; Total Carb (g) = 33; Net Carb (g) = 32; Fat (g) = 19; Protein = 3

🍰 Cake Or Cupcake Pumpkin Without Icing Or Filling ☞ serving size: 1 regular cupcake = 50 g; Calories = 193.5; Total Carb (g) = 20.5; Net Carb (g) = 19.4; Fat (g) = 11.8; Protein = 2.5

🍰 Cake Or Cupcake Raisin-Nut ☞ serving size: 1 regular cupcake = 50 g; Calories = 205.5; Total Carb (g) = 26.1; Net Carb (g) = 25.3; Fat (g) = 10.6; Protein = 3

🍰 Cake Or Cupcake Spice With Icing Or Filling ☞ serving size: 1

regular cupcake = 75 g; Calories = 318; Total Carb (g) = 34.9; Net Carb (g) = 34.1; Fat (g) = 19.4; Protein = 2.9

🍰 Cake Or Cupcake Spice Without Icing Or Filling ☞ serving size: 1 regular cupcake = 50 g; Calories = 204; Total Carb (g) = 22.4; Net Carb (g) = 21.6; Fat (g) = 12.1; Protein = 2.5

🍰 Cake Or Cupcake White Without Icing Or Filling ☞ serving size: 1 regular cupcake = 50 g; Calories = 164.5; Total Carb (g) = 24.8; Net Carb (g) = 24.6; Fat (g) = 6.5; Protein = 1.9

🍰 Cake Or Cupcake Yellow Without Icing Or Filling ☞ serving size: 1 regular cupcake = 50 g; Calories = 172; Total Carb (g) = 22.7; Net Carb (g) = 22.5; Fat (g) = 8; Protein = 2.3

🍰 Cake Or Cupcake Zucchini ☞ serving size: 1 1-layer cake (8" or 9" dia, 1-1/2" high) = 579 g; Calories = 2530.2; Total Carb (g) = 267.3; Net Carb (g) = 260.9; Fat (g) = 157.8; Protein = 24.6

🍰 Cake Pound Bimbo Bakeries Usa Panque Casero Home Baked Style ☞ serving size: 1 slice = 39 g; Calories = 163; Total Carb (g) = 19.1; Net Carb (g) = 18.7; Fat (g) = 8.5; Protein = 2.6

🍰 Cake Pound Chocolate ☞ serving size: 1 loaf (9" x 5" x 3") = 909 g; Calories = 3763.3; Total Carb (g) = 557.9; Net Carb (g) = 543.4; Fat (g) = 166.3; Protein = 49.3

🍰 Cake Pound Commercially Prepared Other Than All Butter Unenriched ☞ serving size: 1 piece (1/10 of 10.6 oz cake) = 30 g; Calories = 116.7; Total Carb (g) = 15.8; Net Carb (g) = 15.5; Fat (g) = 5.4; Protein = 1.6

🍰 Cake Pound Puerto Rican Style ☞ serving size: 1 slice (3-1/2" x 3-1/2" x 1") = 90 g; Calories = 418.5; Total Carb (g) = 40.7; Net Carb (g) = 40.2; Fat (g) = 26.1; Protein = 6.3

🍰 Cake Pound With Icing Or Filling ☞ serving size: 1 loaf (9-1/4" x 5-1/4" x 3-1/8") = 1228 g; Calories = 4948.8; Total Carb (g) = 770.9; Net Carb (g) = 766; Fat (g) = 194.3; Protein = 44.1

🎂 Cake Pudding-Type Carrot Dry Mix ☞ serving size: 1 oz = 28.4 g; Calories = 117.9; Total Carb (g) = 22.5; Net Carb (g) = 22.5; Fat (g) = 2.8; Protein = 1.4

🎂 Cake Pudding-Type Chocolate Dry Mix ☞ serving size: 1 oz = 28.4 g; Calories = 111; Total Carb (g) = 22.8; Net Carb (g) = 22.1; Fat (g) = 2.3; Protein = 1.3

🎂 Cake Pudding-Type White Enriched Dry Mix ☞ serving size: 1 oz = 28.4 g; Calories = 120.1; Total Carb (g) = 23; Net Carb (g) = 22.8; Fat (g) = 2.7; Protein = 1.1

🎂 Cake Pudding-Type White Unenriched Dry Mix ☞ serving size: 1 oz = 28.4 g; Calories = 120.1; Total Carb (g) = 23; Net Carb (g) = 22.8; Fat (g) = 2.7; Protein = 1.1

🎂 Cake Pudding-Type Yellow Dry Mix ☞ serving size: 1 oz = 28.4 g; Calories = 120.1; Total Carb (g) = 22.7; Net Carb (g) = 22.5; Fat (g) = 2.8; Protein = 1.1

🎂 Cake Ravani ☞ serving size: 1 cake = 564 g; Calories = 1545.4; Total Carb (g) = 276.2; Net Carb (g) = 272.3; Fat (g) = 42.1; Protein = 21.5

🎂 Cake Shortcake Biscuit Type With Fruit ☞ serving size: 1 biscuit (2" dia) with fruit = 65 g; Calories = 141.1; Total Carb (g) = 20.1; Net Carb (g) = 19.1; Fat (g) = 5.7; Protein = 2.8

🎂 Cake Shortcake Biscuit Type With Whipped Cream And Fruit ☞ serving size: 1 biscuit (2" dia) with fruit and whipped cream = 74 g; Calories = 162.1; Total Carb (g) = 20.6; Net Carb (g) = 19.6; Fat (g) = 7.7; Protein = 3

🎂 Cake Shortcake Biscuit-Type Prepared From Recipe ☞ serving size: 1 oz = 28.4 g; Calories = 98.3; Total Carb (g) = 13.8; Net Carb (g) = 13.8; Fat (g) = 4; Protein = 1.7

🎂 Cake Shortcake Sponge Type With Fruit ☞ serving size: 1 cake

(3" dia) with fruit = 102 g; Calories = 251.9; Total Carb (g) = 53.7; Net Carb (g) = 52.7; Fat (g) = 2.3; Protein = 4.5

🍰 Cake Shortcake Sponge Type With Whipped Cream And Fruit ☞ serving size: 1 cake (3" dia) with fruit and whipped cream = 118 g; Calories = 285.6; Total Carb (g) = 55.8; Net Carb (g) = 54.8; Fat (g) = 5; Protein = 5

🍰 Cake Shortcake With Whipped Topping And Fruit Diet ☞ serving size: 1 individual cake = 94 g; Calories = 204; Total Carb (g) = 38.1; Net Carb (g) = 37.1; Fat (g) = 4.5; Protein = 3.4

🍰 Cake Snack Cakes Creme-Filled Chocolate With Frosting ☞ serving size: 1 oz = 28.4 g; Calories = 113.3; Total Carb (g) = 17.1; Net Carb (g) = 16.2; Fat (g) = 4.5; Protein = 1

🍰 Cake Snack Cakes Creme-Filled Chocolate With Frosting Low-Fat With Added Fiber ☞ serving size: 1 cake 1 serving = 27 g; Calories = 110.4; Total Carb (g) = 18.7; Net Carb (g) = 14.7; Fat (g) = 3.5; Protein = 1

🍰 Cake Snack Cakes Creme-Filled Sponge ☞ serving size: 1 oz = 28.4 g; Calories = 106.2; Total Carb (g) = 18.2; Net Carb (g) = 17.9; Fat (g) = 3.3; Protein = 1

🍰 Cake Snack Cakes Not Chocolate With Icing Or Filling Low-Fat With Added Fiber ☞ serving size: 1 cake 1 serving = 27 g; Calories = 111.2; Total Carb (g) = 20.1; Net Carb (g) = 16; Fat (g) = 3; Protein = 1

🍰 Cake Sponge Chocolate ☞ serving size: 1 tube cake (10" dia, 4" high) = 790 g; Calories = 2796.6; Total Carb (g) = 525; Net Carb (g) = 519.4; Fat (g) = 69.1; Protein = 32.5

🍰 Cake Sponge Commercially Prepared ☞ serving size: 1 oz = 28.4 g; Calories = 82.4; Total Carb (g) = 17.3; Net Carb (g) = 17.2; Fat (g) = 0.8; Protein = 1.5

🍰 Cake Sponge Prepared From Recipe ☞ serving size: 1 oz = 28.4 g;

Calories = 84.3; Total Carb (g) = 16.4; Net Carb (g) = 16.4; Fat (g) = 1.2; Protein = 2.1

🍰 Cake Sponge With Icing Or Filling ☞ serving size: 1 tube cake (10-1/2" dia, 4-1/4" high) = 1109 g; Calories = 4014.6; Total Carb (g) = 757.3; Net Carb (g) = 754; Fat (g) = 91; Protein = 40.9

🍰 Cake Torte ☞ serving size: 1 torte = 912 g; Calories = 2581; Total Carb (g) = 338.7; Net Carb (g) = 331.4; Fat (g) = 123.8; Protein = 33.6

🍰 Cake Tres Leche ☞ serving size: 1 cake = 1448 g; Calories = 3866.2; Total Carb (g) = 607; Net Carb (g) = 602.7; Fat (g) = 125.5; Protein = 91.9

🍰 Cake White Dry Mix Special Dietary (Includes Lemon-Flavored) ☞ serving size: 1 oz = 28.4 g; Calories = 112.7; Total Carb (g) = 22.6; Net Carb (g) = 22.6; Fat (g) = 2.4; Protein = 0.9

🍰 Cake White Prepared From Recipe Without Frosting ☞ serving size: 1 piece (1/12 of 9 inch dia) = 74 g; Calories = 264.2; Total Carb (g) = 42.3; Net Carb (g) = 41.7; Fat (g) = 9.2; Protein = 4

🍰 Cake Yellow Enriched Dry Mix ☞ serving size: 1 serving = 43 g; Calories = 160.8; Total Carb (g) = 35.2; Net Carb (g) = 34.7; Fat (g) = 1.5; Protein = 1.6

🍰 Cake Yellow Light Dry Mix ☞ serving size: 1 oz = 28.4 g; Calories = 114.7; Total Carb (g) = 23.9; Net Carb (g) = 23.5; Fat (g) = 1.6; Protein = 1.3

🍰 Cake Yellow Prepared From Recipe Without Frosting ☞ serving size: 1 piece (1/12 of 8 inch dia) = 68 g; Calories = 245.5; Total Carb (g) = 36; Net Carb (g) = 35.6; Fat (g) = 9.9; Protein = 3.6

🍰 Cake Yellow Unenriched Dry Mix ☞ serving size: 1 oz = 28.4 g; Calories = 122.7; Total Carb (g) = 22.2; Net Carb (g) = 21.9; Fat (g) = 3.3; Protein = 1.2

🍰 Calzone With Cheese Meatless ☞ serving size: 1 calzone or

stromboli = 424 g; Calories = 1632.4; Total Carb (g) = 122.2; Net Carb (g) = 116.7; Fat (g) = 93.5; Protein = 73.8

📦 Calzone With Meat And Cheese ☞ serving size: 1 calzone or stromboli = 424 g; Calories = 1475.5; Total Carb (g) = 132.1; Net Carb (g) = 126.2; Fat (g) = 77.3; Protein = 60.5

📦 Casabe Cassava Bread ☞ serving size: 1 piece (6" dia) = 100 g; Calories = 299; Total Carb (g) = 71.2; Net Carb (g) = 67.8; Fat (g) = 0.5; Protein = 2.5

📦 Cheese Croissants ☞ serving size: 1 oz = 28.4 g; Calories = 117.6; Total Carb (g) = 13.3; Net Carb (g) = 12.6; Fat (g) = 5.9; Protein = 2.6

📦 Cheese Pastry Puffs ☞ serving size: 1 puff or cheese straw (5" long) = 6 g; Calories = 15.8; Total Carb (g) = 0.8; Net Carb (g) = 0.8; Fat (g) = 1.2; Protein = 0.6

📦 Cheesecake Chocolate ☞ serving size: 1 cake or pie (9" dia, approx 1-1/2" high) = 1533 g; Calories = 5733.4; Total Carb (g) = 499; Net Carb (g) = 483.7; Fat (g) = 395.8; Protein = 91.5

📦 Cheesecake Commercially Prepared ☞ serving size: 1 oz = 28.4 g; Calories = 91.2; Total Carb (g) = 7.2; Net Carb (g) = 7.1; Fat (g) = 6.4; Protein = 1.6

📦 Cheesecake Prepared From Mix No-Bake Type ☞ serving size: 1 oz = 28.4 g; Calories = 77.8; Total Carb (g) = 10.1; Net Carb (g) = 9.5; Fat (g) = 3.6; Protein = 1.6

📦 Cheesecake With Fruit ☞ serving size: 1 cake or pie (9" dia, approx 1-1/2" high) = 1704 g; Calories = 3561.4; Total Carb (g) = 317.3; Net Carb (g) = 300.2; Fat (g) = 237.2; Protein = 61.9

📦 Chocolate Cake ☞ serving size: 1 piece (1/12 of 9 inch dia) = 95 g; Calories = 352.5; Total Carb (g) = 50.7; Net Carb (g) = 49.2; Fat (g) = 14.3; Protein = 5

📦 Chocolate Cake With Frosting ☞ serving size: 1 piece (1/12 of a cake) = 138 g; Calories = 536.8; Total Carb (g) = 72.9; Net Carb (g) = 69.9; Fat (g) = 27.7; Protein = 4.8

🍪 Chocolate Coated Graham Crackers ☞ serving size: 3 pieces = 27 g; Calories = 135; Total Carb (g) = 18; Net Carb (g) = 17.4; Fat (g) = 7; Protein = 1.1

🍪 Chocolate Coated Marshmallows ☞ serving size: 1 oz = 28.4 g; Calories = 119.6; Total Carb (g) = 19.2; Net Carb (g) = 18.7; Fat (g) = 4.8; Protein = 1.1

🍪 Churros ☞ serving size: 1 churro = 26 g; Calories = 125.1; Total Carb (g) = 12.9; Net Carb (g) = 12.7; Fat (g) = 8; Protein = 0.8

🍪 Cinnamon Buns Frosted (Includes Honey Buns) ☞ serving size: 1 bun = 65 g; Calories = 293.8; Total Carb (g) = 31.6; Net Carb (g) = 30.8; Fat (g) = 17.3; Protein = 2.9

🍪 Cinnamon Coffeecake ☞ serving size: 1 oz = 28.4 g; Calories = 118.7; Total Carb (g) = 13.3; Net Carb (g) = 12.7; Fat (g) = 6.6; Protein = 1.9

🍪 Cinnamon Raisin Bagels ☞ serving size: 1 mini bagel (2-1/2 inch dia) = 26 g; Calories = 71.2; Total Carb (g) = 14.4; Net Carb (g) = 13.8; Fat (g) = 0.4; Protein = 2.5

🍪 Cobbler Apple ☞ serving size: 1 cup = 217 g; Calories = 423.2; Total Carb (g) = 79.1; Net Carb (g) = 77.2; Fat (g) = 10.6; Protein = 5

🍪 Cobbler Apricot ☞ serving size: 1 cup = 217 g; Calories = 408; Total Carb (g) = 77.6; Net Carb (g) = 73.7; Fat (g) = 9.5; Protein = 5.7

🍪 Cobbler Berry ☞ serving size: 1 cup = 217 g; Calories = 499.1; Total Carb (g) = 93.4; Net Carb (g) = 89.5; Fat (g) = 12.6; Protein = 6

🍪 Cobbler Cherry ☞ serving size: 1 cup = 217 g; Calories = 421; Total Carb (g) = 77.4; Net Carb (g) = 75.1; Fat (g) = 11.1; Protein = 5.1

🍪 Cobbler Peach ☞ serving size: 1 cup = 217 g; Calories = 431.8; Total Carb (g) = 82.8; Net Carb (g) = 79.7; Fat (g) = 10.1; Protein = 5.4

🍮 Cobbler Pear ☞ serving size: 1 cup = 217 g; Calories = 466.6; Total Carb (g) = 91.4; Net Carb (g) = 86.2; Fat (g) = 10.6; Protein = 4.6

🍮 Cobbler Pineapple ☞ serving size: 1 cup = 217 g; Calories = 414.5; Total Carb (g) = 79.7; Net Carb (g) = 78; Fat (g) = 10; Protein = 4.3

🍮 Cobbler Plum ☞ serving size: 1 cup = 217 g; Calories = 434; Total Carb (g) = 83.2; Net Carb (g) = 80.4; Fat (g) = 10.3; Protein = 4.9

🍮 Cobbler Rhubarb ☞ serving size: 1 cup = 217 g; Calories = 544.7; Total Carb (g) = 101.7; Net Carb (g) = 98.9; Fat (g) = 14.3; Protein = 5.1

🍮 Coconut Cream Cake Puerto Rican Style ☞ serving size: 1 tablespoon = 15 g; Calories = 47.7; Total Carb (g) = 7.1; Net Carb (g) = 6.9; Fat (g) = 2.2; Protein = 0.4

🍮 Coconut Custard Pie ☞ serving size: 1 oz = 28.4 g; Calories = 73.8; Total Carb (g) = 8.6; Net Carb (g) = 8.1; Fat (g) = 3.7; Protein = 1.7

🍮 Coffee Cake Crumb Or Quick-Bread Type ☞ serving size: 1 cake (9" square) = 692 g; Calories = 2643.4; Total Carb (g) = 354.6; Net Carb (g) = 344.2; Fat (g) = 122.6; Protein = 44

🍮 Coffee Cake Crumb Or Quick-Bread Type Cheese-Filled ☞ serving size: 1 cake (8" square) = 568 g; Calories = 2016.4; Total Carb (g) = 252.4; Net Carb (g) = 245; Fat (g) = 98; Protein = 41.1

🍮 Coffee Cake Crumb Or Quick-Bread Type With Fruit ☞ serving size: 1 cake (9" square) = 785 g; Calories = 2441.4; Total Carb (g) = 394.1; Net Carb (g) = 383.9; Fat (g) = 88.7; Protein = 32.3

🍮 Coffeecake Cheese ☞ serving size: 1 oz = 28.4 g; Calories = 96.3; Total Carb (g) = 12.6; Net Carb (g) = 12.3; Fat (g) = 4.3; Protein = 2

🍮 Coffeecake Cinnamon With Crumb Topping Commercially Prepared Unenriched ☞ serving size: 1 oz = 28.4 g; Calories = 118.7; Total Carb (g) = 13.3; Net Carb (g) = 12.7; Fat (g) = 6.6; Protein = 1.9

🍮 Coffeecake Cinnamon With Crumb Topping Dry Mix Prepared

☞ serving size: 1 oz = 28.4 g; Calories = 90.3; Total Carb (g) = 15; Net Carb (g) = 14.7; Fat (g) = 2.7; Protein = 1.6

🔳 Coffeecake Creme-Filled With Chocolate Frosting ☞ serving size: 1 oz = 28.4 g; Calories = 94; Total Carb (g) = 15.3; Net Carb (g) = 14.7; Fat (g) = 3.1; Protein = 1.4

🔳 Coffeecake Fruit ☞ serving size: 1 oz = 28.4 g; Calories = 88.3; Total Carb (g) = 14.6; Net Carb (g) = 13.9; Fat (g) = 2.9; Protein = 1.5

🔳 Continental Mills Krusteaz Almond Poppyseed Muffin Mix Artificially Flavored Dry ☞ serving size: 1 serving = 40 g; Calories = 167.2; Total Carb (g) = 30.2; Net Carb (g) = 29.6; Fat (g) = 4.1; Protein = 2.2

🔳 Cookie Batter Or Dough Raw ☞ serving size: 1 cup = 250 g; Calories = 1077.5; Total Carb (g) = 135.5; Net Carb (g) = 133.2; Fat (g) = 55.5; Protein = 12

🔳 Cookie Biscotti ☞ serving size: 1 cookie = 32 g; Calories = 117.1; Total Carb (g) = 21.3; Net Carb (g) = 20.9; Fat (g) = 2.5; Protein = 2.4

🔳 Cookie Brownie With Icing Or Filling ☞ serving size: 1 small = 40 g; Calories = 160.4; Total Carb (g) = 25.4; Net Carb (g) = 24.8; Fat (g) = 6.8; Protein = 1.2

🔳 Cookie Butter Or Sugar With Chocolate Icing Or Filling ☞ serving size: 3 cookies = 31 g; Calories = 155.9; Total Carb (g) = 21.3; Net Carb (g) = 20.7; Fat (g) = 7.3; Protein = 1.3

🔳 Cookie Butter Or Sugar With Fruit And/or Nuts ☞ serving size: 1 miniature/bite size = 5 g; Calories = 23.3; Total Carb (g) = 3.3; Net Carb (g) = 3.2; Fat (g) = 1; Protein = 0.3

🔳 Cookie Butter Or Sugar With Icing Or Filling Other Than Chocolate ☞ serving size: 1 miniature/bite size = 7 g; Calories = 30.1; Total Carb (g) = 5.1; Net Carb (g) = 5.1; Fat (g) = 1; Protein = 0.2

🔳 Cookie Chocolate Chip Made From Home Recipe Or Purchased At A Bakery ☞ serving size: 1 miniature/bite size = 5 g;

Calories = 24.5; Total Carb (g) = 3; Net Carb (g) = 2.8; Fat (g) = 1.4; Protein = 0.3

🍪 Cookie Chocolate With Icing Or Coating ☞ serving size: 4 cookies = 32 g; Calories = 162.2; Total Carb (g) = 21.7; Net Carb (g) = 21; Fat (g) = 7.7; Protein = 1.4

🍪 Cookie Graham Cracker With Chocolate And Marshmallow ☞ serving size: 1 suddenly s'mores cookie = 19 g; Calories = 88.4; Total Carb (g) = 13.1; Net Carb (g) = 12.6; Fat (g) = 3.5; Protein = 1.2

🍪 Cookie Oatmeal With Chocolate Chips ☞ serving size: 1 miniature/bite size = 5 g; Calories = 22.9; Total Carb (g) = 3.4; Net Carb (g) = 3.2; Fat (g) = 1; Protein = 0.3

🍪 Cookie Peanut Butter With Chocolate ☞ serving size: 1 miniature/bite size = 5 g; Calories = 23.8; Total Carb (g) = 3; Net Carb (g) = 2.8; Fat (g) = 1.3; Protein = 0.4

🍪 Cookie Shortbread With Icing Or Filling ☞ serving size: 1 miniature/bite size = 7 g; Calories = 36.1; Total Carb (g) = 4.4; Net Carb (g) = 4.2; Fat (g) = 2; Protein = 0.4

🍪 Cookie Vanilla With Caramel Coconut And Chocolate Coating ☞ serving size: 2 cookies = 29 g; Calories = 141.8; Total Carb (g) = 18.6; Net Carb (g) = 17.3; Fat (g) = 7.5; Protein = 1

🍪 Cookie With Peanut Butter Filling Chocolate-Coated ☞ serving size: 2 cookies = 25 g; Calories = 140.5; Total Carb (g) = 13.2; Net Carb (g) = 12.4; Fat (g) = 8.8; Protein = 2

🍪 Cookies Animal Crackers (Includes Arrowroot Tea Biscuits) ☞ serving size: 1 oz = 28.4 g; Calories = 126.7; Total Carb (g) = 21; Net Carb (g) = 20.7; Fat (g) = 3.9; Protein = 2

🍪 Cookies Animal With Frosting Or Icing ☞ serving size: 8 cookies 1 serving = 31 g; Calories = 157.8; Total Carb (g) = 21.7; Net Carb (g) = 21.4; Fat (g) = 7.5; Protein = 0.9

🍪 Cookies Brownies Commercially Prepared ☞ serving size: 1 oz =

28.4 g; Calories = 115; Total Carb (g) = 18.1; Net Carb (g) = 17.6; Fat (g) = 4.6; Protein = 1.4

🍪 Cookies Brownies Commercially Prepared Reduced Fat With Added Fiber ☞ serving size: 1 brownie 1 serving = 36 g; Calories = 124.2; Total Carb (g) = 22.2; Net Carb (g) = 18.2; Fat (g) = 3.5; Protein = 1

🍪 Cookies Brownies Dry Mix Regular ☞ serving size: 1 oz = 28.4 g; Calories = 123.3; Total Carb (g) = 21.8; Net Carb (g) = 21.8; Fat (g) = 4.2; Protein = 1.1

🍪 Cookies Brownies Dry Mix Sugar Free ☞ serving size: 1 oz = 28.4 g; Calories = 121; Total Carb (g) = 22.8; Net Carb (g) = 21.6; Fat (g) = 3.6; Protein = 0.8

🍪 Cookies Brownies Prepared From Recipe ☞ serving size: 1 oz = 28.4 g; Calories = 132.3; Total Carb (g) = 14.3; Net Carb (g) = 14.3; Fat (g) = 8.3; Protein = 1.8

🍪 Cookies Butter Commercially Prepared Enriched ☞ serving size: 1 oz = 28.4 g; Calories = 132.6; Total Carb (g) = 19.6; Net Carb (g) = 19.3; Fat (g) = 5.3; Protein = 1.7

🍪 Cookies Butter Commercially Prepared Unenriched ☞ serving size: 1 oz = 28.4 g; Calories = 132.6; Total Carb (g) = 19.6; Net Carb (g) = 19.3; Fat (g) = 5.3; Protein = 1.7

🍪 Cookies Chocolate Chip Commercially Prepared Regular Higher Fat Enriched ☞ serving size: 1 cookie = 12.9 g; Calories = 63.5; Total Carb (g) = 8.4; Net Carb (g) = 8.2; Fat (g) = 3.2; Protein = 0.7

🍪 Cookies Chocolate Chip Commercially Prepared Regular Higher Fat Unenriched ☞ serving size: 1 oz = 28.4 g; Calories = 136.6; Total Carb (g) = 19; Net Carb (g) = 18.3; Fat (g) = 6.4; Protein = 1.5

🍪 Cookies Chocolate Chip Commercially Prepared Regular Lower Fat ☞ serving size: 1 serving 3 cookies = 34 g; Calories = 153.3; Total Carb (g) = 22.9; Net Carb (g) = 21.9; Fat (g) = 6.1; Protein = 2

Cookies Chocolate Chip Commercially Prepared Soft-Type ☞ serving size: 1 cookie = 14.2 g; Calories = 63; Total Carb (g) = 9.3; Net Carb (g) = 9.1; Fat (g) = 2.8; Protein = 0.5

Cookies Chocolate Chip Commercially Prepared Special Dietary ☞ serving size: 1 oz = 28.4 g; Calories = 127.8; Total Carb (g) = 20.8; Net Carb (g) = 20.4; Fat (g) = 4.8; Protein = 1.1

Cookies Chocolate Chip Dry Mix ☞ serving size: 1 oz = 28.4 g; Calories = 141.1; Total Carb (g) = 18.8; Net Carb (g) = 18.8; Fat (g) = 7.2; Protein = 1.3

Cookies Chocolate Chip Prepared From Recipe Made With Butter ☞ serving size: 1 oz = 28.4 g; Calories = 138.6; Total Carb (g) = 16.5; Net Carb (g) = 16.5; Fat (g) = 8.1; Protein = 1.6

Cookies Chocolate Chip Prepared From Recipe Made With Margarine ☞ serving size: 1 oz = 28.4 g; Calories = 138.6; Total Carb (g) = 16.6; Net Carb (g) = 15.8; Fat (g) = 8; Protein = 1.6

Cookies Chocolate Chip Refrigerated Dough ☞ serving size: 1 serving = 33 g; Calories = 148.8; Total Carb (g) = 20.1; Net Carb (g) = 19.6; Fat (g) = 7; Protein = 1.3

Cookies Chocolate Chip Refrigerated Dough Baked ☞ serving size: 1 oz = 28.4 g; Calories = 139.7; Total Carb (g) = 19.4; Net Carb (g) = 18.9; Fat (g) = 6.4; Protein = 1.4

Cookies Chocolate Chip Sandwich With Creme Filling ☞ serving size: 1 cookie = 34 g; Calories = 144.5; Total Carb (g) = 21.6; Net Carb (g) = 21.6; Fat (g) = 6; Protein = 1

Cookies Chocolate Cream Covered Biscuit Sticks ☞ serving size: 1 serving = 40 g; Calories = 178.8; Total Carb (g) = 20.4; Net Carb (g) = 18.4; Fat (g) = 9; Protein = 4

Cookies Chocolate Made With Rice Cereal ☞ serving size: 1 cookie = 62 g; Calories = 272.8; Total Carb (g) = 39.2; Net Carb (g) = 38.2; Fat (g) = 12; Protein = 2

🍪 Cookies Chocolate Sandwich With Creme Filling Reduced Fat ☞ serving size: 1 serving = 34 g; Calories = 148.2; Total Carb (g) = 25.9; Net Carb (g) = 24.9; Fat (g) = 4.5; Protein = 1

🍪 Cookies Chocolate Sandwich With Creme Filling Regular ☞ serving size: 3 cookie = 36 g; Calories = 167; Total Carb (g) = 25.6; Net Carb (g) = 24.5; Fat (g) = 6.9; Protein = 1.9

🍪 Cookies Chocolate Sandwich With Creme Filling Regular Chocolate-Coated ☞ serving size: 1 oz = 28.4 g; Calories = 136.6; Total Carb (g) = 18.9; Net Carb (g) = 17.4; Fat (g) = 7.5; Protein = 1

🍪 Cookies Chocolate Sandwich With Creme Filling Special Dietary ☞ serving size: 1 oz = 28.4 g; Calories = 130.9; Total Carb (g) = 19.3; Net Carb (g) = 18.1; Fat (g) = 6.3; Protein = 1.3

🍪 Cookies Chocolate Sandwich With Extra Creme Filling ☞ serving size: 1 oz = 28.4 g; Calories = 141.1; Total Carb (g) = 19.4; Net Carb (g) = 18.6; Fat (g) = 7; Protein = 1.2

🍪 Cookies Chocolate Wafers ☞ serving size: 1 oz = 28.4 g; Calories = 123; Total Carb (g) = 20.6; Net Carb (g) = 19.7; Fat (g) = 4; Protein = 1.9

🍪 Cookies Coconut Macaroon ☞ serving size: 2 cookie 1 serving = 36 g; Calories = 165.6; Total Carb (g) = 22; Net Carb (g) = 20.2; Fat (g) = 8.1; Protein = 1.1

🍪 Cookies Fudge Cake-Type (Includes Trolley Cakes) ☞ serving size: 1 oz = 28.4 g; Calories = 99.1; Total Carb (g) = 22.2; Net Carb (g) = 21.4; Fat (g) = 1.1; Protein = 1.4

🍪 Cookies Gluten-Free Chocolate Sandwich With Creme Filling ☞ serving size: 3 cookies = 44 g; Calories = 208.6; Total Carb (g) = 33.5; Net Carb (g) = 32.4; Fat (g) = 7.9; Protein = 1

🍪 Cookies Gluten-Free Chocolate Wafer ☞ serving size: 3 cookies = 23 g; Calories = 124.4; Total Carb (g) = 14.4; Net Carb (g) = 14.1; Fat (g) = 7; Protein = 0.9

🍪 Cookies Gluten-Free Lemon Wafer ☞ serving size: 3 cookies = 30 g; Calories = 154.5; Total Carb (g) = 22.3; Net Carb (g) = 22.3; Fat (g) = 7.3; Protein = 0

🍪 Cookies Gluten-Free Vanilla Sandwich With Creme Filling ☞ serving size: 3 cookies = 44 g; Calories = 216.9; Total Carb (g) = 32.8; Net Carb (g) = 32.6; Fat (g) = 9; Protein = 1.2

🍪 Cookies Graham Crackers Plain Or Honey Lowfat ☞ serving size: 1 serving = 35 g; Calories = 135.1; Total Carb (g) = 27.3; Net Carb (g) = 25.3; Fat (g) = 2; Protein = 2

🍪 Cookies Ladyfingers Without Lemon Juice And Rind ☞ serving size: 1 oz = 28.4 g; Calories = 103.1; Total Carb (g) = 17; Net Carb (g) = 16.7; Fat (g) = 2.6; Protein = 3

🍪 Cookies Marie Biscuit ☞ serving size: 5 cookie = 28 g; Calories = 113.7; Total Carb (g) = 19.8; Net Carb (g) = 18.8; Fat (g) = 3; Protein = 2

🍪 Cookies Marshmallow With Rice Cereal And Chocolate Chips ☞ serving size: 1 bar = 22 g; Calories = 95.7; Total Carb (g) = 13.9; Net Carb (g) = 13.9; Fat (g) = 4; Protein = 1

🍪 Cookies Oatmeal Commercially Prepared Soft-Type ☞ serving size: 1 oz = 28.4 g; Calories = 116.2; Total Carb (g) = 18.7; Net Carb (g) = 17.9; Fat (g) = 4.2; Protein = 1.7

🍪 Cookies Oatmeal Commercially Prepared Special Dietary ☞ serving size: 1 oz = 28.4 g; Calories = 127.5; Total Carb (g) = 19.9; Net Carb (g) = 19; Fat (g) = 5.1; Protein = 1.4

🍪 Cookies Oatmeal Dry Mix ☞ serving size: 1 oz = 28.4 g; Calories = 131.2; Total Carb (g) = 19.1; Net Carb (g) = 19.1; Fat (g) = 5.5; Protein = 1.8

🍪 Cookies Oatmeal Prepared From Recipe With Raisins ☞ serving size: 1 oz = 28.4 g; Calories = 125.2; Total Carb (g) = 19.6; Net Carb (g) = 18.6; Fat (g) = 4.5; Protein = 1.7

🍪 Cookies Oatmeal Prepared From Recipe Without Raisins ☞

serving size: 1 oz = 28.4 g; Calories = 126.9; Total Carb (g) = 18.9; Net Carb (g) = 18.9; Fat (g) = 5.1; Protein = 1.9

🍪 Cookies Oatmeal Reduced Fat ☞ serving size: 1 cookie = 25 g; Calories = 91.3; Total Carb (g) = 16.2; Net Carb (g) = 12.1; Fat (g) = 2.5; Protein = 1

🍪 Cookies Oatmeal Refrigerated Dough ☞ serving size: 1 oz = 28.4 g; Calories = 120.4; Total Carb (g) = 16.8; Net Carb (g) = 16.1; Fat (g) = 5.4; Protein = 1.5

🍪 Cookies Oatmeal Refrigerated Dough Baked ☞ serving size: 1 oz = 28.4 g; Calories = 133.8; Total Carb (g) = 18.7; Net Carb (g) = 17.9; Fat (g) = 6; Protein = 1.7

🍪 Cookies Oatmeal Sandwich With Creme Filling ☞ serving size: 1 cookie 1 serving = 38 g; Calories = 151.2; Total Carb (g) = 21.1; Net Carb (g) = 20.1; Fat (g) = 7; Protein = 1

🍪 Cookies Peanut Butter Commercially Prepared Regular ☞ serving size: 1 oz = 28.4 g; Calories = 134.3; Total Carb (g) = 16.5; Net Carb (g) = 15.9; Fat (g) = 6.8; Protein = 2.5

🍪 Cookies Peanut Butter Commercially Prepared Soft-Type ☞ serving size: 1 oz = 28.4 g; Calories = 129.8; Total Carb (g) = 16.4; Net Carb (g) = 15.9; Fat (g) = 6.9; Protein = 1.5

🍪 Cookies Peanut Butter Commercially Prepared Sugar Free ☞ serving size: 1 serving 3 cookies = 29 g; Calories = 151.7; Total Carb (g) = 14.7; Net Carb (g) = 13.7; Fat (g) = 9; Protein = 3

🍪 Cookies Peanut Butter Prepared From Recipe ☞ serving size: 1 oz = 28.4 g; Calories = 134.9; Total Carb (g) = 16.7; Net Carb (g) = 16.7; Fat (g) = 6.8; Protein = 2.6

🍪 Cookies Peanut Butter Refrigerated Dough ☞ serving size: 1 oz = 28.4 g; Calories = 130.1; Total Carb (g) = 14.8; Net Carb (g) = 14.5; Fat (g) = 7.1; Protein = 2.3

🍪 Cookies Peanut Butter Refrigerated Dough Baked ☞ serving

size: 1 oz = 28.4 g; Calories = 142.9; Total Carb (g) = 16.3; Net Carb (g) = 15.9; Fat (g) = 7.8; Protein = 2.6

Cookies Peanut Butter Sandwich Regular ☞ serving size: 1 oz = 28.4 g; Calories = 135.8; Total Carb (g) = 18.6; Net Carb (g) = 18.1; Fat (g) = 6; Protein = 2.5

Cookies Peanut Butter Sandwich Special Dietary ☞ serving size: 1 oz = 28.4 g; Calories = 151.9; Total Carb (g) = 14.4; Net Carb (g) = 14.4; Fat (g) = 9.7; Protein = 2.8

Cookies Raisin Soft-Type ☞ serving size: 1 oz = 28.4 g; Calories = 113.9; Total Carb (g) = 19.3; Net Carb (g) = 19; Fat (g) = 3.9; Protein = 1.2

Cookies Shortbread Commercially Prepared Pecan ☞ serving size: 1 oz = 28.4 g; Calories = 153.9; Total Carb (g) = 16.6; Net Carb (g) = 16; Fat (g) = 9.2; Protein = 1.4

Cookies Shortbread Commercially Prepared Plain ☞ serving size: 1 oz = 28.4 g; Calories = 146; Total Carb (g) = 18.1; Net Carb (g) = 17.7; Fat (g) = 7.4; Protein = 1.5

Cookies Shortbread Reduced Fat ☞ serving size: 1 cookie = 11.8 g; Calories = 53.2; Total Carb (g) = 9; Net Carb (g) = 8.8; Fat (g) = 1.7; Protein = 0.6

Cookies Sugar Commercially Prepared Regular (Includes Vanilla) ☞ serving size: 1 oz = 28.4 g; Calories = 131.8; Total Carb (g) = 19.1; Net Carb (g) = 18.8; Fat (g) = 5.6; Protein = 1.5

Cookies Sugar Refrigerated Dough ☞ serving size: 1 serving = 33 g; Calories = 143.9; Total Carb (g) = 20.2; Net Carb (g) = 19.9; Fat (g) = 6.4; Protein = 1.3

Cookies Sugar Refrigerated Dough Baked ☞ serving size: 1 oz = 28.4 g; Calories = 138.9; Total Carb (g) = 18.6; Net Carb (g) = 18.4; Fat (g) = 6.6; Protein = 1.3

Cookies Sugar Wafer Chocolate-Covered ☞ serving size: 3

cookie = 29 g; Calories = 152.5; Total Carb (g) = 19.1; Net Carb (g) = 18.2; Fat (g) = 8; Protein = 1

🍪 Cookies Sugar Wafer With Creme Filling Sugar Free ☞ serving size: 1 oz = 28.4 g; Calories = 150.8; Total Carb (g) = 18.8; Net Carb (g) = 14.8; Fat (g) = 8.1; Protein = 1

🍪 Cookies Sugar Wafers With Creme Filling Regular ☞ serving size: 3 cookies = 36 g; Calories = 180.7; Total Carb (g) = 25.4; Net Carb (g) = 24.9; Fat (g) = 8.4; Protein = 1.4

🍪 Cookies Vanilla Sandwich With Creme Filling ☞ serving size: 1 oz = 28.4 g; Calories = 137.2; Total Carb (g) = 20.5; Net Carb (g) = 20.1; Fat (g) = 5.7; Protein = 1.3

🍪 Cookies Vanilla Sandwich With Creme Filling Reduced Fat ☞ serving size: 1 serving cookie = 48 g; Calories = 203; Total Carb (g) = 37.5; Net Carb (g) = 36.5; Fat (g) = 5; Protein = 2

🍪 Cookies Vanilla Wafers Higher Fat ☞ serving size: 8 wafers = 30 g; Calories = 136.5; Total Carb (g) = 21.8; Net Carb (g) = 21.3; Fat (g) = 4.9; Protein = 1.5

🍪 Cookies Vanilla Wafers Lower Fat ☞ serving size: 1 oz = 28.4 g; Calories = 125.2; Total Carb (g) = 20.9; Net Carb (g) = 20.4; Fat (g) = 4.3; Protein = 1.4

🍪 Corn Flour Patty Or Tart Fried ☞ serving size: 1 patty = 10 g; Calories = 21.6; Total Carb (g) = 4.1; Net Carb (g) = 3.8; Fat (g) = 0.5; Protein = 0.4

🍪 Corn Muffins ☞ serving size: 1 oz = 28.4 g; Calories = 86.6; Total Carb (g) = 14.5; Net Carb (g) = 13.5; Fat (g) = 2.4; Protein = 1.7

🍪 Corn Pone Baked ☞ serving size: 1 pone (8" dia x 3/4") = 377 g; Calories = 806.8; Total Carb (g) = 149.6; Net Carb (g) = 142.4; Fat (g) = 16.2; Protein = 13.2

🍪 Corn Pone Fried ☞ serving size: 1 piece = 61 g; Calories = 154.9; Total Carb (g) = 23.1; Net Carb (g) = 22; Fat (g) = 6; Protein = 2

Cornbread Made From Home Recipe ☞ serving size: 1 surface inch = 11 g; Calories = 31.1; Total Carb (g) = 4.7; Net Carb (g) = 4.5; Fat (g) = 1; Protein = 0.7

Cornbread Muffin Stick Round Made From Home Recipe ☞ serving size: 1 small = 66 g; Calories = 200; Total Carb (g) = 30.2; Net Carb (g) = 29.2; Fat (g) = 6.7; Protein = 4.5

Cornmeal Dumpling ☞ serving size: 1 cup, cooked = 240 g; Calories = 400.8; Total Carb (g) = 60.9; Net Carb (g) = 58.3; Fat (g) = 11.2; Protein = 12.7

Cornmeal Fritter Puerto Rican Style ☞ serving size: 1 fritter (2-1/2" x 2-1/2" x 1/4") = 40 g; Calories = 106.4; Total Carb (g) = 8.3; Net Carb (g) = 7.9; Fat (g) = 6.9; Protein = 2.7

Cornmeal Stick Puerto Rican Style ☞ serving size: 1 stick (3" x 3/4") = 20 g; Calories = 82; Total Carb (g) = 9.7; Net Carb (g) = 9.2; Fat (g) = 4.1; Protein = 1.4

Cracker Meal ☞ serving size: 1 oz = 28.4 g; Calories = 108.8; Total Carb (g) = 23; Net Carb (g) = 22.2; Fat (g) = 0.5; Protein = 2.6

Crackers Cheese Low Sodium ☞ serving size: 1/2 oz = 14.2 g; Calories = 71.4; Total Carb (g) = 8.3; Net Carb (g) = 7.9; Fat (g) = 3.6; Protein = 1.4

Crackers Cheese Reduced Fat ☞ serving size: 1 serving = 30 g; Calories = 125.4; Total Carb (g) = 20.5; Net Carb (g) = 19.5; Fat (g) = 3.5; Protein = 3

Crackers Cheese Regular ☞ serving size: 1/2 oz = 14.2 g; Calories = 69.4; Total Carb (g) = 8.4; Net Carb (g) = 8.1; Fat (g) = 3.2; Protein = 1.6

Crackers Cheese Sandwich-Type With Cheese Filling ☞ serving size: 6 cracker 1 cracker = 6.5g = 39 g; Calories = 191.1; Total Carb (g) = 22.9; Net Carb (g) = 22.2; Fat (g) = 9.5; Protein = 3.5

Crackers Cheese Sandwich-Type With Peanut Butter Filling ☞

serving size: 1/2 oz = 14.2 g; Calories = 70.4; Total Carb (g) = 8.1; Net Carb (g) = 7.6; Fat (g) = 3.6; Protein = 1.8

🍪 Crackers Cheese Whole Grain ☞ serving size: 1 serving 55 pieces = 31 g; Calories = 127.7; Total Carb (g) = 17.8; Net Carb (g) = 15.8; Fat (g) = 5; Protein = 3

🍪 Crackers Cream Gamesa Sabrosas ☞ serving size: 11 crackers (1 nlea serving) = 31 g; Calories = 150; Total Carb (g) = 20; Net Carb (g) = 19.3; Fat (g) = 6.3; Protein = 2.2

🍪 Crackers Cream La Moderna Rikis Cream Crackers ☞ serving size: 10 crackers (1 nlea serving) = 32 g; Calories = 148.5; Total Carb (g) = 20.8; Net Carb (g) = 20; Fat (g) = 6.2; Protein = 2.3

🍪 Crackers Flavored Fish-Shaped ☞ serving size: 10 goldfish = 5.2 g; Calories = 24.1; Total Carb (g) = 3.4; Net Carb (g) = 3.3; Fat (g) = 0.9; Protein = 0.5

🍪 Crackers Gluten-Free Multi-Seeded And Multigrain ☞ serving size: 3 crackers = 6.1 g; Calories = 27.6; Total Carb (g) = 4; Net Carb (g) = 3.4; Fat (g) = 1; Protein = 0.7

🍪 Crackers Gluten-Free Multigrain And Vegetable Made With Corn Starch And White Rice Flour ☞ serving size: 3 crackers = 10.7 g; Calories = 48.8; Total Carb (g) = 8.2; Net Carb (g) = 7.9; Fat (g) = 1.6; Protein = 0.3

🍪 Crackers Matzo Egg And Onion ☞ serving size: 1/2 oz = 14.2 g; Calories = 55.5; Total Carb (g) = 10.9; Net Carb (g) = 10.2; Fat (g) = 0.6; Protein = 1.4

🍪 Crackers Matzo Whole-Wheat ☞ serving size: 1/2 oz = 14.2 g; Calories = 49.8; Total Carb (g) = 11.2; Net Carb (g) = 9.5; Fat (g) = 0.2; Protein = 1.9

🍪 Crackers Melba Toast Plain Without Salt ☞ serving size: 1/2 oz = 14.2 g; Calories = 55.4; Total Carb (g) = 10.9; Net Carb (g) = 10; Fat (g) = 0.5; Protein = 1.7

Crackers Milk ☞ serving size: 1/2 oz = 14.2 g; Calories = 63.3; Total Carb (g) = 10.2; Net Carb (g) = 9.7; Fat (g) = 2; Protein = 1.1

Crackers Multigrain ☞ serving size: 4 crackers = 14 g; Calories = 67.5; Total Carb (g) = 9.5; Net Carb (g) = 9; Fat (g) = 2.9; Protein = 1

Crackers Rusk Toast ☞ serving size: 1/2 oz = 14.2 g; Calories = 57.8; Total Carb (g) = 10.3; Net Carb (g) = 10.3; Fat (g) = 1; Protein = 1.9

Crackers Rye Sandwich-Type With Cheese Filling ☞ serving size: 1/2 oz = 14.2 g; Calories = 68.3; Total Carb (g) = 8.6; Net Carb (g) = 8.1; Fat (g) = 3.2; Protein = 1.3

Crackers Rye Wafers Plain ☞ serving size: 1/2 oz = 14.2 g; Calories = 47.4; Total Carb (g) = 11.4; Net Carb (g) = 8.2; Fat (g) = 0.1; Protein = 1.4

Crackers Rye Wafers Seasoned ☞ serving size: 1/2 oz = 14.2 g; Calories = 54.1; Total Carb (g) = 10.5; Net Carb (g) = 7.5; Fat (g) = 1.3; Protein = 1.3

Crackers Saltines (Includes Oyster Soda Soup) ☞ serving size: 5 crackers = 14.9 g; Calories = 62.3; Total Carb (g) = 11; Net Carb (g) = 10.6; Fat (g) = 1.3; Protein = 1.4

Crackers Saltines Fat-Free Low-Sodium ☞ serving size: 3 saltines = 15 g; Calories = 59; Total Carb (g) = 12.3; Net Carb (g) = 11.9; Fat (g) = 0.2; Protein = 1.6

Crackers Saltines Low Salt (Includes Oyster Soda Soup) ☞ serving size: 1/2 oz = 14.2 g; Calories = 59.8; Total Carb (g) = 10.6; Net Carb (g) = 10.1; Fat (g) = 1.3; Protein = 1.3

Crackers Saltines Unsalted Tops (Includes Oyster Soda Soup) ☞ serving size: 1/2 oz = 14.2 g; Calories = 61.6; Total Carb (g) = 10.2; Net Carb (g) = 9.7; Fat (g) = 1.7; Protein = 1.3

Crackers Saltines Whole Wheat (Includes Multi-Grain) ☞ serving size: 1 serving = 14 g; Calories = 55.7; Total Carb (g) = 9.6; Net Carb (g) = 8.6; Fat (g) = 1.5; Protein = 1

⬛ Crackers Sandwich-Type Peanut Butter Filled Reduced Fat ☞ serving size: 1 package = 36 g; Calories = 157.3; Total Carb (g) = 22.9; Net Carb (g) = 21.8; Fat (g) = 6; Protein = 3

⬛ Crackers Snack Goya Crackers ☞ serving size: 1 serving (1 nlea serving - about 4 crackers) = 30 g; Calories = 129.9; Total Carb (g) = 19.3; Net Carb (g) = 18.2; Fat (g) = 4; Protein = 4.3

⬛ Crackers Standard Snack-Type Regular ☞ serving size: 5 crackers = 16 g; Calories = 81.6; Total Carb (g) = 9.8; Net Carb (g) = 9.4; Fat (g) = 4.2; Protein = 1.1

⬛ Crackers Standard Snack-Type Regular Low Salt ☞ serving size: 1/2 oz = 14.2 g; Calories = 71.3; Total Carb (g) = 8.7; Net Carb (g) = 8.4; Fat (g) = 3.6; Protein = 1.1

⬛ Crackers Standard Snack-Type Sandwich With Cheese Filling ☞ serving size: 1/2 oz = 14.2 g; Calories = 67.7; Total Carb (g) = 8.8; Net Carb (g) = 8.5; Fat (g) = 3; Protein = 1.3

⬛ Crackers Standard Snack-Type Sandwich With Peanut Butter Filling ☞ serving size: 1/2 oz = 14.2 g; Calories = 70.1; Total Carb (g) = 8.3; Net Carb (g) = 8; Fat (g) = 3.5; Protein = 1.6

⬛ Crackers Standard Snack-Type With Whole Wheat ☞ serving size: 5 crackers 1 serving = 15 g; Calories = 69.5; Total Carb (g) = 10.3; Net Carb (g) = 9.5; Fat (g) = 2.7; Protein = 1.1

⬛ Crackers Toast Thins Low Sodium ☞ serving size: 1 serving = 31 g; Calories = 137; Total Carb (g) = 21; Net Carb (g) = 18; Fat (g) = 5; Protein = 2

⬛ Crackers Water Biscuits ☞ serving size: 4 cracker 1 serving = 14 g; Calories = 53.8; Total Carb (g) = 10.2; Net Carb (g) = 9.2; Fat (g) = 1; Protein = 1

⬛ Crackers Wheat Low Salt ☞ serving size: 1/2 oz = 14.2 g; Calories = 67.2; Total Carb (g) = 9.2; Net Carb (g) = 8.6; Fat (g) = 2.9; Protein = 1.2

Crackers Wheat Reduced Fat ☞ serving size: 1 serving = 29 g; Calories = 128.8; Total Carb (g) = 20.7; Net Carb (g) = 19.8; Fat (g) = 3.9; Protein = 2.7

Crackers Wheat Regular ☞ serving size: 16 crackers 1 serving = 34 g; Calories = 154.7; Total Carb (g) = 24; Net Carb (g) = 21.7; Fat (g) = 5.6; Protein = 2.5

Crackers Wheat Sandwich With Cheese Filling ☞ serving size: 1/2 oz = 14.2 g; Calories = 70.6; Total Carb (g) = 8.3; Net Carb (g) = 7.8; Fat (g) = 3.6; Protein = 1.4

Crackers Wheat Sandwich With Peanut Butter Filling ☞ serving size: 1/2 oz = 14.2 g; Calories = 70.3; Total Carb (g) = 7.6; Net Carb (g) = 7; Fat (g) = 3.8; Protein = 1.9

Crackers Whole Grain Sandwich-Type With Peanut Butter Filling ☞ serving size: 6 cracker 1 serving = 43 g; Calories = 200; Total Carb (g) = 23.5; Net Carb (g) = 19.4; Fat (g) = 9.1; Protein = 6.1

Crackers Whole-Wheat ☞ serving size: 1 serving = 28 g; Calories = 119.6; Total Carb (g) = 19.5; Net Carb (g) = 16.6; Fat (g) = 4; Protein = 3

Crackers Whole-Wheat Low Salt ☞ serving size: 1/2 oz = 14.2 g; Calories = 62.9; Total Carb (g) = 9.7; Net Carb (g) = 8.3; Fat (g) = 2.4; Protein = 1.2

Crackers Whole-Wheat Reduced Fat ☞ serving size: 1 serving = 29 g; Calories = 120.6; Total Carb (g) = 21.9; Net Carb (g) = 18.7; Fat (g) = 2.2; Protein = 3.3

Cream Puff Eclair Custard Or Cream Filled Iced ☞ serving size: 4 oz = 113 g; Calories = 377.4; Total Carb (g) = 42.3; Net Carb (g) = 41.3; Fat (g) = 20.9; Protein = 5

Cream Puff Eclair Custard Or Cream Filled Iced Reduced Fat ☞ serving size: 1 eclair, frozen = 60 g; Calories = 142.2; Total Carb (g) = 25.1; Net Carb (g) = 24.6; Fat (g) = 4.2; Protein = 2.1

🔲 Cream Puff Eclair Custard Or Cream Filled Not Iced ☞ serving size: 1 eclair (5" x 2" x 1-3/4") = 90 g; Calories = 234; Total Carb (g) = 11.2; Net Carb (g) = 10.9; Fat (g) = 19.2; Protein = 4.4

🔲 Cream Puff Eclair Custard Or Cream Filled Ns As To Icing ☞ serving size: 1 eclair (5" x 2" x 1-3/4") = 102 g; Calories = 281.5; Total Carb (g) = 10.7; Net Carb (g) = 10.4; Fat (g) = 24.8; Protein = 4.6

🔲 Cream Puff Shell Prepared From Recipe ☞ serving size: 1 oz = 28.4 g; Calories = 102.2; Total Carb (g) = 6.5; Net Carb (g) = 6.2; Fat (g) = 7.4; Protein = 2.6

🔲 Crisp Apple Apple Dessert ☞ serving size: 1 cup = 246 g; Calories = 386.2; Total Carb (g) = 75.7; Net Carb (g) = 71.8; Fat (g) = 8.5; Protein = 4.8

🔲 Crisp Blueberry ☞ serving size: 1 cup = 246 g; Calories = 629.8; Total Carb (g) = 101.2; Net Carb (g) = 96.6; Fat (g) = 25; Protein = 4.6

🔲 Crisp Cherry ☞ serving size: 1 cup = 246 g; Calories = 647; Total Carb (g) = 116.5; Net Carb (g) = 113.6; Fat (g) = 19.3; Protein = 4.8

🔲 Crisp Peach ☞ serving size: 1 cup = 246 g; Calories = 524; Total Carb (g) = 93; Net Carb (g) = 89.8; Fat (g) = 16.9; Protein = 4.2

🔲 Crisp Rhubarb ☞ serving size: 1 cup = 246 g; Calories = 553.5; Total Carb (g) = 105.4; Net Carb (g) = 101.5; Fat (g) = 16; Protein = 3

🔲 Croissants Apple ☞ serving size: 1 oz = 28.4 g; Calories = 72.1; Total Carb (g) = 10.5; Net Carb (g) = 9.8; Fat (g) = 2.5; Protein = 2.1

🔲 Croutons Seasoned ☞ serving size: 1/2 oz = 14.2 g; Calories = 66; Total Carb (g) = 9; Net Carb (g) = 8.3; Fat (g) = 2.6; Protein = 1.5

🔲 Crumpet ☞ serving size: 1 small (2-1/2" dia) = 20 g; Calories = 38.6; Total Carb (g) = 5.7; Net Carb (g) = 5.3; Fat (g) = 1.1; Protein = 1.4

🔲 Crumpet Toasted ☞ serving size: 1 small (2-1/2" dia) = 18 g; Calories = 39.1; Total Carb (g) = 5.7; Net Carb (g) = 5.4; Fat (g) = 1.1; Protein = 1.5

🍪 Crunchmaster Multi-Grain Crisps Snack Crackers Gluten-Free ☞ serving size: 3 crackers = 3.9 g; Calories = 17.8; Total Carb (g) = 2.6; Net Carb (g) = 2.3; Fat (g) = 0.6; Protein = 0.4

🍪 Danish Pastry Cheese ☞ serving size: 1 oz = 28.4 g; Calories = 106.2; Total Carb (g) = 10.6; Net Carb (g) = 10.3; Fat (g) = 6.2; Protein = 2.3

🍪 Danish Pastry Cinnamon Enriched ☞ serving size: 1 oz = 28.4 g; Calories = 114.5; Total Carb (g) = 12.7; Net Carb (g) = 12.3; Fat (g) = 6.4; Protein = 2

🍪 Danish Pastry Cinnamon Unenriched ☞ serving size: 1 oz = 28.4 g; Calories = 114.5; Total Carb (g) = 12.7; Net Carb (g) = 12.3; Fat (g) = 6.4; Protein = 2

🍪 Danish Pastry Fruit Enriched (Includes Apple Cinnamon Raisin Lemon Raspberry Strawberry) ☞ serving size: 1 oz = 28.4 g; Calories = 105.4; Total Carb (g) = 13.6; Net Carb (g) = 13; Fat (g) = 5.3; Protein = 1.5

🍪 Danish Pastry Fruit Unenriched (Includes Apple Cinnamon Raisin Strawberry) ☞ serving size: 1 oz = 28.4 g; Calories = 105.4; Total Carb (g) = 13.6; Net Carb (g) = 13; Fat (g) = 5.3; Protein = 1.5

🍪 Danish Pastry Lemon Unenriched ☞ serving size: 1 oz = 28.4 g; Calories = 105.4; Total Carb (g) = 13.6; Net Carb (g) = 13; Fat (g) = 5.3; Protein = 1.5

🍪 Danish Pastry Raspberry Unenriched ☞ serving size: 1 oz = 28.4 g; Calories = 105.4; Total Carb (g) = 13.6; Net Carb (g) = 13; Fat (g) = 5.3; Protein = 1.5

🍪 Dessert Pizza ☞ serving size: 1 piece = 108 g; Calories = 225.7; Total Carb (g) = 33.4; Net Carb (g) = 31.7; Fat (g) = 9.7; Protein = 2.1

🍪 Doughnut Cake Type Chocolate Covered Dipped In Peanuts ☞ serving size: 1 doughnut (3-1/4" dia) = 53 g; Calories = 221.5; Total Carb (g) = 25.3; Net Carb (g) = 24.2; Fat (g) = 12.2; Protein = 3

Doughnut Chocolate Cream-Filled ☞ serving size: 1 doughnut = 65 g; Calories = 230.1; Total Carb (g) = 27.1; Net Carb (g) = 25.9; Fat (g) = 11.9; Protein = 3.6

Doughnut Chocolate Raised Or Yeast ☞ serving size: 1 doughnut (approx 3" dia) = 50 g; Calories = 206; Total Carb (g) = 24.2; Net Carb (g) = 22.5; Fat (g) = 11.1; Protein = 3.3

Doughnut Chocolate Raised Or Yeast With Chocolate Icing ☞ serving size: 1 doughnut (approx 3" dia) = 71 g; Calories = 287.6; Total Carb (g) = 38.3; Net Carb (g) = 35.8; Fat (g) = 14; Protein = 4.2

Doughnut Custard-Filled With Icing ☞ serving size: 1 doughnut = 70 g; Calories = 252.7; Total Carb (g) = 38.9; Net Carb (g) = 38; Fat (g) = 9.8; Protein = 2.9

Doughnut Raised Or Yeast Chocolate Covered ☞ serving size: 1 doughnut (approx 3" dia) = 71 g; Calories = 287.6; Total Carb (g) = 37.4; Net Carb (g) = 35.7; Fat (g) = 13.8; Protein = 3.8

Doughnuts Cake-Type Chocolate Sugared Or Glazed ☞ serving size: 1 oz = 28.4 g; Calories = 118.4; Total Carb (g) = 16.3; Net Carb (g) = 15.7; Fat (g) = 5.7; Protein = 1.3

Doughnuts Cake-Type Plain (Includes Unsugared Old-Fashioned) ☞ serving size: 1 donut = 40 g; Calories = 173.6; Total Carb (g) = 18.8; Net Carb (g) = 18.1; Fat (g) = 10; Protein = 2.1

Doughnuts Cake-Type Plain Chocolate-Coated Or Frosted ☞ serving size: 1 oz = 28.4 g; Calories = 128.4; Total Carb (g) = 14.6; Net Carb (g) = 14; Fat (g) = 7.2; Protein = 1.4

Doughnuts Cake-Type Plain Sugared Or Glazed ☞ serving size: 1 oz = 28.4 g; Calories = 121; Total Carb (g) = 14.4; Net Carb (g) = 14; Fat (g) = 6.5; Protein = 1.5

Doughnuts French Crullers Glazed ☞ serving size: 1 oz = 28.4 g; Calories = 117; Total Carb (g) = 16.9; Net Carb (g) = 16.6; Fat (g) = 5.2; Protein = 0.9

Doughnuts Yeast-Leavened Glazed Enriched (Includes Honey Buns) ☞ serving size: 1 oz = 28.4 g; Calories = 119.6; Total Carb (g) = 13.6; Net Carb (g) = 13; Fat (g) = 6.4; Protein = 1.7

Doughnuts Yeast-Leavened Glazed Unenriched (Includes Honey Buns) ☞ serving size: 1 oz = 28.4 g; Calories = 114.5; Total Carb (g) = 12.6; Net Carb (g) = 12.2; Fat (g) = 6.5; Protein = 1.8

Doughnuts Yeast-Leavened With Creme Filling ☞ serving size: 1 oz = 28.4 g; Calories = 102.5; Total Carb (g) = 8.5; Net Carb (g) = 8.3; Fat (g) = 7; Protein = 1.8

Doughnuts Yeast-Leavened With Jelly Filling ☞ serving size: 1 oz = 28.4 g; Calories = 96.6; Total Carb (g) = 11.1; Net Carb (g) = 10.8; Fat (g) = 5.3; Protein = 1.7

Dumpling Plain ☞ serving size: 1 small = 18 g; Calories = 22.3; Total Carb (g) = 3.6; Net Carb (g) = 3.5; Fat (g) = 0.6; Protein = 0.6

Dutch Apple Pie ☞ serving size: 1/8 pie 1 pie (1/8 of 9 inch pie) = 131 g; Calories = 379.9; Total Carb (g) = 58.3; Net Carb (g) = 56.3; Fat (g) = 15.1; Protein = 2.8

Egg Bagel ☞ serving size: 1 oz = 28.4 g; Calories = 79; Total Carb (g) = 15.1; Net Carb (g) = 14.4; Fat (g) = 0.6; Protein = 3

Empanada Mexican Turnover Pumpkin ☞ serving size: 1 cup = 132 g; Calories = 380.2; Total Carb (g) = 55; Net Carb (g) = 52.3; Fat (g) = 15.4; Protein = 6

Empanada Mexican Turnover Fruit-Filled ☞ serving size: 1 cup = 142 g; Calories = 448.7; Total Carb (g) = 56.9; Net Carb (g) = 54; Fat (g) = 21.8; Protein = 6.6

English Muffins ☞ serving size: 1 oz = 28.4 g; Calories = 63.3; Total Carb (g) = 12.7; Net Carb (g) = 11.4; Fat (g) = 0.6; Protein = 2.5

English Muffins Mixed-Grain (Includes Granola) ☞ serving size: 1 oz = 28.4 g; Calories = 66.7; Total Carb (g) = 13.1; Net Carb (g) = 12.4; Fat (g) = 0.5; Protein = 2.6

🔲 English Muffins Plain Enriched With Ca Prop (Includes Sour-dough) ☞ serving size: 1 oz = 28.4 g; Calories = 64.5; Total Carb (g) = 12.5; Net Carb (g) = 11.6; Fat (g) = 0.5; Protein = 2.5

🔲 English Muffins Plain Enriched Without Calcium Propi-onate(Includes Sourdough) ☞ serving size: 1 oz = 28.4 g; Calories = 66.7; Total Carb (g) = 13.1; Net Carb (g) = 12.3; Fat (g) = 0.5; Protein = 2.2

🔲 English Muffins Plain Toasted Enriched With Calcium Propi-onate (Includes Sourdough) ☞ serving size: 1 oz = 28.4 g; Calories = 76.7; Total Carb (g) = 15; Net Carb (g) = 14.2; Fat (g) = 0.6; Protein = 2.9

🔲 English Muffins Plain Unenriched With Calcium Propionate (Includes Sourdough) ☞ serving size: 1 oz = 28.4 g; Calories = 66.7; Total Carb (g) = 13.1; Net Carb (g) = 12.3; Fat (g) = 0.5; Protein = 2.2

🔲 English Muffins Plain Unenriched Without Calcium Propionate (Includes Sourdough) ☞ serving size: 1 oz = 28.4 g; Calories = 66.7; Total Carb (g) = 13.1; Net Carb (g) = 12.3; Fat (g) = 0.5; Protein = 2.2

🔲 English Muffins Raisin-Cinnamon (Includes Apple-Cinnamon) ☞ serving size: 1 oz = 28.4 g; Calories = 68.2; Total Carb (g) = 13.7; Net Carb (g) = 12.9; Fat (g) = 0.5; Protein = 2.2

🔲 English Muffins Raisin-Cinnamon Toasted (Includes Apple-Cinnamon) ☞ serving size: 1 oz = 28.4 g; Calories = 78.4; Total Carb (g) = 15.6; Net Carb (g) = 14.8; Fat (g) = 0.6; Protein = 2.5

🔲 English Muffins Whole Grain White ☞ serving size: 1 muffin 1 serving = 57 g; Calories = 139.7; Total Carb (g) = 28.6; Net Carb (g) = 26.6; Fat (g) = 1; Protein = 4

🔲 English Muffins Whole-Wheat ☞ serving size: 1 oz = 28.4 g; Calories = 57.7; Total Carb (g) = 11.5; Net Carb (g) = 9.6; Fat (g) = 0.6; Protein = 2.5

🔲 Fig Bars ☞ serving size: 1 oz = 28.4 g; Calories = 98.8; Total Carb (g) = 20.1; Net Carb (g) = 18.8; Fat (g) = 2.1; Protein = 1.1

🎲 Focaccia Italian Flatbread Plain ☞ serving size: 1 piece = 57 g; Calories = 141.9; Total Carb (g) = 20.4; Net Carb (g) = 19.4; Fat (g) = 4.5; Protein = 5

🎲 Forunte Cookies ☞ serving size: 1 oz = 28.4 g; Calories = 107.4; Total Carb (g) = 23.9; Net Carb (g) = 23.4; Fat (g) = 0.8; Protein = 1.2

🎲 French Bread ☞ serving size: 1 oz = 28.4 g; Calories = 77.2; Total Carb (g) = 14.7; Net Carb (g) = 14.1; Fat (g) = 0.7; Protein = 3.1

🎲 French Toast Frozen Ready-To-Heat ☞ serving size: 1 oz = 28.4 g; Calories = 60.5; Total Carb (g) = 9.1; Net Carb (g) = 8.8; Fat (g) = 1.7; Protein = 2.1

🎲 French Toast Prepared From Recipe Made With Low Fat (2%) Milk ☞ serving size: 1 oz = 28.4 g; Calories = 65; Total Carb (g) = 7.1; Net Carb (g) = 7.1; Fat (g) = 3.1; Protein = 2.2

🎲 Fritter Apple ☞ serving size: 1 fritter (2-1/2" long x 1-5/8" wide) = 17 g; Calories = 64.8; Total Carb (g) = 5.9; Net Carb (g) = 5.7; Fat (g) = 4.2; Protein = 1.1

🎲 Fritter Banana ☞ serving size: 1 fritter (2" long) = 34 g; Calories = 116.3; Total Carb (g) = 11.7; Net Carb (g) = 11; Fat (g) = 7.3; Protein = 1.7

🎲 Fritter Berry ☞ serving size: 1 fritter (1-1/4" dia) = 24 g; Calories = 82.1; Total Carb (g) = 7.5; Net Carb (g) = 7.1; Fat (g) = 5.3; Protein = 1.3

🎲 Funnel Cake With Sugar ☞ serving size: 1 cake (6" dia) = 90 g; Calories = 314.1; Total Carb (g) = 38.8; Net Carb (g) = 37.9; Fat (g) = 14.6; Protein = 6.9

🎲 Funnel Cake With Sugar And Fruit ☞ serving size: 1 cake (6" dia) = 135 g; Calories = 509; Total Carb (g) = 74.1; Net Carb (g) = 72.9; Fat (g) = 20.9; Protein = 7.7

🎲 Garlic Bread From Fast Food / Restaurant ☞ serving size: 1 small slice = 37 g; Calories = 129.1; Total Carb (g) = 15.4; Net Carb (g) = 14.5; Fat (g) = 6.1; Protein = 3.1

🍱 Garlic Bread Frozen ☞ serving size: 1 slice presliced = 43 g; Calories = 150.5; Total Carb (g) = 17.9; Net Carb (g) = 16.9; Fat (g) = 7.1; Protein = 3.6

🍱 Garlic Bread Nfs ☞ serving size: 1 small slice = 39 g; Calories = 136.1; Total Carb (g) = 16.2; Net Carb (g) = 15.3; Fat (g) = 6.5; Protein = 3.3

🍱 Garlic Bread With Melted Cheese From Fast Food / Restaurant ☞ serving size: 1 small slice = 44 g; Calories = 148.7; Total Carb (g) = 15.2; Net Carb (g) = 14.3; Fat (g) = 7.6; Protein = 5

🍱 Garlic Bread With Melted Cheese From Frozen ☞ serving size: 1 small slice = 44 g; Calories = 150.9; Total Carb (g) = 16.3; Net Carb (g) = 15.3; Fat (g) = 7.5; Protein = 4.6

🍱 Garlic Bread With Parmesan Cheese From Fast Food / Restaurant ☞ serving size: 1 small slice = 39 g; Calories = 136.9; Total Carb (g) = 16; Net Carb (g) = 15.1; Fat (g) = 6.6; Protein = 3.4

🍱 Garlic Bread With Parmesan Cheese From Frozen ☞ serving size: 1 small slice = 39 g; Calories = 136.9; Total Carb (g) = 16.1; Net Carb (g) = 15.1; Fat (g) = 6.6; Protein = 3.4

🍱 George Weston Bakeries Brownberry Sage And Onion Stuffing Mix Dry ☞ serving size: 1 serving = 67 g; Calories = 261.3; Total Carb (g) = 48.7; Net Carb (g) = 45.1; Fat (g) = 3.4; Protein = 8.9

🍱 George Weston Bakeries Thomas English Muffins ☞ serving size: 1 serving = 57 g; Calories = 132.2; Total Carb (g) = 26.2; Net Carb (g) = 26.2; Fat (g) = 1; Protein = 4.6

🍱 Gingerbread Cake ☞ serving size: 1 oz = 28.4 g; Calories = 101.1; Total Carb (g) = 14; Net Carb (g) = 14; Fat (g) = 4.7; Protein = 1.1

🍱 Gingersnaps ☞ serving size: 1 oz = 28.4 g; Calories = 118.1; Total Carb (g) = 21.8; Net Carb (g) = 21.2; Fat (g) = 2.8; Protein = 1.6

🍱 Glutino Gluten Free Cookies Chocolate Vanilla Creme ☞

serving size: 3 cookies = 44 g; Calories = 208.6; Total Carb (g) = 33.5; Net Carb (g) = 32.4; Fat (g) = 7.9; Protein = 1

Glutino Gluten Free Cookies Vanilla Creme ☞ serving size: 3 cookies = 45 g; Calories = 219.2; Total Carb (g) = 34.8; Net Carb (g) = 34.8; Fat (g) = 8.5; Protein = 1

Glutino Gluten Free Wafers Lemon Flavored ☞ serving size: 3 cookies = 30 g; Calories = 154.5; Total Carb (g) = 22.3; Net Carb (g) = 22.3; Fat (g) = 7.3; Protein = 0

Glutino Gluten Free Wafers Milk Chocolate ☞ serving size: 3 cookies = 23 g; Calories = 124.4; Total Carb (g) = 14.4; Net Carb (g) = 14.1; Fat (g) = 7; Protein = 0.9

Heinz Weight Watcher Chocolate Eclair Frozen ☞ serving size: 1 eclair, frozen = 59 g; Calories = 142.2; Total Carb (g) = 23.8; Net Carb (g) = 22.5; Fat (g) = 4.1; Protein = 2.6

Hush Puppies Prepared From Recipe ☞ serving size: 1 oz = 28.4 g; Calories = 95.7; Total Carb (g) = 13.1; Net Carb (g) = 12.3; Fat (g) = 3.8; Protein = 2.2

Ice Cream Cones Cake Or Wafer-Type ☞ serving size: 1 oz = 28.4 g; Calories = 118.4; Total Carb (g) = 22.4; Net Carb (g) = 21.6; Fat (g) = 2; Protein = 2.3

Ice Cream Cones Sugar Rolled-Type ☞ serving size: 1 oz = 28.4 g; Calories = 114.2; Total Carb (g) = 23.9; Net Carb (g) = 23.4; Fat (g) = 1.1; Protein = 2.2

Injera Ethiopian Bread ☞ serving size: 1 cup, pieces = 68 g; Calories = 59.8; Total Carb (g) = 12.5; Net Carb (g) = 10.6; Fat (g) = 0.6; Protein = 2.4

Interstate Brands Corp Wonder Hamburger Rolls ☞ serving size: 1 serving = 43 g; Calories = 117.4; Total Carb (g) = 21.9; Net Carb (g) = 20.7; Fat (g) = 1.8; Protein = 3.5

Johnnycake ☞ serving size: 1 piece = 49 g; Calories = 134.8; Total Carb (g) = 21.5; Net Carb (g) = 20.6; Fat (g) = 3.5; Protein = 3.9

Keebler Keebler Chocolate Graham Selects ☞ serving size: 1 serving = 31 g; Calories = 144.2; Total Carb (g) = 22.3; Net Carb (g) = 22.3; Fat (g) = 5.1; Protein = 2.2

Keikitos (Muffins) Latino Bakery Item ☞ serving size: 1 piece = 42 g; Calories = 196.1; Total Carb (g) = 22.3; Net Carb (g) = 21.8; Fat (g) = 10.6; Protein = 2.9

Kraft Foods Shake N Bake Original Recipe Coating For Pork Dry ☞ serving size: 1 serving = 28 g; Calories = 105.6; Total Carb (g) = 22.3; Net Carb (g) = 22.3; Fat (g) = 1; Protein = 1.7

Kraft Stove Top Stuffing Mix Chicken Flavor ☞ serving size: 1 nlea serving (makes 1/2 cup prepared) = 28 g; Calories = 106.7; Total Carb (g) = 20.5; Net Carb (g) = 19.8; Fat (g) = 1.1; Protein = 3.5

Ladyfingers ☞ serving size: 1 oz = 28.4 g; Calories = 103.7; Total Carb (g) = 17; Net Carb (g) = 16.7; Fat (g) = 2.6; Protein = 3

Leavening Agents Baking Powder Double-Acting Sodium Aluminum Sulfate ☞ serving size: 1 tsp = 4.6 g; Calories = 2.4; Total Carb (g) = 1.3; Net Carb (g) = 1.3; Fat (g) = 0; Protein = 0

Leavening Agents Baking Powder Double-Acting Straight Phosphate ☞ serving size: 1 tsp = 4.6 g; Calories = 2.3; Total Carb (g) = 1.1; Net Carb (g) = 1.1; Fat (g) = 0; Protein = 0

Leavening Agents Baking Powder Low-Sodium ☞ serving size: 1 tsp = 5 g; Calories = 4.9; Total Carb (g) = 2.3; Net Carb (g) = 2.2; Fat (g) = 0; Protein = 0

Leavening Agents Baking Soda ☞ serving size: 1 tsp = 4.6 g; Calories = 0; Total Carb (g) = 0; Net Carb (g) = 0; Fat (g) = 0; Protein = 0

Leavening Agents Cream Of Tartar ☞ serving size: 1 tsp = 3 g;

Calories = 7.7; Total Carb (g) = 1.8; Net Carb (g) = 1.8; Fat (g) = 0; Protein = 0

🍞 Leavening Agents Yeast Bakers Active Dry ☞ serving size: 1 tsp = 4 g; Calories = 13; Total Carb (g) = 1.6; Net Carb (g) = 0.6; Fat (g) = 0.3; Protein = 1.6

🍞 Leavening Agents Yeast Bakers Compressed ☞ serving size: 1 cake (0.6 oz) = 17 g; Calories = 17.9; Total Carb (g) = 3.1; Net Carb (g) = 1.7; Fat (g) = 0.3; Protein = 1.4

🍞 Martha White Foods Martha Whites Buttermilk Biscuit Mix Dry ☞ serving size: 1 serving = 41 g; Calories = 159.1; Total Carb (g) = 24.4; Net Carb (g) = 23.7; Fat (g) = 5.4; Protein = 3.2

🍞 Martha White Foods Martha Whites Chewy Fudge Brownie Mix Dry ☞ serving size: 1 serving = 28 g; Calories = 114; Total Carb (g) = 23.4; Net Carb (g) = 22.6; Fat (g) = 1.7; Protein = 1.2

🍞 Marys Gone Crackers Original Crackers Organic Gluten Free ☞ serving size: 3 crackers = 7.4 g; Calories = 33; Total Carb (g) = 4.8; Net Carb (g) = 3.6; Fat (g) = 1.2; Protein = 0.9

🍞 Matzo Egg Crackers ☞ serving size: 1/2 oz = 14.2 g; Calories = 55.5; Total Carb (g) = 11.2; Net Carb (g) = 10.8; Fat (g) = 0.3; Protein = 1.7

🍞 Mckee Baking Little Debbie Nutty Bars Wafers With Peanut Butter Chocolate Covered ☞ serving size: 1 serving = 57 g; Calories = 312.4; Total Carb (g) = 31.5; Net Carb (g) = 31.5; Fat (g) = 18.7; Protein = 4.6

🍞 Melba Toast ☞ serving size: 1/2 oz = 14.2 g; Calories = 55.4; Total Carb (g) = 10.9; Net Carb (g) = 10; Fat (g) = 0.5; Protein = 1.7

🍞 Mission Foods Mission Flour Tortillas Soft Taco 8 Inch ☞ serving size: 1 serving = 51 g; Calories = 146.4; Total Carb (g) = 25.3; Net Carb (g) = 25.3; Fat (g) = 3.1; Protein = 4.4

🍞 Mixed Fruit Tart Filled With Custard Or Cream Cheese ☞

serving size: 1 tart (9" dia) = 1265 g; Calories = 2188.5; Total Carb (g) = 265.9; Net Carb (g) = 248.2; Fat (g) = 111.3; Protein = 44.3

Molasses Cookies ☞ serving size: 1 oz = 28.4 g; Calories = 122.1; Total Carb (g) = 21; Net Carb (g) = 20.7; Fat (g) = 3.6; Protein = 1.6

Muffin Blueberry Commercially Prepared Low-Fat ☞ serving size: 1 muffin small = 71 g; Calories = 181.1; Total Carb (g) = 35.5; Net Carb (g) = 32.6; Fat (g) = 3; Protein = 3

Muffin English Cheese ☞ serving size: 1 muffin = 58 g; Calories = 136.9; Total Carb (g) = 24.4; Net Carb (g) = 22.5; Fat (g) = 1.9; Protein = 5.6

Muffin English Oat Bran With Raisins ☞ serving size: 1 muffin = 58 g; Calories = 157.8; Total Carb (g) = 29.9; Net Carb (g) = 27.6; Fat (g) = 2.3; Protein = 4.6

Muffin English Wheat Bran With Raisins ☞ serving size: 1 muffin = 58 g; Calories = 134; Total Carb (g) = 28; Net Carb (g) = 25.4; Fat (g) = 1.1; Protein = 4.7

Muffin English Wheat Or Cracked Wheat With Raisins ☞ serving size: 1 muffin = 58 g; Calories = 133.4; Total Carb (g) = 27.8; Net Carb (g) = 25.2; Fat (g) = 1.1; Protein = 4.8

Muffin English Whole Wheat With Raisins ☞ serving size: 1 muffin = 58 g; Calories = 133.4; Total Carb (g) = 27.8; Net Carb (g) = 25.2; Fat (g) = 1.1; Protein = 4.8

Muffin English With Fruit Other Than Raisins ☞ serving size: 1 muffin = 58 g; Calories = 140.9; Total Carb (g) = 27.6; Net Carb (g) = 25.4; Fat (g) = 1; Protein = 5.4

Muffin English With Raisins ☞ serving size: 1 muffin = 58 g; Calories = 135.7; Total Carb (g) = 27.6; Net Carb (g) = 25.6; Fat (g) = 0.9; Protein = 4.8

Muffin Whole Grain ☞ serving size: 1 miniature = 25 g; Calories = 90; Total Carb (g) = 11.4; Net Carb (g) = 11; Fat (g) = 4.4; Protein = 1.7

🟦 Muffins Blueberry Commercially Prepared (Includes Mini-Muffins) ☞ serving size: 1 oz = 28.4 g; Calories = 106.5; Total Carb (g) = 15.1; Net Carb (g) = 14.7; Fat (g) = 4.6; Protein = 1.3

🟦 Muffins Blueberry Dry Mix ☞ serving size: 1 serving = 43 g; Calories = 126; Total Carb (g) = 26.2; Net Carb (g) = 25.6; Fat (g) = 1.4; Protein = 1.5

🟦 Muffins Blueberry Prepared From Recipe Made With Low Fat (2%) Milk ☞ serving size: 1 oz = 28.4 g; Calories = 80.9; Total Carb (g) = 11.6; Net Carb (g) = 11.6; Fat (g) = 3.1; Protein = 1.8

🟦 Muffins Blueberry Toaster-Type ☞ serving size: 1 oz = 28.4 g; Calories = 88.9; Total Carb (g) = 15.1; Net Carb (g) = 14.6; Fat (g) = 2.7; Protein = 1.3

🟦 Muffins Blueberry Toaster-Type Toasted ☞ serving size: 1 oz = 28.4 g; Calories = 94.6; Total Carb (g) = 16.1; Net Carb (g) = 15.6; Fat (g) = 2.9; Protein = 1.4

🟦 Muffins Corn Dry Mix Prepared ☞ serving size: 1 oz = 28.4 g; Calories = 91.2; Total Carb (g) = 13.9; Net Carb (g) = 13.3; Fat (g) = 2.9; Protein = 2.1

🟦 Muffins Corn Prepared From Recipe Made With Low Fat (2%) Milk ☞ serving size: 1 oz = 28.4 g; Calories = 89.7; Total Carb (g) = 12.6; Net Carb (g) = 12.6; Fat (g) = 3.5; Protein = 2

🟦 Muffins Corn Toaster-Type ☞ serving size: 1 oz = 28.4 g; Calories = 98.3; Total Carb (g) = 16.4; Net Carb (g) = 16; Fat (g) = 3.2; Protein = 1.5

🟦 Muffins Oat Bran ☞ serving size: 1 oz = 28.4 g; Calories = 76.7; Total Carb (g) = 13.7; Net Carb (g) = 12.4; Fat (g) = 2.1; Protein = 2

🟦 Muffins Plain Prepared From Recipe Made With Low Fat (2%) Milk ☞ serving size: 1 oz = 28.4 g; Calories = 84.1; Total Carb (g) = 11.8; Net Carb (g) = 11; Fat (g) = 3.2; Protein = 2

🟦 Muffins Wheat Bran Dry Mix ☞ serving size: 1 oz = 28.4 g; Calories = 112.5; Total Carb (g) = 20.7; Net Carb (g) = 20.7; Fat (g) = 3.4; Protein = 2

Muffins Wheat Bran Toaster-Type With Raisins Toasted ☞ serving size: 1 oz = 28.4 g; Calories = 88.9; Total Carb (g) = 15.8; Net Carb (g) = 13.4; Fat (g) = 2.7; Protein = 1.6

Multi-Grain Toast ☞ serving size: 1 oz = 28.4 g; Calories = 81.8; Total Carb (g) = 13.4; Net Carb (g) = 11.1; Fat (g) = 1.3; Protein = 4.1

Naan Indian Flatbread ☞ serving size: 1 piece (1/4 of 10" dia) = 44 g; Calories = 136.8; Total Carb (g) = 22.1; Net Carb (g) = 19.8; Fat (g) = 3.2; Protein = 4.9

Nabisco Nabisco Grahams Crackers ☞ serving size: 1 serving = 28 g; Calories = 118.7; Total Carb (g) = 21.3; Net Carb (g) = 20.4; Fat (g) = 2.8; Protein = 2

Nabisco Nabisco Oreo Crunchies Cookie Crumb Topping ☞ serving size: 1 serving = 11 g; Calories = 52.4; Total Carb (g) = 7.7; Net Carb (g) = 7.4; Fat (g) = 2.4; Protein = 0.5

Nabisco Nabisco Ritz Crackers ☞ serving size: 1 cracker = 3.3 g; Calories = 16.2; Total Carb (g) = 2.1; Net Carb (g) = 2; Fat (g) = 0.8; Protein = 0.2

Nabisco Nabisco Snackwells Fat Free Devils Food Cookie Cakes ☞ serving size: 1 serving = 16 g; Calories = 48.8; Total Carb (g) = 11.9; Net Carb (g) = 11.6; Fat (g) = 0.2; Protein = 0.8

Oatmeal Cookies ☞ serving size: 1 oz = 28.4 g; Calories = 127.8; Total Carb (g) = 19.5; Net Carb (g) = 18.7; Fat (g) = 5.1; Protein = 1.8

Pan Dulce La Ricura Salpora De Arroz Con Azucar Cookie-Like Contains Wheat Flour And Rice Flour ☞ serving size: 1 piece (1 serving) = 42 g; Calories = 186.9; Total Carb (g) = 27.8; Net Carb (g) = 27.3; Fat (g) = 6.8; Protein = 3.7

Pan Dulce With Raisins And Icing ☞ serving size: 1 roll = 93 g;

Calories = 342.2; Total Carb (g) = 54.5; Net Carb (g) = 52.4; Fat (g) = 10.6; Protein = 7.7

Pancakes Blueberry Prepared From Recipe ☞ serving size: 1 oz = 28.4 g; Calories = 63; Total Carb (g) = 8.2; Net Carb (g) = 8.2; Fat (g) = 2.6; Protein = 1.7

Pancakes Buckwheat Dry Mix Incomplete ☞ serving size: 1 oz = 28.4 g; Calories = 96.6; Total Carb (g) = 20.2; Net Carb (g) = 17.8; Fat (g) = 0.8; Protein = 3.1

Pancakes Buttermilk Prepared From Recipe ☞ serving size: 1 oz = 28.4 g; Calories = 64.5; Total Carb (g) = 8.2; Net Carb (g) = 8.2; Fat (g) = 2.6; Protein = 1.9

Pancakes Gluten-Free Frozen Ready-To-Heat ☞ serving size: 1 pancake = 48 g; Calories = 103.2; Total Carb (g) = 19.4; Net Carb (g) = 18.6; Fat (g) = 2.2; Protein = 1.6

Pancakes Plain Dry Mix Complete (Includes Buttermilk) ☞ serving size: 1/ 3 cup = 52 g; Calories = 191.4; Total Carb (g) = 38.3; Net Carb (g) = 36.8; Fat (g) = 1.6; Protein = 5.1

Pancakes Plain Dry Mix Complete Prepared ☞ serving size: 1 oz = 28.4 g; Calories = 55.1; Total Carb (g) = 10.4; Net Carb (g) = 10.1; Fat (g) = 0.7; Protein = 1.5

Pancakes Plain Dry Mix Incomplete (Includes Buttermilk) ☞ serving size: 1 oz = 28.4 g; Calories = 100.8; Total Carb (g) = 20.9; Net Carb (g) = 19.4; Fat (g) = 0.5; Protein = 2.8

Pancakes Plain Dry Mix Incomplete Prepared ☞ serving size: 1 oz = 28.4 g; Calories = 61.9; Total Carb (g) = 8.2; Net Carb (g) = 7.7; Fat (g) = 2.2; Protein = 2.2

Pancakes Plain Frozen Ready-To-Heat (Includes Buttermilk) ☞ serving size: 1 oz = 28.4 g; Calories = 66.2; Total Carb (g) = 10.7; Net Carb (g) = 10.4; Fat (g) = 1.9; Protein = 1.5

Pancakes Plain Frozen Ready-To-Heat Microwave (Includes

Buttermilk) ☞ serving size: 1 oz = 28.4 g; Calories = 67.9; Total Carb (g) = 12.3; Net Carb (g) = 11.6; Fat (g) = 1.3; Protein = 1.7

🍴 Pancakes Plain Prepared From Recipe ☞ serving size: 1 oz = 28.4 g; Calories = 64.5; Total Carb (g) = 8; Net Carb (g) = 8; Fat (g) = 2.8; Protein = 1.8

🍴 Pancakes Plain Reduced Fat ☞ serving size: 1 serving 3 pancakes = 105 g; Calories = 282.5; Total Carb (g) = 60.2; Net Carb (g) = 59.1; Fat (g) = 2; Protein = 6

🍴 Pancakes Special Dietary Dry Mix ☞ serving size: 1 oz = 28.4 g; Calories = 99.1; Total Carb (g) = 21; Net Carb (g) = 21; Fat (g) = 0.4; Protein = 2.5

🍴 Pancakes Whole Wheat Dry Mix Incomplete ☞ serving size: 1/4 cup mix 1 serving = 38 g; Calories = 133; Total Carb (g) = 28.2; Net Carb (g) = 25.2; Fat (g) = 0.5; Protein = 4

🍴 Pancakes Whole-Wheat Dry Mix Incomplete ☞ serving size: 1 oz = 28.4 g; Calories = 97.7; Total Carb (g) = 20.2; Net Carb (g) = 20.2; Fat (g) = 0.4; Protein = 3.6

🍴 Pancakes Whole-Wheat Dry Mix Incomplete Prepared ☞ serving size: 1 oz = 28.4 g; Calories = 59.1; Total Carb (g) = 8.3; Net Carb (g) = 7.6; Fat (g) = 1.8; Protein = 2.4

🍴 Pannetone ☞ serving size: 1 slice = 27 g; Calories = 86.7; Total Carb (g) = 14.5; Net Carb (g) = 13.9; Fat (g) = 2.2; Protein = 2.3

🍴 Pastry Cheese-Filled ☞ serving size: 1 pastry = 28 g; Calories = 75.9; Total Carb (g) = 4.2; Net Carb (g) = 4.1; Fat (g) = 5.5; Protein = 2.3

🍴 Pastry Chinese Made With Rice Flour ☞ serving size: 1 oz = 28 g; Calories = 68; Total Carb (g) = 12.7; Net Carb (g) = 12.4; Fat (g) = 1.7; Protein = 0.7

🍴 Pastry Cookie Type Fried ☞ serving size: 1 pastry = 46 g; Calories = 179.4; Total Carb (g) = 16.3; Net Carb (g) = 15.8; Fat (g) = 11.6; Protein = 2.6

🔳 Pastry Fruit-Filled ☞ serving size: 1 pastry = 78 g; Calories = 264.4; Total Carb (g) = 31.1; Net Carb (g) = 29; Fat (g) = 15; Protein = 3.2

🔳 Pastry Italian With Cheese ☞ serving size: 1 pastry = 85 g; Calories = 234.6; Total Carb (g) = 27.6; Net Carb (g) = 27; Fat (g) = 10.2; Protein = 8.1

🔳 Pastry Made With Bean Or Lotus Seed Paste Filling Baked ☞ serving size: 1 small square moon cake = 51 g; Calories = 169.8; Total Carb (g) = 34.6; Net Carb (g) = 33.2; Fat (g) = 2.1; Protein = 3.5

🔳 Pastry Made With Bean Paste And Salted Egg Yolk Filling Baked ☞ serving size: 1 large square moon cake = 204 g; Calories = 679.3; Total Carb (g) = 116.8; Net Carb (g) = 112.3; Fat (g) = 16.1; Protein = 17.1

🔳 Pastry Pastelitos De Guava (Guava Pastries) ☞ serving size: 1 piece = 86 g; Calories = 325.9; Total Carb (g) = 41.1; Net Carb (g) = 39.2; Fat (g) = 15.9; Protein = 4.7

🔳 Pastry Puff Custard Or Cream Filled Iced Or Not Iced ☞ serving size: 1 cream horn = 57 g; Calories = 233.1; Total Carb (g) = 17; Net Carb (g) = 16.6; Fat (g) = 17; Protein = 3.3

🔳 Pepperidge Farm Goldfish Baked Snack Crackers Cheddar ☞ serving size: 10 goldfish = 5.2 g; Calories = 23.8; Total Carb (g) = 3.4; Net Carb (g) = 3.4; Fat (g) = 0.8; Protein = 0.6

🔳 Pepperidge Farm Goldfish Baked Snack Crackers Explosive Pizza ☞ serving size: 10 goldfish = 5.3 g; Calories = 24.3; Total Carb (g) = 3.6; Net Carb (g) = 3.6; Fat (g) = 0.9; Protein = 0.5

🔳 Pepperidge Farm Goldfish Baked Snack Crackers Original ☞ serving size: 10 goldfish = 5.2 g; Calories = 24.3; Total Carb (g) = 3.4; Net Carb (g) = 3.3; Fat (g) = 1; Protein = 0.5

🔳 Pepperidge Farm Goldfish Baked Snack Crackers Parmesan ☞ serving size: 10 goldfish = 5.3 g; Calories = 24.3; Total Carb (g) = 3.4; Net Carb (g) = 3.2; Fat (g) = 0.9; Protein = 0.6

🔳 Pepperidge Farm Goldfish Baked Snack Crackers Pizza ☞

serving size: 10 goldfish = 5.1 g; Calories = 23.9; Total Carb (g) = 3.3; Net Carb (g) = 3.1; Fat (g) = 1; Protein = 0.5

Phyllo Dough ☞ serving size: 1 oz = 28.4 g; Calories = 84.9; Total Carb (g) = 14.9; Net Carb (g) = 14.4; Fat (g) = 1.7; Protein = 2

Pie Apple Commercially Prepared Enriched Flour ☞ serving size: 1 oz = 28.4 g; Calories = 67.3; Total Carb (g) = 9.7; Net Carb (g) = 9.2; Fat (g) = 3.1; Protein = 0.5

Pie Apple Commercially Prepared Unenriched Flour ☞ serving size: 1 oz = 28.4 g; Calories = 67.3; Total Carb (g) = 9.7; Net Carb (g) = 9.2; Fat (g) = 3.1; Protein = 0.5

Pie Apple Diet ☞ serving size: 1 individual serving = 85 g; Calories = 193; Total Carb (g) = 38; Net Carb (g) = 36.2; Fat (g) = 4.5; Protein = 1.8

Pie Apple One Crust ☞ serving size: 1 pie (9" dia) = 1203 g; Calories = 2911.3; Total Carb (g) = 469.3; Net Carb (g) = 456.1; Fat (g) = 111.5; Protein = 21.7

Pie Apple Prepared From Recipe ☞ serving size: 1 oz = 28.4 g; Calories = 75.3; Total Carb (g) = 10.5; Net Carb (g) = 10.5; Fat (g) = 3.6; Protein = 0.7

Pie Apple-Sour Cream ☞ serving size: 1 pie (9" dia) = 1274 g; Calories = 2611.7; Total Carb (g) = 381.9; Net Carb (g) = 365.4; Fat (g) = 117.5; Protein = 23.4

Pie Apricot Two Crust ☞ serving size: 1 pie (9" dia) = 1203 g; Calories = 3344.3; Total Carb (g) = 470.7; Net Carb (g) = 450.3; Fat (g) = 150.7; Protein = 38

Pie Banana Cream Individual Size Or Tart ☞ serving size: 1 tart = 117 g; Calories = 277.3; Total Carb (g) = 36.3; Net Carb (g) = 35; Fat (g) = 12.7; Protein = 5.3

Pie Banana Cream Prepared From Mix No-Bake Type ☞ serving

size: 1 oz = 28.4 g; Calories = 71.3; Total Carb (g) = 9; Net Carb (g) = 8.8; Fat (g) = 3.7; Protein = 1

Pie Banana Cream Prepared From Recipe ☞ serving size: 1 oz = 28.4 g; Calories = 76.4; Total Carb (g) = 9.3; Net Carb (g) = 9.1; Fat (g) = 3.9; Protein = 1.2

Pie Berry Not Blackberry Blueberry Boysenberry Huckleberry Raspberry Or Strawberry Individual Size Or Tart ☞ serving size: 1 tart = 117 g; Calories = 362.7; Total Carb (g) = 47.6; Net Carb (g) = 45.1; Fat (g) = 18.2; Protein = 3.5

Pie Berry Not Blackberry Blueberry Boysenberry Huckleberry Raspberry Or Strawberry; One Crust ☞ serving size: 1 pie (9" dia) = 1096 g; Calories = 2729; Total Carb (g) = 424.5; Net Carb (g) = 397.1; Fat (g) = 113; Protein = 19.3

Pie Berry Not Blackberry Blueberry Boysenberry Huckleberry Raspberry Or Strawberry; Two Crust ☞ serving size: 1 pie (9" dia) = 1203 g; Calories = 3476.7; Total Carb (g) = 476.6; Net Carb (g) = 451.4; Fat (g) = 165.8; Protein = 31.3

Pie Black Bottom ☞ serving size: 1 pie (9" dia) = 792 g; Calories = 2439.4; Total Carb (g) = 296.8; Net Carb (g) = 287.3; Fat (g) = 123.1; Protein = 43.2

Pie Blackberry Individual Size Or Tart ☞ serving size: 1 tart = 117 g; Calories = 332.3; Total Carb (g) = 43.2; Net Carb (g) = 39.7; Fat (g) = 16.6; Protein = 3.7

Pie Blackberry Two Crust ☞ serving size: 1 pie (10" dia) = 1521 g; Calories = 3985; Total Carb (g) = 543.3; Net Carb (g) = 496.2; Fat (g) = 190.6; Protein = 43

Pie Blueberry Individual Size Or Tart ☞ serving size: 1 tart = 117 g; Calories = 335.8; Total Carb (g) = 45.4; Net Carb (g) = 43.3; Fat (g) = 16.3; Protein = 3.3

Pie Blueberry One Crust ☞ serving size: 1 pie (9" dia) = 1096 g;

Calories = 2334.5; Total Carb (g) = 357.2; Net Carb (g) = 337.5; Fat (g) = 95.6; Protein = 24.3

🍴 Pie Blueberry Prepared From Recipe ☞ serving size: 1 oz = 28.4 g; Calories = 69.6; Total Carb (g) = 9.5; Net Carb (g) = 9.5; Fat (g) = 3.4; Protein = 0.8

🍴 Pie Buttermilk ☞ serving size: 1 pie (9" dia) = 1154 g; Calories = 4385.2; Total Carb (g) = 595.8; Net Carb (g) = 591.2; Fat (g) = 208.6; Protein = 47.8

🍴 Pie Cherry Commercially Prepared ☞ serving size: 1 oz = 28.4 g; Calories = 73.8; Total Carb (g) = 11.3; Net Carb (g) = 11.1; Fat (g) = 3.1; Protein = 0.6

🍴 Pie Cherry Made With Cream Cheese And Sour Cream ☞ serving size: 1 pie (9" dia) = 1274 g; Calories = 3605.4; Total Carb (g) = 509.1; Net Carb (g) = 501.4; Fat (g) = 165; Protein = 39.9

🍴 Pie Cherry One Crust ☞ serving size: 1 pie (9" dia) = 1096 g; Calories = 2498.9; Total Carb (g) = 402.6; Net Carb (g) = 389.4; Fat (g) = 93.8; Protein = 22.8

🍴 Pie Cherry Prepared From Recipe ☞ serving size: 1 oz = 28.4 g; Calories = 76.7; Total Carb (g) = 10.9; Net Carb (g) = 10.9; Fat (g) = 3.5; Protein = 0.8

🍴 Pie Chess ☞ serving size: 1 pie (9" dia) = 714 g; Calories = 2920.3; Total Carb (g) = 381.6; Net Carb (g) = 375.1; Fat (g) = 143.1; Protein = 37.9

🍴 Pie Chiffon Chocolate ☞ serving size: 1 pie (9" dia) = 792 g; Calories = 2574; Total Carb (g) = 328.1; Net Carb (g) = 317; Fat (g) = 118.8; Protein = 50.6

🍴 Pie Chiffon Not Chocolate ☞ serving size: 1 pie (9" dia) = 792 g; Calories = 2296.8; Total Carb (g) = 318.3; Net Carb (g) = 314.3; Fat (g) = 93; Protein = 52.7

🍴 Pie Chocolate Cream Individual Size Or Tart ☞ serving size: 1

tart = 117 g; Calories = 338.1; Total Carb (g) = 42.3; Net Carb (g) = 40.6; Fat (g) = 16.2; Protein = 6.2

🍰 Pie Chocolate Creme Commercially Prepared ☞ serving size: 1 serving .167 pie = 120 g; Calories = 423.6; Total Carb (g) = 46.1; Net Carb (g) = 45.2; Fat (g) = 26.9; Protein = 5

🍰 Pie Chocolate Mousse Prepared From Mix No-Bake Type ☞ serving size: 1 oz = 28.4 g; Calories = 73.8; Total Carb (g) = 8.4; Net Carb (g) = 8.4; Fat (g) = 4.4; Protein = 1

🍰 Pie Chocolate-Marshmallow ☞ serving size: 1 pie (8" dia) = 819 g; Calories = 3194.1; Total Carb (g) = 387.2; Net Carb (g) = 374.1; Fat (g) = 169; Protein = 37.7

🍰 Pie Coconut Cream Individual Size Or Tart ☞ serving size: 1 tart = 117 g; Calories = 263.3; Total Carb (g) = 29.8; Net Carb (g) = 28.9; Fat (g) = 13.2; Protein = 6.4

🍰 Pie Coconut Cream Prepared From Mix No-Bake Type ☞ serving size: 1 oz = 28.4 g; Calories = 78.4; Total Carb (g) = 8.1; Net Carb (g) = 8; Fat (g) = 5; Protein = 0.8

🍰 Pie Coconut Creme Commercially Prepared ☞ serving size: 1 oz = 28.4 g; Calories = 84.6; Total Carb (g) = 10.6; Net Carb (g) = 10.2; Fat (g) = 4.7; Protein = 0.6

🍰 Pie Crust Cookie-Type Chocolate Ready Crust ☞ serving size: 1 crust = 182 g; Calories = 880.9; Total Carb (g) = 117.4; Net Carb (g) = 112.4; Fat (g) = 40.8; Protein = 11.1

🍰 Pie Crust Cookie-Type Graham Cracker Ready Crust ☞ serving size: 1 oz = 28.4 g; Calories = 142.3; Total Carb (g) = 18.3; Net Carb (g) = 17.7; Fat (g) = 7.1; Protein = 1.4

🍰 Pie Crust Cookie-Type Prepared From Recipe Graham Cracker Chilled ☞ serving size: 1 piece (1/8 of 9 inch crust) = 30 g; Calories = 145.2; Total Carb (g) = 19.2; Net Carb (g) = 18.7; Fat (g) = 7.3; Protein = 1.2

🥧 Pie Crust Cookie-Type Prepared From Recipe Vanilla Wafer Chilled ☞ serving size: 1 cup = 129 g; Calories = 685; Total Carb (g) = 64.8; Net Carb (g) = 64.6; Fat (g) = 46.7; Protein = 4.8

🥧 Pie Crust Deep Dish Frozen Baked Made With Enriched Flour ☞ serving size: 1 pie crust (average weight) = 202 g; Calories = 1052.4; Total Carb (g) = 106; Net Carb (g) = 101.3; Fat (g) = 64.3; Protein = 12.3

🥧 Pie Crust Deep Dish Frozen Unbaked Made With Enriched Flour ☞ serving size: 1 pie crust (average weight) = 225 g; Calories = 1053; Total Carb (g) = 105.3; Net Carb (g) = 102.1; Fat (g) = 64.7; Protein = 12.4

🥧 Pie Crust Refrigerated Regular Baked ☞ serving size: 1 pie crust = 198 g; Calories = 1001.9; Total Carb (g) = 115.9; Net Carb (g) = 113.1; Fat (g) = 56.8; Protein = 6.8

🥧 Pie Crust Refrigerated Regular Unbaked ☞ serving size: 1 pie crust (average weight) = 229 g; Calories = 1019.1; Total Carb (g) = 117; Net Carb (g) = 112.9; Fat (g) = 58.3; Protein = 6.8

🥧 Pie Crust Standard-Type Dry Mix ☞ serving size: 1 oz = 28.4 g; Calories = 147.1; Total Carb (g) = 14.8; Net Carb (g) = 14.8; Fat (g) = 8.9; Protein = 2

🥧 Pie Crust Standard-Type Dry Mix Prepared Baked ☞ serving size: 1 piece (1/8 of 9 inch crust) = 20 g; Calories = 100.2; Total Carb (g) = 10.1; Net Carb (g) = 9.7; Fat (g) = 6.1; Protein = 1.3

🥧 Pie Crust Standard-Type Frozen Ready-To-Bake Enriched ☞ serving size: 1 piece (1/8 of 9 inch crust) = 18 g; Calories = 82.3; Total Carb (g) = 8.8; Net Carb (g) = 8.3; Fat (g) = 4.7; Protein = 1.1

🥧 Pie Crust Standard-Type Frozen Ready-To-Bake Enriched Baked ☞ serving size: 1 pie crust (average weight of 1 baked crust) = 154 g; Calories = 782.3; Total Carb (g) = 86.6; Net Carb (g) = 81.5; Fat (g) = 44; Protein = 10

🥧 Pie Crust Standard-Type Frozen Ready-To-Bake Unenriched

☞ serving size: 1 crust, single 9 inch = 142 g; Calories = 648.9; Total Carb (g) = 62.6; Net Carb (g) = 61.3; Fat (g) = 41.5; Protein = 5.5

🍽 Pie Crust Standard-Type Prepared From Recipe Baked ☞ serving size: 1 piece (1/8 of 9 inch crust) = 23 g; Calories = 121.2; Total Carb (g) = 10.9; Net Carb (g) = 10.5; Fat (g) = 8; Protein = 1.5

🍽 Pie Crust Standard-Type Prepared From Recipe Unbaked ☞ serving size: 1 piece (1/8 of 9 inch crust) = 24 g; Calories = 112.6; Total Carb (g) = 10.2; Net Carb (g) = 9.3; Fat (g) = 7.4; Protein = 1.4

🍽 Pie Custard Individual Size Or Tart ☞ serving size: 1 tart = 117 g; Calories = 201.2; Total Carb (g) = 31; Net Carb (g) = 30.4; Fat (g) = 5.5; Protein = 6.7

🍽 Pie Egg Custard Commercially Prepared ☞ serving size: 1 oz = 28.4 g; Calories = 59.6; Total Carb (g) = 5.9; Net Carb (g) = 5.5; Fat (g) = 3.3; Protein = 1.6

🍽 Pie Fried Pies Cherry ☞ serving size: 1 oz = 28.4 g; Calories = 89.7; Total Carb (g) = 12.1; Net Carb (g) = 11.4; Fat (g) = 4.6; Protein = 0.9

🍽 Pie Fried Pies Fruit ☞ serving size: 1 oz = 28.4 g; Calories = 89.7; Total Carb (g) = 12.1; Net Carb (g) = 11.4; Fat (g) = 4.6; Protein = 0.9

🍽 Pie Fried Pies Lemon ☞ serving size: 1 oz = 28.4 g; Calories = 89.7; Total Carb (g) = 12.1; Net Carb (g) = 11.4; Fat (g) = 4.6; Protein = 0.9

🍽 Pie Lemon Cream ☞ serving size: 1 pie (9" dia) = 1154 g; Calories = 3081.2; Total Carb (g) = 446; Net Carb (g) = 441.4; Fat (g) = 124.9; Protein = 53.2

🍽 Pie Lemon Cream Individual Size Or Tart ☞ serving size: 1 tart = 117 g; Calories = 331.1; Total Carb (g) = 45.3; Net Carb (g) = 44.7; Fat (g) = 14.6; Protein = 5.5

🍽 Pie Lemon Meringue Commercially Prepared ☞ serving size: 1

oz = 28.4 g; Calories = 76.1; Total Carb (g) = 13.4; Net Carb (g) = 13.1; Fat (g) = 2.5; Protein = 0.4

🥧 Pie Lemon Meringue Prepared From Recipe ☞ serving size: 1 oz = 28.4 g; Calories = 80.9; Total Carb (g) = 11.1; Net Carb (g) = 11.1; Fat (g) = 3.7; Protein = 1.1

🥧 Pie Lemon Not Cream Or Meringue ☞ serving size: 1 pie (9" dia) = 791 g; Calories = 3037.4; Total Carb (g) = 452.4; Net Carb (g) = 445.3; Fat (g) = 122.8; Protein = 40

🥧 Pie Lemon Not Cream Or Meringue Individual Size Or Tart ☞ serving size: 1 tart = 117 g; Calories = 462.2; Total Carb (g) = 66.5; Net Carb (g) = 65.3; Fat (g) = 19.6; Protein = 6.1

🥧 Pie Mince Individual Size Or Tart ☞ serving size: 1 tart = 117 g; Calories = 358; Total Carb (g) = 49.2; Net Carb (g) = 47.3; Fat (g) = 16.9; Protein = 3.9

🥧 Pie Mince Prepared From Recipe ☞ serving size: 1 oz = 28.4 g; Calories = 82.1; Total Carb (g) = 13.6; Net Carb (g) = 12.9; Fat (g) = 3.1; Protein = 0.7

🥧 Pie Oatmeal ☞ serving size: 1 pie (9" dia) = 915 g; Calories = 3568.5; Total Carb (g) = 550.6; Net Carb (g) = 537.7; Fat (g) = 143.2; Protein = 46.5

🥧 Pie Peach ☞ serving size: 1 oz = 28.4 g; Calories = 63.6; Total Carb (g) = 9.3; Net Carb (g) = 9.1; Fat (g) = 2.8; Protein = 0.5

🥧 Pie Peach Individual Size Or Tart ☞ serving size: 1 tart = 117 g; Calories = 342.8; Total Carb (g) = 45.7; Net Carb (g) = 44.1; Fat (g) = 16.6; Protein = 3.8

🥧 Pie Peach One Crust ☞ serving size: 1 pie (9" dia) = 1203 g; Calories = 2791; Total Carb (g) = 463; Net Carb (g) = 446.2; Fat (g) = 99.5; Protein = 26.7

🥧 Pie Peanut Butter Cream ☞ serving size: 1 pie (9" dia) = 1154 g;

Calories = 3381.2; Total Carb (g) = 393.3; Net Carb (g) = 380.6; Fat (g) = 168.8; Protein = 88.3

🥧 Pie Pear Individual Size Or Tart ☞ serving size: 1 tart = 117 g; Calories = 339.3; Total Carb (g) = 45.7; Net Carb (g) = 43.4; Fat (g) = 16.5; Protein = 3.3

🥧 Pie Pear Two Crust ☞ serving size: 1 pie (9" dia) = 1203 g; Calories = 3212; Total Carb (g) = 457; Net Carb (g) = 433; Fat (g) = 145.8; Protein = 29.7

🥧 Pie Pecan Commercially Prepared ☞ serving size: 1 oz = 28.4 g; Calories = 115.6; Total Carb (g) = 16.9; Net Carb (g) = 16.3; Fat (g) = 4.7; Protein = 1.3

🥧 Pie Pecan Prepared From Recipe ☞ serving size: 1 oz = 28.4 g; Calories = 117; Total Carb (g) = 14.8; Net Carb (g) = 14.8; Fat (g) = 6.3; Protein = 1.4

🥧 Pie Pineapple Cream ☞ serving size: 1 pie (9" dia) = 1154 g; Calories = 2319.5; Total Carb (g) = 344.6; Net Carb (g) = 338.8; Fat (g) = 88.3; Protein = 43

🥧 Pie Pineapple Two Crust ☞ serving size: 1 pie (9" dia) = 1203 g; Calories = 3163.9; Total Carb (g) = 443.9; Net Carb (g) = 431.9; Fat (g) = 145.2; Protein = 30.4

🥧 Pie Plum Two Crust ☞ serving size: 1 pie (9" dia) = 1203 g; Calories = 3512.8; Total Carb (g) = 490; Net Carb (g) = 475.5; Fat (g) = 163.7; Protein = 33.4

🥧 Pie Prune One Crust ☞ serving size: 1 pie (9" dia) = 1203 g; Calories = 3621; Total Carb (g) = 616.5; Net Carb (g) = 599.7; Fat (g) = 116; Protein = 45.1

🥧 Pie Pudding Chocolate With Chocolate Coating Individual Size ☞ serving size: 1 individual pie = 142 g; Calories = 552.4; Total Carb (g) = 61; Net Carb (g) = 58.2; Fat (g) = 31.5; Protein = 6.1

🥧 Pie Pudding Flavors Other Than Chocolate ☞ serving size: 1 pie

(8" dia) = 885 g; Calories = 1982.4; Total Carb (g) = 240; Net Carb (g) = 235.6; Fat (g) = 98.2; Protein = 34.1

🥧 Pie Pudding Flavors Other Than Chocolate Individual Size Or Tart ☞ serving size: 1 small tart = 117 g; Calories = 390.8; Total Carb (g) = 46.6; Net Carb (g) = 44.3; Fat (g) = 20.2; Protein = 5.7

🥧 Pie Pudding Flavors Other Than Chocolate With Chocolate Coating Individual Size ☞ serving size: 1 individual pie = 142 g; Calories = 545.3; Total Carb (g) = 60.8; Net Carb (g) = 58; Fat (g) = 31.1; Protein = 5.8

🥧 Pie Pumpkin Commercially Prepared ☞ serving size: 1 oz = 28.4 g; Calories = 69; Total Carb (g) = 9.9; Net Carb (g) = 9.4; Fat (g) = 2.8; Protein = 1.1

🥧 Pie Pumpkin Prepared From Recipe ☞ serving size: 1 oz = 28.4 g; Calories = 57.9; Total Carb (g) = 7.5; Net Carb (g) = 7.5; Fat (g) = 2.6; Protein = 1.3

🥧 Pie Raisin Individual Size Or Tart ☞ serving size: 1 tart = 117 g; Calories = 339.3; Total Carb (g) = 47.3; Net Carb (g) = 45.8; Fat (g) = 15.8; Protein = 3.7

🥧 Pie Raisin Two Crust ☞ serving size: 1 pie (9" dia) = 1203 g; Calories = 3019.5; Total Carb (g) = 444.3; Net Carb (g) = 431; Fat (g) = 131.8; Protein = 31.5

🥧 Pie Raspberry Cream ☞ serving size: 1 pie (9" dia) = 1154 g; Calories = 2284.9; Total Carb (g) = 266.8; Net Carb (g) = 239.1; Fat (g) = 130.5; Protein = 28.4

🥧 Pie Raspberry One Crust ☞ serving size: 1 pie (9" dia) = 1096 g; Calories = 2630.4; Total Carb (g) = 415.1; Net Carb (g) = 371.2; Fat (g) = 105.4; Protein = 23.3

🥧 Pie Raspberry Two Crust ☞ serving size: 1 pie (9" dia) = 1203 g; Calories = 3380.4; Total Carb (g) = 462.9; Net Carb (g) = 420.8; Fat (g) = 161.4; Protein = 34.2

🎂 Pie Rhubarb Individual Size Or Tart ☞ serving size: 1 tart = 117 g; Calories = 372.1; Total Carb (g) = 44.2; Net Carb (g) = 42.5; Fat (g) = 20; Protein = 4.2

🎂 Pie Rhubarb One Crust ☞ serving size: 1 pie (9" dia) = 1096 g; Calories = 2685.2; Total Carb (g) = 390; Net Carb (g) = 372.4; Fat (g) = 117.2; Protein = 26.5

🎂 Pie Rhubarb Two Crust ☞ serving size: 1 pie (9" dia) = 1203 g; Calories = 3560.9; Total Carb (g) = 442.7; Net Carb (g) = 424.7; Fat (g) = 184.5; Protein = 39.1

🎂 Pie Shoo-Fly ☞ serving size: 1 pie (9" dia) = 915 g; Calories = 3239.1; Total Carb (g) = 555.7; Net Carb (g) = 547.4; Fat (g) = 101; Protein = 35.8

🎂 Pie Sour Cream Raisin ☞ serving size: 1 pie (9" dia) = 1154 g; Calories = 4085.2; Total Carb (g) = 398.7; Net Carb (g) = 382.6; Fat (g) = 261.7; Protein = 58.3

🎂 Pie Squash ☞ serving size: 1 pie (9" dia) = 1235 g; Calories = 2334.2; Total Carb (g) = 319.6; Net Carb (g) = 303.6; Fat (g) = 98.8; Protein = 51.4

🎂 Pie Strawberry Cream ☞ serving size: 1 pie (10" dia) = 1449 g; Calories = 2956; Total Carb (g) = 381.2; Net Carb (g) = 365.3; Fat (g) = 155.2; Protein = 23.9

🎂 Pie Strawberry Cream Individual Size Or Tart ☞ serving size: 1 tart = 117 g; Calories = 280.8; Total Carb (g) = 33.6; Net Carb (g) = 32.3; Fat (g) = 15.6; Protein = 2.6

🎂 Pie Strawberry Individual Size Or Tart ☞ serving size: 1 tart = 117 g; Calories = 310.1; Total Carb (g) = 42.5; Net Carb (g) = 40.5; Fat (g) = 14.6; Protein = 3.3

🎂 Pie Strawberry One Crust ☞ serving size: 1 pie (9" dia) = 1343 g; Calories = 3088.9; Total Carb (g) = 464.7; Net Carb (g) = 440.5; Fat (g) = 128.7; Protein = 30.8

Pie Strawberry-Rhubarb Two Crust ☞ serving size: 1 pie (10" dia) = 1521 g; Calories = 4274; Total Carb (g) = 542.1; Net Carb (g) = 517.7; Fat (g) = 217.7; Protein = 47.2

Pie Sweet Potato ☞ serving size: 1 pie (10" dia) = 1530 g; Calories = 3978; Total Carb (g) = 444.2; Net Carb (g) = 415.1; Fat (g) = 230.4; Protein = 49.9

Pie Tofu With Fruit ☞ serving size: 1 pie (9" dia) = 1154 g; Calories = 2411.9; Total Carb (g) = 261.3; Net Carb (g) = 252; Fat (g) = 138.8; Protein = 54.7

Pie Toll House Chocolate Chip ☞ serving size: 1 pie (9" dia) = 915 g; Calories = 4895.3; Total Carb (g) = 409.1; Net Carb (g) = 388.1; Fat (g) = 358.8; Protein = 53.6

Pie Vanilla Cream Prepared From Recipe ☞ serving size: 1 oz = 28.4 g; Calories = 79; Total Carb (g) = 9.3; Net Carb (g) = 9.1; Fat (g) = 4.1; Protein = 1.4

Pie Yogurt Frozen ☞ serving size: 1 pie (9" dia) = 1154 g; Calories = 2850.4; Total Carb (g) = 315.8; Net Carb (g) = 308.9; Fat (g) = 164.1; Protein = 37.9

Pillsbury Buttermilk Biscuits Artificial Flavor Refrigerated Dough ☞ serving size: 1 biscuit = 64 g; Calories = 151; Total Carb (g) = 30.1; Net Carb (g) = 29.1; Fat (g) = 1.8; Protein = 4.1

Pillsbury Chocolate Chip Cookies Refrigerated Dough ☞ serving size: 1 serving 2 cookies = 38 g; Calories = 171; Total Carb (g) = 23.1; Net Carb (g) = 22.4; Fat (g) = 8.1; Protein = 1.5

Pillsbury Cinnamon Rolls With Icing Refrigerated Dough ☞ serving size: 1 serving 1 roll with icing = 44 g; Calories = 145.2; Total Carb (g) = 23.5; Net Carb (g) = 22.9; Fat (g) = 5; Protein = 1.9

Pillsbury Crusty French Loaf Refrigerated Dough ☞ serving size: 1 serving = 52 g; Calories = 126.4; Total Carb (g) = 24.1; Net Carb (g) = 22.8; Fat (g) = 1.5; Protein = 4.5

Pillsbury Golden Layer Buttermilk Biscuits Artificial Flavor Refrigerated Dough ☞ serving size: 1 serving = 34 g; Calories = 104.4; Total Carb (g) = 14; Net Carb (g) = 13.6; Fat (g) = 4.5; Protein = 2

Pillsbury Grands Buttermilk Biscuits Refrigerated Dough ☞ serving size: 1 biscuit = 34 g; Calories = 99.6; Total Carb (g) = 14.4; Net Carb (g) = 13.9; Fat (g) = 3.9; Protein = 2.1

Pita Bread ☞ serving size: 1 pita, large (6-1/2 inch dia) = 60 g; Calories = 165; Total Carb (g) = 33.4; Net Carb (g) = 32.1; Fat (g) = 0.7; Protein = 5.5

Pizza Cheese And Vegetables Gluten-Free Thick Crust ☞ serving size: 1 piece, nfs = 149 g; Calories = 339.7; Total Carb (g) = 39.2; Net Carb (g) = 35.1; Fat (g) = 16.2; Protein = 9.6

Pizza Cheese And Vegetables Gluten-Free Thin Crust ☞ serving size: 1 piece, nfs = 133 g; Calories = 296.6; Total Carb (g) = 29.5; Net Carb (g) = 26.3; Fat (g) = 16; Protein = 9.1

Pizza Cheese And Vegetables Whole Wheat Thick Crust ☞ serving size: 1 piece, nfs = 149 g; Calories = 353.1; Total Carb (g) = 43.6; Net Carb (g) = 37.4; Fat (g) = 14.9; Protein = 13.5

Pizza Cheese And Vegetables Whole Wheat Thin Crust ☞ serving size: 1 piece, nfs = 133 g; Calories = 307.2; Total Carb (g) = 32.7; Net Carb (g) = 27.9; Fat (g) = 15.1; Protein = 12

Pizza Cheese From School Lunch Medium Crust ☞ serving size: 1 piece, nfs = 147 g; Calories = 367.5; Total Carb (g) = 43.7; Net Carb (g) = 38.7; Fat (g) = 12.6; Protein = 20.1

Pizza Cheese Gluten-Free Thick Crust ☞ serving size: 1 piece, nfs = 132 g; Calories = 344.5; Total Carb (g) = 39.6; Net Carb (g) = 35.8; Fat (g) = 16.2; Protein = 9.9

Pizza Cheese Gluten-Free Thin Crust ☞ serving size: 1 piece, nfs = 119 g; Calories = 314.2; Total Carb (g) = 30.7; Net Carb (g) = 27.8; Fat (g) = 16.9; Protein = 9.9

Pizza Cheese Whole Wheat Thick Crust ☞ serving size: 1 piece, nfs = 132 g; Calories = 359; Total Carb (g) = 44.3; Net Carb (g) = 38.3; Fat (g) = 14.9; Protein = 14.1

Pizza Cheese Whole Wheat Thin Crust ☞ serving size: 1 piece, nfs = 119 g; Calories = 324.9; Total Carb (g) = 34.4; Net Carb (g) = 29.5; Fat (g) = 15.8; Protein = 13.1

Pizza Cheese With Fruit Medium Crust ☞ serving size: 1 piece, nfs = 137 g; Calories = 327.4; Total Carb (g) = 42.5; Net Carb (g) = 39.5; Fat (g) = 11.5; Protein = 13.6

Pizza Cheese With Fruit Thick Crust ☞ serving size: 1 piece, nfs = 150 g; Calories = 369; Total Carb (g) = 46.6; Net Carb (g) = 43.4; Fat (g) = 13.9; Protein = 14.4

Pizza Cheese With Fruit Thin Crust ☞ serving size: 1 piece, nfs = 104 g; Calories = 270.4; Total Carb (g) = 29.6; Net Carb (g) = 27.2; Fat (g) = 12; Protein = 11.1

Pizza Cheese With Vegetables From Frozen Thick Crust ☞ serving size: 1 piece, nfs = 143 g; Calories = 350.4; Total Carb (g) = 44.8; Net Carb (g) = 41.3; Fat (g) = 11.8; Protein = 16.6

Pizza Cheese With Vegetables From Frozen Thin Crust ☞ serving size: 1 piece, nfs = 109 g; Calories = 261.6; Total Carb (g) = 28.9; Net Carb (g) = 26.6; Fat (g) = 11.8; Protein = 10.1

Pizza Cheese With Vegetables From Restaurant Or Fast Food Medium Crust ☞ serving size: 1 piece, nfs = 133 g; Calories = 321.9; Total Carb (g) = 40.8; Net Carb (g) = 37.9; Fat (g) = 11.6; Protein = 13.7

Pizza Cheese With Vegetables From Restaurant Or Fast Food Thick Crust ☞ serving size: 1 piece, nfs = 149 g; Calories = 365.1; Total Carb (g) = 45.3; Net Carb (g) = 42.2; Fat (g) = 14; Protein = 14.5

Pizza Cheese With Vegetables From Restaurant Or Fast Food Thin Crust ☞ serving size: 1 piece, nfs = 100 g; Calories = 265; Total Carb (g) = 28; Net Carb (g) = 25.7; Fat (g) = 12; Protein = 11.2

Pizza Extra Cheese Thick Crust ☞ serving size: 1 piece, nfs = 141 g; Calories = 383.5; Total Carb (g) = 45; Net Carb (g) = 42; Fat (g) = 15.5; Protein = 16.1

Pizza Extra Cheese Thin Crust ☞ serving size: 1 piece, nfs = 92 g; Calories = 277.8; Total Carb (g) = 27.4; Net Carb (g) = 25.2; Fat (g) = 13.1; Protein = 12.4

Pizza No Cheese Thick Crust ☞ serving size: 1 piece, nfs = 124 g; Calories = 362.1; Total Carb (g) = 47.1; Net Carb (g) = 44.5; Fat (g) = 15; Protein = 9.2

Pizza No Cheese Thin Crust ☞ serving size: 1 piece, nfs = 75 g; Calories = 207; Total Carb (g) = 23.1; Net Carb (g) = 21.6; Fat (g) = 10.2; Protein = 5.5

Pizza Rolls ☞ serving size: 1 cup = 119 g; Calories = 410.6; Total Carb (g) = 63.5; Net Carb (g) = 62; Fat (g) = 12.5; Protein = 10.9

Pizza With Beans And Vegetables Thick Crust ☞ serving size: 1 piece, nfs = 173 g; Calories = 389.3; Total Carb (g) = 49.3; Net Carb (g) = 44.4; Fat (g) = 14.2; Protein = 16.3

Pizza With Beans And Vegetables Thin Crust ☞ serving size: 1 piece, nfs = 129 g; Calories = 291.5; Total Carb (g) = 32.5; Net Carb (g) = 28.3; Fat (g) = 12.2; Protein = 13.2

Pizza With Cheese And Extra Vegetables Medium Crust ☞ serving size: 1 piece, nfs = 152 g; Calories = 334.4; Total Carb (g) = 42; Net Carb (g) = 38.7; Fat (g) = 12.5; Protein = 14

Pizza With Cheese And Extra Vegetables Thick Crust ☞ serving size: 1 piece, nfs = 155 g; Calories = 372; Total Carb (g) = 45.7; Net Carb (g) = 42.3; Fat (g) = 14.6; Protein = 14.7

Pizza With Cheese And Extra Vegetables Thin Crust ☞ serving size: 1 piece, nfs = 120 g; Calories = 279.6; Total Carb (g) = 29.4; Net Carb (g) = 26.5; Fat (g) = 13; Protein = 11.6

Pizza With Extra Meat And Extra Vegetables Medium Crust ☞

serving size: 1 piece, nfs = 159 g; Calories = 372.1; Total Carb (g) = 41.5; Net Carb (g) = 38.3; Fat (g) = 14.8; Protein = 18.3

🍕 Pizza With Extra Meat And Extra Vegetables Thick Crust ☞ serving size: 1 piece, nfs = 173 g; Calories = 415.2; Total Carb (g) = 45.9; Net Carb (g) = 42.4; Fat (g) = 17.3; Protein = 19.1

🍕 Pizza With Extra Meat And Extra Vegetables Thin Crust ☞ serving size: 1 piece, nfs = 129 g; Calories = 319.9; Total Carb (g) = 28.9; Net Carb (g) = 26.2; Fat (g) = 15.6; Protein = 16.2

🍕 Pizza With Extra Meat Medium Crust ☞ serving size: 1 piece, nfs = 150 g; Calories = 415.5; Total Carb (g) = 40.1; Net Carb (g) = 37.4; Fat (g) = 18.7; Protein = 21.1

🍕 Pizza With Extra Meat Thick Crust ☞ serving size: 1 piece, nfs = 166 g; Calories = 464.8; Total Carb (g) = 44.4; Net Carb (g) = 41.4; Fat (g) = 21.7; Protein = 22.5

🍕 Pizza With Extra Meat Thin Crust ☞ serving size: 1 piece, nfs = 120 g; Calories = 367.2; Total Carb (g) = 27.4; Net Carb (g) = 25.3; Fat (g) = 19.8; Protein = 19.2

🍕 Pizza With Meat And Fruit Medium Crust ☞ serving size: 1 piece, nfs = 150 g; Calories = 351; Total Carb (g) = 42.5; Net Carb (g) = 39.5; Fat (g) = 12.9; Protein = 16.5

🍕 Pizza With Meat And Fruit Thick Crust ☞ serving size: 1 piece, nfs = 157 g; Calories = 384.7; Total Carb (g) = 45.9; Net Carb (g) = 42.8; Fat (g) = 14.9; Protein = 16.6

🍕 Pizza With Meat And Fruit Thin Crust ☞ serving size: 1 piece, nfs = 115 g; Calories = 292.1; Total Carb (g) = 29.4; Net Carb (g) = 27.1; Fat (g) = 13.2; Protein = 13.8

🍕 Pizza With Meat And Vegetables From Restaurant Or Fast Food Thick Crust ☞ serving size: 1 piece, nfs = 149 g; Calories = 387.4; Total Carb (g) = 44.9; Net Carb (g) = 42; Fat (g) = 15.7; Protein = 16.3

🍕 Pizza With Meat And Vegetables From Restaurant Or Fast Food

Thin Crust ☞ serving size: 1 piece, nfs = 113 g; Calories = 306.2; Total Carb (g) = 28.4; Net Carb (g) = 26; Fat (g) = 14.9; Protein = 14.4

Pizza With Meat Gluten-Free Thick Crust ☞ serving size: 1 piece, nfs = 139 g; Calories = 393.4; Total Carb (g) = 35.9; Net Carb (g) = 32.4; Fat (g) = 21.8; Protein = 12.9

Pizza With Meat Gluten-Free Thin Crust ☞ serving size: 1 piece, nfs = 124 g; Calories = 359.6; Total Carb (g) = 26.8; Net Carb (g) = 24.2; Fat (g) = 22.2; Protein = 12.8

Pizza With Meat Other Than Pepperoni From Frozen Medium Crust ☞ serving size: 1 piece, nfs = 102 g; Calories = 271.3; Total Carb (g) = 29.9; Net Carb (g) = 27.2; Fat (g) = 11.2; Protein = 12.8

Pizza With Meat Other Than Pepperoni From Frozen Thick Crust ☞ serving size: 1 piece, nfs = 144 g; Calories = 380.2; Total Carb (g) = 45.3; Net Carb (g) = 41.9; Fat (g) = 14; Protein = 18.3

Pizza With Meat Other Than Pepperoni From Frozen Thin Crust ☞ serving size: 1 piece, nfs = 97 g; Calories = 260.9; Total Carb (g) = 26.3; Net Carb (g) = 23.6; Fat (g) = 11.8; Protein = 12

Pizza With Meat Other Than Pepperoni From School Lunch Medium Crust ☞ serving size: 1 piece, nfs = 147 g; Calories = 373.4; Total Carb (g) = 46.2; Net Carb (g) = 40.3; Fat (g) = 12.4; Protein = 19

Pizza With Meat Other Than Pepperoni Stuffed Crust ☞ serving size: 1 piece, nfs = 164 g; Calories = 460.8; Total Carb (g) = 45.1; Net Carb (g) = 42.6; Fat (g) = 21.6; Protein = 21.2

Pizza With Meat Whole Wheat Thick Crust ☞ serving size: 1 piece, nfs = 139 g; Calories = 405.9; Total Carb (g) = 40.1; Net Carb (g) = 34.8; Fat (g) = 20.6; Protein = 16.7

Pizza With Meat Whole Wheat Thin Crust ☞ serving size: 1 piece, nfs = 124 g; Calories = 368.3; Total Carb (g) = 29.8; Net Carb (g) = 25.7; Fat (g) = 21.4; Protein = 15.6

Pizza With Pepperoni From Frozen Medium Crust ☞ serving

size: 1 piece, nfs = 102 g; Calories = 276.4; Total Carb (g) = 30.3; Net Carb (g) = 27.6; Fat (g) = 11.6; Protein = 12.7

🍕 Pizza With Pepperoni From Frozen Thick Crust ☞ serving size: 1 piece, nfs = 144 g; Calories = 385.9; Total Carb (g) = 45.8; Net Carb (g) = 42.4; Fat (g) = 14.5; Protein = 18.1

🍕 Pizza With Pepperoni From Frozen Thin Crust ☞ serving size: 1 piece, nfs = 97 g; Calories = 265.8; Total Carb (g) = 26.7; Net Carb (g) = 23.9; Fat (g) = 12.3; Protein = 11.9

🍕 Pizza With Pepperoni From School Lunch Medium Crust ☞ serving size: 1 piece, nfs = 147 g; Calories = 376.3; Total Carb (g) = 43.8; Net Carb (g) = 37.4; Fat (g) = 13.6; Protein = 19.9

🍕 Pizza With Pepperoni Stuffed Crust ☞ serving size: 1 piece, nfs = 164 g; Calories = 485.4; Total Carb (g) = 44.6; Net Carb (g) = 42.1; Fat (g) = 24.6; Protein = 21.2

🍕 Plain Buttermilk Biscuits ☞ serving size: 1 oz = 28.4 g; Calories = 95.1; Total Carb (g) = 13.7; Net Carb (g) = 13.2; Fat (g) = 3.4; Protein = 2.1

🍕 Plain Croutons ☞ serving size: 1/2 oz = 14.2 g; Calories = 57.8; Total Carb (g) = 10.4; Net Carb (g) = 9.7; Fat (g) = 0.9; Protein = 1.7

🍕 Plain Graham Crackers ☞ serving size: 1 oz = 28.4 g; Calories = 122.1; Total Carb (g) = 22.1; Net Carb (g) = 21.1; Fat (g) = 3; Protein = 1.9

🍕 Plain Matzo Crackers ☞ serving size: 1/2 oz = 14.2 g; Calories = 56.1; Total Carb (g) = 11.9; Net Carb (g) = 11.5; Fat (g) = 0.2; Protein = 1.4

🍕 Popover ☞ serving size: 1 popover = 31 g; Calories = 82.2; Total Carb (g) = 10.8; Net Carb (g) = 10.4; Fat (g) = 2.7; Protein = 3.4

🍕 Popovers Dry Mix Enriched ☞ serving size: 1 oz = 28.4 g; Calories = 105.4; Total Carb (g) = 20.2; Net Carb (g) = 20.2; Fat (g) = 1.2; Protein = 3

🍘 Popovers Dry Mix Unenriched ☞ serving size: 1 oz = 28.4 g; Calories = 105.4; Total Carb (g) = 20.2; Net Carb (g) = 20.2; Fat (g) = 1.2; Protein = 3

🍘 Puff Pastry ☞ serving size: 1 oz = 28.4 g; Calories = 156.5; Total Carb (g) = 12.8; Net Carb (g) = 12.4; Fat (g) = 10.8; Protein = 2.1

🍘 Puff Pastry Frozen Ready-To-Bake Baked ☞ serving size: 1 oz = 28.4 g; Calories = 158.5; Total Carb (g) = 13; Net Carb (g) = 12.6; Fat (g) = 10.9; Protein = 2.1

🍘 Pumpernickel Melba Rye Toast ☞ serving size: 1/2 oz = 14.2 g; Calories = 55.2; Total Carb (g) = 11; Net Carb (g) = 9.8; Fat (g) = 0.5; Protein = 1.6

🍘 Roll Cheese ☞ serving size: 1 roll = 41 g; Calories = 129.2; Total Carb (g) = 20.3; Net Carb (g) = 19.6; Fat (g) = 3.2; Protein = 4.7

🍘 Roll Sweet Frosted ☞ serving size: 1 small = 54 g; Calories = 216; Total Carb (g) = 27.5; Net Carb (g) = 26.1; Fat (g) = 10.8; Protein = 3

🍘 Roll Sweet With Fruit Frosted ☞ serving size: 1 small = 54 g; Calories = 204.7; Total Carb (g) = 28.9; Net Carb (g) = 27.8; Fat (g) = 8.8; Protein = 2.8

🍘 Rolls Dinner Egg ☞ serving size: 1 oz = 28.4 g; Calories = 87.2; Total Carb (g) = 14.8; Net Carb (g) = 13.7; Fat (g) = 1.8; Protein = 2.7

🍘 Rolls Dinner Oat Bran ☞ serving size: 1 oz = 28.4 g; Calories = 67; Total Carb (g) = 11.4; Net Carb (g) = 10.3; Fat (g) = 1.3; Protein = 2.7

🍘 Rolls Dinner Plain Commercially Prepared (Includes Brown-And-Serve) ☞ serving size: 1 roll (1 oz) = 28 g; Calories = 86.8; Total Carb (g) = 14.6; Net Carb (g) = 14; Fat (g) = 1.8; Protein = 3

🍘 Rolls Dinner Plain Prepared From Recipe Made With Low Fat (2%) Milk ☞ serving size: 1 oz = 28.4 g; Calories = 89.7; Total Carb (g) = 15.2; Net Carb (g) = 14.6; Fat (g) = 2.1; Protein = 2.4

🍘 Rolls Dinner Rye ☞ serving size: 1 large (approx 3-1/2 inch to 4 inch dia) = 43 g; Calories = 123; Total Carb (g) = 22.8; Net Carb (g) = 20.7; Fat (g) = 1.5; Protein = 4.4

Rolls Dinner Sweet ☞ serving size: 1 roll = 30 g; Calories = 96.3; Total Carb (g) = 16.1; Net Carb (g) = 15.1; Fat (g) = 2.2; Protein = 3

Rolls Dinner Wheat ☞ serving size: 1 roll (1 oz) = 28 g; Calories = 76.4; Total Carb (g) = 12.9; Net Carb (g) = 11.8; Fat (g) = 1.8; Protein = 2.4

Rolls Dinner Whole-Wheat ☞ serving size: 1 roll (1 oz) = 28 g; Calories = 74.5; Total Carb (g) = 14.3; Net Carb (g) = 12.2; Fat (g) = 1.3; Protein = 2.4

Rolls French ☞ serving size: 1 oz = 28.4 g; Calories = 78.7; Total Carb (g) = 14.3; Net Carb (g) = 13.3; Fat (g) = 1.2; Protein = 2.4

Rolls Gluten-Free White Made With Brown Rice Flour Tapioca Starch And Potato Starch ☞ serving size: 1 roll = 36 g; Calories = 111.6; Total Carb (g) = 19.8; Net Carb (g) = 18.5; Fat (g) = 2.3; Protein = 2.9

Rolls Gluten-Free White Made With Brown Rice Flour Tapioca Starch And Sorghum Flour ☞ serving size: 1 roll = 69 g; Calories = 177.3; Total Carb (g) = 27.8; Net Carb (g) = 25.8; Fat (g) = 5.7; Protein = 3.9

Rolls Gluten-Free White Made With Rice Flour Rice Starch And Corn Starch ☞ serving size: 1 roll = 78 g; Calories = 186.4; Total Carb (g) = 39.4; Net Carb (g) = 35.4; Fat (g) = 2.1; Protein = 2.6

Rolls Gluten-Free Whole Grain Made With Tapioca Starch And Brown Rice Flour ☞ serving size: 1 roll = 44 g; Calories = 144.8; Total Carb (g) = 19.5; Net Carb (g) = 14.6; Fat (g) = 5.1; Protein = 5.2

Rolls Hamburger Or Hot Dog Wheat/cracked Wheat ☞ serving size: 1 roll = 51 g; Calories = 137.2; Total Carb (g) = 24.1; Net Carb (g) = 22; Fat (g) = 1.8; Protein = 6

Rolls Hamburger Or Hot Dog Whole Wheat ☞ serving size: 1

roll = 56 g; Calories = 150.6; Total Carb (g) = 25.2; Net Carb (g) = 21.7; Fat (g) = 2.5; Protein = 6.9

🍞 Rolls Hamburger Or Hotdog Mixed-Grain ☞ serving size: 1 oz = 28.4 g; Calories = 74.7; Total Carb (g) = 12.7; Net Carb (g) = 11.6; Fat (g) = 1.7; Protein = 2.7

🍞 Rolls Hamburger Or Hotdog Plain ☞ serving size: 1 roll 1 serving = 44 g; Calories = 122.8; Total Carb (g) = 22.1; Net Carb (g) = 21.3; Fat (g) = 1.7; Protein = 4.3

🍞 Rolls Hamburger Whole Grain White Calcium-Fortified ☞ serving size: 1 piece roll = 43 g; Calories = 109.7; Total Carb (g) = 20; Net Carb (g) = 19; Fat (g) = 1.5; Protein = 4

🍞 Rolls Hard (Includes Kaiser) ☞ serving size: 1 oz = 28.4 g; Calories = 83.2; Total Carb (g) = 15; Net Carb (g) = 14.3; Fat (g) = 1.2; Protein = 2.8

🍞 Rolls Pumpernickel ☞ serving size: 1 medium (2-1/2 inch dia) = 36 g; Calories = 99.4; Total Carb (g) = 18.7; Net Carb (g) = 16.7; Fat (g) = 1; Protein = 3.9

🍞 Rudis Gluten-Free Bakery Original Sandwich Bread ☞ serving size: 1 slice = 34 g; Calories = 108.8; Total Carb (g) = 18; Net Carb (g) = 16.8; Fat (g) = 3.6; Protein = 1.1

🍞 Rye Bread ☞ serving size: 1 oz = 28.4 g; Calories = 73.6; Total Carb (g) = 13.7; Net Carb (g) = 12.1; Fat (g) = 0.9; Protein = 2.4

🍞 Rye Crispbread ☞ serving size: 1/2 oz = 14.2 g; Calories = 52; Total Carb (g) = 11.7; Net Carb (g) = 9.3; Fat (g) = 0.2; Protein = 1.1

🍞 Sage Valley Gluten Free Vanilla Sandwich Cookies ☞ serving size: 3 cookies = 44 g; Calories = 219.6; Total Carb (g) = 31.6; Net Carb (g) = 31.2; Fat (g) = 9.7; Protein = 1.4

🍞 Schar Gluten-Free Classic White Rolls ☞ serving size: 1 roll = 78 g; Calories = 186.4; Total Carb (g) = 39.4; Net Carb (g) = 35.4; Fat (g) = 2.1; Protein = 2.6

Scone ☞ serving size: 1 scone = 42 g; Calories = 148.3; Total Carb (g) = 19; Net Carb (g) = 18.4; Fat (g) = 6.2; Protein = 3.8

Scone With Fruit ☞ serving size: 1 scone = 42 g; Calories = 147.8; Total Carb (g) = 20.9; Net Carb (g) = 20.2; Fat (g) = 5.6; Protein = 3.6

Sopaipilla With Syrup Or Honey ☞ serving size: 1 sopaipilla (1 1/2" x 1 1/2") = 12 g; Calories = 43.2; Total Carb (g) = 6.2; Net Carb (g) = 6.1; Fat (g) = 1.9; Protein = 0.5

Sopaipilla Without Syrup Or Honey ☞ serving size: 1 sopaipilla (1 1/2" x 1 1/2") = 10 g; Calories = 36.6; Total Carb (g) = 4.1; Net Carb (g) = 4; Fat (g) = 2; Protein = 0.5

Spoonbread ☞ serving size: 1 cup = 187 g; Calories = 306.7; Total Carb (g) = 34.6; Net Carb (g) = 33.3; Fat (g) = 12.9; Protein = 12.4

Strudel Berry ☞ serving size: 1 piece (approx 2" - 2-1/2" square) = 64 g; Calories = 159.4; Total Carb (g) = 29.7; Net Carb (g) = 28.1; Fat (g) = 4; Protein = 2.2

Strudel Cheese ☞ serving size: 1 piece (approx 2" - 2-1/2" square) = 64 g; Calories = 195.2; Total Carb (g) = 24.1; Net Carb (g) = 23.6; Fat (g) = 8.2; Protein = 6.5

Strudel Cheese And Fruit ☞ serving size: 1 piece (approx 2" - 2-1/2" square) = 64 g; Calories = 140.8; Total Carb (g) = 19.1; Net Carb (g) = 18.5; Fat (g) = 5.4; Protein = 4.4

Strudel Cherry ☞ serving size: 1 piece (approx 2" - 2-1/2" square) = 64 g; Calories = 179.2; Total Carb (g) = 28.8; Net Carb (g) = 27.5; Fat (g) = 6.5; Protein = 2.8

Strudel Peach ☞ serving size: 1 piece (approx 2" - 2-1/2" square) = 64 g; Calories = 130.6; Total Carb (g) = 24.1; Net Carb (g) = 22.9; Fat (g) = 3.3; Protein = 2

Strudel Pineapple ☞ serving size: 1 piece (approx 2" - 2-1/2" square) = 64 g; Calories = 159.4; Total Carb (g) = 30.8; Net Carb (g) = 30; Fat (g) = 3.6; Protein = 1.8

Sweet Bread Dough Filled With Bean Paste Meatless Steamed ☞ serving size: 1 manapua = 103 g; Calories = 273; Total Carb (g) = 55.6; Net Carb (g) = 52.1; Fat (g) = 3; Protein = 6.8

Sweet Rolls Cheese ☞ serving size: 1 oz = 28.4 g; Calories = 102.2; Total Carb (g) = 12.4; Net Carb (g) = 12.1; Fat (g) = 5.2; Protein = 2

Sweet Rolls Cinnamon Commercially Prepared With Raisins ☞ serving size: 1 oz = 28.4 g; Calories = 105.6; Total Carb (g) = 14.5; Net Carb (g) = 13.8; Fat (g) = 4.7; Protein = 1.8

Sweet Rolls Cinnamon Refrigerated Dough With Frosting ☞ serving size: 1 oz = 28.4 g; Calories = 94.6; Total Carb (g) = 14.7; Net Carb (g) = 14.7; Fat (g) = 3.5; Protein = 1.4

Sweet Rolls Cinnamon Refrigerated Dough With Frosting Baked ☞ serving size: 1 oz = 28.4 g; Calories = 102.8; Total Carb (g) = 15.9; Net Carb (g) = 15.9; Fat (g) = 3.7; Protein = 1.5

Taco Shells Baked ☞ serving size: 1 shell = 12.9 g; Calories = 61.4; Total Carb (g) = 8.2; Net Carb (g) = 7.3; Fat (g) = 2.8; Protein = 0.8

Taco Shells Baked Without Added Salt ☞ serving size: 1 oz = 28.4 g; Calories = 132.9; Total Carb (g) = 17.7; Net Carb (g) = 15.6; Fat (g) = 6.4; Protein = 2

Tamale Sweet ☞ serving size: 1 tamale = 34 g; Calories = 87.4; Total Carb (g) = 12.1; Net Carb (g) = 11.3; Fat (g) = 4.3; Protein = 0.8

Tamale Sweet With Fruit ☞ serving size: 1 tamale = 49 g; Calories = 98; Total Carb (g) = 15.3; Net Carb (g) = 14.3; Fat (g) = 4.2; Protein = 0.9

Tiramisu ☞ serving size: 1 piece = 174 g; Calories = 616; Total Carb (g) = 51.5; Net Carb (g) = 50.8; Fat (g) = 42.2; Protein = 10.3

Toasted Bagels ☞ serving size: 1 mini bagel (2-1/2 inch dia) = 24 g; Calories = 68.9; Total Carb (g) = 13.8; Net Carb (g) = 13.3; Fat (g) = 0.3; Protein = 2.7

Toasted Cinnamon Raisin Bagels ☞ serving size: 1 mini bagel (2-1/2 inch dia) = 24 g; Calories = 70.6; Total Carb (g) = 14.2; Net Carb (g) = 13.6; Fat (g) = 0.4; Protein = 2.5

Toasted White Bread ☞ serving size: 1 oz = 28.4 g; Calories = 82.4; Total Carb (g) = 15.5; Net Carb (g) = 14.7; Fat (g) = 1.1; Protein = 2.6

Toasted Whole Wheat Bread ☞ serving size: 1 oz = 28.4 g; Calories = 86.9; Total Carb (g) = 14.5; Net Carb (g) = 12.4; Fat (g) = 1.2; Protein = 4.6

Toaster Pastries Brown-Sugar-Cinnamon ☞ serving size: 1 oz = 28.4 g; Calories = 105.1; Total Carb (g) = 20.6; Net Carb (g) = 20; Fat (g) = 2.3; Protein = 1.2

Toaster Pastries Fruit (Includes Apple Blueberry Cherry Strawberry) ☞ serving size: 1 oz = 28.4 g; Calories = 110.2; Total Carb (g) = 20; Net Carb (g) = 19.7; Fat (g) = 2.8; Protein = 1.2

Toaster Pastries Fruit Frosted (Include Apples Blueberry Cherry Strawberry) ☞ serving size: 1 piece = 53 g; Calories = 204.1; Total Carb (g) = 38.1; Net Carb (g) = 37.1; Fat (g) = 4.8; Protein = 2.1

Toaster Pastries Fruit Toasted (Include Apple Blueberry Cherry Strawberry) ☞ serving size: 1 pastry = 51 g; Calories = 208.6; Total Carb (g) = 37.1; Net Carb (g) = 36.6; Fat (g) = 5.6; Protein = 2.4

Topping From Cheese Pizza ☞ serving size: topping from 1 piece = 40 g; Calories = 91.2; Total Carb (g) = 3.2; Net Carb (g) = 2.8; Fat (g) = 5.7; Protein = 6.8

Topping From Meat And Vegetable Pizza ☞ serving size: topping from 1 piece = 51 g; Calories = 155.6; Total Carb (g) = 4.3; Net Carb (g) = 3.8; Fat (g) = 11.3; Protein = 9.1

Topping From Meat Pizza ☞ serving size: topping from 1 piece = 41 g; Calories = 134.5; Total Carb (g) = 2.7; Net Carb (g) = 2.4; Fat (g) = 10.1; Protein = 8

Topping From Vegetable Pizza ☞ serving size: topping from 1 piece = 49 g; Calories = 120.5; Total Carb (g) = 6.2; Net Carb (g) = 5; Fat (g) = 7.5; Protein = 7.6

Tortillas Ready-To-Bake Or -Fry Corn ☞ serving size: 1 oz = 28.4 g; Calories = 61.9; Total Carb (g) = 12.7; Net Carb (g) = 10.9; Fat (g) = 0.8; Protein = 1.6

Tortillas Ready-To-Bake Or -Fry Corn Without Added Salt ☞ serving size: 1 oz = 28.4 g; Calories = 63; Total Carb (g) = 13.2; Net Carb (g) = 11.8; Fat (g) = 0.7; Protein = 1.6

Tortillas Ready-To-Bake Or -Fry Flour Refrigerated ☞ serving size: 1 tortilla = 48 g; Calories = 146.9; Total Carb (g) = 23.7; Net Carb (g) = 22; Fat (g) = 3.8; Protein = 3.9

Tortillas Ready-To-Bake Or -Fry Flour Shelf Stable ☞ serving size: 1 tortilla = 49 g; Calories = 145.5; Total Carb (g) = 24.1; Net Carb (g) = 23; Fat (g) = 3.7; Protein = 3.9

Tortillas Ready-To-Bake Or -Fry Flour Without Added Calcium ☞ serving size: 1 oz = 28.4 g; Calories = 92.3; Total Carb (g) = 15.8; Net Carb (g) = 14.9; Fat (g) = 2; Protein = 2.5

Tortillas Ready-To-Bake Or -Fry Whole Wheat ☞ serving size: 1 tortilla 1 serving = 41 g; Calories = 127.1; Total Carb (g) = 18.8; Net Carb (g) = 14.8; Fat (g) = 4; Protein = 4

Tostada Shells Corn ☞ serving size: 1 piece = 12.3 g; Calories = 58.3; Total Carb (g) = 7.9; Net Carb (g) = 7.2; Fat (g) = 2.9; Protein = 0.8

Turnover Guava ☞ serving size: 1 turnover = 78 g; Calories = 239.5; Total Carb (g) = 29.2; Net Carb (g) = 26.7; Fat (g) = 12.7; Protein = 3.1

Turnover Or Dumpling Apple ☞ serving size: 1 turnover = 82 g; Calories = 285.4; Total Carb (g) = 35.8; Net Carb (g) = 34.7; Fat (g) = 14.8; Protein = 3

Turnover Or Dumpling Berry ☞ serving size: 1 turnover = 78 g; Calories = 275.3; Total Carb (g) = 35.5; Net Carb (g) = 34; Fat (g) = 13.8; Protein = 3

Turnover Or Dumpling Cherry ☞ serving size: 1 turnover = 78 g; Calories = 238.7; Total Carb (g) = 31.2; Net Carb (g) = 30.2; Fat (g) = 11.8; Protein = 2.6

Turnover Or Dumpling Lemon ☞ serving size: 1 turnover = 78 g; Calories = 234.8; Total Carb (g) = 28.9; Net Carb (g) = 28.4; Fat (g) = 12.2; Protein = 2.7

Turnover Or Dumpling Peach ☞ serving size: 1 turnover = 78 g; Calories = 261.3; Total Carb (g) = 33.7; Net Carb (g) = 32.4; Fat (g) = 12.9; Protein = 3.1

Turnover Pumpkin ☞ serving size: 1 turnover = 78 g; Calories = 195.8; Total Carb (g) = 19.9; Net Carb (g) = 18.6; Fat (g) = 11.2; Protein = 4.3

Udis Gluten Free Classic French Dinner Rolls ☞ serving size: 1 roll = 36 g; Calories = 111.6; Total Carb (g) = 19.8; Net Carb (g) = 18.5; Fat (g) = 2.3; Protein = 2.9

Udis Gluten Free Soft & Delicious White Sandwich Bread ☞ serving size: 1 slice = 28 g; Calories = 83.4; Total Carb (g) = 14.3; Net Carb (g) = 12.8; Fat (g) = 2.2; Protein = 1.5

Udis Gluten Free Soft & Hearty Whole Grain Bread ☞ serving size: 1 slice = 25 g; Calories = 77.3; Total Carb (g) = 12.3; Net Carb (g) = 11; Fat (g) = 2.3; Protein = 1.8

Udis Gluten Free Whole Grain Dinner Rolls ☞ serving size: 1 roll = 44 g; Calories = 144.8; Total Carb (g) = 19.5; Net Carb (g) = 14.6; Fat (g) = 5.1; Protein = 5.2

Upside-Down Pineapple Cake ☞ serving size: 1 oz = 28.4 g; Calories = 90.6; Total Carb (g) = 14.3; Net Carb (g) = 14.1; Fat (g) = 3.4; Protein = 1

🍶 Vans Gluten Free Totally Original Pancakes ☞ serving size: 1 pancake = 48 g; Calories = 103.2; Total Carb (g) = 19.4; Net Carb (g) = 18.6; Fat (g) = 2.2; Protein = 1.6

🍶 Vans Gluten Free Totally Original Waffles ☞ serving size: 1 waffle = 47 g; Calories = 116.6; Total Carb (g) = 19.1; Net Carb (g) = 19.1; Fat (g) = 3.9; Protein = 1.4

🍶 Vans The Perfect 10 Crispy Six Whole Grain + Four Seed Baked Crackers Gluten Free ☞ serving size: 3 crackers = 8.4 g; Calories = 39.6; Total Carb (g) = 5.7; Net Carb (g) = 5.7; Fat (g) = 1.6; Protein = 0.6

🍶 Waffle Buttermilk Frozen Ready-To-Heat Microwaved ☞ serving size: 1 waffle = 35 g; Calories = 101.2; Total Carb (g) = 15.5; Net Carb (g) = 14.6; Fat (g) = 3.3; Protein = 2.4

🍶 Waffle Buttermilk Frozen Ready-To-Heat Toasted ☞ serving size: 1 oz = 28 g; Calories = 86.5; Total Carb (g) = 13.5; Net Carb (g) = 12.8; Fat (g) = 2.7; Protein = 2.1

🍶 Waffle Plain Frozen Ready-To-Heat Microwave ☞ serving size: 1 waffle, round (4 inchdia) = 32 g; Calories = 95.4; Total Carb (g) = 14.5; Net Carb (g) = 13.8; Fat (g) = 3.2; Protein = 2.1

🍶 Waffles Buttermilk Frozen Ready-To-Heat ☞ serving size: 1 waffle, square = 39 g; Calories = 106.5; Total Carb (g) = 16; Net Carb (g) = 15.2; Fat (g) = 3.6; Protein = 2.6

🍶 Waffles Chocolate Chip Frozen Ready-To-Heat ☞ serving size: 2 waffles = 70 g; Calories = 207.9; Total Carb (g) = 32; Net Carb (g) = 30.9; Fat (g) = 7.1; Protein = 4.1

🍶 Waffles Gluten-Free Frozen Ready-To-Heat ☞ serving size: 1 waffle = 45 g; Calories = 118.4; Total Carb (g) = 19.4; Net Carb (g) = 18.7; Fat (g) = 4; Protein = 1.2

🍶 Waffles Plain Frozen Ready -To-Heat Toasted ☞ serving size: 1 oz = 28.4 g; Calories = 88.6; Total Carb (g) = 14; Net Carb (g) = 13.3; Fat (g) = 2.7; Protein = 2

Waffles Plain Frozen Ready-To-Heat ☞ serving size: 1 oz = 28.4 g; Calories = 80.9; Total Carb (g) = 12.2; Net Carb (g) = 11.6; Fat (g) = 2.8; Protein = 1.8

Waffles Plain Prepared From Recipe ☞ serving size: 1 oz = 28.4 g; Calories = 82.6; Total Carb (g) = 9.3; Net Carb (g) = 9.3; Fat (g) = 4; Protein = 2.2

Waffles Whole Wheat Lowfat Frozen Ready-To-Heat ☞ serving size: 1 serving 2 waffles = 70 g; Calories = 179.9; Total Carb (g) = 34.4; Net Carb (g) = 31.4; Fat (g) = 2.5; Protein = 5

Wheat Bread ☞ serving size: 1 oz = 28.4 g; Calories = 77.8; Total Carb (g) = 13.5; Net Carb (g) = 12.4; Fat (g) = 1.3; Protein = 3

Wheat Flour Fritter Without Syrup ☞ serving size: 1 fritter = 22 g; Calories = 105.2; Total Carb (g) = 4.3; Net Carb (g) = 4.1; Fat (g) = 9.1; Protein = 1.7

Wheat Melba Toast Crackers ☞ serving size: 1/2 oz = 14.2 g; Calories = 53.1; Total Carb (g) = 10.8; Net Carb (g) = 9.8; Fat (g) = 0.3; Protein = 1.8

White Bread ☞ serving size: 1 slice = 29 g; Calories = 77.1; Total Carb (g) = 14.3; Net Carb (g) = 13.5; Fat (g) = 1; Protein = 2.6

White Cake With Coconut Frosting ☞ serving size: 1 oz = 28.4 g; Calories = 101.1; Total Carb (g) = 17.9; Net Carb (g) = 17.7; Fat (g) = 2.9; Protein = 1.2

White Pizza Cheese Thick Crust ☞ serving size: 1 piece, nfs = 141 g; Calories = 407.5; Total Carb (g) = 45.3; Net Carb (g) = 42.5; Fat (g) = 17.7; Protein = 16.2

White Pizza Cheese Thin Crust ☞ serving size: 1 piece, nfs = 92 g; Calories = 270.5; Total Carb (g) = 25.3; Net Carb (g) = 23.7; Fat (g) = 13.7; Protein = 11.2

White Pizza Cheese With Meat And Vegetables Thick Crust ☞

serving size: 1 piece, nfs = 155 g; Calories = 432.5; Total Carb (g) = 39.9; Net Carb (g) = 37.3; Fat (g) = 22.1; Protein = 17.8

White Pizza Cheese With Meat And Vegetables Thin Crust ☞ serving size: 1 piece, nfs = 118 g; Calories = 331.6; Total Carb (g) = 25; Net Carb (g) = 23.4; Fat (g) = 19.2; Protein = 14.2

White Pizza Cheese With Meat Thick Crust ☞ serving size: 1 piece, nfs = 154 g; Calories = 472.8; Total Carb (g) = 42.6; Net Carb (g) = 40; Fat (g) = 24.4; Protein = 19.5

White Pizza Cheese With Meat Thin Crust ☞ serving size: 1 piece, nfs = 100 g; Calories = 314; Total Carb (g) = 23; Net Carb (g) = 21.6; Fat (g) = 18.5; Protein = 13.5

White Pizza Cheese With Vegetables Thick Crust ☞ serving size: 1 piece, nfs = 155 g; Calories = 390.6; Total Carb (g) = 43.6; Net Carb (g) = 40.5; Fat (g) = 17.2; Protein = 15.1

White Pizza Cheese With Vegetables Thin Crust ☞ serving size: 1 piece, nfs = 106 g; Calories = 262.9; Total Carb (g) = 24.9; Net Carb (g) = 23.1; Fat (g) = 13.4; Protein = 10.5

Whole Wheat Bread ☞ serving size: 1 slice = 32 g; Calories = 80.6; Total Carb (g) = 13.7; Net Carb (g) = 11.7; Fat (g) = 1.1; Protein = 4

Whole Wheat Pita ☞ serving size: 1 pita, large (6-1/2 inch dia) = 64 g; Calories = 167.7; Total Carb (g) = 35.8; Net Carb (g) = 31.9; Fat (g) = 1.1; Protein = 6.3

Wonton Wrappers (Includes Egg Roll Wrappers) ☞ serving size: 1 oz = 28.4 g; Calories = 82.6; Total Carb (g) = 16.4; Net Carb (g) = 15.9; Fat (g) = 0.4; Protein = 2.8

Yam Buns; Puerto Rican Style ☞ serving size: 1 cup = 153 g; Calories = 462.1; Total Carb (g) = 45.5; Net Carb (g) = 40.2; Fat (g) = 29.1; Protein = 5.3

Yellow Cake With Chocolate Frosting ☞ serving size: 1 piece

(1/12 of a cake) = 144 g; Calories = 545.8; Total Carb (g) = 79.7; Net Carb (g) = 77.6; Fat (g) = 25.6; Protein = 4.6

Yellow Cake With Vanilla Frosting ☞ serving size: 1 serving = 67 g; Calories = 262; Total Carb (g) = 37.7; Net Carb (g) = 37.5; Fat (g) = 12; Protein = 2

12

BEANS AND LENTILS

🫘 Adzuki Beans ☞ serving size: 1 cup, diced = 130 g; Calories = 294.4; Total Carb (g) = 11.1; Net Carb (g) = 5.5; Fat (g) = 16.6; Protein = 27.7

🫘 Bacon Bits Meatless ☞ serving size: 1 cup = 262 g; Calories = 33.3; Total Carb (g) = 41.8; Net Carb (g) = 41.3; Fat (g) = 4.7; Protein = 9.2

🫘 Baked Beans ☞ serving size: 1 cup = 253 g; Calories = 392.2; Total Carb (g) = 51.8; Net Carb (g) = 37.9; Fat (g) = 1; Protein = 12.1

🫘 Bean Cake ☞ serving size: 1 cup = 165 g; Calories = 130.6; Total Carb (g) = 33.5; Net Carb (g) = 25.3; Fat (g) = 0.6; Protein = 5.2

🫘 Beans Adzuki Mature Seed Cooked Boiled With Salt ☞ serving size: 1 cup = 155 g; Calories = 294.4; Total Carb (g) = 13.8; Net Carb (g) = 5.8; Fat (g) = 8.1; Protein = 18.5

🫘 Beans Adzuki Mature Seeds Canned Sweetened ☞ serving size: 1 cup = 126 g; Calories = 701.5; Total Carb (g) = 22.2; Net Carb (g) = 12.8; Fat (g) = 0.9; Protein = 10

🫘 Beans Adzuki Mature Seeds Raw ☞ serving size: 1 cup = 253 g;

Calories = 648.1; Total Carb (g) = 42.8; Net Carb (g) = 32.1; Fat (g) = 2.5; Protein = 12.7

Beans And Franks ☞ serving size: 1 slice, thin = 14 g; Calories = 357.4; Total Carb (g) = 0.6; Net Carb (g) = 0.5; Fat (g) = 1.6; Protein = 2.5

Beans And Tomatoes Fat Added In Cooking ☞ serving size: 1 cup = 144 g; Calories = 341.2; Total Carb (g) = 11.5; Net Carb (g) = 4.9; Fat (g) = 13; Protein = 30.2

Beans And Tomatoes Fat Not Added In Cooking ☞ serving size: 1 fillet = 85 g; Calories = 244.4; Total Carb (g) = 7.7; Net Carb (g) = 2.5; Fat (g) = 15.3; Protein = 19.6

Beans And Tomatoes Ns As To Fat Added In Cooking ☞ serving size: 1 tbsp = 15 g; Calories = 341.2; Total Carb (g) = 1.4; Net Carb (g) = 0.9; Fat (g) = 1.4; Protein = 1.2

Beans Baked Canned No Salt Added ☞ serving size: 1 cup = 225 g; Calories = 265.7; Total Carb (g) = 15.5; Net Carb (g) = 15.5; Fat (g) = 18.2; Protein = 28.1

Beans Baked Canned With Franks ☞ serving size: 1 cup = 256 g; Calories = 367.8; Total Carb (g) = 28.3; Net Carb (g) = 17.5; Fat (g) = 17.4; Protein = 33.2

Beans Baked Canned With Pork ☞ serving size: 1 cup = 180 g; Calories = 268.2; Total Carb (g) = 19.9; Net Carb (g) = 12.3; Fat (g) = 11.5; Protein = 22.2

Beans Baked Canned With Pork And Sweet Sauce ☞ serving size: 1 tbsp = 16 g; Calories = 261.5; Total Carb (g) = 3.5; Net Carb (g) = 2.4; Fat (g) = 8; Protein = 3.8

Beans Baked Canned With Pork And Tomato Sauce ☞ serving size: 1 cup = 140 g; Calories = 231.2; Total Carb (g) = 115.3; Net Carb (g) = 109.8; Fat (g) = 0.1; Protein = 0.1

Beans Black Mature Seeds Canned Low Sodium ☞ serving size:

1 cup = 240 g; Calories = 218.4; Total Carb (g) = 6.7; Net Carb (g) = 6.5; Fat (g) = 7.7; Protein = 4.3

🫘 Beans Black Mature Seeds Cooked Boiled With Salt ☞ serving size: 1 cup = 168 g; Calories = 227; Total Carb (g) = 6.1; Net Carb (g) = 0.1; Fat (g) = 21.4; Protein = 39.7

🫘 Beans Black Mature Seeds Raw ☞ serving size: 1 cup, sliced = 140 g; Calories = 661.5; Total Carb (g) = 10.8; Net Carb (g) = 5.3; Fat (g) = 19.2; Protein = 27.5

🫘 Beans Black Turtle Mature Seeds Canned ☞ serving size: 1 slice = 56 g; Calories = 218.4; Total Carb (g) = 4.5; Net Carb (g) = 1.9; Fat (g) = 5; Protein = 11.8

🫘 Beans Black Turtle Mature Seeds Cooked Boiled With Salt ☞ serving size: 1 tbsp = 7 g; Calories = 240.5; Total Carb (g) = 2; Net Carb (g) = 1.3; Fat (g) = 1.8; Protein = 2.2

🫘 Beans Canned Drained Ns As To Type And As To Fat Added In Cooking ☞ serving size: 1 cup = 192 g; Calories = 340.2; Total Carb (g) = 121.6; Net Carb (g) = 101.1; Fat (g) = 2; Protein = 47.3

🫘 Beans Canned Drained Ns As To Type Fat Added In Cooking ☞ serving size: 1 cup = 198 g; Calories = 340.2; Total Carb (g) = 39.9; Net Carb (g) = 24.2; Fat (g) = 0.8; Protein = 17.9

🫘 Beans Canned Drained Ns As To Type Fat Not Added In Cooking ☞ serving size: 1 cup = 182 g; Calories = 246.6; Total Carb (g) = 42.4; Net Carb (g) = 28.4; Fat (g) = 0.7; Protein = 14.6

🫘 Beans Chili Barbecue Ranch Style Cooked ☞ serving size: 1 cup = 180 g; Calories = 245.4; Total Carb (g) = 72.7; Net Carb (g) = 38.7; Fat (g) = 17.5; Protein = 65.1

🫘 Beans Cranberry (Roman) Mature Seeds Cooked Boiled With Salt ☞ serving size: 1 cup = 166 g; Calories = 240.7; Total Carb (g) = 16.4; Net Carb (g) = 11.8; Fat (g) = 4.9; Protein = 25.9

🫘 Beans Cranberry (Roman) Mature Seeds Raw ☞ serving size: 1

cup = 196 g; Calories = 653.3; Total Carb (g) = 120.6; Net Carb (g) = 120.6; Fat (g) = 3.2; Protein = 45

👉 Beans Dry Cooked Ns As To Type And As To Fat Added In Cooking ☞ serving size: 1 cup = 177 g; Calories = 354.6; Total Carb (g) = 37.1; Net Carb (g) = 37.1; Fat (g) = 1; Protein = 13.8

👉 Beans Dry Cooked Ns As To Type Fat Added In Cooking ☞ serving size: 1 cup = 180 g; Calories = 354.6; Total Carb (g) = 33; Net Carb (g) = 21.5; Fat (g) = 1; Protein = 13.6

👉 Beans Dry Cooked Ns As To Type Fat Not Added In Cooking ☞ serving size: 1 cup = 197 g; Calories = 255.6; Total Carb (g) = 121.4; Net Carb (g) = 77.7; Fat (g) = 7.7; Protein = 45.6

👉 Beans Dry Cooked With Ground Beef ☞ serving size: 1 cup = 196 g; Calories = 540; Total Carb (g) = 41.4; Net Carb (g) = 25.1; Fat (g) = 0.8; Protein = 16.4

👉 Beans Dry Cooked With Pork ☞ serving size: 1 oz = 28.4 g; Calories = 336.4; Total Carb (g) = 4.6; Net Carb (g) = 2.2; Fat (g) = 14; Protein = 7.3

👉 Beans French Mature Seeds Cooked Boiled With Salt ☞ serving size: 1 cup = 147 g; Calories = 228.3; Total Carb (g) = 25.7; Net Carb (g) = 12.6; Fat (g) = 72.1; Protein = 41.2

👉 Beans French Mature Seeds Cooked Boiled Without Salt ☞ serving size: 1 cup = 146 g; Calories = 228.3; Total Carb (g) = 30.5; Net Carb (g) = 17.8; Fat (g) = 69.5; Protein = 36.6

👉 Beans French Mature Seeds Raw ☞ serving size: 1 cup = 144 g; Calories = 631.1; Total Carb (g) = 23.5; Net Carb (g) = 10.7; Fat (g) = 73.8; Protein = 38.9

👉 Beans Great Northern Mature Seeds Canned ☞ serving size: 1 cup = 146 g; Calories = 298.7; Total Carb (g) = 24.2; Net Carb (g) = 11.7; Fat (g) = 71.2; Protein = 36.8

👉 Beans Great Northern Mature Seeds Canned Low Sodium ☞

serving size: 1 cup = 60 g; Calories = 298.7; Total Carb (g) = 18.8; Net Carb (g) = 9.3; Fat (g) = 13.1; Protein = 20.3

🫘 Beans Great Northern Mature Seeds Cooked Boiled With Salt ☞ serving size: 1 cup = 205 g; Calories = 208.9; Total Carb (g) = 128.7; Net Carb (g) = 98; Fat (g) = 3.1; Protein = 44.5

🫘 Beans Great Northern Mature Seeds Raw ☞ serving size: 1 cup = 168 g; Calories = 620.4; Total Carb (g) = 39.1; Net Carb (g) = 27.8; Fat (g) = 0.6; Protein = 11.4

🫘 Beans Kidney All Types Mature Seeds Cooked Boiled With Salt ☞ serving size: 1 cup = 238 g; Calories = 224.8; Total Carb (g) = 32.3; Net Carb (g) = 23.4; Fat (g) = 4.8; Protein = 11.9

🫘 Beans Kidney All Types Mature Seeds Raw ☞ serving size: 1 cup = 144 g; Calories = 612.7; Total Carb (g) = 7.7; Net Carb (g) = 3.9; Fat (g) = 42.5; Protein = 16.8

🫘 Beans Kidney California Red Mature Seeds Cooked Boiled With Salt ☞ serving size: 1 cup = 172 g; Calories = 219.5; Total Carb (g) = 52; Net Carb (g) = 21.5; Fat (g) = 43.7; Protein = 66.3

🫘 Beans Kidney California Red Mature Seeds Raw ☞ serving size: 1 cup = 93 g; Calories = 607.2; Total Carb (g) = 27; Net Carb (g) = 19.4; Fat (g) = 20.1; Protein = 40.3

🫘 Beans Kidney Red Mature Seeds Canned Drained Solids ☞ serving size: 1 tbsp = 17 g; Calories = 329.8; Total Carb (g) = 4.3; Net Carb (g) = 3.4; Fat (g) = 1; Protein = 2.2

🫘 Beans Kidney Red Mature Seeds Canned Drained Solids Rinsed In Tap Water ☞ serving size: 1 cup = 175 g; Calories = 191.2; Total Carb (g) = 22.2; Net Carb (g) = 12.7; Fat (g) = 19.3; Protein = 34

🫘 Beans Kidney Red Mature Seeds Canned Solids And Liquid Low Sodium ☞ serving size: 1 cup, stirred = 88 g; Calories = 207.4; Total Carb (g) = 27; Net Carb (g) = 12.9; Fat (g) = 7.8; Protein = 43.8

🫘 Beans Kidney Red Mature Seeds Cooked Boiled With Salt ☞

serving size: 1 cup = 122 g; Calories = 224.8; Total Carb (g) = 43.8; Net Carb (g) = 43.8; Fat (g) = 2.9; Protein = 60

🫘 Beans Kidney Red Mature Seeds Raw ☞ serving size: 1 cup = 243 g; Calories = 620.1; Total Carb (g) = 15.3; Net Carb (g) = 13.8; Fat (g) = 4.3; Protein = 8

🫘 Beans Kidney Royal Red Mature Seeds Cooked Boiled With Salt ☞ serving size: 1 oz = 28.4 g; Calories = 217.7; Total Carb (g) = 7.2; Net Carb (g) = 5.7; Fat (g) = 0.1; Protein = 18.1

🫘 Beans Kidney Royal Red Mature Seeds Raw ☞ serving size: 1/2 cup = 126 g; Calories = 605.4; Total Carb (g) = 3.6; Net Carb (g) = 2.5; Fat (g) = 5.3; Protein = 11.4

🫘 Beans Liquid From Stewed Kidney Beans ☞ serving size: 1 piece (2-1/2 inch x 2-3/4 inch x 1 inch) = 120 g; Calories = 112.8; Total Carb (g) = 1.4; Net Carb (g) = 1.2; Fat (g) = 4.4; Protein = 8.6

🫘 Beans Navy Mature Seeds Cooked Boiled With Salt ☞ serving size: 1 piece = 17 g; Calories = 254.8; Total Carb (g) = 1.7; Net Carb (g) = 0.5; Fat (g) = 5.2; Protein = 8.9

🫘 Beans Navy Mature Seeds Raw ☞ serving size: 1 oz = 28.4 g; Calories = 701; Total Carb (g) = 2.5; Net Carb (g) = 1.4; Fat (g) = 5.7; Protein = 5.3

🫘 Beans Pink Mature Seeds Cooked Boiled With Salt ☞ serving size: 1 cup = 122 g; Calories = 251.8; Total Carb (g) = 14.9; Net Carb (g) = 14.9; Fat (g) = 2.1; Protein = 4.3

🫘 Beans Pink Mature Seeds Cooked Boiled Without Salt ☞ serving size: 1 cup = 172 g; Calories = 251.8; Total Carb (g) = 25.7; Net Carb (g) = 25.7; Fat (g) = 10; Protein = 18.3

🫘 Beans Pink Mature Seeds Raw ☞ serving size: 1 tablespoon = 15 g; Calories = 720.3; Total Carb (g) = 3; Net Carb (g) = 2.4; Fat (g) = 1.3; Protein = 0.7

🫘 Beans Pinto Canned Drained Solids ☞ serving size: 1 patty

(approx 2-1/4 inch dia) = 17 g; Calories = 315.8; Total Carb (g) = 5.4; Net Carb (g) = 5.4; Fat (g) = 3; Protein = 2.3

🫘 Beans Pinto Mature Seeds Canned Drained Solids Rinsed In Tap Water ☞ serving size: 1 cup = 243 g; Calories = 197.7; Total Carb (g) = 12; Net Carb (g) = 11.5; Fat (g) = 3.6; Protein = 6.3

🫘 Beans Pinto Mature Seeds Canned Solids And Liquids ☞ serving size: 2 tbsp = 31 g; Calories = 196.8; Total Carb (g) = 4.4; Net Carb (g) = 2; Fat (g) = 17; Protein = 7.7

🫘 Beans Pinto Mature Seeds Canned Solids And Liquids Low Sodium ☞ serving size: 2 tablespoon = 36 g; Calories = 196.8; Total Carb (g) = 12.8; Net Carb (g) = 11; Fat (g) = 12.2; Protein = 9.3

🫘 Beans Pinto Mature Seeds Cooked Boiled With Salt ☞ serving size: 2 tbsp = 32 g; Calories = 244.5; Total Carb (g) = 6; Net Carb (g) = 4.2; Fat (g) = 16.3; Protein = 8.2

🫘 Beans Pinto Mature Seeds Raw ☞ serving size: 2 tbsp = 32 g; Calories = 669.7; Total Carb (g) = 5.7; Net Carb (g) = 3.8; Fat (g) = 16.5; Protein = 8.3

🫘 Beans Small White Mature Seeds Cooked Boiled With Salt ☞ serving size: 1 slice = 84 g; Calories = 254.2; Total Carb (g) = 2; Net Carb (g) = 1.9; Fat (g) = 2.3; Protein = 5.8

🫘 Beans Small White Mature Seeds Raw ☞ serving size: 1 slice = 84 g; Calories = 722.4; Total Carb (g) = 1.7; Net Carb (g) = 1.6; Fat (g) = 1.6; Protein = 6.2

🫘 Beans White Mature Seeds Canned ☞ serving size: 1 slice = 84 g; Calories = 298.7; Total Carb (g) = 0.9; Net Carb (g) = 0.9; Fat (g) = 0.7; Protein = 5.3

🫘 Beans White Mature Seeds Cooked Boiled With Salt ☞ serving size: 1 slice = 84 g; Calories = 248.8; Total Carb (g) = 0.8; Net Carb (g) = 0.8; Fat (g) = 0.6; Protein = 5.9

🫘 Beans White Mature Seeds Raw ☞ serving size: 1 cup = 231 g;

Calories = 672.7; Total Carb (g) = 31.2; Net Carb (g) = 20.3; Fat (g) = 1; Protein = 12.3

🖐 Beans Yellow Mature Seeds Cooked Boiled With Salt ☞ serving size: 1 cup = 233 g; Calories = 254.9; Total Carb (g) = 36.1; Net Carb (g) = 25.1; Fat (g) = 16.2; Protein = 11.7

🖐 Beans Yellow Mature Seeds Raw ☞ serving size: 1/5 package = 79 g; Calories = 676.2; Total Carb (g) = 1; Net Carb (g) = 0.6; Fat (g) = 1.3; Protein = 6.6

🖐 Black Bean Salad ☞ serving size: 2 tbsp = 32 g; Calories = 251.8; Total Carb (g) = 6.9; Net Carb (g) = 4.3; Fat (g) = 16; Protein = 7.7

🖐 Black Beans ☞ serving size: 2 tbsp = 32 g; Calories = 227; Total Carb (g) = 7.1; Net Carb (g) = 5.5; Fat (g) = 16.4; Protein = 7.1

🖐 Black Beans Cuban Style ☞ serving size: 1 tbsp = 16 g; Calories = 294.3; Total Carb (g) = 2.7; Net Carb (g) = 1.7; Fat (g) = 8.7; Protein = 3.9

🖐 Black Brown Or Bayo Beans Canned Drained Fat Added In Cooking Ns As To Type Of Fat ☞ serving size: 1 cup = 168 g; Calories = 336.6; Total Carb (g) = 39.1; Net Carb (g) = 27.8; Fat (g) = 0.6; Protein = 11.4

🖐 Black Brown Or Bayo Beans Canned Drained Fat Not Added In Cooking ☞ serving size: 1 tbsp = 14.2 g; Calories = 241.2; Total Carb (g) = 0.8; Net Carb (g) = 0.7; Fat (g) = 0; Protein = 1.3

🖐 Black Brown Or Bayo Beans Canned Drained Low Sodium Fat Added In Cooking ☞ serving size: 1 tbsp = 15 g; Calories = 336.6; Total Carb (g) = 2.2; Net Carb (g) = 2.1; Fat (g) = 0.1; Protein = 1.2

🖐 Black Brown Or Bayo Beans Canned Drained Low Sodium Fat Not Added In Cooking ☞ serving size: 1/2 cup = 126 g; Calories = 241.2; Total Carb (g) = 3.5; Net Carb (g) = 0.6; Fat (g) = 11; Protein = 21.8

🖐 Black Brown Or Bayo Beans Canned Drained Low Sodium Ns As To Fat Added In Cooking ☞ serving size: 1/2 cup = 124 g; Calories = 336.6; Total Carb (g) = 2.3; Net Carb (g) = 2; Fat (g) = 5.9; Protein = 10

🫘 Black Brown Or Bayo Beans Canned Drained Made With Animal Fat Or Meat Drippings ☞ serving size: 1 cup = 172 g; Calories = 325.8; Total Carb (g) = 25.7; Net Carb (g) = 25.7; Fat (g) = 10; Protein = 18.3

🫘 Black Brown Or Bayo Beans Canned Drained Made With Margarine ☞ serving size: 1 cup = 197 g; Calories = 293.4; Total Carb (g) = 123.9; Net Carb (g) = 98.9; Fat (g) = 1; Protein = 39.1

🫘 Black Brown Or Bayo Beans Canned Drained Made With Oil ☞ serving size: 1 cup = 230 g; Calories = 336.6; Total Carb (g) = 57; Net Carb (g) = 40.2; Fat (g) = 0.2; Protein = 17.3

🫘 Black Brown Or Bayo Beans Canned Drained Ns As To Fat Added In Cooking ☞ serving size: 1 cup = 296 g; Calories = 336.6; Total Carb (g) = 162.8; Net Carb (g) = 162.8; Fat (g) = 0.1; Protein = 11.3

🫘 Black Brown Or Bayo Beans Dry Cooked Fat Added In Cooking Ns As To Type Of Fat ☞ serving size: 1 slice = 14 g; Calories = 331.2; Total Carb (g) = 8.5; Net Carb (g) = 8.5; Fat (g) = 0; Protein = 0.5

🫘 Black Brown Or Bayo Beans Dry Cooked Fat Not Added In Cooking ☞ serving size: 1 cup = 253 g; Calories = 235.8; Total Carb (g) = 54.7; Net Carb (g) = 40.8; Fat (g) = 13; Protein = 14

🫘 Black Brown Or Bayo Beans Dry Cooked Made With Animal Fat Or Meat Drippings ☞ serving size: 1 cup = 249 g; Calories = 320.4; Total Carb (g) = 53.7; Net Carb (g) = 42.8; Fat (g) = 2.2; Protein = 11.3

🫘 Black Brown Or Bayo Beans Dry Cooked Made With Margarine ☞ serving size: 1 cup = 246 g; Calories = 289.8; Total Carb (g) = 46; Net Carb (g) = 36.1; Fat (g) = 2.3; Protein = 12.7

🫘 Black Brown Or Bayo Beans Dry Cooked Made With Oil ☞ serving size: 1 cup = 194 g; Calories = 334.8; Total Carb (g) = 121; Net Carb (g) = 90.9; Fat (g) = 2.8; Protein = 41.9

🫘 Black Brown Or Bayo Beans Dry Cooked Ns As To Fat Added In Cooking ☞ serving size: 1 cup = 172 g; Calories = 331.2; Total Carb (g) = 40.8; Net Carb (g) = 25.8; Fat (g) = 0.9; Protein = 15.2

🫘 Black Turtle Beans ☞ serving size: 1 cup = 177 g; Calories = 240.5; Total Carb (g) = 43.3; Net Carb (g) = 28.1; Fat (g) = 0.8; Protein = 16.5

🫘 Black-Eyed Peas (Cowpeas) ☞ serving size: 1 cup = 260 g; Calories = 198.4; Total Carb (g) = 39.3; Net Carb (g) = 22.9; Fat (g) = 0.7; Protein = 14.4

🫘 Boiled Lupin Beans ☞ serving size: 1 cup = 184 g; Calories = 197.5; Total Carb (g) = 118; Net Carb (g) = 71.6; Fat (g) = 3.7; Protein = 34.6

🫘 Boiled Red Kidney Beans ☞ serving size: 1 cup = 177 g; Calories = 217.7; Total Carb (g) = 42.5; Net Carb (g) = 25.9; Fat (g) = 1.4; Protein = 12.5

🫘 Boiled Soybeans (Edamame) ☞ serving size: 1 cup = 177 g; Calories = 295.8; Total Carb (g) = 40.4; Net Carb (g) = 29; Fat (g) = 0.9; Protein = 15.4

🫘 Broad Beans (Fava) ☞ serving size: 1 cup = 256 g; Calories = 187; Total Carb (g) = 37.1; Net Carb (g) = 26.1; Fat (g) = 1.5; Protein = 13.4

🫘 Broadbeans (Fava Beans) Mature Seeds Canned ☞ serving size: 1 cup = 184 g; Calories = 181.8; Total Carb (g) = 110; Net Carb (g) = 64.2; Fat (g) = 0.5; Protein = 44.8

🫘 Broadbeans (Fava Beans) Mature Seeds Cooked Boiled With Salt ☞ serving size: 1 cup = 177 g; Calories = 187; Total Carb (g) = 39.7; Net Carb (g) = 23.2; Fat (g) = 0.2; Protein = 16.2

🫘 Broadbeans (Fava Beans) Mature Seeds Raw ☞ serving size: 1 cup = 184 g; Calories = 511.5; Total Carb (g) = 112.8; Net Carb (g) = 84.8; Fat (g) = 2; Protein = 41.5

🫘 California Red Kidney Beans ☞ serving size: 1 cup = 208 g; Calories = 219.5; Total Carb (g) = 126.4; Net Carb (g) = 94.5; Fat (g) = 3.1; Protein = 46.5

🫘 Canned Baked Beans ☞ serving size: 1 cup = 182 g; Calories = 238.8; Total Carb (g) = 47.4; Net Carb (g) = 28.3; Fat (g) = 1.1; Protein = 15

🫘 Canned Baked Beans With Beef ☞ serving size: 1 cup = 262 g; Calories = 321.9; Total Carb (g) = 53.6; Net Carb (g) = 40.2; Fat (g) = 1.1; Protein = 19.7

🫘 Canned Chili With Beans ☞ serving size: 1 cup = 210 g; Calories = 263.7; Total Carb (g) = 134.8; Net Carb (g) = 108.1; Fat (g) = 2.4; Protein = 44

🫘 Canned Cranberry Beans ☞ serving size: 1 cup = 215 g; Calories = 215.8; Total Carb (g) = 133.8; Net Carb (g) = 80.3; Fat (g) = 2.5; Protein = 45.4

🫘 Canned Kidney Beans ☞ serving size: 1 cup = 179 g; Calories = 215; Total Carb (g) = 46.2; Net Carb (g) = 27.6; Fat (g) = 1.2; Protein = 16.1

🫘 Canned Mature (White) Lima Beans ☞ serving size: 1 cup = 196 g; Calories = 190.4; Total Carb (g) = 119; Net Carb (g) = 69.8; Fat (g) = 5.1; Protein = 43.1

🫘 Canned Navy Beans ☞ serving size: 1 cup = 177 g; Calories = 296.1; Total Carb (g) = 44.8; Net Carb (g) = 26.3; Fat (g) = 1.9; Protein = 16.2

🫘 Canned Red Kidney Beans ☞ serving size: 1 cup = 170 g; Calories = 207.4; Total Carb (g) = 33.4; Net Carb (g) = 24.2; Fat (g) = 0.7; Protein = 12.9

🫘 Canned Refried Beans ☞ serving size: 1 cup = 256 g; Calories = 200.9; Total Carb (g) = 31.8; Net Carb (g) = 22.3; Fat (g) = 0.6; Protein = 14

🫘 Carob Flour ☞ serving size: 1 cup = 103 g; Calories = 228.7; Total Carb (g) = 91.6; Net Carb (g) = 50.6; Fat (g) = 0.7; Protein = 4.8

🫘 Chicken Meatless ☞ serving size: 1 cup = 200 g; Calories = 376.3;

Total Carb (g) = 125.9; Net Carb (g) = 101.5; Fat (g) = 12.1; Protein = 40.9

🥩 Chicken Meatless Breaded Fried ☞ serving size: 1 cup = 164 g; Calories = 304.2; Total Carb (g) = 45; Net Carb (g) = 32.5; Fat (g) = 4.3; Protein = 14.5

🥩 Chickpea Flour (Besan) ☞ serving size: 1 cup = 167 g; Calories = 356; Total Carb (g) = 100.3; Net Carb (g) = 82.6; Fat (g) = 2.1; Protein = 39.3

🥩 Chickpeas (Garbanzo Beans Bengal Gram) Mature Seeds Canned Drained Rinsed In Tap Water ☞ serving size: 1 cup = 171 g; Calories = 350.5; Total Carb (g) = 35.5; Net Carb (g) = 24.4; Fat (g) = 0.9; Protein = 13.2

🥩 Chickpeas (Garbanzo Beans Bengal Gram) Mature Seeds Canned Drained Solids ☞ serving size: 1 cup = 240 g; Calories = 351.7; Total Carb (g) = 32.7; Net Carb (g) = 24.8; Fat (g) = 1.3; Protein = 11.4

🥩 Chickpeas (Garbanzo Beans Bengal Gram) Mature Seeds Canned Solids And Liquids ☞ serving size: 1 cup = 240 g; Calories = 211.2; Total Carb (g) = 39.7; Net Carb (g) = 31.8; Fat (g) = 3.8; Protein = 6.6

🥩 Chickpeas (Garbanzo Beans Bengal Gram) Mature Seeds Canned Solids And Liquids Low Sodium ☞ serving size: 1/5 package = 79 g; Calories = 211.2; Total Carb (g) = 2.1; Net Carb (g) = 1; Fat (g) = 4.1; Protein = 8

🥩 Chickpeas (Garbanzo Beans Bengal Gram) Mature Seeds Cooked Boiled With Salt ☞ serving size: 1/5 package = 79 g; Calories = 269; Total Carb (g) = 1.8; Net Carb (g) = 1.2; Fat (g) = 3.5; Protein = 7

🥩 Chickpeas (Garbanzo Beans Bengal Gram) Mature Seeds Raw ☞ serving size: 1/5 package = 91 g; Calories = 756; Total Carb (g) = 1.3; Net Carb (g) = 1; Fat (g) = 2.3; Protein = 4.4

Chickpeas (Garbanzo Beans) (Cooked) ☞ serving size: 1 cup = 243 g; Calories = 269; Total Carb (g) = 8.4; Net Carb (g) = 7.4; Fat (g) = 4.8; Protein = 7.1

Chickpeas Canned Drained Fat Added In Cooking Ns As To Type Of Fat ☞ serving size: 1 cup = 243 g; Calories = 356.4; Total Carb (g) = 8.5; Net Carb (g) = 7.8; Fat (g) = 1.9; Protein = 5.8

Chickpeas Canned Drained Fat Not Added In Cooking ☞ serving size: 1 cup = 243 g; Calories = 262.8; Total Carb (g) = 20; Net Carb (g) = 18.3; Fat (g) = 1.6; Protein = 5.1

Chickpeas Canned Drained Low Sodium Fat Added In Cooking ☞ serving size: 1 cup = 243 g; Calories = 358.2; Total Carb (g) = 9.4; Net Carb (g) = 7.9; Fat (g) = 2.1; Protein = 6.4

Chickpeas Canned Drained Low Sodium Fat Not Added In Cooking ☞ serving size: 1 cup = 243 g; Calories = 264.6; Total Carb (g) = 17.5; Net Carb (g) = 15.6; Fat (g) = 1.5; Protein = 4

Chickpeas Canned Drained Low Sodium Ns As To Fat Added In Cooking ☞ serving size: 1 cup = 243 g; Calories = 358.2; Total Carb (g) = 23; Net Carb (g) = 21.1; Fat (g) = 3.5; Protein = 5

Chickpeas Canned Drained Made With Oil ☞ serving size: 1 cup = 243 g; Calories = 356.4; Total Carb (g) = 8; Net Carb (g) = 7; Fat (g) = 2; Protein = 6

Chickpeas Canned Drained Ns As To Fat Added In Cooking ☞ serving size: 1 cup = 243 g; Calories = 356.4; Total Carb (g) = 10; Net Carb (g) = 9; Fat (g) = 2; Protein = 6

Chickpeas Dry Cooked Fat Added In Cooking Ns As To Type Of Fat ☞ serving size: 1 cup = 243 g; Calories = 392.4; Total Carb (g) = 22; Net Carb (g) = 20.1; Fat (g) = 1.5; Protein = 5

Chickpeas Dry Cooked Fat Not Added In Cooking ☞ serving size: 1 cup = 243 g; Calories = 293.4; Total Carb (g) = 19; Net Carb (g) = 18; Fat (g) = 4; Protein = 6

🫛 Chickpeas Dry Cooked Made With Animal Fat Or Meat Drippings ☞ serving size: 1/2 cup = 122 g; Calories = 381.6; Total Carb (g) = 15; Net Carb (g) = 15; Fat (g) = 2; Protein = 3

🫛 Chickpeas Dry Cooked Made With Margarine ☞ serving size: 1 cup = 243 g; Calories = 347.4; Total Carb (g) = 19; Net Carb (g) = 19; Fat (g) = 3.5; Protein = 6

🫛 Chickpeas Dry Cooked Made With Oil ☞ serving size: 1 cup = 243 g; Calories = 392.4; Total Carb (g) = 22; Net Carb (g) = 22; Fat (g) = 3.5; Protein = 5

🫛 Chickpeas Dry Cooked Ns As To Fat Added In Cooking ☞ serving size: 1 container = 170 g; Calories = 392.4; Total Carb (g) = 30; Net Carb (g) = 29; Fat (g) = 2; Protein = 4

🫛 Chickpeas Stewed With Pig's Feet Puerto Rican Style ☞ serving size: 1 container = 170 g; Calories = 305; Total Carb (g) = 32; Net Carb (g) = 31; Fat (g) = 2; Protein = 4

🫛 Chili With Beans Without Meat ☞ serving size: 1 container = 170 g; Calories = 106.3; Total Carb (g) = 29; Net Carb (g) = 28; Fat (g) = 2; Protein = 4

🫛 Cooked Blackeyed Peas ☞ serving size: 1 container = 170 g; Calories = 160.1; Total Carb (g) = 29; Net Carb (g) = 28; Fat (g) = 2; Protein = 4

🫛 Cooked Catjang Beans ☞ serving size: 1/5 package = 79 g; Calories = 200.1; Total Carb (g) = 0.6; Net Carb (g) = 0.1; Fat (g) = 2.8; Protein = 6.9

🫛 Cooked Green Soybeans ☞ serving size: 1/5 package = 91 g; Calories = 253.8; Total Carb (g) = 0; Net Carb (g) = 0; Fat (g) = 1; Protein = 7.5

🫛 Cooked Large White Beans ☞ serving size: 3 oz = 85 g; Calories = 248.8; Total Carb (g) = 1.6; Net Carb (g) = 0.7; Fat (g) = 4.2; Protein = 8.7

🫘 Cooked Red Kidney Beans ☞ serving size: 1/5 package = 91 g; Calories = 224.8; Total Carb (g) = 0.5; Net Carb (g) = 0.4; Fat (g) = 2.2; Protein = 4.4

🫘 Cooked Small White Beans ☞ serving size: 2 oz = 56 g; Calories = 254.2; Total Carb (g) = 1.2; Net Carb (g) = 0.8; Fat (g) = 1.5; Protein = 3.6

🫘 Cowpeas Catjang Mature Seeds Cooked Boiled With Salt ☞ serving size: 2 oz = 56 g; Calories = 200.1; Total Carb (g) = 0.5; Net Carb (g) = 0; Fat (g) = 2.4; Protein = 6.1

🫘 Cowpeas Catjang Mature Seeds Raw ☞ serving size: 1 cup = 230 g; Calories = 572.8; Total Carb (g) = 57; Net Carb (g) = 40.2; Fat (g) = 0.2; Protein = 17.3

🫘 Cowpeas Common (Blackeyes Crowder Southern) Mature Seeds Canned Plain ☞ serving size: 1 cup = 177 g; Calories = 184.8; Total Carb (g) = 37.3; Net Carb (g) = 24.9; Fat (g) = 0.8; Protein = 14.7

🫘 Cowpeas Common (Blackeyes Crowder Southern) Mature Seeds Canned With Pork ☞ serving size: 1 cup = 262 g; Calories = 199.2; Total Carb (g) = 55.1; Net Carb (g) = 42.2; Fat (g) = 1; Protein = 19.3

🫘 Cowpeas Common (Blackeyes Crowder Southern) Mature Seeds Cooked Boiled With Salt ☞ serving size: 1 cup = 177 g; Calories = 198.4; Total Carb (g) = 40.4; Net Carb (g) = 29; Fat (g) = 0.9; Protein = 15.4

🫘 Cowpeas Common (Blackeyes Crowder Southern) Mature Seeds Raw ☞ serving size: 1 cup = 177 g; Calories = 561.1; Total Carb (g) = 39.7; Net Carb (g) = 23.2; Fat (g) = 0.2; Protein = 16.2

🫘 Cowpeas Dry Cooked Fat Added In Cooking ☞ serving size: 1 cup = 182 g; Calories = 309.6; Total Carb (g) = 47.4; Net Carb (g) = 28.3; Fat (g) = 1.1; Protein = 15

🫘 Cowpeas Dry Cooked Fat Not Added In Cooking ☞ serving size:

1 cup = 169 g; Calories = 207; Total Carb (g) = 47.2; Net Carb (g) = 38.2; Fat (g) = 0.8; Protein = 15.3

🫘 Cowpeas Dry Cooked Ns As To Fat Added In Cooking ☞ serving size: 1 cup = 171 g; Calories = 309.6; Total Carb (g) = 44.8; Net Carb (g) = 29.5; Fat (g) = 1.1; Protein = 15.4

🫘 Cowpeas Dry Cooked With Pork ☞ serving size: 1 cup = 169 g; Calories = 309.7; Total Carb (g) = 35.1; Net Carb (g) = 35.1; Fat (g) = 1.6; Protein = 11.9

🫘 Cranberry Beans (Roman Beans) ☞ serving size: 1 cup = 170 g; Calories = 240.7; Total Carb (g) = 33.4; Net Carb (g) = 24.2; Fat (g) = 0.7; Protein = 12.9

🫘 Dry-Roasted Soybeans ☞ serving size: 1 cup = 164 g; Calories = 417.6; Total Carb (g) = 45; Net Carb (g) = 32.5; Fat (g) = 4.3; Protein = 14.5

🫘 Edamame ☞ serving size: 1 can drained = 253 g; Calories = 187.6; Total Carb (g) = 57; Net Carb (g) = 40.8; Fat (g) = 7; Protein = 17.8

🫘 Extra Firm Fortified Tofu ☞ serving size: 1 can drained, rinsed = 254 g; Calories = 78.2; Total Carb (g) = 58.1; Net Carb (g) = 42.1; Fat (g) = 6.3; Protein = 17.9

🫘 Falafel ☞ serving size: 1 cup = 188 g; Calories = 56.6; Total Carb (g) = 39.3; Net Carb (g) = 26.1; Fat (g) = 0.7; Protein = 14.7

🫘 Fava Beans (Raw) ☞ serving size: 1 cup = 182 g; Calories = 110.9; Total Carb (g) = 42.4; Net Carb (g) = 28.4; Fat (g) = 0.7; Protein = 14.6

🫘 Fava Beans Canned Drained Fat Added In Cooking ☞ serving size: 1 cup = 166 g; Calories = 293.4; Total Carb (g) = 15.4; Net Carb (g) = 10.8; Fat (g) = 4.9; Protein = 25.9

🫘 Fava Beans Dry Cooked Fat Added In Cooking ☞ serving size: 1 cup = 177 g; Calories = 300.6; Total Carb (g) = 37.1; Net Carb (g) = 37.1; Fat (g) = 1; Protein = 13.8

🫘 Fava Beans Dry Cooked Fat Not Added In Cooking ☞ serving size: 1 cup = 147 g; Calories = 196.2; Total Carb (g) = 25.7; Net Carb (g) = 12.6; Fat (g) = 72.1; Protein = 41.2

🫘 Fava Beans Dry Cooked Ns As To Fat Added In Cooking ☞ serving size: 1 cup = 144 g; Calories = 300.6; Total Carb (g) = 23.5; Net Carb (g) = 10.7; Fat (g) = 73.8; Protein = 38.9

🫘 Firm Tofu ☞ serving size: 1 cup = 143 g; Calories = 181.4; Total Carb (g) = 28.4; Net Carb (g) = 15.7; Fat (g) = 69.5; Protein = 37

🫘 Firm Tofu (With Calcium And Magnesium) ☞ serving size: 1 cup = 178 g; Calories = 98.3; Total Carb (g) = 112.8; Net Carb (g) = 79; Fat (g) = 1.2; Protein = 38.2

🫘 Fortified Chocolate Soy Milk ☞ serving size: 1 cup = 188 g; Calories = 153.1; Total Carb (g) = 39.3; Net Carb (g) = 26.1; Fat (g) = 0.7; Protein = 14.7

🫘 Fortified Silken Tofu ☞ serving size: 1 cup = 241 g; Calories = 39.1; Total Carb (g) = 35.9; Net Carb (g) = 24.4; Fat (g) = 0.4; Protein = 11.9

🫘 Frankfurter Meatless ☞ serving size: 1 cup = 202 g; Calories = 326.2; Total Carb (g) = 126.9; Net Carb (g) = 85.3; Fat (g) = 1.9; Protein = 41.7

🫘 Fried Chickpeas With Bacon Puerto Rican Style ☞ serving size: 1 cup = 207 g; Calories = 370.8; Total Carb (g) = 129.6; Net Carb (g) = 95.9; Fat (g) = 2.4; Protein = 49.4

🫘 Frijoles Rojos Volteados (Refried Beans Red Canned) ☞ serving size: 1 cup = 202 g; Calories = 335.5; Total Carb (g) = 38.7; Net Carb (g) = 23.3; Fat (g) = 0.8; Protein = 14.2

🫘 Great Northern Beans ☞ serving size: 1 cup = 140 g; Calories = 208.9; Total Carb (g) = 120.5; Net Carb (g) = 119.8; Fat (g) = 0.1; Protein = 0.2

🫘 Green Or Yellow Split Peas Dry Cooked Fat Added In Cooking

Ns As To Type Of Fat ☞ serving size: 1 cup = 207 g; Calories = 300.6; Total Carb (g) = 122.1; Net Carb (g) = 84.2; Fat (g) = 3.4; Protein = 52.2

🫘 Green Or Yellow Split Peas Dry Cooked Fat Not Added In Cooking ☞ serving size: 1 cup in shell, edible yield = 63 g; Calories = 210.6; Total Carb (g) = 13.4; Net Carb (g) = 7.9; Fat (g) = 13.9; Protein = 8.5

🫘 Green Or Yellow Split Peas Dry Cooked Made With Animal Fat Or Meat Drippings ☞ serving size: 1 cup, chopped = 144 g; Calories = 291.6; Total Carb (g) = 22; Net Carb (g) = 8.4; Fat (g) = 75.6; Protein = 40.4

🫘 Green Or Yellow Split Peas Dry Cooked Made With Margarine ☞ serving size: 1 oz = 28.4 g; Calories = 262.8; Total Carb (g) = 6; Net Carb (g) = 3.7; Fat (g) = 14.1; Protein = 6.9

🫘 Green Or Yellow Split Peas Dry Cooked Made With Oil ☞ serving size: 1 cup = 146 g; Calories = 300.6; Total Carb (g) = 23.1; Net Carb (g) = 9.2; Fat (g) = 72.4; Protein = 38.2

🫘 Green Or Yellow Split Peas Dry Cooked Ns As To Fat Added In Cooking ☞ serving size: 1 cup = 143 g; Calories = 300.6; Total Carb (g) = 28.4; Net Carb (g) = 15.7; Fat (g) = 69.5; Protein = 37

🫘 Green Soybeans ☞ serving size: 2 tbsp = 32 g; Calories = 376.3; Total Carb (g) = 6.9; Net Carb (g) = 4.3; Fat (g) = 16; Protein = 7.7

🫘 House Foods Premium Firm Tofu ☞ serving size: 2 tbsp = 32 g; Calories = 47.6; Total Carb (g) = 7.1; Net Carb (g) = 5.5; Fat (g) = 16.4; Protein = 7.1

🫘 House Foods Premium Soft Tofu ☞ serving size: 1 cup = 60 g; Calories = 33; Total Carb (g) = 20.8; Net Carb (g) = 11.3; Fat (g) = 0.3; Protein = 31.3

🫘 Hummus (Commercial) ☞ serving size: 1 cup = 88 g; Calories = 35.6; Total Carb (g) = 30.5; Net Carb (g) = 15.1; Fat (g) = 2.6; Protein = 36.7

🦪 Hummus (Homemade) ☞ serving size: 1 link = 25 g; Calories = 26.6; Total Carb (g) = 2; Net Carb (g) = 1.3; Fat (g) = 4.5; Protein = 5.1

🦪 Hyacinth Beans Mature Seeds Cooked Boiled With Salt ☞ serving size: 1 cup = 186 g; Calories = 227; Total Carb (g) = 56.1; Net Carb (g) = 38.8; Fat (g) = 37.1; Protein = 67.9

🦪 Hyacinth Beans Mature Seeds Cooked Boiled Without Salt ☞ serving size: 1 cup = 172 g; Calories = 227; Total Carb (g) = 14.4; Net Carb (g) = 4.1; Fat (g) = 15.4; Protein = 31.3

🦪 Hyacinth Beans Mature Seeds Raw ☞ serving size: 1 cup = 166 g; Calories = 722.4; Total Carb (g) = 12.7; Net Carb (g) = 12.7; Fat (g) = 17.9; Protein = 33.7

🦪 Kidney Beans ☞ serving size: 1 cup, stirred = 84 g; Calories = 224.8; Total Carb (g) = 26.8; Net Carb (g) = 18.8; Fat (g) = 17.4; Protein = 31.8

🦪 Lentils (Cooked) ☞ serving size: 1 cup, stirred = 85 g; Calories = 229.7; Total Carb (g) = 25.8; Net Carb (g) = 17.6; Fat (g) = 18.6; Protein = 32.4

🦪 Lentils Dry Cooked Fat Added In Cooking Ns As To Type Of Fat ☞ serving size: 1 cup = 105 g; Calories = 297; Total Carb (g) = 35.6; Net Carb (g) = 17.2; Fat (g) = 1.3; Protein = 54

🦪 Lentils Dry Cooked Fat Not Added In Cooking ☞ serving size: 1 oz = 28.4 g; Calories = 207; Total Carb (g) = 0; Net Carb (g) = 0; Fat (g) = 1; Protein = 25.1

🦪 Lentils Dry Cooked Made With Animal Fat Or Meat Drippings ☞ serving size: 1 tbsp = 16 g; Calories = 286.2; Total Carb (g) = 0.8; Net Carb (g) = 0.7; Fat (g) = 0.1; Protein = 1.3

🦪 Lentils Dry Cooked Made With Margarine ☞ serving size: 1 tbsp = 18 g; Calories = 257.4; Total Carb (g) = 1; Net Carb (g) = 0.9; Fat (g) = 0; Protein = 1.9

🦪 Lentils Dry Cooked Made With Oil ☞ serving size: 1 tbsp = 18 g;

Calories = 297; Total Carb (g) = 1.4; Net Carb (g) = 1.3; Fat (g) = 0.1; Protein = 1.3

🫘 Lentils Dry Cooked Ns As To Fat Added In Cooking ☞ serving size: 1 block = 11 g; Calories = 297; Total Carb (g) = 0.5; Net Carb (g) = 0.5; Fat (g) = 0.9; Protein = 1

🫘 Lentils Mature Seeds Cooked Boiled With Salt ☞ serving size: 1 cup = 167 g; Calories = 225.7; Total Carb (g) = 103.4; Net Carb (g) = 85; Fat (g) = 2.2; Protein = 40.6

🫘 Lentils Pink Or Red Raw ☞ serving size: 1 cup = 171 g; Calories = 687.4; Total Carb (g) = 36.1; Net Carb (g) = 29.6; Fat (g) = 0.8; Protein = 14.2

🫘 Lentils Raw ☞ serving size: 1 cup = 182 g; Calories = 675.8; Total Carb (g) = 75.9; Net Carb (g) = 28.8; Fat (g) = 29.7; Protein = 54

🫘 Lima Beans ☞ serving size: 1 cup = 192 g; Calories = 216.2; Total Carb (g) = 121.2; Net Carb (g) = 100.4; Fat (g) = 4.2; Protein = 45.9

🫘 Lima Beans Dry Cooked Fat Added In Cooking Ns As To Type Of Fat ☞ serving size: 1 can drained solids = 266 g; Calories = 298.8; Total Carb (g) = 57.2; Net Carb (g) = 42.5; Fat (g) = 2.8; Protein = 21.2

🫘 Lima Beans Dry Cooked Fat Not Added In Cooking ☞ serving size: 1 can drained solids = 277 g; Calories = 205.2; Total Carb (g) = 56; Net Carb (g) = 40.8; Fat (g) = 2.5; Protein = 19.4

🫘 Lima Beans Dry Cooked Made With Animal Fat Or Meat Drippings ☞ serving size: 1 pattie = 70 g; Calories = 289.8; Total Carb (g) = 10; Net Carb (g) = 6.6; Fat (g) = 4.4; Protein = 11

🫘 Lima Beans Dry Cooked Made With Margarine ☞ serving size: 1 cup = 92 g; Calories = 259.2; Total Carb (g) = 53.2; Net Carb (g) = 43.3; Fat (g) = 6.2; Protein = 20.6

🫘 Lima Beans Dry Cooked Made With Oil ☞ serving size: 1 tbsp = 15 g; Calories = 298.8; Total Carb (g) = 2.3; Net Carb (g) = 1.4; Fat (g) = 2.7; Protein = 1.2

🫘 Lima Beans Dry Cooked Ns As To Fat Added In Cooking ☞ serving size: 1/5 block = 91 g; Calories = 298.8; Total Carb (g) = 1.1; Net Carb (g) = 0.2; Fat (g) = 4.8; Protein = 9.1

🫘 Lima Beans Large Mature Seeds Cooked Boiled With Salt ☞ serving size: 1/4 block = 122 g; Calories = 216.2; Total Carb (g) = 5.4; Net Carb (g) = 4.6; Fat (g) = 12.2; Protein = 15.5

🫘 Lima Beans Large Mature Seeds Raw ☞ serving size: 1 slice = 84 g; Calories = 601.6; Total Carb (g) = 2.4; Net Carb (g) = 2.4; Fat (g) = 2.3; Protein = 4

🫘 Lima Beans Thin Seeded (Baby) Mature Seeds Cooked Boiled With Salt ☞ serving size: 1 cup = 243 g; Calories = 229.3; Total Carb (g) = 24.2; Net Carb (g) = 23.2; Fat (g) = 3.7; Protein = 5.5

🫘 Lima Beans Thin Seeded (Baby) Mature Seeds Cooked Boiled Without Salt ☞ serving size: 2 tbsp = 32 g; Calories = 229.3; Total Carb (g) = 7.7; Net Carb (g) = 5.9; Fat (g) = 15.9; Protein = 7

🫘 Lima Beans Thin Seeded (Baby) Mature Seeds Raw ☞ serving size: 1 cup = 243 g; Calories = 676.7; Total Carb (g) = 24.2; Net Carb (g) = 23.2; Fat (g) = 3.7; Protein = 5.5

🫘 Loaf Lentil ☞ serving size: 1 cup = 242 g; Calories = 33.8; Total Carb (g) = 32.7; Net Carb (g) = 21.3; Fat (g) = 2.1; Protein = 12.8

🫘 Luncheon Slices Meatless ☞ serving size: 1/5 package = 79 g; Calories = 26.5; Total Carb (g) = 2.2; Net Carb (g) = 0.6; Fat (g) = 5; Protein = 9.8

🫘 Lupin Beans (Cooked) ☞ serving size: 1 cup = 238 g; Calories = 192.6; Total Carb (g) = 32.3; Net Carb (g) = 23.4; Fat (g) = 4.8; Protein = 11.9

🫘 Lupins Mature Seeds Raw ☞ serving size: 1 cup = 172 g; Calories = 667.8; Total Carb (g) = 14.4; Net Carb (g) = 4.1; Fat (g) = 15.4; Protein = 31.3

🌰 Meat Extender ☞ serving size: 1 cup = 172 g; Calories = 273.7; Total Carb (g) = 52; Net Carb (g) = 21.5; Fat (g) = 43.7; Protein = 66.3

🌰 Meat Substitute Cereal- And Vegetable Protein-Based Fried ☞ serving size: 1 oz = 28.4 g; Calories = 487.6; Total Carb (g) = 7.2; Net Carb (g) = 5.7; Fat (g) = 0.1; Protein = 18.1

🌰 Meatballs Meatless ☞ serving size: 1 oz = 28.4 g; Calories = 283.7; Total Carb (g) = 0.7; Net Carb (g) = 0.7; Fat (g) = 0.2; Protein = 25.1

🌰 Miso ☞ serving size: 1 piece = 17 g; Calories = 33.7; Total Carb (g) = 1.4; Net Carb (g) = 1.2; Fat (g) = 5.2; Protein = 8.9

🌰 Mori-Nu Tofu Silken Extra Firm ☞ serving size: 1 piece = 13 g; Calories = 46.2; Total Carb (g) = 1.2; Net Carb (g) = 0.6; Fat (g) = 2.6; Protein = 2.5

🌰 Mori-Nu Tofu Silken Firm ☞ serving size: 1 block = 11 g; Calories = 52.1; Total Carb (g) = 0.6; Net Carb (g) = 0.6; Fat (g) = 0.9; Protein = 0.9

🌰 Mori-Nu Tofu Silken Lite Extra Firm ☞ serving size: 1 cup = 171 g; Calories = 31.9; Total Carb (g) = 36.1; Net Carb (g) = 29.6; Fat (g) = 0.8; Protein = 14.2

🌰 Mori-Nu Tofu Silken Lite Firm ☞ serving size: 1 cup = 254 g; Calories = 31.1; Total Carb (g) = 53.7; Net Carb (g) = 43.3; Fat (g) = 0.9; Protein = 12.1

🌰 Mori-Nu Tofu Silken Soft ☞ serving size: 1 cup = 266 g; Calories = 46.2; Total Carb (g) = 45; Net Carb (g) = 45; Fat (g) = 9.2; Protein = 17

🌰 Mothbeans Mature Seeds Cooked Boiled With Salt ☞ serving size: 1 cup = 259 g; Calories = 207.1; Total Carb (g) = 39.9; Net Carb (g) = 22; Fat (g) = 17; Protein = 17.5

🌰 Mothbeans Mature Seeds Cooked Boiled Without Salt ☞ serving size: 1 cup = 253 g; Calories = 207.1; Total Carb (g) = 50.6; Net Carb (g) = 36.7; Fat (g) = 3.9; Protein = 13.1

🫘 Mothbeans Mature Seeds Raw ☞ serving size: 1 cup = 184 g; Calories = 672.3; Total Carb (g) = 116.4; Net Carb (g) = 87.9; Fat (g) = 1.7; Protein = 39.1

🫘 Mung Beans (Cooked) ☞ serving size: 1 cup = 185 g; Calories = 212.1; Total Carb (g) = 45.1; Net Carb (g) = 29.7; Fat (g) = 0.7; Protein = 15.1

🫘 Mung Beans Canned Drained Ns As To Fat Added In Cooking ☞ serving size: 1 cup = 240 g; Calories = 286.2; Total Carb (g) = 39.7; Net Carb (g) = 23.2; Fat (g) = 0.7; Protein = 14.5

🫘 Mung Beans Dry Cooked Fat Added In Cooking ☞ serving size: 1 cup = 195 g; Calories = 277.2; Total Carb (g) = 117.1; Net Carb (g) = 68.9; Fat (g) = 2.4; Protein = 44.9

🫘 Mung Beans Dry Cooked Fat Not Added In Cooking ☞ serving size: 1 cup = 183 g; Calories = 187.2; Total Carb (g) = 114.1; Net Carb (g) = 77.2; Fat (g) = 2.1; Protein = 40

🫘 Mung Beans Dry Cooked Ns As To Fat Added In Cooking ☞ serving size: 1 cup = 177 g; Calories = 277.2; Total Carb (g) = 37.3; Net Carb (g) = 24.9; Fat (g) = 0.8; Protein = 14.7

🫘 Mung Beans Mature Seeds Cooked Boiled With Salt ☞ serving size: 1 cup = 262 g; Calories = 212.1; Total Carb (g) = 55.1; Net Carb (g) = 42.2; Fat (g) = 1; Protein = 19.3

🫘 Mung Beans Mature Seeds Raw ☞ serving size: 1 cup = 184 g; Calories = 718.3; Total Carb (g) = 110.4; Net Carb (g) = 64.6; Fat (g) = 1.5; Protein = 43.4

🫘 Mungo Beans (Cooked) ☞ serving size: 1 cup = 177 g; Calories = 189; Total Carb (g) = 40.4; Net Carb (g) = 27.3; Fat (g) = 0.9; Protein = 15.4

🫘 Mungo Beans Mature Seeds Cooked Boiled With Salt ☞ serving size: 1 cup = 256 g; Calories = 189; Total Carb (g) = 38; Net Carb (g) = 27; Fat (g) = 0.9; Protein = 13.4

🍢 Mungo Beans Mature Seeds Raw ☞ serving size: 1 cup = 184 g; Calories = 705.9; Total Carb (g) = 107.3; Net Carb (g) = 61.5; Fat (g) = 0.8; Protein = 46.6

🍢 Natto ☞ serving size: 1 cup = 177 g; Calories = 369.3; Total Carb (g) = 38.7; Net Carb (g) = 22.2; Fat (g) = 0.3; Protein = 16.8

🍢 Navy Beans ☞ serving size: 1 cup = 169 g; Calories = 254.8; Total Carb (g) = 47.2; Net Carb (g) = 38.2; Fat (g) = 0.8; Protein = 15.3

🍢 Noodles Chinese Cellophane Or Long Rice (Mung Beans) Dehydrated ☞ serving size: 1 cup = 193 g; Calories = 491.4; Total Carb (g) = 120.7; Net Carb (g) = 90.8; Fat (g) = 2.4; Protein = 41.3

🍢 Okara ☞ serving size: 1 cup = 171 g; Calories = 92.7; Total Carb (g) = 44.8; Net Carb (g) = 29.5; Fat (g) = 1.1; Protein = 15.4

🍢 Peanut Butter (Chunk Style) ☞ serving size: 1 cup = 202 g; Calories = 188.5; Total Carb (g) = 121.8; Net Carb (g) = 91; Fat (g) = 1.7; Protein = 47.2

🍢 Peanut Butter (Smooth) ☞ serving size: 1 cup = 179 g; Calories = 188.2; Total Carb (g) = 44.9; Net Carb (g) = 33.6; Fat (g) = 0.6; Protein = 17.4

🍢 Peanut Butter Chunk Style With Salt ☞ serving size: 1 cup = 262 g; Calories = 188.5; Total Carb (g) = 55.5; Net Carb (g) = 43; Fat (g) = 0.8; Protein = 19

🍢 Peanut Butter Chunky Vitamin And Mineral Fortified ☞ serving size: 1 cup = 150 g; Calories = 189.8; Total Carb (g) = 87.4; Net Carb (g) = 49.9; Fat (g) = 2.3; Protein = 39.2

🍢 Peanut Butter Reduced Sodium ☞ serving size: 1 cup = 240 g; Calories = 94.4; Total Carb (g) = 32.4; Net Carb (g) = 21.8; Fat (g) = 4.7; Protein = 11.8

🍢 Peanut Butter Smooth Reduced Fat ☞ serving size: 1 cup = 256 g; Calories = 187.2; Total Carb (g) = 33.9; Net Carb (g) = 25.5; Fat (g) = 9.6; Protein = 15.7

🥜 Peanut Butter Smooth Style With Salt ☞ serving size: 1 cup = 167 g; Calories = 191.4; Total Carb (g) = 99.6; Net Carb (g) = 81.7; Fat (g) = 3.5; Protein = 39.8

🥜 Peanut Butter Smooth Vitamin And Mineral Fortified ☞ serving size: 1 cup = 171 g; Calories = 189.1; Total Carb (g) = 34.8; Net Carb (g) = 28.6; Fat (g) = 1.2; Protein = 13.9

🥜 Peanut Butter With Omega-3 Creamy ☞ serving size: 1 cup = 210 g; Calories = 97.3; Total Carb (g) = 127.6; Net Carb (g) = 73.8; Fat (g) = 3.6; Protein = 50.2

🥜 Peanut Flour Defatted ☞ serving size: 1 cup = 194 g; Calories = 196.2; Total Carb (g) = 40.1; Net Carb (g) = 40.1; Fat (g) = 1.1; Protein = 15.8

🥜 Peanut Flour Low Fat ☞ serving size: 1 cup = 243 g; Calories = 256.8; Total Carb (g) = 10.9; Net Carb (g) = 10; Fat (g) = 3.9; Protein = 7.1

🥜 Peanut Spread Reduced Sugar ☞ serving size: 1 cup = 243 g; Calories = 201.5; Total Carb (g) = 10.9; Net Carb (g) = 10; Fat (g) = 4.4; Protein = 7.8

🥜 Peanuts All Types Cooked Boiled With Salt ☞ serving size: 1 cup = 243 g; Calories = 200.3; Total Carb (g) = 10; Net Carb (g) = 9.7; Fat (g) = 2; Protein = 3.9

🥜 Peanuts All Types Dry-Roasted With Salt ☞ serving size: 1 cup = 243 g; Calories = 166.7; Total Carb (g) = 4.2; Net Carb (g) = 3; Fat (g) = 3.9; Protein = 7

🥜 Peanuts All Types Oil-Roasted With Salt ☞ serving size: 1 cup = 243 g; Calories = 862.6; Total Carb (g) = 10.1; Net Carb (g) = 9.6; Fat (g) = 0.1; Protein = 6

🥜 Peanuts All Types Oil-Roasted Without Salt ☞ serving size: 1 cup = 243 g; Calories = 862.6; Total Carb (g) = 20.7; Net Carb (g) = 20.2; Fat (g) = 0.1; Protein = 6

🥜 Peanuts Spanish Oil-Roasted With Salt ☞ serving size: 1 cup = 243 g; Calories = 851.1; Total Carb (g) = 8; Net Carb (g) = 7; Fat (g) = 4; Protein = 7

🥜 Peanuts Spanish Oil-Roasted Without Salt ☞ serving size: 1 cup = 243 g; Calories = 851.1; Total Carb (g) = 10; Net Carb (g) = 9; Fat (g) = 3.5; Protein = 6

🥜 Peanuts Spanish Raw ☞ serving size: 1 cup = 243 g; Calories = 832.2; Total Carb (g) = 8; Net Carb (g) = 7; Fat (g) = 5; Protein = 7

🥜 Peanuts Valencia Oil-Roasted With Salt ☞ serving size: 1 cup = 243 g; Calories = 848.2; Total Carb (g) = 11; Net Carb (g) = 9.1; Fat (g) = 3.5; Protein = 6

🥜 Peanuts Valencia Oil-Roasted Without Salt ☞ serving size: 1 cup = 243 g; Calories = 848.2; Total Carb (g) = 14; Net Carb (g) = 8.9; Fat (g) = 3.5; Protein = 6

🥜 Peanuts Valencia Raw ☞ serving size: 1 cup = 243 g; Calories = 832.2; Total Carb (g) = 4; Net Carb (g) = 3; Fat (g) = 4; Protein = 7

🥜 Peanuts Virginia Oil-Roasted With Salt ☞ serving size: 1 cup = 243 g; Calories = 826.5; Total Carb (g) = 25; Net Carb (g) = 25; Fat (g) = 3.5; Protein = 5

🥜 Peanuts Virginia Oil-Roasted Without Salt ☞ serving size: 1 container = 227 g; Calories = 826.5; Total Carb (g) = 31; Net Carb (g) = 30.1; Fat (g) = 4; Protein = 6

🥜 Peanuts Virginia Raw ☞ serving size: 1 container = 170 g; Calories = 822; Total Carb (g) = 25; Net Carb (g) = 24; Fat (g) = 3; Protein = 5

🥜 Peas Dry Cooked With Pork ☞ serving size: 1 container = 227 g; Calories = 332.9; Total Carb (g) = 22; Net Carb (g) = 21.1; Fat (g) = 4; Protein = 6

🥜 Peas Green Split Mature Seeds Raw ☞ serving size: 1 container =

170 g; Calories = 717.1; Total Carb (g) = 31; Net Carb (g) = 30; Fat (g) = 2; Protein = 4

🫛 Peas Split Mature Seeds Cooked Boiled With Salt ☞ serving size: 1 container = 170 g; Calories = 227.4; Total Carb (g) = 30; Net Carb (g) = 29; Fat (g) = 2; Protein = 4

🫛 Pigeon Peas (Red Gram) Mature Seeds Cooked Boiled With Salt ☞ serving size: 1 container = 170 g; Calories = 203.3; Total Carb (g) = 29; Net Carb (g) = 28; Fat (g) = 2; Protein = 4

🫛 Pigeon Peas (Red Gram) Mature Seeds Cooked Boiled Without Salt ☞ serving size: 1 tbsp = 15 g; Calories = 203.3; Total Carb (g) = 1; Net Carb (g) = 1; Fat (g) = 1; Protein = 0

🫛 Pigeon Peas (Red Gram) Mature Seeds Raw ☞ serving size: 1 tbsp = 15 g; Calories = 703.2; Total Carb (g) = 3; Net Carb (g) = 3; Fat (g) = 1; Protein = 0

🫛 Pink Beans Canned Drained Fat Added In Cooking ☞ serving size: 3 oz = 85 g; Calories = 360; Total Carb (g) = 1.5; Net Carb (g) = 0.8; Fat (g) = 2.9; Protein = 7.8

🫛 Pink Beans Canned Drained Fat Not Added In Cooking ☞ serving size: 3 oz = 85 g; Calories = 266.4; Total Carb (g) = 1.8; Net Carb (g) = 0.8; Fat (g) = 5; Protein = 11.3

🫛 Pink Beans Dry Cooked Fat Added In Cooking ☞ serving size: 1/5 package = 79 g; Calories = 365.4; Total Carb (g) = 1.2; Net Carb (g) = 0.5; Fat (g) = 3.6; Protein = 8

🫛 Pink Beans Dry Cooked Fat Not Added In Cooking ☞ serving size: 1/5 package = 79 g; Calories = 266.4; Total Carb (g) = 1.2; Net Carb (g) = 0.7; Fat (g) = 3.3; Protein = 7.2

🫛 Pink Beans Dry Cooked Ns As To Fat Added In Cooking ☞ serving size: 1 cup = 172 g; Calories = 365.4; Total Carb (g) = 40.8; Net Carb (g) = 25.8; Fat (g) = 0.9; Protein = 15.2

🫛 Pinto Beans (Cooked) ☞ serving size: 1 cup = 240 g; Calories =

244.5; Total Carb (g) = 39.7; Net Carb (g) = 23.2; Fat (g) = 0.7; Protein = 14.5

🫘 Pinto Calico Or Red Mexican Beans Canned Drained Fat Added In Cooking Ns As To Type Of Fat ☞ serving size: 1 cup = 185 g; Calories = 340.2; Total Carb (g) = 45.1; Net Carb (g) = 29.7; Fat (g) = 0.7; Protein = 15.1

🫘 Pinto Calico Or Red Mexican Beans Canned Drained Fat Not Added In Cooking ☞ serving size: 1 cup = 177 g; Calories = 246.6; Total Carb (g) = 43.3; Net Carb (g) = 28.1; Fat (g) = 0.8; Protein = 16.5

🫘 Pinto Calico Or Red Mexican Beans Canned Drained Low Sodium Fat Added In Cooking ☞ serving size: 1 cup = 177 g; Calories = 336.4; Total Carb (g) = 42.5; Net Carb (g) = 25.9; Fat (g) = 1.4; Protein = 12.5

🫘 Pinto Calico Or Red Mexican Beans Canned Drained Low Sodium Fat Not Added In Cooking ☞ serving size: 1 cup = 177 g; Calories = 237; Total Carb (g) = 40.4; Net Carb (g) = 27.3; Fat (g) = 0.9; Protein = 15.4

🫘 Pinto Calico Or Red Mexican Beans Canned Drained Low Sodium Ns As To Fat Added In Cooking ☞ serving size: 1 cup cup rinsed solids = 158 g; Calories = 336.4; Total Carb (g) = 32.9; Net Carb (g) = 23.4; Fat (g) = 1.5; Protein = 12.8

🫘 Pinto Calico Or Red Mexican Beans Canned Drained Made With Animal Fat Or Meat Drippings ☞ serving size: 1 cup = 177 g; Calories = 329.4; Total Carb (g) = 38.7; Net Carb (g) = 22.2; Fat (g) = 0.3; Protein = 16.8

🫘 Pinto Calico Or Red Mexican Beans Canned Drained Made With Margarine ☞ serving size: 1 cup = 256 g; Calories = 298.8; Total Carb (g) = 38; Net Carb (g) = 24.4; Fat (g) = 0.9; Protein = 13.4

🫘 Pinto Calico Or Red Mexican Beans Canned Drained Made With Oil ☞ serving size: 1 cup = 179 g; Calories = 340.2; Total Carb (g) = 46.2; Net Carb (g) = 27.6; Fat (g) = 1.2; Protein = 16.1

🫘 Pinto Calico Or Red Mexican Beans Canned Drained Ns As To Fat Added In Cooking ☞ serving size: 1 cup = 240 g; Calories = 340.2; Total Carb (g) = 36.4; Net Carb (g) = 25.4; Fat (g) = 1.3; Protein = 11

🫘 Pinto Calico Or Red Mexican Beans Dry Cooked Fat Added In Cooking Ns As To Type Of Fat ☞ serving size: 1 cup = 177 g; Calories = 354.6; Total Carb (g) = 44.8; Net Carb (g) = 26.3; Fat (g) = 1.9; Protein = 16.2

🫘 Pinto Calico Or Red Mexican Beans Dry Cooked Fat Not Added In Cooking ☞ serving size: 1 cup = 179 g; Calories = 255.6; Total Carb (g) = 44.9; Net Carb (g) = 33.6; Fat (g) = 0.6; Protein = 17.4

🫘 Pinto Calico Or Red Mexican Beans Dry Cooked Made With Animal Fat Or Meat Drippings ☞ serving size: 1 cup = 240 g; Calories = 343.8; Total Carb (g) = 32.4; Net Carb (g) = 21.8; Fat (g) = 4.7; Protein = 11.8

🫘 Pinto Calico Or Red Mexican Beans Dry Cooked Made With Margarine ☞ serving size: 1 cup = 171 g; Calories = 309.6; Total Carb (g) = 34.8; Net Carb (g) = 28.6; Fat (g) = 1.2; Protein = 13.9

🫘 Pinto Calico Or Red Mexican Beans Dry Cooked Made With Oil ☞ serving size: 1 cup = 171 g; Calories = 354.6; Total Carb (g) = 35.5; Net Carb (g) = 24.4; Fat (g) = 0.9; Protein = 13.2

🫘 Pinto Calico Or Red Mexican Beans Dry Cooked Ns As To Fat Added In Cooking ☞ serving size: 1 cup = 194 g; Calories = 354.6; Total Carb (g) = 40.2; Net Carb (g) = 40.2; Fat (g) = 1.1; Protein = 15.8

🫘 Raw Peanuts ☞ serving size: 1 cup = 198 g; Calories = 161; Total Carb (g) = 38.7; Net Carb (g) = 23.1; Fat (g) = 0.8; Protein = 17.9

🫘 Red Kidney Beans Canned Drained Fat Added In Cooking Ns As To Type Of Fat ☞ serving size: 1 cup = 202 g; Calories = 338.4; Total Carb (g) = 38.7; Net Carb (g) = 23.3; Fat (g) = 0.8; Protein = 14.2

🫘 Red Kidney Beans Canned Drained Fat Not Added In Cooking

☞ serving size: 1 cup = 180 g; Calories = 243; Total Carb (g) = 33; Net Carb (g) = 21.5; Fat (g) = 1; Protein = 13.6

🫘 Red Kidney Beans Canned Drained Low Sodium Fat Added In Cooking ☞ serving size: 1 cup = 196 g; Calories = 338.4; Total Carb (g) = 40.2; Net Carb (g) = 23.9; Fat (g) = 0.8; Protein = 16.4

🫘 Red Kidney Beans Canned Drained Low Sodium Fat Not Added In Cooking ☞ serving size: 1 cup, = 144 g; Calories = 243; Total Carb (g) = 22; Net Carb (g) = 8.4; Fat (g) = 75.6; Protein = 40.4

🫘 Red Kidney Beans Canned Drained Low Sodium Ns As To Fat Added In Cooking ☞ serving size: 1 cup = 180 g; Calories = 338.4; Total Carb (g) = 43.5; Net Carb (g) = 28.5; Fat (g) = 14.3; Protein = 14.9

🫘 Red Kidney Beans Canned Drained Made With Oil ☞ serving size: 1 cup = 180 g; Calories = 338.4; Total Carb (g) = 43.5; Net Carb (g) = 28.5; Fat (g) = 14.3; Protein = 14.9

🫘 Red Kidney Beans Dry Cooked Fat Added In Cooking Ns As To Type Of Fat ☞ serving size: 1 cup = 180 g; Calories = 324; Total Carb (g) = 46.9; Net Carb (g) = 30.9; Fat (g) = 1.2; Protein = 16.1

🫘 Red Kidney Beans Dry Cooked Fat Not Added In Cooking ☞ serving size: 1 cup = 180 g; Calories = 226.8; Total Carb (g) = 42.3; Net Carb (g) = 29.5; Fat (g) = 14.2; Protein = 12.8

🫘 Red Kidney Beans Dry Cooked Made With Animal Fat Or Meat Drippings ☞ serving size: 1 cup = 180 g; Calories = 313.2; Total Carb (g) = 42.3; Net Carb (g) = 29.5; Fat (g) = 14.2; Protein = 12.8

🫘 Red Kidney Beans Dry Cooked Made With Margarine ☞ serving size: 1 cup = 180 g; Calories = 282.6; Total Carb (g) = 45.5; Net Carb (g) = 31.6; Fat (g) = 1.7; Protein = 13.8

🫘 Red Kidney Beans Dry Cooked Made With Oil ☞ serving size: 1 cup = 180 g; Calories = 324; Total Carb (g) = 41.8; Net Carb (g) = 31.3; Fat (g) = 13.3; Protein = 16.2

🫘 Red Kidney Beans Dry Cooked Ns As To Fat Added In Cooking

☞ serving size: 1 cup = 180 g; Calories = 324; Total Carb (g) = 41.8; Net Carb (g) = 31.3; Fat (g) = 13.3; Protein = 16.2

🔴 Refried Beans Canned Fat-Free ☞ serving size: 1 cup = 180 g; Calories = 182.5; Total Carb (g) = 41.8; Net Carb (g) = 31.3; Fat (g) = 13.3; Protein = 16.2

🔴 Refried Beans Canned Traditional Reduced Sodium ☞ serving size: 1 cup = 180 g; Calories = 211.8; Total Carb (g) = 41.9; Net Carb (g) = 31.5; Fat (g) = 11.6; Protein = 16.5

🔴 Refried Beans Canned Traditional Style (Includes USDA Commodity) ☞ serving size: 1 cup = 180 g; Calories = 214.2; Total Carb (g) = 41.7; Net Carb (g) = 31.3; Fat (g) = 8.5; Protein = 16.2

🔴 Refried Beans Fat Added In Cooking Ns As To Type Of Fat ☞ serving size: 1 cup = 180 g; Calories = 364.3; Total Carb (g) = 44.9; Net Carb (g) = 33.6; Fat (g) = 0.6; Protein = 17.4

🔴 Refried Beans Made With Animal Fat Or Meat Drippings ☞ serving size: 1 cup = 180 g; Calories = 354.2; Total Carb (g) = 51.7; Net Carb (g) = 39.7; Fat (g) = 13.6; Protein = 18.1

🔴 Refried Beans Made With Margarine ☞ serving size: 1 cup = 180 g; Calories = 326.4; Total Carb (g) = 51.7; Net Carb (g) = 39.7; Fat (g) = 13.6; Protein = 18.1

🔴 Refried Beans Made With Oil ☞ serving size: 1 cup = 180 g; Calories = 364.3; Total Carb (g) = 55.6; Net Carb (g) = 42.7; Fat (g) = 1; Protein = 19.5

🔴 Refried Beans Ns As To Fat Added In Cooking ☞ serving size: 1 cup, nfs = 180 g; Calories = 364.3; Total Carb (g) = 51.7; Net Carb (g) = 39.7; Fat (g) = 13.6; Protein = 18.1

🔴 Refried Beans With Cheese ☞ serving size: 1 cup = 180 g; Calories = 270.7; Total Carb (g) = 51.7; Net Carb (g) = 39.7; Fat (g) = 13.6; Protein = 18.1

🔴 Refried Beans With Meat ☞ serving size: 1 cup = 180 g; Calories

= 293.5; Total Carb (g) = 55.6; Net Carb (g) = 42.7; Fat (g) = 1; Protein = 19.5

🥟 Sandwich Spread Meatless ☞ serving size: 1 cup = 180 g; Calories = 22.4; Total Carb (g) = 39.5; Net Carb (g) = 25.1; Fat (g) = 13.5; Protein = 14.7

🥟 Sausage Meatless ☞ serving size: 1 cup = 180 g; Calories = 63.8; Total Carb (g) = 39.5; Net Carb (g) = 25.1; Fat (g) = 13.5; Protein = 14.7

🥟 Silk (Soy Milk) ☞ serving size: 1 cup = 180 g; Calories = 99.6; Total Carb (g) = 39.3; Net Carb (g) = 24.9; Fat (g) = 14; Protein = 14.7

🥟 Silk Banana-Strawberry Soy Yogurt ☞ serving size: 1 cup = 180 g; Calories = 149.6; Total Carb (g) = 39.6; Net Carb (g) = 25.1; Fat (g) = 11.9; Protein = 15.1

🥟 Silk Black Cherry Soy Yogurt ☞ serving size: 1 cup = 180 g; Calories = 149.6; Total Carb (g) = 39.4; Net Carb (g) = 25; Fat (g) = 8.8; Protein = 14.7

🥟 Silk Blueberry Soy Yogurt ☞ serving size: 1 cup = 180 g; Calories = 149.6; Total Carb (g) = 42.4; Net Carb (g) = 26.8; Fat (g) = 1; Protein = 15.9

🥟 Silk Chai Soy Milk ☞ serving size: 1 cup = 180 g; Calories = 128.8; Total Carb (g) = 40.7; Net Carb (g) = 23.8; Fat (g) = 13.4; Protein = 14.8

🥟 Silk Chocolate Soy Milk ☞ serving size: 1 cup = 180 g; Calories = 140.9; Total Carb (g) = 40.7; Net Carb (g) = 23.8; Fat (g) = 13.4; Protein = 14.8

🥟 Silk Coffee Soy Milk ☞ serving size: 1 cup = 180 g; Calories = 150.7; Total Carb (g) = 40.7; Net Carb (g) = 23.8; Fat (g) = 13.4; Protein = 14.8

🥟 Silk French Vanilla Creamer ☞ serving size: 1 cup = 180 g; Calories = 20; Total Carb (g) = 40.9; Net Carb (g) = 23.8; Fat (g) = 11.7; Protein = 15.2

● Silk Hazelnut Creamer ☞ serving size: 1 cup = 180 g; Calories = 20; Total Carb (g) = 40.7; Net Carb (g) = 23.8; Fat (g) = 8.6; Protein = 14.8

● Silk Key Lime Soy Yogurt ☞ serving size: 1 cup = 180 g; Calories = 149.6; Total Carb (g) = 43.8; Net Carb (g) = 25.6; Fat (g) = 0.8; Protein = 16

● Silk Light Chocolate Soy Milk ☞ serving size: 1 cup = 180 g; Calories = 119.1; Total Carb (g) = 40.7; Net Carb (g) = 23.8; Fat (g) = 13.4; Protein = 14.8

● Silk Light Plain Soy Milk ☞ serving size: 1 cup = 180 g; Calories = 70.5; Total Carb (g) = 40.7; Net Carb (g) = 23.8; Fat (g) = 13.4; Protein = 14.8

● Silk Light Vanilla Soy Milk ☞ serving size: 1 cup = 180 g; Calories = 80.2; Total Carb (g) = 43.8; Net Carb (g) = 25.6; Fat (g) = 0.8; Protein = 16

● Silk Mocha Soy Milk ☞ serving size: 1 cup = 180 g; Calories = 140.9; Total Carb (g) = 32.6; Net Carb (g) = 23.6; Fat (g) = 14; Protein = 12.6

● Silk Nog Soy Milk ☞ serving size: 1 cup = 180 g; Calories = 90.3; Total Carb (g) = 32.6; Net Carb (g) = 23.6; Fat (g) = 14; Protein = 12.6

● Silk Original Creamer ☞ serving size: 1 cup = 180 g; Calories = 15; Total Carb (g) = 35.2; Net Carb (g) = 25.5; Fat (g) = 0.7; Protein = 13.6

● Silk Peach Soy Yogurt ☞ serving size: 1 cup = 180 g; Calories = 159.8; Total Carb (g) = 32.6; Net Carb (g) = 23.6; Fat (g) = 13.2; Protein = 12.6

● Silk Plain Soy Yogurt ☞ serving size: 1 cup = 180 g; Calories = 149.8; Total Carb (g) = 34.9; Net Carb (g) = 23.2; Fat (g) = 12.7; Protein = 13

● Silk Plus Fiber Soy Milk ☞ serving size: 1 cup = 180 g; Calories =

99.6; Total Carb (g) = 34.9; Net Carb (g) = 23.2; Fat (g) = 12.7; Protein = 13

🍃 Silk Plus For Bone Health Soy Milk ☞ serving size: 1 cup = 180 g; Calories = 99.6; Total Carb (g) = 34.9; Net Carb (g) = 23.2; Fat (g) = 12.7; Protein = 13

🍃 Silk Plus Omega-3 Dha Soy Milk ☞ serving size: 1 cup = 180 g; Calories = 109.4; Total Carb (g) = 35; Net Carb (g) = 23.3; Fat (g) = 11.2; Protein = 13.3

🍃 Silk Raspberry Soy Yogurt ☞ serving size: 1 cup = 180 g; Calories = 149.6; Total Carb (g) = 34.9; Net Carb (g) = 23.2; Fat (g) = 8.2; Protein = 13

🍃 Silk Strawberry Soy Yogurt ☞ serving size: 1 cup = 180 g; Calories = 159.8; Total Carb (g) = 37.4; Net Carb (g) = 24.8; Fat (g) = 0.7; Protein = 14

🍃 Silk Vanilla Soy Milk ☞ serving size: 1 cup = 180 g; Calories = 99.6; Total Carb (g) = 46.2; Net Carb (g) = 37.4; Fat (g) = 14.2; Protein = 15

🍃 Silk Vanilla Soy Yogurt (Family Size) ☞ serving size: 1 cup = 180 g; Calories = 179.3; Total Carb (g) = 50; Net Carb (g) = 40.4; Fat (g) = 0.9; Protein = 16.2

🍃 Silk Vanilla Soy Yogurt (Single Serving Size) ☞ serving size: 1 cup = 180 g; Calories = 149.6; Total Carb (g) = 46.2; Net Carb (g) = 37.4; Fat (g) = 14.2; Protein = 15

🍃 Silk Very Vanilla Soy Milk ☞ serving size: 1 cup = 180 g; Calories = 128.8; Total Carb (g) = 46.3; Net Carb (g) = 37.5; Fat (g) = 13.5; Protein = 15

🍃 Soft Tofu ☞ serving size: 1 cup = 180 g; Calories = 73.2; Total Carb (g) = 49.8; Net Carb (g) = 40.3; Fat (g) = 0.9; Protein = 16.2

🍃 Soy Flour Defatted ☞ serving size: 1 cup = 180 g; Calories =

343.4; Total Carb (g) = 43.5; Net Carb (g) = 28.5; Fat (g) = 14.3; Protein = 14.9

🍀 Soy Flour Full-Fat Raw ☞ serving size: 1 cup = 180 g; Calories = 364.6; Total Carb (g) = 43.5; Net Carb (g) = 28.5; Fat (g) = 14.3; Protein = 14.9

🍀 Soy Flour Full-Fat Roasted ☞ serving size: 1 cup = 180 g; Calories = 373.2; Total Carb (g) = 43.5; Net Carb (g) = 28.5; Fat (g) = 14.3; Protein = 14.9

🍀 Soy Flour Low-Fat ☞ serving size: 1 cup = 180 g; Calories = 327.4; Total Carb (g) = 43.7; Net Carb (g) = 28.7; Fat (g) = 12.6; Protein = 15.3

🍀 Soy Meal Defatted Raw ☞ serving size: 1 cup = 180 g; Calories = 411.1; Total Carb (g) = 43.4; Net Carb (g) = 28.5; Fat (g) = 9.3; Protein = 14.9

🍀 Soy Milk ☞ serving size: 1 cup = 180 g; Calories = 80.2; Total Carb (g) = 46.9; Net Carb (g) = 30.9; Fat (g) = 1.2; Protein = 16.1

🍀 Soy Milk (All Flavors) Enhanced ☞ serving size: 1 cup = 180 g; Calories = 109.4; Total Carb (g) = 42.3; Net Carb (g) = 29.5; Fat (g) = 14.2; Protein = 12.8

🍀 Soy Milk (All Flavors) Lowfat With Added Calcium Vitamins A And D ☞ serving size: 1 cup = 180 g; Calories = 104.5; Total Carb (g) = 42.3; Net Carb (g) = 29.5; Fat (g) = 14.2; Protein = 12.8

🍀 Soy Milk (All Flavors) Nonfat With Added Calcium Vitamins A And D ☞ serving size: 1 cup = 180 g; Calories = 68; Total Carb (g) = 42.3; Net Carb (g) = 29.5; Fat (g) = 14.2; Protein = 12.8

🍀 Soy Milk Chocolate And Other Flavors Light With Added Calcium Vitamins A And D ☞ serving size: 1 cup = 180 g; Calories = 114.2; Total Carb (g) = 42.5; Net Carb (g) = 29.5; Fat (g) = 12.6; Protein = 13.1

🍀 Soy Milk Chocolate Nonfat With Added Calcium Vitamins A

And D ☞ serving size: 1 cup = 180 g; Calories = 106.9; Total Carb (g) = 42.3; Net Carb (g) = 29.5; Fat (g) = 9.5; Protein = 12.8

🌰 Soy Milk Chocolate Unfortified ☞ serving size: 1 cup = 180 g; Calories = 153.1; Total Carb (g) = 45.5; Net Carb (g) = 31.6; Fat (g) = 1.7; Protein = 13.8

🌰 Soy Milk Original And Vanilla Light Unsweetened With Added Calcium Vitamins A And D ☞ serving size: 1 cup = 178 g; Calories = 82.6; Total Carb (g) = 41.9; Net Carb (g) = 29.2; Fat (g) = 14.1; Protein = 12.7

🌰 Soy Milk Original And Vanilla Light With Added Calcium Vitamins A And D ☞ serving size: 1 cup = 178 g; Calories = 72.9; Total Carb (g) = 41.9; Net Carb (g) = 29.2; Fat (g) = 14.1; Protein = 12.7

🌰 Soy Milk Original And Vanilla With Added Calcium Vitamins A And D ☞ serving size: 1 cup = 173 g; Calories = 104.5; Total Carb (g) = 43.8; Net Carb (g) = 30.5; Fat (g) = 1.6; Protein = 13.3

🌰 Soy Protein Concentrate Produced By Acid Wash ☞ serving size: 1 cup = 180 g; Calories = 93.2; Total Carb (g) = 37.9; Net Carb (g) = 25.7; Fat (g) = 13.6; Protein = 14.4

🌰 Soy Protein Concentrate Produced By Alcohol Extraction ☞ serving size: 1 cup = 180 g; Calories = 93.2; Total Carb (g) = 37.9; Net Carb (g) = 25.7; Fat (g) = 13.6; Protein = 14.4

🌰 Soy Protein Isolate Potassium Type ☞ serving size: 1 cup = 180 g; Calories = 91.2; Total Carb (g) = 37.9; Net Carb (g) = 25.7; Fat (g) = 13.6; Protein = 14.4

🌰 Soy Protein Powder (Isolate) ☞ serving size: 1 cup = 180 g; Calories = 95.1; Total Carb (g) = 38.1; Net Carb (g) = 25.7; Fat (g) = 12; Protein = 14.7

🌰 Soy Sauce ☞ serving size: 1 cup = 180 g; Calories = 8.5; Total Carb (g) = 37.9; Net Carb (g) = 25.7; Fat (g) = 8.8; Protein = 14.4

🌰 Soy Sauce Made From Hydrolyzed Vegetable Protein ☞ serving size: 1 cup = 180 g; Calories = 10.8; Total Carb (g) = 40.8; Net Carb (g) = 27.5; Fat (g) = 0.9; Protein = 15.5

🍢 Soy Sauce Made From Soy And Wheat (Shoyu) Low Sodium ☞ serving size: 1 cup = 180 g; Calories = 8.1; Total Carb (g) = 41.4; Net Carb (g) = 28; Fat (g) = 13.6; Protein = 14.6

🍢 Soy Sauce Reduced Sodium Made From Hydrolyzed Vegetable Protein ☞ serving size: 1 cup = 180 g; Calories = 13.5; Total Carb (g) = 41.4; Net Carb (g) = 28; Fat (g) = 13.6; Protein = 14.6

🍢 Soybean Curd Breaded Fried ☞ serving size: 1 cup = 180 g; Calories = 43.5; Total Carb (g) = 44.5; Net Carb (g) = 30.1; Fat (g) = 1.1; Protein = 15.7

🍢 Soybean Curd Cheese ☞ serving size: 1 cup = 180 g; Calories = 339.8; Total Carb (g) = 41.4; Net Carb (g) = 26.6; Fat (g) = 13.7; Protein = 14.6

🍢 Soybeans Dry Cooked Fat Added In Cooking ☞ serving size: 1 cup = 180 g; Calories = 401.4; Total Carb (g) = 41.4; Net Carb (g) = 26.6; Fat (g) = 13.7; Protein = 14.6

🍢 Soybeans Dry Cooked Fat Not Added In Cooking ☞ serving size: 1 cup = 180 g; Calories = 307.8; Total Carb (g) = 44.5; Net Carb (g) = 28.7; Fat (g) = 1.1; Protein = 15.7

🍢 Soybeans Dry Cooked Ns As To Fat Added In Cooking ☞ serving size: 1 cup = 180 g; Calories = 401.4; Total Carb (g) = 42.1; Net Carb (g) = 24.8; Fat (g) = 14.4; Protein = 15.3

🍢 Soybeans Mature Seeds Cooked Boiled With Salt ☞ serving size: 1 cup = 180 g; Calories = 295.8; Total Carb (g) = 42.1; Net Carb (g) = 24.8; Fat (g) = 14.4; Protein = 15.3

🍢 Soybeans Mature Seeds Raw ☞ serving size: 1 cup = 180 g; Calories = 829.6; Total Carb (g) = 42.1; Net Carb (g) = 24.8; Fat (g) = 14.4; Protein = 15.3

🍢 Soybeans Mature Seeds Roasted No Salt Added ☞ serving size:

1 cup = 180 g; Calories = 806.7; Total Carb (g) = 42.3; Net Carb (g) = 24.8; Fat (g) = 12.8; Protein = 15.6

🫘 Soybeans Mature Seeds Roasted Salted ☞ serving size: 1 cup = 180 g; Calories = 806.7; Total Carb (g) = 42.1; Net Carb (g) = 24.8; Fat (g) = 9.7; Protein = 15.2

🫘 Soyburger Meatless With Cheese On Bun ☞ serving size: 1 cup = 180 g; Calories = 291.2; Total Carb (g) = 45.3; Net Carb (g) = 26.7; Fat (g) = 1.9; Protein = 16.4

🫘 Split Peas ☞ serving size: 1 cup = 180 g; Calories = 231.3; Total Carb (g) = 42; Net Carb (g) = 24.7; Fat (g) = 14.4; Protein = 15.2

🫘 Stewed Beans With Pork Tomatoes And Chili Peppers Mexican Style ☞ serving size: 1 cup = 180 g; Calories = 329.1; Total Carb (g) = 15; Net Carb (g) = 4.2; Fat (g) = 16.1; Protein = 32.6

🫘 Stewed Chickpeas Puerto Rican Style ☞ serving size: 1 cup = 180 g; Calories = 231.4; Total Carb (g) = 13.9; Net Carb (g) = 4; Fat (g) = 28; Protein = 30.2

🫘 Stewed Chickpeas With Potatoes Puerto Rican Style ☞ serving size: 1 cup = 180 g; Calories = 416; Total Carb (g) = 13.9; Net Carb (g) = 4; Fat (g) = 28; Protein = 30.2

🫘 Stewed Chickpeas With Spanish Sausages Puerto Rican Style ☞ serving size: 1 cup = 180 g; Calories = 530; Total Carb (g) = 34.3; Net Carb (g) = 20.6; Fat (g) = 0.7; Protein = 12.6

🫘 Stewed Pink Beans With Pig's Feet Puerto Rican Style ☞ serving size: 1 cup = 180 g; Calories = 288.9; Total Carb (g) = 32.2; Net Carb (g) = 19.4; Fat (g) = 12; Protein = 11.8

🫘 Stewed Pink Beans With White Potatoes And Ham Puerto Rican Style ☞ serving size: 1 cup = 180 g; Calories = 219.3; Total Carb (g) = 32.2; Net Carb (g) = 19.4; Fat (g) = 12; Protein = 11.8

🫘 Stewed Red Beans Puerto Rican Style ☞ serving size: 1 cup = 180 g; Calories = 210; Total Carb (g) = 31.8; Net Carb (g) = 19.2; Fat (g) = 13.2; Protein = 11.7

🍃 Stewed Red Beans With Pig's Feet And Potatoes Puerto Rican Style ☞ serving size: 1 cup = 242 g; Calories = 332.2; Total Carb (g) = 43.3; Net Carb (g) = 28.6; Fat (g) = 13.3; Protein = 14.7

🍃 Stewed Red Beans With Pig's Feet Puerto Rican Style ☞ serving size: 1 cup = 242 g; Calories = 286.8; Total Carb (g) = 45.9; Net Carb (g) = 30.4; Fat (g) = 1.2; Protein = 15.2

🍃 Stinky Tofu ☞ serving size: 1 cup = 242 g; Calories = 12.8; Total Carb (g) = 43.3; Net Carb (g) = 28.6; Fat (g) = 13.3; Protein = 14.7

🍃 Swiss Steak With Gravy Meatless ☞ serving size: 1 cup = 231 g; Calories = 165.6; Total Carb (g) = 36.2; Net Carb (g) = 26.9; Fat (g) = 9; Protein = 9.1

🍃 Tamari ☞ serving size: 1 cup = 253 g; Calories = 10.8; Total Carb (g) = 45; Net Carb (g) = 31.4; Fat (g) = 14.5; Protein = 15.5

🍃 Tempeh ☞ serving size: 1 cup = 253 g; Calories = 318.7; Total Carb (g) = 45; Net Carb (g) = 31.4; Fat (g) = 14.5; Protein = 15.5

🍃 Tofu Dried-Frozen (Koyadofu) ☞ serving size: 1 cup = 253 g; Calories = 81.1; Total Carb (g) = 45; Net Carb (g) = 31.4; Fat (g) = 10.3; Protein = 15.5

🍃 Tofu Dried-Frozen (Koyadofu) Prepared With Calcium Sulfate ☞ serving size: 1 cup = 253 g; Calories = 79.9; Total Carb (g) = 45; Net Carb (g) = 31.4; Fat (g) = 14.5; Protein = 15.5

🍃 Tofu Extra Firm Prepared With Nigari ☞ serving size: 1 cup = 253 g; Calories = 75.5; Total Carb (g) = 32.9; Net Carb (g) = 24; Fat (g) = 9.3; Protein = 15

🍃 Tofu Fried ☞ serving size: 1 cup = 253 g; Calories = 76.7; Total Carb (g) = 44; Net Carb (g) = 30.8; Fat (g) = 5.5; Protein = 18.4

🍃 Tofu Fried Prepared With Calcium Sulfate ☞ serving size: 1 cup

= 259 g; Calories = 35.1; Total Carb (g) = 44.8; Net Carb (g) = 36.2; Fat (g) = 13.5; Protein = 17.5

🍃 Tofu Hard Prepared With Nigari ☞ serving size: 1 cup = 266 g; Calories = 176.9; Total Carb (g) = 50.6; Net Carb (g) = 37.8; Fat (g) = 24.1; Protein = 31.8

🍃 Tofu Prepared With Calcium ☞ serving size: 1 cup = 178 g; Calories = 94.2; Total Carb (g) = 35.2; Net Carb (g) = 26.7; Fat (g) = 14; Protein = 18.4

🍃 Tofu Salted And Fermented (Fuyu) Prepared With Calcium Sulfate ☞ serving size: 1 cake = 32 g; Calories = 12.8; Total Carb (g) = 15.9; Net Carb (g) = 14.9; Fat (g) = 6.8; Protein = 1.8

🍃 Tofu Yogurt ☞ serving size: 1 cup = 242 g; Calories = 246.3; Total Carb (g) = 23.4; Net Carb (g) = 18.8; Fat (g) = 20.5; Protein = 13.3

🍃 Unsalted Peanut Butter (Smooth) ☞ serving size: 1 cup = 250 g; Calories = 191.4; Total Carb (g) = 25.6; Net Carb (g) = 19.6; Fat (g) = 7.6; Protein = 10.7

🍃 Unsweetened Soy Milk ☞ serving size: 1 cup = 255 g; Calories = 80.2; Total Carb (g) = 26.9; Net Carb (g) = 20.8; Fat (g) = 7.8; Protein = 10.6

🍃 Vanilla Soy Milk ☞ serving size: 1 cup, with bone (yield after bone removed) = 202 g; Calories = 131.2; Total Carb (g) = 16; Net Carb (g) = 12.5; Fat (g) = 16.7; Protein = 18.5

🍃 Vegetarian Chili Made With Meat Substitute ☞ serving size: 1 cup, with bone (yield after bone removed) = 202 g; Calories = 271.8; Total Carb (g) = 15.7; Net Carb (g) = 12.3; Fat (g) = 16.7; Protein = 18.8

🍃 Vegetarian Fillets ☞ serving size: 1 cup, with bone (yield after bone removed) = 220 g; Calories = 246.5; Total Carb (g) = 21.3; Net Carb (g) = 16.9; Fat (g) = 18.2; Protein = 20.8

🍃 Vegetarian Meatloaf Or Patties ☞ serving size: 1 cup = 270 g;

Calories = 110.3; Total Carb (g) = 49.6; Net Carb (g) = 37.8; Fat (g) = 4.2; Protein = 16.2

🖋 Vegetarian Pot Pie ☞ serving size: 1 cup = 253 g; Calories = 508.5; Total Carb (g) = 20.7; Net Carb (g) = 13.9; Fat (g) = 0.8; Protein = 6.1

🖋 Vegetarian Stew ☞ serving size: 1 cup = 180 g; Calories = 76.6; Total Carb (g) = 34.4; Net Carb (g) = 23.6; Fat (g) = 14; Protein = 12.8

🖋 Vegetarian Stroganoff ☞ serving size: 1 cup = 180 g; Calories = 773.6; Total Carb (g) = 34.4; Net Carb (g) = 23.6; Fat (g) = 14; Protein = 12.8

🖋 Veggie Burgers ☞ serving size: 1 cup = 180 g; Calories = 123.9; Total Carb (g) = 37.2; Net Carb (g) = 25.5; Fat (g) = 1; Protein = 13.8

🖋 Vermicelli Made From Soy ☞ serving size: 1 cup = 180 g; Calories = 463.4; Total Carb (g) = 45.3; Net Carb (g) = 32.7; Fat (g) = 18; Protein = 14.7

🖋 Vitasoy Usa Azumaya Extra Firm Tofu ☞ serving size: 1 cup = 180 g; Calories = 69.5; Total Carb (g) = 45.3; Net Carb (g) = 32.7; Fat (g) = 18; Protein = 14.7

🖋 Vitasoy Usa Azumaya Firm Tofu ☞ serving size: 1 cup = 180 g; Calories = 63.2; Total Carb (g) = 45.3; Net Carb (g) = 32.7; Fat (g) = 18; Protein = 14.7

🖋 Vitasoy Usa Azumaya Silken Tofu ☞ serving size: 1 cup = 180 g; Calories = 39.1; Total Carb (g) = 45.5; Net Carb (g) = 32.9; Fat (g) = 16.3; Protein = 15

🖋 Vitasoy Usa Nasoya Lite Firm Tofu ☞ serving size: 1 cup = 180 g; Calories = 42.7; Total Carb (g) = 45.3; Net Carb (g) = 32.7; Fat (g) = 12.9; Protein = 14.6

🖋 Vitasoy Usa Organic Nasoya Extra Firm Tofu ☞ serving size: 1 cup = 180 g; Calories = 77.4; Total Carb (g) = 49.1; Net Carb (g) = 35.4; Fat (g) = 4.6; Protein = 15.9

🥄 Vitasoy Usa Organic Nasoya Firm Tofu ☞ serving size: 1 cup = 180 g; Calories = 66.4; Total Carb (g) = 37.6; Net Carb (g) = 25.3; Fat (g) = 18.1; Protein = 13.7

🥄 Vitasoy Usa Organic Nasoya Silken Tofu ☞ serving size: 1 cup = 180 g; Calories = 42.8; Total Carb (g) = 37.6; Net Carb (g) = 25.3; Fat (g) = 18.1; Protein = 13.7

🥄 Vitasoy Usa Organic Nasoya Soft Tofu ☞ serving size: 1 cup = 180 g; Calories = 55.3; Total Carb (g) = 37.6; Net Carb (g) = 25.3; Fat (g) = 18.1; Protein = 13.7

🥄 Vitasoy Usa Organic Nasoya Sprouted Tofu Plus Super Firm ☞ serving size: 1 cup = 180 g; Calories = 97.8; Total Carb (g) = 40.4; Net Carb (g) = 27.3; Fat (g) = 5.8; Protein = 14.7

🥄 Vitasoy Usa Organic Nasoya Super Firm Cubed Tofu ☞ serving size: 1 cup = 180 g; Calories = 93.2; Total Carb (g) = 37.6; Net Carb (g) = 25.4; Fat (g) = 18.1; Protein = 13.7

🥄 Vitasoy Usa Organic Nasoya Tofu Plus Firm ☞ serving size: 1 cup = 180 g; Calories = 62.9; Total Carb (g) = 37.6; Net Carb (g) = 25.4; Fat (g) = 18.1; Protein = 13.7

🥄 Vitasoy Usa Vitasoy Light Vanilla Soy Milk ☞ serving size: 1 cup = 180 g; Calories = 72.9; Total Carb (g) = 40.5; Net Carb (g) = 27.3; Fat (g) = 5.9; Protein = 14.8

🥄 Vitasoy Usa Vitasoy Organic Classic Original Soy Milk ☞ serving size: 1 cup = 180 g; Calories = 114.2; Total Carb (g) = 37.8; Net Carb (g) = 22.8; Fat (g) = 0.7; Protein = 14.9

🥄 Vitasoy Usa Vitasoy Organic Creamy Original Soy Milk ☞ serving size: 1 cup = 180 g; Calories = 106.9; Total Carb (g) = 35.4; Net Carb (g) = 21.5; Fat (g) = 12.3; Protein = 14

🥄 White Beans Canned Drained Fat Added In Cooking Ns As To Type Of Fat ☞ serving size: 1 cup = 180 g; Calories = 392.4; Total Carb (g) = 35.4; Net Carb (g) = 21.5; Fat (g) = 12.3; Protein = 14

🫘 White Beans Canned Drained Fat Not Added In Cooking ☞ serving size: 1 cup = 180 g; Calories = 302.4; Total Carb (g) = 35.5; Net Carb (g) = 21.4; Fat (g) = 10.8; Protein = 14.3

🫘 White Beans Canned Drained Low Sodium Fat Added In Cooking ☞ serving size: 1 cup = 180 g; Calories = 392.4; Total Carb (g) = 35.3; Net Carb (g) = 21.5; Fat (g) = 7.9; Protein = 14

🫘 White Beans Canned Drained Low Sodium Fat Not Added In Cooking ☞ serving size: 1 cup = 180 g; Calories = 302.4; Total Carb (g) = 35.4; Net Carb (g) = 21.5; Fat (g) = 12.3; Protein = 14

🫘 White Beans Canned Drained Low Sodium Ns As To Fat Added In Cooking ☞ serving size: 1 cup = 197 g; Calories = 392.4; Total Carb (g) = 33.6; Net Carb (g) = 21; Fat (g) = 14.6; Protein = 18.2

🫘 White Beans Canned Drained Made With Oil ☞ serving size: 1 cup = 179 g; Calories = 392.4; Total Carb (g) = 29.3; Net Carb (g) = 20.5; Fat (g) = 14.8; Protein = 15.9

🫘 White Beans Dry Cooked Fat Added In Cooking Ns As To Type Of Fat ☞ serving size: 1 cup = 180 g; Calories = 343.8; Total Carb (g) = 33.7; Net Carb (g) = 20.4; Fat (g) = 12.2; Protein = 15.1

🫘 White Beans Dry Cooked Fat Not Added In Cooking ☞ serving size: 1 cup = 180 g; Calories = 248.4; Total Carb (g) = 33.7; Net Carb (g) = 20.4; Fat (g) = 12.2; Protein = 15.1

🫘 White Beans Dry Cooked Made With Animal Fat Or Meat Drippings ☞ serving size: 1 cup = 180 g; Calories = 333; Total Carb (g) = 33.7; Net Carb (g) = 20.4; Fat (g) = 12.2; Protein = 15.1

🫘 White Beans Dry Cooked Made With Margarine ☞ serving size: 1 cup = 180 g; Calories = 300.6; Total Carb (g) = 33.9; Net Carb (g) = 20.6; Fat (g) = 10.7; Protein = 15.4

🫘 White Beans Dry Cooked Made With Oil ☞ serving size: 1 cup = 180 g; Calories = 343.8; Total Carb (g) = 33.7; Net Carb (g) = 20.6; Fat (g) = 7.9; Protein = 15.1

White Beans Dry Cooked Ns As To Fat Added In Cooking ☞ serving size: 1 cup = 180 g; Calories = 343.8; Total Carb (g) = 36.1; Net Carb (g) = 21.8; Fat (g) = 0.7; Protein = 16.2

Winged Beans Mature Seeds Cooked Boiled With Salt ☞ serving size: 1 slice (3/4" thick) = 47 g; Calories = 252.8; Total Carb (g) = 5; Net Carb (g) = 4.3; Fat (g) = 1.1; Protein = 1

Winged Beans Mature Seeds Cooked Boiled Without Salt ☞ serving size: 1 cup = 260 g; Calories = 252.8; Total Carb (g) = 25.5; Net Carb (g) = 20.6; Fat (g) = 10.2; Protein = 10.7

Winged Beans Mature Seeds Raw ☞ serving size: 1 cup = 260 g; Calories = 744.4; Total Carb (g) = 56.3; Net Carb (g) = 45.6; Fat (g) = 13.3; Protein = 20.2

Yardlong Beans Mature Seeds Cooked Boiled With Salt ☞ serving size: 1 cup, with bone (yield after bone removed) = 202 g; Calories = 201.8; Total Carb (g) = 16.4; Net Carb (g) = 13.3; Fat (g) = 18.3; Protein = 19.1

Yardlong Beans Mature Seeds Cooked Boiled Without Salt ☞ serving size: 1 cup = 250 g; Calories = 201.8; Total Carb (g) = 31; Net Carb (g) = 24.8; Fat (g) = 39.1; Protein = 16.1

Yardlong Beans Mature Seeds Raw ☞ serving size: 1 cup = 120 g; Calories = 579.5; Total Carb (g) = 28.2; Net Carb (g) = 22.8; Fat (g) = 22.9; Protein = 14.4

Yellow Canary Or Peruvian Beans Canned Drained Fat Added In Cooking Ns As To Type Of Fat ☞ serving size: 1 slice (2-3/4" x 1" x 1/2") = 29 g; Calories = 351; Total Carb (g) = 2.5; Net Carb (g) = 2.3; Fat (g) = 2.8; Protein = 2.4

Yellow Canary Or Peruvian Beans Dry Cooked Fat Added In Cooking Ns As To Type Of Fat ☞ serving size: 1 steak with gravy = 92 g; Calories = 351; Total Carb (g) = 13; Net Carb (g) = 9.3; Fat (g) = 7.4; Protein = 11.7

🫘 Yellow Canary Or Peruvian Beans Dry Cooked Fat Not Added In Cooking ☞ serving size: 1 pie = 227 g; Calories = 257.4; Total Carb (g) = 38.6; Net Carb (g) = 33.6; Fat (g) = 31.7; Protein = 17.5

🫘 Yellow Canary Or Peruvian Beans Dry Cooked Made With Animal Fat Or Meat Drippings ☞ serving size: 1 cup = 254 g; Calories = 340.2; Total Carb (g) = 35.3; Net Carb (g) = 24.1; Fat (g) = 7.4; Protein = 18.9

🫘 Yellow Canary Or Peruvian Beans Dry Cooked Made With Margarine ☞ serving size: 1 cup = 247 g; Calories = 309.6; Total Carb (g) = 7.4; Net Carb (g) = 4.6; Fat (g) = 5.3; Protein = 2

🫘 Yellow Canary Or Peruvian Beans Dry Cooked Made With Oil ☞ serving size: 1 box (3.2 oz), dry, yields = 466 g; Calories = 351; Total Carb (g) = 54.2; Net Carb (g) = 42; Fat (g) = 47.4; Protein = 35.3

🫘 Yellow Canary Or Peruvian Beans Dry Cooked Ns As To Fat Added In Cooking ☞ serving size: 1 sandwich = 140 g; Calories = 351; Total Carb (g) = 34.7; Net Carb (g) = 30.3; Fat (g) = 9.3; Protein = 17.2

🫘 Yokan Prepared From Adzuki Beans And Sugar ☞ serving size: 1 cup, cubes = 146 g; Calories = 36.4; Total Carb (g) = 90.3; Net Carb (g) = 77.2; Fat (g) = 10.3; Protein = 16.5

13

BEVERAGES

100 Proof Liquor ☞ serving size: 1 fl oz = 27.8 g; Calories = 82; Total Carb (g) = 0; Net Carb (g) = 0; Fat (g) = 0; Protein = 0

86 Proof Liquor ☞ serving size: 1 fl oz = 27.8 g; Calories = 69.5; Total Carb (g) = 0; Net Carb (g) = 0; Fat (g) = 0; Protein = 0

90 Proof Liquor ☞ serving size: 1 fl oz = 27.8 g; Calories = 73.1; Total Carb (g) = 0; Net Carb (g) = 0; Fat (g) = 0; Protein = 0

94 Proof Liquor ☞ serving size: 1 fl oz = 27.8 g; Calories = 76.5; Total Carb (g) = 0; Net Carb (g) = 0; Fat (g) = 0; Protein = 0

Abbott Eas Soy Protein Powder ☞ serving size: 1 scoop = 44 g; Calories = 178.2; Total Carb (g) = 19.3; Net Carb (g) = 19.3; Fat (g) = 1.6; Protein = 21

Abbott Eas Whey Protein Powder ☞ serving size: 2 scoop = 39 g; Calories = 150.2; Total Carb (g) = 7; Net Carb (g) = 7; Fat (g) = 2; Protein = 26

Abbott Ensure Nutritional Shake Ready-To-Drink ☞ serving size: 8 fl oz = 254 g; Calories = 266.7; Total Carb (g) = 42.9; Net Carb (g) = 42.9; Fat (g) = 6.4; Protein = 9.7

Abbott Ensure Plus Ready-To-Drink ☞ serving size: 1 cup = 252 g; Calories = 355.3; Total Carb (g) = 50.1; Net Carb (g) = 50.1; Fat (g) = 11.4; Protein = 13

Acai Berry Drink Fortified ☞ serving size: 8 fl oz = 266 g; Calories = 164.9; Total Carb (g) = 34.1; Net Carb (g) = 30.9; Fat (g) = 2.2; Protein = 2.2

Alcoholic Beverage Beer Light Budweiser Select ☞ serving size: 1 fl oz = 29.5 g; Calories = 8.3; Total Carb (g) = 0.3; Net Carb (g) = 0.3; Fat (g) = 0; Protein = 0.1

Alcoholic Beverage Beer Light Higher Alcohol ☞ serving size: 12 fl oz = 356 g; Calories = 163.8; Total Carb (g) = 2.7; Net Carb (g) = 2.7; Fat (g) = 0; Protein = 0.9

Alcoholic Beverage Beer Light Low Carb ☞ serving size: 1 fl oz = 29.5 g; Calories = 8; Total Carb (g) = 0.2; Net Carb (g) = 0.2; Fat (g) = 0; Protein = 0.1

Alcoholic Beverage Creme De Menthe 72 Proof ☞ serving size: 1 fl oz = 33.6 g; Calories = 124.7; Total Carb (g) = 14; Net Carb (g) = 14; Fat (g) = 0.1; Protein = 0

Alcoholic Beverage Daiquiri Prepared-From-Recipe ☞ serving size: 1 fl oz = 30.2 g; Calories = 56.2; Total Carb (g) = 2.1; Net Carb (g) = 2.1; Fat (g) = 0; Protein = 0

Alcoholic Beverage Distilled All (Gin Rum Vodka Whiskey) 80 Proof ☞ serving size: 1 fl oz = 27.8 g; Calories = 64.2; Total Carb (g) = 0; Net Carb (g) = 0; Fat (g) = 0; Protein = 0

Alcoholic Beverage Liqueur Coffee 63 Proof ☞ serving size: 1 fl oz = 34.8 g; Calories = 107.2; Total Carb (g) = 11.2; Net Carb (g) = 11.2; Fat (g) = 0.1; Protein = 0

Alcoholic Beverage Malt Beer Hard Lemonade ☞ serving size: fl oz = 335 g; Calories = 227.8; Total Carb (g) = 33.7; Net Carb (g) = 33.7; Fat (g) = 0; Protein = 0

Alcoholic Beverage Pina Colada Canned ☞ serving size: 1 fl oz = 32.6 g; Calories = 77.3; Total Carb (g) = 9; Net Carb (g) = 9; Fat (g) = 2.5; Protein = 0.2

Alcoholic Beverage Pina Colada Prepared-From-Recipe ☞ serving size: 1 fl oz = 31.4 g; Calories = 54.6; Total Carb (g) = 7.1; Net Carb (g) = 7; Fat (g) = 0.6; Protein = 0.1

Alcoholic Beverage Rice (Sake) ☞ serving size: 1 fl oz = 29.1 g; Calories = 39; Total Carb (g) = 1.5; Net Carb (g) = 1.5; Fat (g) = 0; Protein = 0.2

Alcoholic Beverage Whiskey Sour ☞ serving size: 1 fl oz = 30.4 g; Calories = 45.3; Total Carb (g) = 4; Net Carb (g) = 4; Fat (g) = 0; Protein = 0

Alcoholic Beverage Whiskey Sour Canned ☞ serving size: 1 fl oz = 30.8 g; Calories = 36.7; Total Carb (g) = 4.1; Net Carb (g) = 4.1; Fat (g) = 0; Protein = 0

Alcoholic Beverage Whiskey Sour Prepared From Item 14028 ☞ serving size: 1 fl oz = 30.4 g; Calories = 46.5; Total Carb (g) = 3.9; Net Carb (g) = 3.9; Fat (g) = 0; Protein = 0

Alcoholic Beverage Whiskey Sour Prepared With Water Whiskey And Powder Mix ☞ serving size: 1 fl oz = 29.4 g; Calories = 48.2; Total Carb (g) = 4.7; Net Carb (g) = 4.7; Fat (g) = 0; Protein = 0

Alcoholic Beverage Wine Cooking ☞ serving size: 1 tsp = 4.9 g; Calories = 2.5; Total Carb (g) = 0.3; Net Carb (g) = 0.3; Fat (g) = 0; Protein = 0

Alcoholic Beverage Wine Light ☞ serving size: 1 fl oz = 29.5 g; Calories = 14.5; Total Carb (g) = 0.4; Net Carb (g) = 0.4; Fat (g) = 0; Protein = 0

Alcoholic Beverage Wine Table White Muller Thurgau ☞ serving size: 1 fl oz = 29.5 g; Calories = 22.4; Total Carb (g) = 1; Net Carb (g) = 1; Fat (g) = 0; Protein = 0

Alcoholic Malt Beverage Higher Alcohol Sweetened ☞ serving size: 1 fl oz = 30 g; Calories = 26.4; Total Carb (g) = 2.7; Net Carb (g) = 2.7; Fat (g) = 0; Protein = 0

Aloe Vera Juice Drink Fortified With Vitamin C ☞ serving size: 8 fl oz = 240 g; Calories = 36; Total Carb (g) = 9; Net Carb (g) = 9; Fat (g) = 0; Protein = 0

Amber Hard Cider ☞ serving size: 12 fl oz = 355 g; Calories = 198.8; Total Carb (g) = 21; Net Carb (g) = 21; Fat (g) = 0; Protein = 0

Arizona Tea Ready-To-Drink Lemon ☞ serving size: 1 fl oz = 30.6 g; Calories = 11.9; Total Carb (g) = 3; Net Carb (g) = 3; Fat (g) = 0; Protein = 0

Barbera ☞ serving size: 1 fl oz = 29.4 g; Calories = 25; Total Carb (g) = 0.8; Net Carb (g) = 0.8; Fat (g) = 0; Protein = 0

Beer ☞ serving size: 1 fl oz = 29.7 g; Calories = 12.8; Total Carb (g) = 1.1; Net Carb (g) = 1.1; Fat (g) = 0; Protein = 0.1

Black Tea (Brewed) ☞ serving size: 1 fl oz = 29.6 g; Calories = 0.3; Total Carb (g) = 0.1; Net Carb (g) = 0.1; Fat (g) = 0; Protein = 0

Black Tea (Ready To Drink) ☞ serving size: 16 fl oz = 473 g; Calories = 0; Total Carb (g) = 0; Net Carb (g) = 0; Fat (g) = 0; Protein = 0

Bottled Water ☞ serving size: 1 fl oz = 29.6 g; Calories = 0; Total Carb (g) = 0; Net Carb (g) = 0; Fat (g) = 0; Protein = 0

Brandy And Cola ☞ serving size: 1 fl oz = 30 g; Calories = 26.7; Total Carb (g) = 2.3; Net Carb (g) = 2.3; Fat (g) = 0.1; Protein = 0

Budweiser Beer ☞ serving size: 1 fl oz = 29.8 g; Calories = 12.2; Total Carb (g) = 0.9; Net Carb (g) = 0.9; Fat (g) = 0; Protein = 0.1

Budweiser Light Beer ☞ serving size: 1 fl oz = 29.5 g; Calories = 8.6; Total Carb (g) = 0.4; Net Carb (g) = 0.4; Fat (g) = 0; Protein = 0.1

Burgundy ☞ serving size: 1 fl oz = 29.5 g; Calories = 25.4; Total Carb (g) = 1.1; Net Carb (g) = 1.1; Fat (g) = 0; Protein = 0

Cabernet Franc ☞ serving size: 1 fl oz = 29.4 g; Calories = 24.4; Total Carb (g) = 0.7; Net Carb (g) = 0.7; Fat (g) = 0; Protein = 0

Cabernet Sauvignon ☞ serving size: 1 fl oz = 29.4 g; Calories = 24.4; Total Carb (g) = 0.8; Net Carb (g) = 0.8; Fat (g) = 0; Protein = 0

Caffeine Free Cola ☞ serving size: 1 fl oz = 30.7 g; Calories = 12.6; Total Carb (g) = 3.3; Net Carb (g) = 3.3; Fat (g) = 0; Protein = 0

Carbonated Beverage Chocolate-Flavored Soda ☞ serving size: 1 fl oz = 31 g; Calories = 13; Total Carb (g) = 3.3; Net Carb (g) = 3.3; Fat (g) = 0; Protein = 0

Carbonated Beverage Low Calorie Other Than Cola Or Pepper With Sodium Saccharin Without Caffeine ☞ serving size: 1 fl oz = 29.6 g; Calories = 0; Total Carb (g) = 0; Net Carb (g) = 0; Fat (g) = 0; Protein = 0

Carbonated Cola Fast-Food Cola ☞ serving size: 1 serving child 12 fl oz, without ice = 258 g; Calories = 95.5; Total Carb (g) = 24.7; Net Carb (g) = 24.7; Fat (g) = 0.1; Protein = 0.2

Carbonated Lemon-Lime Soda No Caffeine ☞ serving size: 1 fl oz = 30.8 g; Calories = 12.6; Total Carb (g) = 3.2; Net Carb (g) = 3.2; Fat (g) = 0; Protein = 0

Carbonated Limeade High Caffeine ☞ serving size: 1 cup = 253 g; Calories = 43; Total Carb (g) = 10.4; Net Carb (g) = 10.4; Fat (g) = 0.3; Protein = 0

Carbonated Low Calorie Cola Or Pepper-Type With Aspartame Contains Caffeine ☞ serving size: 1 fl oz = 29.6 g; Calories = 0.6; Total Carb (g) = 0.1; Net Carb (g) = 0.1; Fat (g) = 0; Protein = 0

Carbonated Low Calorie Other Than Cola Or Pepper Without Caffeine ☞ serving size: 1 fl oz = 29.6 g; Calories = 0; Total Carb (g) = 0; Net Carb (g) = 0; Fat (g) = 0; Protein = 0

Carbonated Low Calorie Other Than Cola Or Pepper With Aspartame Contains Caffeine ☞ serving size: 1 fl oz = 29.6 g;

Calories = 0; Total Carb (g) = 0; Net Carb (g) = 0; Fat (g) = 0; Protein = 0

🔲 Carignane ☞ serving size: 1 fl oz = 29.4 g; Calories = 21.8; Total Carb (g) = 0.7; Net Carb (g) = 0.7; Fat (g) = 0; Protein = 0

🔲 Carob-Flavor Beverage Mix Powder ☞ serving size: 1 tbsp = 12 g; Calories = 44.6; Total Carb (g) = 11.2; Net Carb (g) = 10.2; Fat (g) = 0; Protein = 0.2

🔲 Carob-Flavor Beverage Mix Powder Prepared With Whole Milk ☞ serving size: 1 cup (8 fl oz) = 256 g; Calories = 192; Total Carb (g) = 22.2; Net Carb (g) = 21.2; Fat (g) = 8; Protein = 8.1

🔲 Cereal Beverage ☞ serving size: 1 fl oz = 30 g; Calories = 1.5; Total Carb (g) = 0.3; Net Carb (g) = 0.2; Fat (g) = 0; Protein = 0

🔲 Cereal Beverage With Beet Roots From Powdered Instant ☞ serving size: 1 fl oz = 30 g; Calories = 1.5; Total Carb (g) = 0.3; Net Carb (g) = 0.2; Fat (g) = 0; Protein = 0

🔲 Champagne Punch ☞ serving size: 1 fl oz = 30 g; Calories = 38.4; Total Carb (g) = 3.7; Net Carb (g) = 3.6; Fat (g) = 0; Protein = 0.1

🔲 Chardonnay ☞ serving size: 1 fl oz = 29.3 g; Calories = 24.6; Total Carb (g) = 0.6; Net Carb (g) = 0.6; Fat (g) = 0; Protein = 0

🔲 Chenin Blanc ☞ serving size: 1 fl oz = 29.5 g; Calories = 23.6; Total Carb (g) = 1; Net Carb (g) = 1; Fat (g) = 0; Protein = 0

🔲 Chicory Beverage ☞ serving size: 1 fl oz = 30 g; Calories = 2.1; Total Carb (g) = 0.4; Net Carb (g) = 0.4; Fat (g) = 0; Protein = 0.1

🔲 Chocolate Almond Milk ☞ serving size: 8 fl oz = 240 g; Calories = 120; Total Carb (g) = 22.5; Net Carb (g) = 21.6; Fat (g) = 3; Protein = 1.5

🔲 Chocolate Drink Powder ☞ serving size: 2 tbsp = 11 g; Calories = 38.5; Total Carb (g) = 7.5; Net Carb (g) = 6.5; Fat (g) = 0.5; Protein = 1

🔲 Chocolate Malt Powder Prepared With 1% Milk Fortified ☞

serving size: 1 cup dry mix = 98 g; Calories = 55.9; Total Carb (g) = 8.6; Net Carb (g) = 8.6; Fat (g) = 1; Protein = 3.3

Chocolate Malt Powder Prepared With Fat Free Milk ☞ serving size: 1 serving = 256 g; Calories = 125.4; Total Carb (g) = 22.1; Net Carb (g) = 22.1; Fat (g) = 0.4; Protein = 8.3

Chocolate Syrup ☞ serving size: 1 serving 2 tbsp = 39 g; Calories = 108.8; Total Carb (g) = 25.4; Net Carb (g) = 24.4; Fat (g) = 0.4; Protein = 0.8

Chocolate Syrup Prepared With Whole Milk ☞ serving size: 1 cup (8 fl oz) = 282 g; Calories = 253.8; Total Carb (g) = 36; Net Carb (g) = 35.2; Fat (g) = 8.4; Protein = 8.7

Chocolate-Flavor Beverage Mix For Milk Powder With Added Nutrients ☞ serving size: 1 serving = 22 g; Calories = 88; Total Carb (g) = 19.9; Net Carb (g) = 18.9; Fat (g) = 0.5; Protein = 1

Chocolate-Flavor Beverage Mix For Milk Powder With Added Nutrients Prepared With Whole Milk ☞ serving size: 1 serving = 266 g; Calories = 236.7; Total Carb (g) = 31.6; Net Carb (g) = 30.5; Fat (g) = 8.4; Protein = 8.7

Chocolate-Flavor Beverage Mix Powder Prepared With Whole Milk ☞ serving size: 1 cup (8 fl oz) = 266 g; Calories = 226.1; Total Carb (g) = 31.8; Net Carb (g) = 30.8; Fat (g) = 8.6; Protein = 8.6

Chocolate-Flavored Drink Whey And Milk Based ☞ serving size: 1 cup = 244 g; Calories = 119.6; Total Carb (g) = 26.1; Net Carb (g) = 24.6; Fat (g) = 1; Protein = 1.6

Citrus Energy Drink ☞ serving size: 8 fl oz = 240 g; Calories = 108; Total Carb (g) = 27.1; Net Carb (g) = 27.1; Fat (g) = 0; Protein = 0

Citrus Fruit Juice Drink Frozen Concentrate ☞ serving size: 1 fl oz = 35.2 g; Calories = 57; Total Carb (g) = 14.2; Net Carb (g) = 14.1; Fat (g) = 0; Protein = 0.4

Citrus Fruit Juice Drink Frozen Concentrate Prepared With

Water ☞ serving size: 1 fl oz = 31 g; Calories = 14.3; Total Carb (g) = 3.5; Net Carb (g) = 3.5; Fat (g) = 0; Protein = 0.1

Citrus Green Tea ☞ serving size: 1 cup = 265 g; Calories = 2.7; Total Carb (g) = 0.8; Net Carb (g) = 0.8; Fat (g) = 0; Protein = 0

Clam And Tomato Juice Canned ☞ serving size: 1 fl oz = 30.2 g; Calories = 14.5; Total Carb (g) = 3.3; Net Carb (g) = 3.2; Fat (g) = 0.1; Protein = 0.2

Claret ☞ serving size: 1 fl oz = 29.4 g; Calories = 24.4; Total Carb (g) = 0.9; Net Carb (g) = 0.9; Fat (g) = 0; Protein = 0

Club Soda ☞ serving size: 1 fl oz = 29.6 g; Calories = 0; Total Carb (g) = 0; Net Carb (g) = 0; Fat (g) = 0; Protein = 0

Coca-Cola Powerade Lemon-Lime Flavored Ready-To-Drink ☞ serving size: 1 fl oz = 30.5 g; Calories = 9.8; Total Carb (g) = 2.4; Net Carb (g) = 2.4; Fat (g) = 0; Protein = 0

Cocktail Mix Non-Alcoholic Concentrated Frozen ☞ serving size: 1 fl oz = 36 g; Calories = 103.3; Total Carb (g) = 25.8; Net Carb (g) = 25.8; Fat (g) = 0; Protein = 0

Cocoa Mix Low Calorie Powder With Added Calcium Phosphorus Aspartame Without Added Sodium Or Vitamin A ☞ serving size: 1 envelope swiss miss (.53 oz) = 15 g; Calories = 53.9; Total Carb (g) = 8.7; Net Carb (g) = 8.5; Fat (g) = 0.5; Protein = 3.8

Cocoa Mix Nestle Hot Cocoa Mix Rich Chocolate With Marshmallows ☞ serving size: 1 serving 1 envelope = 20 g; Calories = 80; Total Carb (g) = 15; Net Carb (g) = 14.3; Fat (g) = 3; Protein = 0.6

Cocoa Mix Nestle Rich Chocolate Hot Cocoa Mix ☞ serving size: 1 serving 1 envelope = 20 g; Calories = 80; Total Carb (g) = 15; Net Carb (g) = 14.2; Fat (g) = 3; Protein = 0.6

Cocoa Mix No Sugar Added Powder ☞ serving size: 1 envelope alba (.675 oz) = 19 g; Calories = 71.6; Total Carb (g) = 13.7; Net Carb (g) = 12.2; Fat (g) = 0.6; Protein = 2.9

🍵 Cocoa Mix Powder ☞ serving size: 1 serving (3 heaping tsp or 1 envelope) = 28 g; Calories = 111.4; Total Carb (g) = 23.4; Net Carb (g) = 22.4; Fat (g) = 1.1; Protein = 1.9

🍵 Cocoa Mix Powder Prepared With Water ☞ serving size: 1 fl oz = 34.3 g; Calories = 18.9; Total Carb (g) = 4; Net Carb (g) = 3.8; Fat (g) = 0.2; Protein = 0.3

🍵 Cocoa Mix With Aspartame Powder Prepared With Water ☞ serving size: 1 fl oz = 32.1 g; Calories = 9.3; Total Carb (g) = 1.8; Net Carb (g) = 1.6; Fat (g) = 0.1; Protein = 0.4

🍵 Coconut Milk Sweetened Fortified With Calcium Vitamins A B12 D2 ☞ serving size: 1 cup = 240 g; Calories = 74.4; Total Carb (g) = 7; Net Carb (g) = 7; Fat (g) = 5; Protein = 0.5

🍵 Coconut Water Ready-To-Drink Unsweetened ☞ serving size: 1 cup = 245 g; Calories = 44.1; Total Carb (g) = 10.4; Net Carb (g) = 10.4; Fat (g) = 0; Protein = 0.5

🍵 Coffee ☞ serving size: 1 fl oz = 29.6 g; Calories = 0.3; Total Carb (g) = 0; Net Carb (g) = 0; Fat (g) = 0; Protein = 0

🍵 Coffee And Cocoa Instant Decaffeinated With Whitener And Low Calorie Sweetener ☞ serving size: 1 tsp dry = 6.4 g; Calories = 28.2; Total Carb (g) = 4.6; Net Carb (g) = 4.3; Fat (g) = 0.9; Protein = 0.6

🍵 Coffee Bottled/canned Light ☞ serving size: 1 fl oz = 30 g; Calories = 10.5; Total Carb (g) = 1.8; Net Carb (g) = 1.8; Fat (g) = 0.2; Protein = 0.4

🍵 Coffee Brewed Blend Of Regular And Decaffeinated ☞ serving size: 1 fl oz = 30 g; Calories = 0; Total Carb (g) = 0; Net Carb (g) = 0; Fat (g) = 0; Protein = 0

🍵 Coffee Brewed Breakfast Blend ☞ serving size: 1 cup = 248 g; Calories = 5; Total Carb (g) = 0.4; Net Carb (g) = 0.4; Fat (g) = 0; Protein = 0.7

Coffee Brewed Espresso Restaurant-Prepared Decaffeinated ☞ serving size: 1 fl oz = 29.6 g; Calories = 2.7; Total Carb (g) = 0.5; Net Carb (g) = 0.5; Fat (g) = 0.1; Protein = 0

Coffee Cafe Con Leche ☞ serving size: 1 fl oz = 31 g; Calories = 12.1; Total Carb (g) = 1.8; Net Carb (g) = 1.8; Fat (g) = 0.3; Protein = 0.5

Coffee Cafe Con Leche Decaffeinated ☞ serving size: 1 fl oz = 31 g; Calories = 12.1; Total Carb (g) = 1.8; Net Carb (g) = 1.8; Fat (g) = 0.3; Protein = 0.5

Coffee Cafe Mocha ☞ serving size: 1 fl oz = 31 g; Calories = 19.8; Total Carb (g) = 3.2; Net Carb (g) = 3.2; Fat (g) = 0.5; Protein = 0.8

Coffee Cafe Mocha Decaffeinated ☞ serving size: 1 fl oz = 31 g; Calories = 19.8; Total Carb (g) = 3.2; Net Carb (g) = 3.2; Fat (g) = 0.5; Protein = 0.8

Coffee Cafe Mocha Decaffeinated Nonfat ☞ serving size: 1 fl oz = 31 g; Calories = 16.1; Total Carb (g) = 3.2; Net Carb (g) = 3.2; Fat (g) = 0; Protein = 0.8

Coffee Cafe Mocha Decaffeinated With Non-Dairy Milk ☞ serving size: 1 fl oz = 31 g; Calories = 17.7; Total Carb (g) = 3.4; Net Carb (g) = 3.3; Fat (g) = 0.3; Protein = 0.4

Coffee Cafe Mocha Nonfat ☞ serving size: 1 fl oz = 31 g; Calories = 16.1; Total Carb (g) = 3.2; Net Carb (g) = 3.2; Fat (g) = 0; Protein = 0.8

Coffee Cafe Mocha With Non-Dairy Milk ☞ serving size: 1 fl oz = 31 g; Calories = 17.7; Total Carb (g) = 3.4; Net Carb (g) = 3.3; Fat (g) = 0.3; Protein = 0.4

Coffee Cappuccino ☞ serving size: 1 fl oz = 30 g; Calories = 8.1; Total Carb (g) = 0.8; Net Carb (g) = 0.8; Fat (g) = 0.3; Protein = 0.5

Coffee Cappuccino Decaffeinated ☞ serving size: 1 fl oz = 30 g; Calories = 8.1; Total Carb (g) = 0.8; Net Carb (g) = 0.8; Fat (g) = 0.3; Protein = 0.5

Coffee Cappuccino Decaffeinated Nonfat ☞ serving size: 1 fl oz = 30 g; Calories = 5.7; Total Carb (g) = 0.8; Net Carb (g) = 0.8; Fat (g) = 0; Protein = 0.5

Coffee Cappuccino Decaffeinated With Non-Dairy Milk ☞ serving size: 1 fl oz = 30 g; Calories = 6.6; Total Carb (g) = 1; Net Carb (g) = 0.9; Fat (g) = 0.2; Protein = 0.2

Coffee Cappuccino Nonfat ☞ serving size: 1 fl oz = 30 g; Calories = 5.7; Total Carb (g) = 0.8; Net Carb (g) = 0.8; Fat (g) = 0; Protein = 0.5

Coffee Cappuccino With Non-Dairy Milk ☞ serving size: 1 fl oz = 30 g; Calories = 6.6; Total Carb (g) = 1; Net Carb (g) = 0.9; Fat (g) = 0.2; Protein = 0.2

Coffee Cream Liqueur ☞ serving size: 1 fl oz = 31.1 g; Calories = 101.7; Total Carb (g) = 6.5; Net Carb (g) = 6.5; Fat (g) = 4.9; Protein = 0.9

Coffee Cuban ☞ serving size: 1 fl oz = 31 g; Calories = 10.2; Total Carb (g) = 2.4; Net Carb (g) = 2.4; Fat (g) = 0.1; Protein = 0

Coffee Decaffeinated Pre-Lightened ☞ serving size: 1 fl oz = 30 g; Calories = 4.2; Total Carb (g) = 0.6; Net Carb (g) = 0.6; Fat (g) = 0.2; Protein = 0.1

Coffee Decaffeinated Pre-Lightened And Pre-Sweetened With Low Calorie Sweetener ☞ serving size: 1 fl oz = 30 g; Calories = 4.8; Total Carb (g) = 0.7; Net Carb (g) = 0.7; Fat (g) = 0.2; Protein = 0.1

Coffee Decaffeinated Pre-Lightened And Pre-Sweetened With Sugar ☞ serving size: 1 fl oz = 31 g; Calories = 8.1; Total Carb (g) = 1.6; Net Carb (g) = 1.6; Fat (g) = 0.2; Protein = 0

Coffee Decaffeinated Pre-Sweetened With Low Calorie Sweetener ☞ serving size: 1 fl oz = 30 g; Calories = 1.5; Total Carb (g) = 0.3; Net Carb (g) = 0.3; Fat (g) = 0; Protein = 0

Coffee Decaffeinated Pre-Sweetened With Sugar ☞ serving size:

1 fl oz = 31 g; Calories = 5; Total Carb (g) = 1.2; Net Carb (g) = 1.2; Fat (g) = 0; Protein = 0

🍶 Coffee Iced Cafe Mocha ☞ serving size: 1 fl oz = 31 g; Calories = 15.5; Total Carb (g) = 2.8; Net Carb (g) = 2.8; Fat (g) = 0.3; Protein = 0.5

🍶 Coffee Iced Cafe Mocha Decaffeinated ☞ serving size: 1 fl oz = 31 g; Calories = 15.8; Total Carb (g) = 2.8; Net Carb (g) = 2.8; Fat (g) = 0.3; Protein = 0.5

🍶 Coffee Iced Cafe Mocha Decaffeinated Nonfat ☞ serving size: 1 fl oz = 31 g; Calories = 13.3; Total Carb (g) = 2.8; Net Carb (g) = 2.8; Fat (g) = 0; Protein = 0.5

🍶 Coffee Iced Cafe Mocha Decaffeinated With Non-Dairy Milk ☞ serving size: 1 fl oz = 31 g; Calories = 14.3; Total Carb (g) = 2.9; Net Carb (g) = 2.9; Fat (g) = 0.2; Protein = 0.2

🍶 Coffee Iced Cafe Mocha Nonfat ☞ serving size: 1 fl oz = 31 g; Calories = 13.3; Total Carb (g) = 2.8; Net Carb (g) = 2.8; Fat (g) = 0; Protein = 0.5

🍶 Coffee Iced Cafe Mocha With Non-Dairy Milk ☞ serving size: 1 fl oz = 31 g; Calories = 14.3; Total Carb (g) = 2.9; Net Carb (g) = 2.9; Fat (g) = 0.2; Protein = 0.2

🍶 Coffee Iced Latte ☞ serving size: 1 fl oz = 30 g; Calories = 8.1; Total Carb (g) = 0.8; Net Carb (g) = 0.8; Fat (g) = 0.3; Protein = 0.5

🍶 Coffee Iced Latte Decaffeinated ☞ serving size: 1 fl oz = 30 g; Calories = 8.1; Total Carb (g) = 0.8; Net Carb (g) = 0.8; Fat (g) = 0.3; Protein = 0.5

🍶 Coffee Iced Latte Decaffeinated Flavored ☞ serving size: 1 fl oz = 31 g; Calories = 12.4; Total Carb (g) = 1.9; Net Carb (g) = 1.9; Fat (g) = 0.3; Protein = 0.5

🍶 Coffee Iced Latte Decaffeinated Nonfat ☞ serving size: 1 fl oz = 30 g; Calories = 5.7; Total Carb (g) = 0.9; Net Carb (g) = 0.9; Fat (g) = 0; Protein = 0.5

🍶 Coffee Iced Latte Decaffeinated Nonfat Flavored ☞ serving size: 1 fl oz = 31 g; Calories = 9.9; Total Carb (g) = 1.9; Net Carb (g) = 1.9; Fat (g) = 0; Protein = 0.5

🍶 Coffee Iced Latte Decaffeinated With Non-Dairy Milk ☞ serving size: 1 fl oz = 30 g; Calories = 6.9; Total Carb (g) = 1; Net Carb (g) = 0.9; Fat (g) = 0.2; Protein = 0.2

🍶 Coffee Iced Latte Decaffeinated With Non-Dairy Milk Flavored ☞ serving size: 1 fl oz = 31 g; Calories = 10.9; Total Carb (g) = 2; Net Carb (g) = 2; Fat (g) = 0.2; Protein = 0.2

🍶 Coffee Iced Latte Flavored ☞ serving size: 1 fl oz = 31 g; Calories = 12.1; Total Carb (g) = 1.9; Net Carb (g) = 1.9; Fat (g) = 0.3; Protein = 0.5

🍶 Coffee Iced Latte Nonfat ☞ serving size: 1 fl oz = 30 g; Calories = 5.7; Total Carb (g) = 0.9; Net Carb (g) = 0.9; Fat (g) = 0; Protein = 0.5

🍶 Coffee Iced Latte Nonfat Flavored ☞ serving size: 1 fl oz = 31 g; Calories = 9.9; Total Carb (g) = 1.9; Net Carb (g) = 1.9; Fat (g) = 0; Protein = 0.5

🍶 Coffee Iced Latte With Non-Dairy Milk ☞ serving size: 1 fl oz = 30 g; Calories = 6.6; Total Carb (g) = 1; Net Carb (g) = 0.9; Fat (g) = 0.2; Protein = 0.2

🍶 Coffee Iced Latte With Non-Dairy Milk Flavored ☞ serving size: 1 fl oz = 31 g; Calories = 10.9; Total Carb (g) = 2; Net Carb (g) = 2; Fat (g) = 0.2; Protein = 0.2

🍶 Coffee Instant 50% Less Caffeine Reconstituted ☞ serving size: 1 fl oz = 30 g; Calories = 0.9; Total Carb (g) = 0.2; Net Carb (g) = 0.2; Fat (g) = 0; Protein = 0

🍶 Coffee Instant Chicory ☞ serving size: 1 fl oz = 29.9 g; Calories = 0.9; Total Carb (g) = 0.2; Net Carb (g) = 0.2; Fat (g) = 0; Protein = 0

🍶 Coffee Instant Decaffeinated Powder ☞ serving size: 1 tsp

rounded = 1.8 g; Calories = 6.3; Total Carb (g) = 1.4; Net Carb (g) = 1.4; Fat (g) = 0; Protein = 0.2

Coffee Instant Decaffeinated Pre-Lightened And Pre-Sweetened With Low Calorie Sweetener Reconstituted ☞ serving size: 1 fl oz = 30 g; Calories = 4.8; Total Carb (g) = 0.7; Net Carb (g) = 0.7; Fat (g) = 0.2; Protein = 0.1

Coffee Instant Decaffeinated Pre-Lightened And Pre-Sweetened With Sugar Reconsititued ☞ serving size: 1 fl oz = 31 g; Calories = 8.1; Total Carb (g) = 1.6; Net Carb (g) = 1.6; Fat (g) = 0.2; Protein = 0

Coffee Instant Decaffeinated Prepared With Water ☞ serving size: 1 fl oz = 29.9 g; Calories = 0.6; Total Carb (g) = 0.1; Net Carb (g) = 0.1; Fat (g) = 0; Protein = 0

Coffee Instant Decaffeinated Reconstituted ☞ serving size: 1 fl oz = 30 g; Calories = 0.9; Total Carb (g) = 0.2; Net Carb (g) = 0.2; Fat (g) = 0; Protein = 0

Coffee Instant Mocha Sweetened ☞ serving size: 1 serving 2 tbsp = 13 g; Calories = 59.8; Total Carb (g) = 9.6; Net Carb (g) = 9.4; Fat (g) = 2.1; Protein = 0.7

Coffee Instant Pre-Lightened And Pre-Sweetened With Low Calorie Sweetener Reconstituted ☞ serving size: 1 fl oz = 30 g; Calories = 4.8; Total Carb (g) = 0.7; Net Carb (g) = 0.7; Fat (g) = 0.2; Protein = 0.1

Coffee Instant Pre-Lightened And Pre-Sweetened With Sugar Reconstituted ☞ serving size: 1 fl oz = 31 g; Calories = 8.4; Total Carb (g) = 1.6; Net Carb (g) = 1.6; Fat (g) = 0.2; Protein = 0.1

Coffee Instant Pre-Sweetened With Sugar Reconstituted ☞ serving size: 1 fl oz = 31 g; Calories = 5; Total Carb (g) = 1.2; Net Carb (g) = 1.2; Fat (g) = 0; Protein = 0

Coffee Instant Reconstituted ☞ serving size: 1 fl oz = 30 g; Calories = 0.9; Total Carb (g) = 0.2; Net Carb (g) = 0.2; Fat (g) = 0; Protein = 0

🔲 Coffee Instant Regular Half The Caffeine ☞ serving size: 1 tsp = 1 g; Calories = 3.5; Total Carb (g) = 0.7; Net Carb (g) = 0.7; Fat (g) = 0; Protein = 0.1

🔲 Coffee Instant Regular Powder ☞ serving size: 1 tsp = 1 g; Calories = 3.5; Total Carb (g) = 0.8; Net Carb (g) = 0.8; Fat (g) = 0; Protein = 0.1

🔲 Coffee Instant Vanilla Sweetened Decaffeinated With Non Dairy Creamer ☞ serving size: 1 serving = 15 g; Calories = 69.8; Total Carb (g) = 12.9; Net Carb (g) = 12.9; Fat (g) = 2; Protein = 0

🔲 Coffee Instant With Chicory ☞ serving size: 1 tsp, rounded = 1.8 g; Calories = 6.4; Total Carb (g) = 1.4; Net Carb (g) = 1.4; Fat (g) = 0; Protein = 0.2

🔲 Coffee Instant With Whitener Reduced Calorie ☞ serving size: 1 tsp dry = 1.7 g; Calories = 8.7; Total Carb (g) = 1; Net Carb (g) = 1; Fat (g) = 0.5; Protein = 0

🔲 Coffee Latte ☞ serving size: 1 fl oz = 30 g; Calories = 12.9; Total Carb (g) = 1.3; Net Carb (g) = 1.3; Fat (g) = 0.5; Protein = 0.8

🔲 Coffee Latte Decaffeinated ☞ serving size: 1 fl oz = 30 g; Calories = 12.9; Total Carb (g) = 1.3; Net Carb (g) = 1.3; Fat (g) = 0.5; Protein = 0.8

🔲 Coffee Latte Decaffeinated Flavored ☞ serving size: 1 fl oz = 31 g; Calories = 17.1; Total Carb (g) = 2.3; Net Carb (g) = 2.3; Fat (g) = 0.5; Protein = 0.8

🔲 Coffee Latte Decaffeinated Nonfat ☞ serving size: 1 fl oz = 30 g; Calories = 9; Total Carb (g) = 1.3; Net Carb (g) = 1.3; Fat (g) = 0; Protein = 0.9

🔲 Coffee Latte Decaffeinated Nonfat Flavored ☞ serving size: 1 fl oz = 31 g; Calories = 13; Total Carb (g) = 2.4; Net Carb (g) = 2.4; Fat (g) = 0; Protein = 0.9

◻ Coffee Latte Decaffeinated With Non-Dairy Milk ☞ serving size: 1 fl oz = 30 g; Calories = 10.5; Total Carb (g) = 1.5; Net Carb (g) = 1.4; Fat (g) = 0.3; Protein = 0.4

◻ Coffee Latte Decaffeinated With Non-Dairy Milk Flavored ☞ serving size: 1 fl oz = 31 g; Calories = 14.6; Total Carb (g) = 2.6; Net Carb (g) = 2.5; Fat (g) = 0.3; Protein = 0.4

◻ Coffee Latte Flavored ☞ serving size: 1 fl oz = 31 g; Calories = 16.7; Total Carb (g) = 2.3; Net Carb (g) = 2.3; Fat (g) = 0.5; Protein = 0.8

◻ Coffee Latte Nonfat ☞ serving size: 1 fl oz = 30 g; Calories = 9; Total Carb (g) = 1.3; Net Carb (g) = 1.3; Fat (g) = 0; Protein = 0.9

◻ Coffee Latte Nonfat Flavored ☞ serving size: 1 fl oz = 31 g; Calories = 13; Total Carb (g) = 2.3; Net Carb (g) = 2.3; Fat (g) = 0; Protein = 0.9

◻ Coffee Latte With Non-Dairy Milk ☞ serving size: 1 fl oz = 30 g; Calories = 10.5; Total Carb (g) = 1.5; Net Carb (g) = 1.5; Fat (g) = 0.3; Protein = 0.4

◻ Coffee Latte With Non-Dairy Milk Flavored ☞ serving size: 1 fl oz = 31 g; Calories = 14.6; Total Carb (g) = 2.5; Net Carb (g) = 2.5; Fat (g) = 0.3; Protein = 0.4

◻ Coffee Liqueur ☞ serving size: 1 fl oz = 34.8 g; Calories = 116.9; Total Carb (g) = 16.3; Net Carb (g) = 16.3; Fat (g) = 0.1; Protein = 0

◻ Coffee Macchiato ☞ serving size: 1 fl oz = 30 g; Calories = 6.9; Total Carb (g) = 0.8; Net Carb (g) = 0.8; Fat (g) = 0.2; Protein = 0.4

◻ Coffee Macchiato Sweetened ☞ serving size: 1 fl oz = 31 g; Calories = 11.8; Total Carb (g) = 2.1; Net Carb (g) = 2.1; Fat (g) = 0.2; Protein = 0.3

◻ Coffee Mocha Instant Decaffeinated Pre-Lightened And Pre-

Sweetened With Low Calorie Sweetener Reconstituted ☞ serving size: 1 fl oz = 30 g; Calories = 4.2; Total Carb (g) = 0.7; Net Carb (g) = 0.6; Fat (g) = 0.1; Protein = 0.1

🍵 Coffee Mocha Instant Pre-Lightened And Pre-Sweetened With Low Calorie Sweetener Reconstituted ☞ serving size: 1 fl oz = 30 g; Calories = 4.5; Total Carb (g) = 0.7; Net Carb (g) = 0.7; Fat (g) = 0.1; Protein = 0.1

🍵 Coffee Mocha Instant Pre-Lightened And Pre-Sweetened With Sugar Reconstituted ☞ serving size: 1 fl oz = 31 g; Calories = 13.6; Total Carb (g) = 2; Net Carb (g) = 2; Fat (g) = 0.6; Protein = 0.1

🍵 Coffee Pre-Lightened ☞ serving size: 1 fl oz = 30 g; Calories = 4.2; Total Carb (g) = 0.6; Net Carb (g) = 0.6; Fat (g) = 0.2; Protein = 0.1

🍵 Coffee Pre-Lightened And Pre-Sweetened With Low Calorie Sweetener ☞ serving size: 1 fl oz = 30 g; Calories = 4.8; Total Carb (g) = 0.7; Net Carb (g) = 0.7; Fat (g) = 0.2; Protein = 0.1

🍵 Coffee Pre-Lightened And Pre-Sweetened With Sugar ☞ serving size: 1 fl oz = 31 g; Calories = 8.4; Total Carb (g) = 1.6; Net Carb (g) = 1.6; Fat (g) = 0.2; Protein = 0.1

🍵 Coffee Pre-Sweetened With Low Calorie Sweetener ☞ serving size: 1 fl oz = 30 g; Calories = 1.5; Total Carb (g) = 0.3; Net Carb (g) = 0.3; Fat (g) = 0; Protein = 0

🍵 Coffee Pre-Sweetened With Sugar ☞ serving size: 1 fl oz = 31 g; Calories = 5; Total Carb (g) = 1.2; Net Carb (g) = 1.2; Fat (g) = 0; Protein = 0

🍵 Coffee Ready To Drink Milk Based Sweetened ☞ serving size: 1 cup = 262 g; Calories = 186; Total Carb (g) = 33; Net Carb (g) = 33; Fat (g) = 3.6; Protein = 5.2

🍵 Coffee Ready To Drink Vanilla Light Milk Based Sweetened ☞ serving size: fl oz = 281 g; Calories = 101.2; Total Carb (g) = 12; Net Carb (g) = 12; Fat (g) = 3; Protein = 6

🍶 Coffee Substitute Cereal Grain Beverage Powder ☞ serving size: 1 tsp (1 serving) = 3 g; Calories = 10.8; Total Carb (g) = 2.4; Net Carb (g) = 1.7; Fat (g) = 0.1; Protein = 0.2

🍶 Coffee Substitute Cereal Grain Beverage Powder Prepared With Whole Milk ☞ serving size: 6 fl oz = 185 g; Calories = 120.3; Total Carb (g) = 10.4; Net Carb (g) = 10.2; Fat (g) = 6.1; Protein = 6.1

🍶 Coffee Substitute Cereal Grain Beverage Prepared With Water ☞ serving size: 1 fl oz = 30.1 g; Calories = 1.8; Total Carb (g) = 0.4; Net Carb (g) = 0.3; Fat (g) = 0; Protein = 0

🍶 Coffee Turkish ☞ serving size: 1 fl oz = 31 g; Calories = 8.1; Total Carb (g) = 2; Net Carb (g) = 2; Fat (g) = 0; Protein = 0

🍶 Cola Soft Drink ☞ serving size: 1 fl oz = 30.7 g; Calories = 12.9; Total Carb (g) = 3.2; Net Carb (g) = 3.2; Fat (g) = 0.1; Protein = 0

🍶 Corn Beverage ☞ serving size: 1 fl oz = 30 g; Calories = 13.2; Total Carb (g) = 2.8; Net Carb (g) = 2.7; Fat (g) = 0.1; Protein = 0.3

🍶 Cornmeal Beverage ☞ serving size: 1 cup = 248 g; Calories = 208.3; Total Carb (g) = 40.7; Net Carb (g) = 40.2; Fat (g) = 3.8; Protein = 4.1

🍶 Cranberry Juice Cocktail ☞ serving size: 1 cup = 271 g; Calories = 140.9; Total Carb (g) = 33.2; Net Carb (g) = 33.2; Fat (g) = 0.9; Protein = 0

🍶 Cranberry Juice Cocktail Bottled ☞ serving size: 1 fl oz = 31.6 g; Calories = 17.1; Total Carb (g) = 4.3; Net Carb (g) = 4.3; Fat (g) = 0; Protein = 0

🍶 Cranberry Juice Cocktail Bottled Low Calorie With Calcium Saccharin And Corn Sweetener ☞ serving size: 1 fl oz = 29.6 g; Calories = 5.6; Total Carb (g) = 1.4; Net Carb (g) = 1.4; Fat (g) = 0; Protein = 0

🍶 Cranberry Juice Cocktail Frozen Concentrate ☞ serving size: 1 fl oz = 36.2 g; Calories = 72.8; Total Carb (g) = 18.6; Net Carb (g) = 18.6; Fat (g) = 0; Protein = 0

🍶 Cranberry Juice Cocktail Frozen Concentrate Prepared With Water ☞ serving size: 1 fl oz = 29.6 g; Calories = 13.9; Total Carb (g) = 3.5; Net Carb (g) = 3.5; Fat (g) = 0; Protein = 0

🍶 Cranberry-Apple Juice Drink Bottled ☞ serving size: 1 fl oz = 30.6 g; Calories = 19.3; Total Carb (g) = 4.9; Net Carb (g) = 4.9; Fat (g) = 0; Protein = 0

🍶 Cranberry-Apple Juice Drink Low Calorie With Vitamin C Added ☞ serving size: 1 cup (8 fl oz) = 240 g; Calories = 45.6; Total Carb (g) = 11.3; Net Carb (g) = 11; Fat (g) = 0; Protein = 0.2

🍶 Cranberry-Apricot Juice Drink Bottled ☞ serving size: 1 fl oz = 30.6 g; Calories = 19.6; Total Carb (g) = 5; Net Carb (g) = 4.9; Fat (g) = 0; Protein = 0.1

🍶 Cranberry-Grape Juice Drink Bottled ☞ serving size: 1 fl oz = 30.6 g; Calories = 17.1; Total Carb (g) = 4.3; Net Carb (g) = 4.3; Fat (g) = 0; Protein = 0.1

🍶 Cream Soda ☞ serving size: 1 fl oz = 30.9 g; Calories = 15.8; Total Carb (g) = 4.1; Net Carb (g) = 4.1; Fat (g) = 0; Protein = 0

🍶 Cytosport Muscle Milk Ready-To-Drink ☞ serving size: 14 fl oz = 414 g; Calories = 215.3; Total Carb (g) = 9.4; Net Carb (g) = 8.6; Fat (g) = 9; Protein = 24.3

🍶 Daiquiri ☞ serving size: 1 fl oz = 30.5 g; Calories = 38.1; Total Carb (g) = 4.8; Net Carb (g) = 4.8; Fat (g) = 0; Protein = 0

🍶 Dairy Drink Mix Chocolate Reduced Calorie With Aspartame Powder Prepared With Water And Ice ☞ serving size: 1 serving = 243 g; Calories = 70.5; Total Carb (g) = 11; Net Carb (g) = 9; Fat (g) = 0.6; Protein = 5.3

🍶 Dairy Drink Mix Chocolate Reduced Calorie With Low-Calorie Sweeteners Powder ☞ serving size: 1 packet (.75 oz) = 21 g; Calories =

69.1; Total Carb (g) = 10.8; Net Carb (g) = 8.8; Fat (g) = 0.6; Protein = 5.3

🍶 Decaf Coffee ☞ serving size: 1 fl oz = 29.6 g; Calories = 0; Total Carb (g) = 0; Net Carb (g) = 0; Fat (g) = 0; Protein = 0

🍶 Diet Cola ☞ serving size: 1 fl oz = 29.6 g; Calories = 5.9; Total Carb (g) = 1.5; Net Carb (g) = 1.5; Fat (g) = 0; Protein = 0

🍶 Diet Green Tea ☞ serving size: 1 cup = 269 g; Calories = 10.8; Total Carb (g) = 2.5; Net Carb (g) = 2.5; Fat (g) = 0; Protein = 0

🍶 Diet Pepper Cola ☞ serving size: 1 fl oz = 29.6 g; Calories = 0.3; Total Carb (g) = 0; Net Carb (g) = 0; Fat (g) = 0; Protein = 0

🍶 Drink Mix Quaker Oats Gatorade Orange Flavor Powder ☞ serving size: 1 scoop powder = 23 g; Calories = 89.2; Total Carb (g) = 21.7; Net Carb (g) = 21.7; Fat (g) = 0.3; Protein = 0

🍶 Dry Dessert Wine ☞ serving size: 1 fl oz = 29.5 g; Calories = 44.8; Total Carb (g) = 3.4; Net Carb (g) = 3.4; Fat (g) = 0; Protein = 0.1

🍶 Eggnog Alcoholic ☞ serving size: 1 fl oz = 30 g; Calories = 33.9; Total Carb (g) = 2; Net Carb (g) = 2; Fat (g) = 1; Protein = 1.1

🍶 Eggnog-Flavor Mix Powder Prepared With Whole Milk ☞ serving size: 1 cup (8 fl oz) = 272 g; Calories = 258.4; Total Carb (g) = 38.6; Net Carb (g) = 38.6; Fat (g) = 8.2; Protein = 8

🍶 Energy Drink ☞ serving size: 8 fl oz = 240 g; Calories = 148.8; Total Carb (g) = 36; Net Carb (g) = 36; Fat (g) = 0; Protein = 1

🍶 Energy Drink Amp ☞ serving size: 1 serving = 240 g; Calories = 110.4; Total Carb (g) = 29; Net Carb (g) = 29; Fat (g) = 0.2; Protein = 0.6

🍶 Energy Drink Amp Sugar Free ☞ serving size: 8 fl oz = 240 g; Calories = 4.8; Total Carb (g) = 2.5; Net Carb (g) = 2.5; Fat (g) = 0; Protein = 0

🍶 Energy Drink Full Throttle ☞ serving size: 1 serving 8 fluid oz =

240 g; Calories = 110.4; Total Carb (g) = 29; Net Carb (g) = 29; Fat (g) = 0.2; Protein = 0.6

🍶 Energy Drink Monster Fortified With Vitamins C B2 B3 B6 B12 ☞ serving size: 1 serving = 240 g; Calories = 112.8; Total Carb (g) = 27.1; Net Carb (g) = 27.1; Fat (g) = 0; Protein = 1.1

🍶 Energy Drink Red Bull ☞ serving size: 1 can 8.4 fl oz = 258 g; Calories = 110.9; Total Carb (g) = 26.4; Net Carb (g) = 26.4; Fat (g) = 0; Protein = 1.2

🍶 Energy Drink Red Bull Sugar Free With Added Caffeine Niacin Pantothenic Acid Vitamins B6 And B12 ☞ serving size: 1 serving 8.3 fl oz can = 250 g; Calories = 12.5; Total Carb (g) = 1.8; Net Carb (g) = 1.8; Fat (g) = 0.2; Protein = 0.6

🍶 Energy Drink Rockstar ☞ serving size: 1 fl oz = 31 g; Calories = 18; Total Carb (g) = 3.9; Net Carb (g) = 3.9; Fat (g) = 0.1; Protein = 0.1

🍶 Energy Drink Rockstar Sugar Free ☞ serving size: 8 fl oz = 240 g; Calories = 9.6; Total Carb (g) = 1.7; Net Carb (g) = 1.7; Fat (g) = 0.2; Protein = 0.6

🍶 Energy Drink Sugar Free ☞ serving size: 8 fl oz = 240 g; Calories = 9.6; Total Carb (g) = 1; Net Carb (g) = 1; Fat (g) = 0; Protein = 1

🍶 Energy Drink Vault Citrus Flavor ☞ serving size: 1 oz = 31 g; Calories = 15.2; Total Carb (g) = 4; Net Carb (g) = 4; Fat (g) = 0; Protein = 0

🍶 Energy Drink Vault Zero Sugar-Free Citrus Flavor ☞ serving size: 1 serving (8 fl oz) = 246 g; Calories = 2.5; Total Carb (g) = 1.7; Net Carb (g) = 1.7; Fat (g) = 0.2; Protein = 0.6

🍶 Espresso ☞ serving size: 1 fl oz = 29.6 g; Calories = 2.7; Total Carb (g) = 0.5; Net Carb (g) = 0.5; Fat (g) = 0.1; Protein = 0

🍶 Fluid Replacement 5% Glucose In Water ☞ serving size: 1 cup = 240 g; Calories = 43.2; Total Carb (g) = 12; Net Carb (g) = 12; Fat (g) = 0; Protein = 0

⬜ Frozen Coffee Drink ☞ serving size: 1 fl oz = 31 g; Calories = 20.8; Total Carb (g) = 4.2; Net Carb (g) = 4.2; Fat (g) = 0.3; Protein = 0.5

⬜ Frozen Coffee Drink Decaffeinated ☞ serving size: 1 fl oz = 31 g; Calories = 20.8; Total Carb (g) = 4.2; Net Carb (g) = 4.2; Fat (g) = 0.3; Protein = 0.5

⬜ Frozen Coffee Drink Decaffeinated Nonfat ☞ serving size: 1 fl oz = 31 g; Calories = 18.6; Total Carb (g) = 4.2; Net Carb (g) = 4.2; Fat (g) = 0; Protein = 0.5

⬜ Frozen Coffee Drink Decaffeinated Nonfat With Whipped Cream ☞ serving size: 1 fl oz = 31 g; Calories = 23.3; Total Carb (g) = 4; Net Carb (g) = 4; Fat (g) = 0.6; Protein = 0.5

⬜ Frozen Coffee Drink Decaffeinated With Non-Dairy Milk ☞ serving size: 1 fl oz = 31 g; Calories = 19.8; Total Carb (g) = 4.2; Net Carb (g) = 4.2; Fat (g) = 0.2; Protein = 0.4

⬜ Frozen Coffee Drink Decaffeinated With Non-Dairy Milk And Whipped Cream ☞ serving size: 1 fl oz = 31 g; Calories = 23.9; Total Carb (g) = 4.1; Net Carb (g) = 4.1; Fat (g) = 0.8; Protein = 0.3

⬜ Frozen Coffee Drink Decaffeinated With Whipped Cream ☞ serving size: 1 fl oz = 31 g; Calories = 25.1; Total Carb (g) = 4; Net Carb (g) = 4; Fat (g) = 0.9; Protein = 0.5

⬜ Frozen Coffee Drink Nonfat ☞ serving size: 1 fl oz = 31 g; Calories = 18.3; Total Carb (g) = 4.2; Net Carb (g) = 4.2; Fat (g) = 0; Protein = 0.5

⬜ Frozen Coffee Drink Nonfat With Whipped Cream ☞ serving size: 1 fl oz = 31 g; Calories = 22.9; Total Carb (g) = 4; Net Carb (g) = 4; Fat (g) = 0.6; Protein = 0.5

⬜ Frozen Coffee Drink With Non-Dairy Milk ☞ serving size: 1 fl oz = 31 g; Calories = 19.2; Total Carb (g) = 4.3; Net Carb (g) = 4.3; Fat (g) = 0.2; Protein = 0.2

⬜ Frozen Coffee Drink With Non-Dairy Milk And Whipped

Cream ☞ serving size: 1 fl oz = 31 g; Calories = 23.9; Total Carb (g) = 4.1; Net Carb (g) = 4.1; Fat (g) = 0.8; Protein = 0.3

🥤 Frozen Coffee Drink With Whipped Cream ☞ serving size: 1 fl oz = 31 g; Calories = 25.1; Total Carb (g) = 4; Net Carb (g) = 4; Fat (g) = 0.9; Protein = 0.5

🥤 Frozen Daiquiri ☞ serving size: 1 fl oz = 30 g; Calories = 38.1; Total Carb (g) = 5.3; Net Carb (g) = 5.3; Fat (g) = 0; Protein = 0

🥤 Frozen Daiquiri Mix From Frozen Concentrate Reconstituted ☞ serving size: 1 fl oz = 29 g; Calories = 19.1; Total Carb (g) = 4.8; Net Carb (g) = 4.8; Fat (g) = 0; Protein = 0

🥤 Frozen Margarita ☞ serving size: 1 fl oz = 30 g; Calories = 36.6; Total Carb (g) = 4.8; Net Carb (g) = 4.8; Fat (g) = 0; Protein = 0

🥤 Frozen Mocha Coffee Drink ☞ serving size: 1 fl oz = 31 g; Calories = 20.5; Total Carb (g) = 4; Net Carb (g) = 4; Fat (g) = 0.3; Protein = 0.5

🥤 Frozen Mocha Coffee Drink Decaffeinated ☞ serving size: 1 fl oz = 31 g; Calories = 20.5; Total Carb (g) = 4.1; Net Carb (g) = 4.1; Fat (g) = 0.3; Protein = 0.5

🥤 Frozen Mocha Coffee Drink Decaffeinated Nonfat ☞ serving size: 1 fl oz = 31 g; Calories = 18.3; Total Carb (g) = 4.1; Net Carb (g) = 4.1; Fat (g) = 0; Protein = 0.5

🥤 Frozen Mocha Coffee Drink Decaffeinated Nonfat With Whipped Cream ☞ serving size: 1 fl oz = 31 g; Calories = 22.6; Total Carb (g) = 3.9; Net Carb (g) = 3.9; Fat (g) = 0.6; Protein = 0.5

🥤 Frozen Mocha Coffee Drink Decaffeinated With Non-Dairy Milk ☞ serving size: 1 fl oz = 31 g; Calories = 19.2; Total Carb (g) = 4.2; Net Carb (g) = 4.2; Fat (g) = 0.2; Protein = 0.2

🥤 Frozen Mocha Coffee Drink Decaffeinated With Non-Dairy Milk And Whipped Cream ☞ serving size: 1 fl oz = 31 g; Calories = 23.6; Total Carb (g) = 4; Net Carb (g) = 4; Fat (g) = 0.8; Protein = 0.3

Frozen Mocha Coffee Drink Decaffeinated With Whipped Cream ☞ serving size: 1 fl oz = 31 g; Calories = 24.8; Total Carb (g) = 3.9; Net Carb (g) = 3.9; Fat (g) = 0.9; Protein = 0.5

Frozen Mocha Coffee Drink Nonfat ☞ serving size: 1 fl oz = 31 g; Calories = 18.3; Total Carb (g) = 4.1; Net Carb (g) = 4.1; Fat (g) = 0; Protein = 0.5

Frozen Mocha Coffee Drink Nonfat With Whipped Cream ☞ serving size: 1 fl oz = 31 g; Calories = 22.6; Total Carb (g) = 3.9; Net Carb (g) = 3.9; Fat (g) = 0.6; Protein = 0.5

Frozen Mocha Coffee Drink With Non-Dairy Milk ☞ serving size: 1 fl oz = 31 g; Calories = 18.9; Total Carb (g) = 4.2; Net Carb (g) = 4.1; Fat (g) = 0.2; Protein = 0.2

Frozen Mocha Coffee Drink With Non-Dairy Milk And Whipped Cream ☞ serving size: 1 fl oz = 31 g; Calories = 23.6; Total Carb (g) = 4; Net Carb (g) = 4; Fat (g) = 0.8; Protein = 0.3

Frozen Mocha Coffee Drink With Whipped Cream ☞ serving size: 1 fl oz = 31 g; Calories = 24.8; Total Carb (g) = 3.9; Net Carb (g) = 3.9; Fat (g) = 0.8; Protein = 0.5

Fruit And Vegetable Smoothie ☞ serving size: 1 fl oz = 27 g; Calories = 16.2; Total Carb (g) = 3.6; Net Carb (g) = 3.2; Fat (g) = 0.2; Protein = 0.5

Fruit And Vegetable Smoothie Added Protein ☞ serving size: 1 fl oz = 27 g; Calories = 22.4; Total Carb (g) = 3.4; Net Carb (g) = 3; Fat (g) = 0.2; Protein = 2.1

Fruit Flavored Drink Containing Less Than 3% Fruit Juice With High Vitamin C ☞ serving size: 1 cup (8 fl oz) = 238 g; Calories = 64.3; Total Carb (g) = 15.9; Net Carb (g) = 15.9; Fat (g) = 0; Protein = 0

Fruit Flavored Drink Less Than 3% Juice Not Fortified With Vitamin C ☞ serving size: 1 cup (8 fl oz) = 238 g; Calories = 152.3; Total Carb (g) = 38.2; Net Carb (g) = 38.2; Fat (g) = 0; Protein = 0

🍹 Fruit Flavored Drink Reduced Sugar Greater Than 3% Fruit Juice High Vitamin C Added Calcium ☞ serving size: 8 fl oz = 240 g; Calories = 69.6; Total Carb (g) = 16; Net Carb (g) = 16; Fat (g) = 0.9; Protein = 0

🍹 Fruit Flavored Drink With High Vitamin C Powdered Reconstituted ☞ serving size: 1 fl oz (no ice) = 31 g; Calories = 12.7; Total Carb (g) = 3.2; Net Carb (g) = 3.2; Fat (g) = 0; Protein = 0

🍹 Fruit Flavored Smoothie Drink Frozen Light No Dairy ☞ serving size: 1 fl oz = 30 g; Calories = 3.6; Total Carb (g) = 1; Net Carb (g) = 1; Fat (g) = 0; Protein = 0

🍹 Fruit Flavored Smoothie Drink Frozen No Dairy ☞ serving size: 1 fl oz = 30 g; Calories = 8.4; Total Carb (g) = 2.3; Net Carb (g) = 2.3; Fat (g) = 0; Protein = 0

🍹 Fruit Juice Drink Citrus Carbonated ☞ serving size: 1 fl oz (no ice) = 31 g; Calories = 9.3; Total Carb (g) = 2.2; Net Carb (g) = 2.1; Fat (g) = 0; Protein = 0.2

🍹 Fruit Juice Drink Diet ☞ serving size: 1 fl oz (no ice) = 30 g; Calories = 0.3; Total Carb (g) = 0.1; Net Carb (g) = 0.1; Fat (g) = 0; Protein = 0

🍹 Fruit Juice Drink Greater Than 3% Fruit Juice High Vitamin C And Added Thiamin ☞ serving size: 8 fl oz = 237 g; Calories = 128; Total Carb (g) = 31.2; Net Carb (g) = 31; Fat (g) = 0; Protein = 0.3

🍹 Fruit Juice Drink Greater Than 3% Juice High Vitamin C ☞ serving size: 1 cup (8 fl oz) = 238 g; Calories = 109.5; Total Carb (g) = 27; Net Carb (g) = 26.8; Fat (g) = 0.3; Protein = 0.3

🍹 Fruit Juice Drink Noncitrus Carbonated ☞ serving size: 1 fl oz (no ice) = 31 g; Calories = 10.2; Total Carb (g) = 2.6; Net Carb (g) = 2.6; Fat (g) = 0; Protein = 0.1

🍹 Fruit Juice Drink Reduced Sugar (Sunny D) ☞ serving size: 1 fl oz (no ice) = 31 g; Calories = 0.6; Total Carb (g) = 0.3; Net Carb (g) = 0.3; Fat (g) = 0; Protein = 0

Fruit Juice Drink Reduced Sugar With Vitamin E Added ☞ serving size: 1 container = 209 g; Calories = 81.5; Total Carb (g) = 20.9; Net Carb (g) = 20.9; Fat (g) = 0.2; Protein = 0

Fruit Punch Drink Frozen Concentrate ☞ serving size: 1 fl oz = 34.8 g; Calories = 56.4; Total Carb (g) = 14.4; Net Carb (g) = 14.3; Fat (g) = 0; Protein = 0.1

Fruit Punch Drink Frozen Concentrate Prepared With Water ☞ serving size: 1 fl oz = 30.9 g; Calories = 14.2; Total Carb (g) = 3.6; Net Carb (g) = 3.6; Fat (g) = 0; Protein = 0

Fruit Punch Drink With Added Nutrients Canned ☞ serving size: 1 fl oz = 31 g; Calories = 14.6; Total Carb (g) = 3.7; Net Carb (g) = 3.6; Fat (g) = 0; Protein = 0

Fruit Punch Drink Without Added Nutrients Canned ☞ serving size: 6 (3/4) fl oz = 210 g; Calories = 100.8; Total Carb (g) = 25.1; Net Carb (g) = 25.1; Fat (g) = 0; Protein = 0

Fruit Punch Juice Drink Frozen Concentrate ☞ serving size: 1 fl oz = 35.2 g; Calories = 61.6; Total Carb (g) = 15.2; Net Carb (g) = 15.1; Fat (g) = 0.3; Protein = 0.1

Fruit Punch Juice Drink Frozen Concentrate Prepared With Water ☞ serving size: 1 fl oz = 29.3 g; Calories = 12.3; Total Carb (g) = 3.3; Net Carb (g) = 3.3; Fat (g) = 0.1; Protein = 0

Fruit Punch-Flavor Drink Powder Without Added Sodium Prepared With Water ☞ serving size: 1 fl oz = 32.7 g; Calories = 12.1; Total Carb (g) = 3.1; Net Carb (g) = 3.1; Fat (g) = 0; Protein = 0

Fruit Smoothie Juice Drink No Dairy ☞ serving size: 1 fl oz = 27 g; Calories = 13.5; Total Carb (g) = 3.4; Net Carb (g) = 3; Fat (g) = 0; Protein = 0.2

Fruit Smoothie Light ☞ serving size: 1 fl oz = 27 g; Calories = 14; Total Carb (g) = 2.6; Net Carb (g) = 2.3; Fat (g) = 0.2; Protein = 0.7

Fruit Smoothie Nfs ☞ serving size: 1 fl oz = 27 g; Calories = 17; Total Carb (g) = 3.2; Net Carb (g) = 2.8; Fat (g) = 0.3; Protein = 0.6

Fruit Smoothie With Whole Fruit And Dairy ☞ serving size: 1 fl oz = 27 g; Calories = 17; Total Carb (g) = 3.2; Net Carb (g) = 2.8; Fat (g) = 0.3; Protein = 0.6

Fruit Smoothie With Whole Fruit And Dairy Added Protein ☞ serving size: 1 fl oz = 27 g; Calories = 20.8; Total Carb (g) = 2.6; Net Carb (g) = 2.3; Fat (g) = 0.3; Protein = 2

Fruit Smoothie With Whole Fruit No Dairy ☞ serving size: 1 fl oz = 27 g; Calories = 14.3; Total Carb (g) = 3.5; Net Carb (g) = 3.1; Fat (g) = 0.1; Protein = 0.2

Fruit Smoothie With Whole Fruit No Dairy Added Protein ☞ serving size: 1 fl oz = 27 g; Calories = 20.3; Total Carb (g) = 3.4; Net Carb (g) = 2.9; Fat (g) = 0.1; Protein = 1.7

Fruit-Flavored Drink Dry Powdered Mix Low Calorie With Aspartame ☞ serving size: 1 tsp = 8 g; Calories = 17.4; Total Carb (g) = 7; Net Carb (g) = 7; Fat (g) = 0; Protein = 0

Fruit-Flavored Drink Powder With High Vitamin C With Other Added Vitamins Low Calorie ☞ serving size: 1 tsp = 2 g; Calories = 4.5; Total Carb (g) = 1.8; Net Carb (g) = 1.8; Fat (g) = 0; Protein = 0

Fume Blanc ☞ serving size: 1 fl oz = 29.3 g; Calories = 24; Total Carb (g) = 0.7; Net Carb (g) = 0.7; Fat (g) = 0; Protein = 0

Fuze Orange Mango Fortified With Vitamins A C E B6 ☞ serving size: 1 bottle = 500 g; Calories = 190; Total Carb (g) = 46; Net Carb (g) = 45; Fat (g) = 0.3; Protein = 3.4

Gamay (Red Wine) ☞ serving size: 1 fl oz = 29.4 g; Calories = 22.9; Total Carb (g) = 0.7; Net Carb (g) = 0.7; Fat (g) = 0; Protein = 0

Gelatin Shot Alcoholic ☞ serving size: 1 shot = 42 g; Calories = 69.3; Total Carb (g) = 7.5; Net Carb (g) = 7.5; Fat (g) = 0; Protein = 0.7

Gerolsteiner Brunnen Gmbh & Co. Kggerolsteiner Naturally Sparkling Mineral Water ☞ serving size: 8 fl oz = 240 g; Calories = 0; Total Carb (g) = 0; Net Carb (g) = 0; Fat (g) = 0; Protein = 0

Gewurztraminer ☞ serving size: 1 fl oz = 29.5 g; Calories = 23.9; Total Carb (g) = 0.8; Net Carb (g) = 0.8; Fat (g) = 0; Protein = 0

Gewurztraminer (Late Harvest) ☞ serving size: 1 fl oz = 30.5 g; Calories = 32.9; Total Carb (g) = 3.5; Net Carb (g) = 3.5; Fat (g) = 0; Protein = 0

Ginger Ale ☞ serving size: 1 fl oz = 30.5 g; Calories = 10.4; Total Carb (g) = 2.7; Net Carb (g) = 2.7; Fat (g) = 0; Protein = 0

Grape Drink Canned ☞ serving size: 1 fl oz = 31.3 g; Calories = 19.1; Total Carb (g) = 4.9; Net Carb (g) = 4.9; Fat (g) = 0; Protein = 0

Grape Juice Drink Canned ☞ serving size: 1 fl oz = 31.3 g; Calories = 17.8; Total Carb (g) = 4.6; Net Carb (g) = 4.5; Fat (g) = 0; Protein = 0

Grape Juice Drink Light ☞ serving size: 1 fl oz (no ice) = 30 g; Calories = 6.3; Total Carb (g) = 1.6; Net Carb (g) = 1.5; Fat (g) = 0; Protein = 0

Grape Soda ☞ serving size: 1 fl oz = 31 g; Calories = 13.3; Total Carb (g) = 3.5; Net Carb (g) = 3.5; Fat (g) = 0; Protein = 0

Green Tea ☞ serving size: 16 fl oz = 473 g; Calories = 0; Total Carb (g) = 0; Net Carb (g) = 0; Fat (g) = 0; Protein = 0

Greyhound ☞ serving size: 1 fl oz = 30 g; Calories = 24.9; Total Carb (g) = 1.8; Net Carb (g) = 1.6; Fat (g) = 0; Protein = 0.1

High Alcohol Beer ☞ serving size: 1 fl oz = 30.6 g; Calories = 17.7; Total Carb (g) = 0.1; Net Carb (g) = 0.1; Fat (g) = 0; Protein = 0.3

🥛 Horchata ☞ serving size: 1 cup = 228 g; Calories = 123.1; Total Carb (g) = 26.3; Net Carb (g) = 26.3; Fat (g) = 1.6; Protein = 1.1

🥛 Horchata Beverage Made With Milk ☞ serving size: 1 cup = 248 g; Calories = 223.2; Total Carb (g) = 48.9; Net Carb (g) = 47.9; Fat (g) = 1.5; Protein = 3.5

🥛 Horchata Beverage Made With Water ☞ serving size: 1 cup = 248 g; Calories = 215.8; Total Carb (g) = 50.8; Net Carb (g) = 49.6; Fat (g) = 0.3; Protein = 2.7

🥛 Ice Mocha ☞ serving size: 1 cup = 265 g; Calories = 159; Total Carb (g) = 30.3; Net Carb (g) = 30.3; Fat (g) = 2.6; Protein = 3.9

🥛 Iced Coffee Brewed ☞ serving size: 1 fl oz = 30 g; Calories = 0.3; Total Carb (g) = 0; Net Carb (g) = 0; Fat (g) = 0; Protein = 0

🥛 Iced Coffee Brewed Decaffeinated ☞ serving size: 1 fl oz = 30 g; Calories = 0; Total Carb (g) = 0; Net Carb (g) = 0; Fat (g) = 0; Protein = 0

🥛 Iced Coffee Pre-Lightened And Pre-Sweetened ☞ serving size: 1 fl oz = 31 g; Calories = 9.3; Total Carb (g) = 1.5; Net Carb (g) = 1.5; Fat (g) = 0.3; Protein = 0.1

🥛 Iced Tea / Lemonade Juice Drink ☞ serving size: 1 fl oz (no ice) = 30 g; Calories = 9.9; Total Carb (g) = 2.8; Net Carb (g) = 2.7; Fat (g) = 0; Protein = 0.1

🥛 Iced Tea / Lemonade Juice Drink Diet ☞ serving size: 1 fl oz (no ice) = 30 g; Calories = 0.6; Total Carb (g) = 0.2; Net Carb (g) = 0.2; Fat (g) = 0; Protein = 0

🥛 Iced Tea / Lemonade Juice Drink Light ☞ serving size: 1 fl oz (no ice) = 30 g; Calories = 6.3; Total Carb (g) = 1.8; Net Carb (g) = 1.8; Fat (g) = 0; Protein = 0.1

🥛 Instant Coffee (Prepared With Water) ☞ serving size: 1 fl oz = 29.8 g; Calories = 0.6; Total Carb (g) = 0.1; Net Carb (g) = 0.1; Fat (g) = 0; Protein = 0

Irish Coffee ☞ serving size: 1 fl oz = 30 g; Calories = 26.4; Total Carb (g) = 0.6; Net Carb (g) = 0.6; Fat (g) = 0.7; Protein = 0.1

Jagerbomb ☞ serving size: 1 fl oz = 30 g; Calories = 37.5; Total Carb (g) = 5.4; Net Carb (g) = 5.4; Fat (g) = 0; Protein = 0.1

Kiwi Strawberry Juice Drink ☞ serving size: 16 fl oz = 473 g; Calories = 222.3; Total Carb (g) = 58; Net Carb (g) = 58; Fat (g) = 0; Protein = 0

Kraft Coffee Instant French Vanilla Cafe ☞ serving size: 1 nlea serving = 14 g; Calories = 67.3; Total Carb (g) = 10.4; Net Carb (g) = 10.3; Fat (g) = 2.7; Protein = 0.4

Late Harvest White Wine ☞ serving size: 1 fl oz = 30.8 g; Calories = 34.5; Total Carb (g) = 4.1; Net Carb (g) = 4.1; Fat (g) = 0; Protein = 0

Lemberger ☞ serving size: 1 fl oz = 29.4 g; Calories = 23.5; Total Carb (g) = 0.7; Net Carb (g) = 0.7; Fat (g) = 0; Protein = 0

Lemonade Frozen Concentrate Pink ☞ serving size: 1 fl oz = 36.4 g; Calories = 69.9; Total Carb (g) = 17.8; Net Carb (g) = 17.7; Fat (g) = 0.3; Protein = 0.1

Lemonade Frozen Concentrate Pink Prepared With Water ☞ serving size: 1 fl oz = 30.9 g; Calories = 13.3; Total Carb (g) = 3.3; Net Carb (g) = 3.3; Fat (g) = 0.1; Protein = 0

Lemonade Frozen Concentrate White ☞ serving size: 1 fl oz = 36.5 g; Calories = 71.5; Total Carb (g) = 18.2; Net Carb (g) = 18.1; Fat (g) = 0.3; Protein = 0.1

Lemonade Frozen Concentrate White Prepared With Water ☞ serving size: 1 fl oz = 30.9 g; Calories = 12.4; Total Carb (g) = 3.2; Net Carb (g) = 3.2; Fat (g) = 0; Protein = 0

Lemonade Fruit Flavored Drink ☞ serving size: 1 fl oz (no ice) = 31 g; Calories = 7.8; Total Carb (g) = 2; Net Carb (g) = 2; Fat (g) = 0; Protein = 0

Lemonade Fruit Juice Drink Light Fortified With Vitamin E And C ☞ serving size: 8 fl oz = 240 g; Calories = 50.4; Total Carb (g) = 12; Net Carb (g) = 12; Fat (g) = 0; Protein = 0

Lemonade Powder ☞ serving size: 1 serving = 18 g; Calories = 67.7; Total Carb (g) = 17.6; Net Carb (g) = 17.5; Fat (g) = 0.2; Protein = 0

Lemonade Powder Prepared With Water ☞ serving size: 1 fl oz = 33 g; Calories = 4.6; Total Carb (g) = 1.2; Net Carb (g) = 1.2; Fat (g) = 0; Protein = 0

Lemonade-Flavor Drink Powder ☞ serving size: 1 serving = 18 g; Calories = 68.4; Total Carb (g) = 17.6; Net Carb (g) = 17.6; Fat (g) = 0.2; Protein = 0

Lemonade-Flavor Drink Powder Prepared With Water ☞ serving size: 1 fl oz = 31.8 g; Calories = 8.6; Total Carb (g) = 2.2; Net Carb (g) = 2.2; Fat (g) = 0; Protein = 0

Licuado Or Batido ☞ serving size: 1 fl oz = 27 g; Calories = 19.2; Total Carb (g) = 3.5; Net Carb (g) = 3.4; Fat (g) = 0.4; Protein = 0.6

Light Beer ☞ serving size: 1 fl oz = 29.5 g; Calories = 8.6; Total Carb (g) = 0.5; Net Carb (g) = 0.5; Fat (g) = 0; Protein = 0.1

Limeade Frozen Concentrate Prepared With Water ☞ serving size: 1 fl oz = 30.9 g; Calories = 16.1; Total Carb (g) = 4.3; Net Carb (g) = 4.3; Fat (g) = 0; Protein = 0

Lipton Brisk Tea Black Ready-To-Drink Lemon ☞ serving size: 1 fl oz = 30.6 g; Calories = 10.7; Total Carb (g) = 2.7; Net Carb (g) = 2.7; Fat (g) = 0; Protein = 0

Low Calorie Cola ☞ serving size: 1 fl oz = 29.6 g; Calories = 0; Total Carb (g) = 0; Net Carb (g) = 0; Fat (g) = 0; Protein = 0

Low Carb Monster Energy Drink ☞ serving size: 8 fl oz = 240 g; Calories = 12; Total Carb (g) = 3.3; Net Carb (g) = 3.3; Fat (g) = 0; Protein = 0

🍺 Malt Beverage Includes Non-Alcoholic Beer ☞ serving size: 1 fl oz = 29.6 g; Calories = 11; Total Carb (g) = 2.4; Net Carb (g) = 2.4; Fat (g) = 0; Protein = 0.1

🍺 Malt Liquor Beverage ☞ serving size: 1 bottle = 1184 g; Calories = 473.6; Total Carb (g) = 0; Net Carb (g) = 0; Fat (g) = 0; Protein = 4.1

🍺 Malted Drink Mix Chocolate Powder ☞ serving size: 1 serving (3 heaping tsp or 1 envelope) = 21 g; Calories = 86.3; Total Carb (g) = 18.3; Net Carb (g) = 17.3; Fat (g) = 1; Protein = 1.1

🍺 Malted Drink Mix Chocolate Powder Prepared With Whole Milk ☞ serving size: 1 cup (8 fl oz) = 265 g; Calories = 225.3; Total Carb (g) = 29.7; Net Carb (g) = 28.4; Fat (g) = 8.7; Protein = 8.9

🍺 Malted Drink Mix Chocolate With Added Nutrients Powder Prepared With Whole Milk ☞ serving size: 1 cup (8 fl oz) = 265 g; Calories = 230.6; Total Carb (g) = 29.7; Net Carb (g) = 28.6; Fat (g) = 8.6; Protein = 8.7

🍺 Malted Drink Mix Natural Powder Dairy Based. ☞ serving size: 1 serving (3 heaping tsp or 1 envelope) = 21 g; Calories = 89.9; Total Carb (g) = 15; Net Carb (g) = 14.9; Fat (g) = 2; Protein = 3

🍺 Malted Drink Mix Natural Powder Prepared With Whole Milk ☞ serving size: 1 cup (8 fl oz) = 265 g; Calories = 233.2; Total Carb (g) = 27.1; Net Carb (g) = 26.8; Fat (g) = 9.6; Protein = 10.2

🍺 Malted Drink Mix Natural With Added Nutrients Powder Prepared With Whole Milk ☞ serving size: 1 cup (8 fl oz) = 265 g; Calories = 227.9; Total Carb (g) = 28.3; Net Carb (g) = 28.3; Fat (g) = 8.5; Protein = 9.7

🍺 Martini Flavored ☞ serving size: 1 fl oz = 30 g; Calories = 56.7; Total Carb (g) = 2; Net Carb (g) = 2; Fat (g) = 0; Protein = 0

🍺 Meal Supplement Drink Canned Peanut Flavor ☞ serving size: 1 cup = 158 g; Calories = 159.6; Total Carb (g) = 23.3; Net Carb (g) = 23.3; Fat (g) = 4.9; Protein = 5.5

◌ Merlot ☞ serving size: 1 fl oz = 29.4 g; Calories = 24.4; Total Carb (g) = 0.7; Net Carb (g) = 0.7; Fat (g) = 0; Protein = 0

◌ Milk And Soy Chocolate Drink ☞ serving size: 8 fl oz = 237 g; Calories = 239.4; Total Carb (g) = 41; Net Carb (g) = 37.9; Fat (g) = 4; Protein = 10

◌ Milk Beverage Reduced Fat Flavored And Sweetened Ready-To-Drink Added Calcium Vitamin A And Vitamin D ☞ serving size: 1 cup = 244 g; Calories = 187.9; Total Carb (g) = 29.5; Net Carb (g) = 28.5; Fat (g) = 4.5; Protein = 7.4

◌ Minute Maid Lemonada Limeade ☞ serving size: 8 fl oz = 240 g; Calories = 120; Total Carb (g) = 33; Net Carb (g) = 33; Fat (g) = 0; Protein = 0

◌ Minute Maid Lemonade ☞ serving size: 8 fl oz = 240 g; Calories = 110.4; Total Carb (g) = 29; Net Carb (g) = 29; Fat (g) = 0; Protein = 0

◌ Mixed Berry Powerade Zero ☞ serving size: 12 fl oz = 360 g; Calories = 0; Total Carb (g) = 0.5; Net Carb (g) = 0.5; Fat (g) = 0; Protein = 0

◌ Mixed Vegetable And Fruit Juice Drink With Added Nutrients ☞ serving size: 8 fl oz = 247 g; Calories = 71.6; Total Carb (g) = 18.5; Net Carb (g) = 18.5; Fat (g) = 0; Protein = 0.1

◌ Motts Light Apple Juice ☞ serving size: 8 fl oz = 240 g; Calories = 52.8; Total Carb (g) = 12.2; Net Carb (g) = 12.2; Fat (g) = 0.2; Protein = 0

◌ Mouvedre Wine ☞ serving size: 1 fl oz = 29.4 g; Calories = 25.9; Total Carb (g) = 0.8; Net Carb (g) = 0.8; Fat (g) = 0; Protein = 0

◌ Muscat Wine ☞ serving size: 1 fl oz = 30 g; Calories = 24.6; Total Carb (g) = 1.6; Net Carb (g) = 1.6; Fat (g) = 0; Protein = 0

◌ Nestea ☞ serving size: 1 fl oz = 30.6 g; Calories = 11; Total Carb (g) = 2.8; Net Carb (g) = 2.8; Fat (g) = 0; Protein = 0

◌ Nestle Boost Plus Nutritional Drink Ready-To-Drink ☞ serving size: 1 bottle = 237 g; Calories = 327.1; Total Carb (g) = 41; Net Carb (g) = 38.1; Fat (g) = 12.8; Protein = 12.8

Nutritional Drink Or Shake High Protein Ready-To-Drink (Slim Fast) ☞ serving size: 1 cup = 248 g; Calories = 143.8; Total Carb (g) = 2.1; Net Carb (g) = 1.1; Fat (g) = 7.1; Protein = 16.3

Nutritional Drink Or Shake High Protein Ready-To-Drink Nfs ☞ serving size: 1 cup = 256 g; Calories = 148.5; Total Carb (g) = 2.2; Net Carb (g) = 1.2; Fat (g) = 7.4; Protein = 16.9

Nutritional Drink Or Shake Ready-To-Drink (Carnation Instant Breakfast) ☞ serving size: 1 cup = 248 g; Calories = 225.7; Total Carb (g) = 32.1; Net Carb (g) = 31.8; Fat (g) = 4.9; Protein = 13.5

Nutritional Drink Or Shake Ready-To-Drink (Kellogg's Special K Protein) ☞ serving size: 1 fl oz = 32 g; Calories = 20.5; Total Carb (g) = 2.9; Net Carb (g) = 2.4; Fat (g) = 0.5; Protein = 1

Nutritional Drink Or Shake Ready-To-Drink (Muscle Milk) ☞ serving size: 1 cup = 256 g; Calories = 125.4; Total Carb (g) = 5.3; Net Carb (g) = 4.8; Fat (g) = 5.2; Protein = 15

Nutritional Drink Or Shake Ready-To-Drink Light (Muscle Milk) ☞ serving size: 1 cup = 256 g; Calories = 97.3; Total Carb (g) = 5.4; Net Carb (g) = 4.9; Fat (g) = 2.9; Protein = 12.2

Nutritional Shake Mix High Protein Powder ☞ serving size: 1 tbsp = 10 g; Calories = 39.2; Total Carb (g) = 2; Net Carb (g) = 2; Fat (g) = 1.1; Protein = 5.4

Oatmeal Beverage With Milk ☞ serving size: 1 cup = 248 g; Calories = 203.4; Total Carb (g) = 38.7; Net Carb (g) = 38.2; Fat (g) = 3.9; Protein = 4.2

Oatmeal Beverage With Water ☞ serving size: 1 fl oz = 31 g; Calories = 13.3; Total Carb (g) = 3.3; Net Carb (g) = 3.2; Fat (g) = 0; Protein = 0.1

Ocean Spray Cran Cherry ☞ serving size: 8 fl oz = 248 g; Calo-

ries = 114.1; Total Carb (g) = 31.6; Net Carb (g) = 30.2; Fat (g) = 0; Protein = 0.5

Ocean Spray Cran Grape ☞ serving size: 8 fl oz = 240 g; Calories = 129.6; Total Carb (g) = 31.6; Net Carb (g) = 30.1; Fat (g) = 0; Protein = 0.5

Ocean Spray Cran Lemonade ☞ serving size: 8 fl oz = 247 g; Calories = 111.2; Total Carb (g) = 27.5; Net Carb (g) = 26; Fat (g) = 0; Protein = 0.2

Ocean Spray Cran Pomegranate ☞ serving size: 8 fl oz = 248 g; Calories = 116.6; Total Carb (g) = 31.2; Net Carb (g) = 29.7; Fat (g) = 0; Protein = 0.2

Ocean Spray Cran Raspberry Juice Drink ☞ serving size: 8 fl oz = 248 g; Calories = 121.5; Total Carb (g) = 29.7; Net Carb (g) = 28.2; Fat (g) = 0; Protein = 0.7

Ocean Spray Cran-Energy Cranberry Energy Juice Drink ☞ serving size: 1 can = 250 g; Calories = 37.5; Total Carb (g) = 9.4; Net Carb (g) = 9.4; Fat (g) = 0; Protein = 0

Ocean Spray Cranberry-Apple Juice Drink Bottled ☞ serving size: 8 fl oz = 249 g; Calories = 139.4; Total Carb (g) = 34.1; Net Carb (g) = 32.6; Fat (g) = 0; Protein = 0.7

Ocean Spray Diet Cran Cherry ☞ serving size: 8 fl oz = 237 g; Calories = 9.5; Total Carb (g) = 1.7; Net Carb (g) = 0.2; Fat (g) = 0; Protein = 0.5

Ocean Spray Diet Cranberry Juice ☞ serving size: 8 fl oz = 237 g; Calories = 9.5; Total Carb (g) = 1.9; Net Carb (g) = 0.5; Fat (g) = 0; Protein = 0.2

Ocean Spray Light Cranberry ☞ serving size: 8 fl oz = 248 g; Calories = 47.1; Total Carb (g) = 11.7; Net Carb (g) = 10; Fat (g) = 0; Protein = 0.6

Ocean Spray Light Cranberry And Raspberry Flavored Juice ☞

serving size: 8 fl oz = 242 g; Calories = 62.9; Total Carb (g) = 14; Net Carb (g) = 12.3; Fat (g) = 0; Protein = 1.8

Ocean Spray Light Cranberry Concord Grape ☞ serving size: 8 fl oz = 248 g; Calories = 57; Total Carb (g) = 14.3; Net Carb (g) = 12.6; Fat (g) = 0.1; Protein = 0.9

Ocean Spray Ruby Red Cranberry ☞ serving size: 8 fl oz = 227 g; Calories = 102.2; Total Carb (g) = 26.3; Net Carb (g) = 24.9; Fat (g) = 0; Protein = 0.2

Ocean Spray White Cranberry Peach ☞ serving size: 8 fl oz = 247 g; Calories = 111.2; Total Carb (g) = 29.3; Net Carb (g) = 27.9; Fat (g) = 0; Protein = 0.3

Ocean Spray White Cranberry Strawberry Flavored Juice Drink ☞ serving size: 8 fl oz = 247 g; Calories = 121; Total Carb (g) = 29.6; Net Carb (g) = 28.1; Fat (g) = 0; Protein = 0.5

Orange And Apricot Juice Drink Canned ☞ serving size: 1 fl oz = 31.2 g; Calories = 15.9; Total Carb (g) = 4; Net Carb (g) = 3.9; Fat (g) = 0; Protein = 0.1

Orange Blossom ☞ serving size: 1 fl oz = 30 g; Calories = 29.7; Total Carb (g) = 3.1; Net Carb (g) = 3; Fat (g) = 0; Protein = 0.2

Orange Breakfast Drink Ready-To-Drink With Added Nutrients ☞ serving size: 1 fl oz = 31.6 g; Calories = 16.7; Total Carb (g) = 4.2; Net Carb (g) = 4.1; Fat (g) = 0; Protein = 0

Orange Drink Breakfast Type With Juice And Pulp Frozen Concentrate ☞ serving size: 1 fl oz = 36.3 g; Calories = 55.5; Total Carb (g) = 14.2; Net Carb (g) = 14.1; Fat (g) = 0; Protein = 0.2

Orange Drink Breakfast Type With Juice And Pulp Frozen Concentrate Prepared With Water ☞ serving size: 1 fl oz = 31.3 g; Calories = 14.1; Total Carb (g) = 3.5; Net Carb (g) = 3.5; Fat (g) = 0; Protein = 0

Orange Drink Canned With Added Vitamin C ☞ serving size: 1

fl oz = 31 g; Calories = 15.2; Total Carb (g) = 3.8; Net Carb (g) = 3.8; Fat (g) = 0; Protein = 0

🍷 Orange Juice Drink ☞ serving size: 1 cup = 249 g; Calories = 134.5; Total Carb (g) = 33.4; Net Carb (g) = 32.9; Fat (g) = 0; Protein = 0.5

🍷 Orange Juice Light No Pulp ☞ serving size: 8 fl oz = 240 g; Calories = 50.4; Total Carb (g) = 13; Net Carb (g) = 13; Fat (g) = 0; Protein = 0.5

🍷 Orange Soda ☞ serving size: 1 fl oz = 31 g; Calories = 14.9; Total Carb (g) = 3.8; Net Carb (g) = 3.8; Fat (g) = 0; Protein = 0

🍷 Orange-Flavor Drink Breakfast Type Low Calorie Powder ☞ serving size: 1 portion, amount of dry mix to make 8 fl oz prepared = 2.5 g; Calories = 5.4; Total Carb (g) = 2.2; Net Carb (g) = 2.1; Fat (g) = 0; Protein = 0.1

🍷 Orange-Flavor Drink Breakfast Type Powder ☞ serving size: 1 serving 2 tbsp = 26 g; Calories = 100.4; Total Carb (g) = 25.7; Net Carb (g) = 25.6; Fat (g) = 0; Protein = 0

🍷 Orange-Flavor Drink Breakfast Type Powder Prepared With Water ☞ serving size: 1 fl oz = 33.9 g; Calories = 16.6; Total Carb (g) = 4.3; Net Carb (g) = 4.3; Fat (g) = 0; Protein = 0

🍷 Orange-Flavor Drink Breakfast Type With Pulp Frozen Concentrate Prepared With Water ☞ serving size: 1 fl oz = 31 g; Calories = 15.2; Total Carb (g) = 3.8; Net Carb (g) = 3.8; Fat (g) = 0; Protein = 0

🍷 Orange-Flavor Drink Breakfast Type With Pulp Frozen Concentrate. Not Manufactured Anymore. ☞ serving size: 1 fl oz = 35.3 g; Calories = 60.7; Total Carb (g) = 15.1; Net Carb (g) = 15.1; Fat (g) = 0.2; Protein = 0

🍷 Ovaltine Chocolate Malt Powder ☞ serving size: 1 cup = 78 g; Calories = 290.2; Total Carb (g) = 72.5; Net Carb (g) = 72.5; Fat (g) = 0; Protein = 0

🍶 Ovaltine Classic Malt Powder ☞ serving size: 1 serving (4 tbsp or 1 envelope) = 21 g; Calories = 78.1; Total Carb (g) = 19.6; Net Carb (g) = 19.6; Fat (g) = 0; Protein = 0

🍶 Pepper Soda ☞ serving size: 1 fl oz = 30.7 g; Calories = 12.6; Total Carb (g) = 3.2; Net Carb (g) = 3.2; Fat (g) = 0; Protein = 0

🍶 Pepsico Quaker Gatorade G Performance O 2 Ready-To-Drink. ☞ serving size: 1 fl oz = 30.5 g; Calories = 7.9; Total Carb (g) = 2; Net Carb (g) = 2; Fat (g) = 0; Protein = 0

🍶 Pepsico Quaker Gatorade G2 Low Calorie ☞ serving size: 8 fl oz = 237 g; Calories = 19; Total Carb (g) = 4.6; Net Carb (g) = 4.6; Fat (g) = 0; Protein = 0.1

🍶 Petite Sirah ☞ serving size: 1 fl oz = 29.5 g; Calories = 25.1; Total Carb (g) = 0.8; Net Carb (g) = 0.8; Fat (g) = 0; Protein = 0

🍶 Pina Colada Nonalcoholic ☞ serving size: 1 fl oz = 30 g; Calories = 27.6; Total Carb (g) = 5.1; Net Carb (g) = 4.9; Fat (g) = 0.9; Protein = 0.1

🍶 Pineapple And Grapefruit Juice Drink Canned ☞ serving size: 1 fl oz = 31.3 g; Calories = 14.7; Total Carb (g) = 3.6; Net Carb (g) = 3.6; Fat (g) = 0; Protein = 0.1

🍶 Pineapple And Orange Juice Drink Canned ☞ serving size: 1 fl oz = 31.3 g; Calories = 15.7; Total Carb (g) = 3.7; Net Carb (g) = 3.7; Fat (g) = 0; Protein = 0.4

🍶 Pinot Blanc ☞ serving size: 1 fl oz = 29.3 g; Calories = 23.7; Total Carb (g) = 0.6; Net Carb (g) = 0.6; Fat (g) = 0; Protein = 0

🍶 Pinot Gris (Grigio) ☞ serving size: 1 fl oz = 29.3 g; Calories = 24.3; Total Carb (g) = 0.6; Net Carb (g) = 0.6; Fat (g) = 0; Protein = 0

🍶 Pinot Noir ☞ serving size: 1 fl oz = 29.4 g; Calories = 24.1; Total Carb (g) = 0.7; Net Carb (g) = 0.7; Fat (g) = 0; Protein = 0

🍶 Powerade Zero Ion4 Calorie-Free Assorted Flavors ☞ serving

size: 8 fl oz = 237 g; Calories = 0; Total Carb (g) = 0; Net Carb (g) = 0;
Fat (g) = 0; Protein = 0

🛢 Propel Zero Fruit-Flavored Non-Carbonated ☞ serving size: 1 fl
oz = 29.6 g; Calories = 1.5; Total Carb (g) = 0.3; Net Carb (g) = 0.3; Fat
(g) = 0; Protein = 0

🛢 Protein Powder Soy Based ☞ serving size: 1 scoop = 45 g; Calories = 174.6; Total Carb (g) = 13; Net Carb (g) = 10; Fat (g) = 2.5; Protein
= 25

🛢 Protein Powder Whey Based ☞ serving size: 1/3 cup = 32 g; Calories = 112.6; Total Carb (g) = 2; Net Carb (g) = 1; Fat (g) = 0.5; Protein = 25

🛢 Red Wine ☞ serving size: 1 fl oz = 29.4 g; Calories = 25; Total
Carb (g) = 0.8; Net Carb (g) = 0.8; Fat (g) = 0; Protein = 0

🛢 Rich Chocolate Powder ☞ serving size: 2 tbsp = 11 g; Calories =
40.9; Total Carb (g) = 10.2; Net Carb (g) = 10.2; Fat (g) = 0; Protein = 0

🛢 Riesling ☞ serving size: 1 fl oz = 29.6 g; Calories = 23.7; Total
Carb (g) = 1.1; Net Carb (g) = 1.1; Fat (g) = 0; Protein = 0

🛢 Root Beer ☞ serving size: 1 fl oz = 30.8 g; Calories = 12.6; Total
Carb (g) = 3.3; Net Carb (g) = 3.3; Fat (g) = 0; Protein = 0

🛢 Rose Wine ☞ serving size: 1 fl oz = 30.3 g; Calories = 25.1; Total
Carb (g) = 1.2; Net Carb (g) = 1.2; Fat (g) = 0; Protein = 0.1

🛢 Rum ☞ serving size: 1 fl oz = 27.8 g; Calories = 64.2; Total Carb (g)
= 0; Net Carb (g) = 0; Fat (g) = 0; Protein = 0

🛢 Rum And Diet Cola ☞ serving size: 1 fl oz = 30 g; Calories = 18;
Total Carb (g) = 0.1; Net Carb (g) = 0.1; Fat (g) = 0; Protein = 0

🛢 Rum Hot Buttered ☞ serving size: 1 fl oz = 30 g; Calories = 47.7;
Total Carb (g) = 1.5; Net Carb (g) = 1.5; Fat (g) = 1.3; Protein = 0

🛢 Sangiovese ☞ serving size: 1 fl oz = 29.4 g; Calories = 25.3; Total
Carb (g) = 0.8; Net Carb (g) = 0.8; Fat (g) = 0; Protein = 0

🍷 Sangria Red ☞ serving size: 1 fl oz = 30 g; Calories = 28.8; Total Carb (g) = 2.5; Net Carb (g) = 2.5; Fat (g) = 0; Protein = 0

🍷 Sangria White ☞ serving size: 1 fl oz = 30 g; Calories = 28.2; Total Carb (g) = 2.5; Net Carb (g) = 2.5; Fat (g) = 0; Protein = 0

🍷 Sauvignon Blanc ☞ serving size: 1 fl oz = 29.3 g; Calories = 23.7; Total Carb (g) = 0.6; Net Carb (g) = 0.6; Fat (g) = 0; Protein = 0

🍷 Semillon ☞ serving size: 1 fl oz = 29.5 g; Calories = 24.2; Total Carb (g) = 0.9; Net Carb (g) = 0.9; Fat (g) = 0; Protein = 0

🍷 Shake Fast Food Strawberry ☞ serving size: 1 fl oz = 23.5 g; Calories = 26.6; Total Carb (g) = 4.4; Net Carb (g) = 4.4; Fat (g) = 0.7; Protein = 0.8

🍷 Shake Fast Food Vanilla ☞ serving size: 1 fl oz = 20.8 g; Calories = 30.8; Total Carb (g) = 4.1; Net Carb (g) = 3.9; Fat (g) = 1.4; Protein = 0.7

🍷 Slimfast Meal Replacement High Protein Shake Ready-To-Drink 3-2-1 Plan ☞ serving size: 1 bottle = 295 g; Calories = 180; Total Carb (g) = 2.5; Net Carb (g) = 1.3; Fat (g) = 10; Protein = 19.4

🍷 Soft Drink Fruit Flavored Caffeine Containing ☞ serving size: 1 fl oz (no ice) = 31 g; Calories = 15.2; Total Carb (g) = 4; Net Carb (g) = 4; Fat (g) = 0; Protein = 0

🍷 Sprite ☞ serving size: 1 fl oz = 30.8 g; Calories = 12.3; Total Carb (g) = 3.1; Net Carb (g) = 3.1; Fat (g) = 0; Protein = 0

🍷 Strawberry-Flavor Beverage Mix Powder ☞ serving size: 1 serving (2-3 heaping tsp) = 22 g; Calories = 85.6; Total Carb (g) = 21.8; Net Carb (g) = 21.8; Fat (g) = 0; Protein = 0

🍷 Strawberry-Flavor Beverage Mix Powder Prepared With Whole Milk ☞ serving size: 1 cup (8 fl oz) = 266 g; Calories = 234.1; Total Carb (g) = 32.7; Net Carb (g) = 32.7; Fat (g) = 8.3; Protein = 8

Sweet Dessert Wine ☞ serving size: 1 fl oz = 29.5 g; Calories = 47.2; Total Carb (g) = 4; Net Carb (g) = 4; Fat (g) = 0; Protein = 0.1

Sweetened Vanilla Almond Milk ☞ serving size: 8 fl oz = 240 g; Calories = 91.2; Total Carb (g) = 15.8; Net Carb (g) = 14.9; Fat (g) = 2.5; Protein = 1

Syrah ☞ serving size: 1 fl oz = 29.4 g; Calories = 24.4; Total Carb (g) = 0.8; Net Carb (g) = 0.8; Fat (g) = 0; Protein = 0

Table Wine ☞ serving size: 1 serving (5 fl oz) = 148 g; Calories = 122.8; Total Carb (g) = 4; Net Carb (g) = 4; Fat (g) = 0; Protein = 0.1

Tap Water ☞ serving size: 1 fl oz = 29.6 g; Calories = 0; Total Carb (g) = 0; Net Carb (g) = 0; Fat (g) = 0; Protein = 0

Tea Black Brewed Prepared With Distilled Water ☞ serving size: 1 fl oz = 29.6 g; Calories = 0.3; Total Carb (g) = 0.1; Net Carb (g) = 0.1; Fat (g) = 0; Protein = 0

Tea Black Brewed Prepared With Tap Water Decaffeinated ☞ serving size: 1 fl oz = 29.6 g; Calories = 0.3; Total Carb (g) = 0.1; Net Carb (g) = 0.1; Fat (g) = 0; Protein = 0

Tea Black Ready To Drink Decaffeinated ☞ serving size: 1 cup = 240 g; Calories = 91.2; Total Carb (g) = 21; Net Carb (g) = 21; Fat (g) = 0; Protein = 0

Tea Black Ready To Drink Decaffeinated Diet ☞ serving size: 1 cup = 240 g; Calories = 0; Total Carb (g) = 2; Net Carb (g) = 2; Fat (g) = 0; Protein = 0

Tea Black Ready-To-Drink Lemon Diet ☞ serving size: 1 cup = 265 g; Calories = 2.7; Total Carb (g) = 0.6; Net Carb (g) = 0.6; Fat (g) = 0; Protein = 0

Tea Black Ready-To-Drink Lemon Sweetened ☞ serving size: 1 cup = 271 g; Calories = 122; Total Carb (g) = 29.3; Net Carb (g) = 29.3; Fat (g) = 0.6; Protein = 0

🍵 Tea Black Ready-To-Drink Peach Diet ☞ serving size: 1 cup = 268 g; Calories = 2.7; Total Carb (g) = 0.7; Net Carb (g) = 0.7; Fat (g) = 0; Protein = 0

🍵 Tea Green Brewed Decaffeinated ☞ serving size: ml = 240 g; Calories = 0; Total Carb (g) = 0; Net Carb (g) = 0; Fat (g) = 0; Protein = 0

🍵 Tea Green Brewed Regular ☞ serving size: 1 cup = 245 g; Calories = 2.5; Total Carb (g) = 0; Net Carb (g) = 0; Fat (g) = 0; Protein = 0.5

🍵 Tea Green Instant Decaffeinated Lemon Unsweetened Fortified With Vitamin C ☞ serving size: 2 tbsp = 4.5 g; Calories = 17; Total Carb (g) = 4.3; Net Carb (g) = 4.3; Fat (g) = 0; Protein = 0

🍵 Tea Green Ready To Drink Ginseng And Honey Sweetened ☞ serving size: 1 cup = 260 g; Calories = 78; Total Carb (g) = 18.6; Net Carb (g) = 18.6; Fat (g) = 0.5; Protein = 0

🍵 Tea Green Ready-To-Drink Sweetened ☞ serving size: 1 cup = 270 g; Calories = 72.9; Total Carb (g) = 16.7; Net Carb (g) = 16.7; Fat (g) = 0.6; Protein = 0

🍵 Tea Herb Brewed Chamomile ☞ serving size: 1 fl oz = 29.6 g; Calories = 0.3; Total Carb (g) = 0.1; Net Carb (g) = 0.1; Fat (g) = 0; Protein = 0

🍵 Tea Herb Other Than Chamomile Brewed ☞ serving size: 1 fl oz = 29.6 g; Calories = 0.3; Total Carb (g) = 0.1; Net Carb (g) = 0.1; Fat (g) = 0; Protein = 0

🍵 Tea Hibiscus Brewed ☞ serving size: 8 fl oz = 237 g; Calories = 0; Total Carb (g) = 0; Net Carb (g) = 0; Fat (g) = 0; Protein = 0

🍵 Tea Hot Chai With Milk ☞ serving size: 1 fl oz = 30 g; Calories = 15; Total Carb (g) = 2.7; Net Carb (g) = 2.7; Fat (g) = 0.3; Protein = 0.5

🍵 Tea Iced Brewed Black Decaffeinated Pre-Sweetened With Low

Calorie Sweetener ☞ serving size: 1 fl oz (no ice) = 30 g; Calories = 0.6; Total Carb (g) = 0.2; Net Carb (g) = 0.2; Fat (g) = 0; Protein = 0

⬤ Tea Iced Brewed Black Decaffeinated Pre-Sweetened With Sugar ☞ serving size: 1 fl oz (no ice) = 31 g; Calories = 9.6; Total Carb (g) = 2.5; Net Carb (g) = 2.5; Fat (g) = 0; Protein = 0

⬤ Tea Iced Brewed Black Pre-Sweetened With Low Calorie Sweetener ☞ serving size: 1 fl oz (no ice) = 30 g; Calories = 0.6; Total Carb (g) = 0.2; Net Carb (g) = 0.2; Fat (g) = 0; Protein = 0

⬤ Tea Iced Brewed Black Pre-Sweetened With Sugar ☞ serving size: 1 fl oz (no ice) = 31 g; Calories = 9.6; Total Carb (g) = 2.5; Net Carb (g) = 2.5; Fat (g) = 0; Protein = 0

⬤ Tea Iced Brewed Green Decaffeinated Pre-Sweetened With Low Calorie Sweetener ☞ serving size: 1 fl oz (no ice) = 30 g; Calories = 0.3; Total Carb (g) = 0.1; Net Carb (g) = 0.1; Fat (g) = 0; Protein = 0

⬤ Tea Iced Brewed Green Decaffeinated Pre-Sweetened With Sugar ☞ serving size: 1 fl oz (no ice) = 31 g; Calories = 9.3; Total Carb (g) = 2.4; Net Carb (g) = 2.4; Fat (g) = 0; Protein = 0

⬤ Tea Iced Brewed Green Pre-Sweetened With Low Calorie Sweetener ☞ serving size: 1 fl oz (no ice) = 30 g; Calories = 0.6; Total Carb (g) = 0.1; Net Carb (g) = 0.1; Fat (g) = 0; Protein = 0.1

⬤ Tea Iced Brewed Green Pre-Sweetened With Sugar ☞ serving size: 1 fl oz (no ice) = 31 g; Calories = 9.6; Total Carb (g) = 2.4; Net Carb (g) = 2.4; Fat (g) = 0; Protein = 0.1

⬤ Tea Instant Decaffeinated Lemon Diet ☞ serving size: 2 tsp = 1.6 g; Calories = 5.4; Total Carb (g) = 1.4; Net Carb (g) = 1.4; Fat (g) = 0; Protein = 0.1

⬤ Tea Instant Decaffeinated Lemon Sweetened ☞ serving size: 1 serving (3 heaping tsp) = 23 g; Calories = 92.2; Total Carb (g) = 22.7; Net Carb (g) = 22.7; Fat (g) = 0.2; Protein = 0

⬤ Tea Instant Decaffeinated Unsweetened ☞ serving size: 1

serving 2 tsp = 0.7 g; Calories = 2.2; Total Carb (g) = 0.4; Net Carb (g) = 0.4; Fat (g) = 0; Protein = 0.1

🫖 Tea Instant Lemon Diet ☞ serving size: 1 fl oz = 29.8 g; Calories = 0.6; Total Carb (g) = 0.1; Net Carb (g) = 0.1; Fat (g) = 0; Protein = 0

🫖 Tea Instant Lemon Sweetened Powder ☞ serving size: 1 serving (3 heaping tsp) = 23 g; Calories = 92.2; Total Carb (g) = 22.7; Net Carb (g) = 22.5; Fat (g) = 0.2; Protein = 0

🫖 Tea Instant Lemon Sweetened Prepared With Water ☞ serving size: 1 cup (8 fl oz) = 259 g; Calories = 90.7; Total Carb (g) = 22.3; Net Carb (g) = 22; Fat (g) = 0.2; Protein = 0

🫖 Tea Instant Lemon Unsweetened ☞ serving size: 1 tsp, rounded = 1.4 g; Calories = 4.8; Total Carb (g) = 1.1; Net Carb (g) = 1; Fat (g) = 0; Protein = 0.1

🫖 Tea Instant Lemon With Added Ascorbic Acid ☞ serving size: 1 serving (3 heaping tsp) = 23 g; Calories = 88.6; Total Carb (g) = 22.5; Net Carb (g) = 22.5; Fat (g) = 0.1; Protein = 0.1

🫖 Tea Instant Sweetened With Sodium Saccharin Lemon-Flavored Powder ☞ serving size: 2 tsp = 1.6 g; Calories = 5.4; Total Carb (g) = 1.4; Net Carb (g) = 1.4; Fat (g) = 0; Protein = 0.1

🫖 Tea Instant Unsweetened Powder ☞ serving size: 1 serving 1 tsp = 0.7 g; Calories = 2.2; Total Carb (g) = 0.4; Net Carb (g) = 0.4; Fat (g) = 0; Protein = 0.1

🫖 Tea Instant Unsweetened Prepared With Water ☞ serving size: 1 fl oz = 29.7 g; Calories = 0.3; Total Carb (g) = 0.1; Net Carb (g) = 0.1; Fat (g) = 0; Protein = 0

🫖 Tea Ready-To-Drink Lemon Diet ☞ serving size: 1 cup = 266 g; Calories = 5.3; Total Carb (g) = 1.1; Net Carb (g) = 1.1; Fat (g) = 0; Protein = 0

🫖 Tequila Sunrise ☞ serving size: 1 fl oz = 31.1 g; Calories = 34.2; Total Carb (g) = 3.5; Net Carb (g) = 3.5; Fat (g) = 0; Protein = 0.1

The Coca-Cola Company Dasani Water Bottled Non-Carbonated ☞ serving size: 1 fl oz = 29.6 g; Calories = 0; Total Carb (g) = 0; Net Carb (g) = 0; Fat (g) = 0; Protein = 0

The Coca-Cola Company Glaceau Vitamin Water Revive Fruit Punch Fortified ☞ serving size: 20 fl oz = 591 g; Calories = 0; Total Carb (g) = 0; Net Carb (g) = 0; Fat (g) = 0; Protein = 0

The Coca-Cola Company Hi-C Flashin Fruit Punch ☞ serving size: 6 (3/4) fl oz = 200 g; Calories = 90; Total Carb (g) = 25; Net Carb (g) = 25; Fat (g) = 0; Protein = 0

The Coca-Cola Company Nos Energy Drink Original Grape Loaded Cherry Charged Citrus Fortified With Vitamins B6 And B12 ☞ serving size: 16 fl oz = 480 g; Calories = 211.2; Total Carb (g) = 54; Net Carb (g) = 54; Fat (g) = 0; Protein = 0

The Coca-Cola Company Nos Zero Energy Drink Sugar-Free With Guarana Fortified With Vitamins B6 And B12 ☞ serving size: 16 fl oz = 480 g; Calories = 19.2; Total Carb (g) = 4.9; Net Carb (g) = 4.9; Fat (g) = 0; Protein = 0

Tonic Water ☞ serving size: 1 fl oz = 30.5 g; Calories = 10.4; Total Carb (g) = 2.7; Net Carb (g) = 2.7; Fat (g) = 0; Protein = 0

Tropical Punch Ready-To-Drink ☞ serving size: 1 nlea serving = 210 g; Calories = 21; Total Carb (g) = 5.3; Net Carb (g) = 5.3; Fat (g) = 0; Protein = 0

Unilever Slimfast Meal Replacement Regular Ready-To-Drink 3-2-1 Plan ☞ serving size: 1 bottle = 295 g; Calories = 168.2; Total Carb (g) = 22.8; Net Carb (g) = 18.1; Fat (g) = 5.7; Protein = 9.8

Unilever Slimfast Shake Mix High Protein Whey Powder 3-2-1 Plan ☞ serving size: 1 scoop = 26 g; Calories = 112.6; Total Carb (g) = 13; Net Carb (g) = 8.3; Fat (g) = 3.5; Protein = 7.3

Unilever Slimfast Shake Mix Powder 3-2-1 Plan ☞ serving size: 1

scoop = 26 g; Calories = 116.5; Total Carb (g) = 19.2; Net Carb (g) = 14.5; Fat (g) = 3.5; Protein = 2.1

Unsweetened Almond Milk ☞ serving size: 1 cup = 262 g; Calories = 39.3; Total Carb (g) = 3.4; Net Carb (g) = 2.9; Fat (g) = 2.5; Protein = 1.1

Unsweetened Chocolate Almond Milk ☞ serving size: 1 cup = 240 g; Calories = 50.4; Total Carb (g) = 3; Net Carb (g) = 2; Fat (g) = 3.5; Protein = 2

Unsweetened Rice Milk ☞ serving size: 8 fl oz (approximate weight, 1 serving) = 240 g; Calories = 112.8; Total Carb (g) = 22; Net Carb (g) = 21.3; Fat (g) = 2.3; Protein = 0.7

V8 Splash Juice Drinks Berry Blend ☞ serving size: 1 serving 8 oz = 243 g; Calories = 70.5; Total Carb (g) = 18; Net Carb (g) = 18; Fat (g) = 0; Protein = 0

V8 Splash Juice Drinks Diet Berry Blend ☞ serving size: 8 fl oz = 243 g; Calories = 9.7; Total Carb (g) = 3; Net Carb (g) = 3; Fat (g) = 0; Protein = 0

V8 Splash Juice Drinks Diet Fruit Medley ☞ serving size: 1 serving 8 oz = 238 g; Calories = 9.5; Total Carb (g) = 3; Net Carb (g) = 3; Fat (g) = 0; Protein = 0

V8 Splash Juice Drinks Diet Strawberry Kiwi ☞ serving size: 1 serving = 238 g; Calories = 9.5; Total Carb (g) = 3; Net Carb (g) = 3; Fat (g) = 0; Protein = 0

V8 Splash Juice Drinks Diet Tropical Blend ☞ serving size: 1 serving 8 oz = 238 g; Calories = 9.5; Total Carb (g) = 3; Net Carb (g) = 3; Fat (g) = 0; Protein = 0

V8 Splash Juice Drinks Fruit Medley ☞ serving size: 1 serving 8 oz = 243 g; Calories = 80.2; Total Carb (g) = 19; Net Carb (g) = 19; Fat (g) = 0; Protein = 0

V8 Splash Juice Drinks Guava Passion Fruit ☞ serving size: 1

serving 8 oz = 243 g; Calories = 80.2; Total Carb (g) = 19; Net Carb (g) = 19; Fat (g) = 0; Protein = 0

V8 Splash Juice Drinks Mango Peach ☞ serving size: 1 serving 8 oz = 243 g; Calories = 80.2; Total Carb (g) = 20; Net Carb (g) = 20; Fat (g) = 0; Protein = 0

V8 Splash Juice Drinks Orange Pineapple ☞ serving size: 1 serving 8 oz = 243 g; Calories = 70.5; Total Carb (g) = 18; Net Carb (g) = 18; Fat (g) = 0; Protein = 0

V8 Splash Juice Drinks Orchard Blend ☞ serving size: 1 serving 8 oz = 243 g; Calories = 80.2; Total Carb (g) = 19; Net Carb (g) = 19; Fat (g) = 0; Protein = 0

V8 Splash Juice Drinks Strawberry Banana ☞ serving size: 1 serving 8 oz = 243 g; Calories = 70.5; Total Carb (g) = 18; Net Carb (g) = 18; Fat (g) = 0; Protein = 0

V8 Splash Juice Drinks Strawberry Kiwi ☞ serving size: 1 serving 8 oz = 243 g; Calories = 70.5; Total Carb (g) = 18; Net Carb (g) = 18; Fat (g) = 0; Protein = 0

V8 Splash Juice Drinks Tropical Blend ☞ serving size: 1 serving 8 oz = 243 g; Calories = 70.5; Total Carb (g) = 18; Net Carb (g) = 18; Fat (g) = 0; Protein = 0

V8 Splash Smoothies Peach Mango ☞ serving size: 1 serving 8 oz = 245 g; Calories = 90.7; Total Carb (g) = 19; Net Carb (g) = 19; Fat (g) = 0; Protein = 3

V8 Splash Smoothies Strawberry Banana ☞ serving size: 1 serving 8 oz = 245 g; Calories = 90.7; Total Carb (g) = 20; Net Carb (g) = 20; Fat (g) = 0; Protein = 3

V8 Splash Smoothies Tropical Colada ☞ serving size: 1 serving 8 oz = 246 g; Calories = 100.9; Total Carb (g) = 21; Net Carb (g) = 20; Fat (g) = 0; Protein = 3

V8 V- Fusion Juices Acai Berry ☞ serving size: 1 serving 8 oz =

246 g; Calories = 110.7; Total Carb (g) = 27; Net Carb (g) = 27; Fat (g) = 0; Protein = 0

🍺 V8 V-Fusion Juices Peach Mango ☞ serving size: 1 serving 8 oz = 246 g; Calories = 120.5; Total Carb (g) = 28; Net Carb (g) = 28; Fat (g) = 0; Protein = 1

🍺 V8 V-Fusion Juices Strawberry Banana ☞ serving size: 1 serving 8 oz = 246 g; Calories = 120.5; Total Carb (g) = 29; Net Carb (g) = 29; Fat (g) = 0; Protein = 1

🍺 V8 V-Fusion Juices Tropical ☞ serving size: 1 serving 8 oz = 246 g; Calories = 120.5; Total Carb (g) = 28; Net Carb (g) = 28; Fat (g) = 0; Protein = 1

🍺 Vegetable And Fruit Juice Blend 100% Juice With Added Vitamins A C E ☞ serving size: 1 serving 8 oz = 246 g; Calories = 113.2; Total Carb (g) = 27.4; Net Carb (g) = 27.4; Fat (g) = 0; Protein = 0.7

🍺 Vegetable And Fruit Juice Drink Reduced Calorie With Low-Calorie Sweetener Added Vitamin C ☞ serving size: 1 serving = 238 g; Calories = 9.5; Total Carb (g) = 2.6; Net Carb (g) = 2.6; Fat (g) = 0; Protein = 0

🍺 Vitamin Fortified Water ☞ serving size: 8 fl oz = 240 g; Calories = 12; Total Carb (g) = 3; Net Carb (g) = 3; Fat (g) = 0; Protein = 0

🍺 Vodka ☞ serving size: 1 fl oz = 27.8 g; Calories = 64.2; Total Carb (g) = 0; Net Carb (g) = 0; Fat (g) = 0; Protein = 0

🍺 Vodka And Cola ☞ serving size: 1 fl oz = 30 g; Calories = 26.7; Total Carb (g) = 2.3; Net Carb (g) = 2.3; Fat (g) = 0.1; Protein = 0

🍺 Vodka And Diet Cola ☞ serving size: 1 fl oz = 30 g; Calories = 18; Total Carb (g) = 0.1; Net Carb (g) = 0.1; Fat (g) = 0; Protein = 0

🍺 Vodka And Energy Drink ☞ serving size: 1 fl oz = 30 g; Calories = 27; Total Carb (g) = 2.3; Net Carb (g) = 2.3; Fat (g) = 0; Protein = 0.1

Vodka And Lemonade ☞ serving size: 1 fl oz = 30 g; Calories = 27.9; Total Carb (g) = 2.7; Net Carb (g) = 2.7; Fat (g) = 0; Protein = 0

Vodka And Soda ☞ serving size: 1 fl oz = 30 g; Calories = 17.7; Total Carb (g) = 0; Net Carb (g) = 0; Fat (g) = 0; Protein = 0

Vodka And Tonic ☞ serving size: 1 fl oz = 30 g; Calories = 25.2; Total Carb (g) = 2; Net Carb (g) = 2; Fat (g) = 0; Protein = 0

Vodka And Water ☞ serving size: 1 fl oz = 30 g; Calories = 17.7; Total Carb (g) = 0; Net Carb (g) = 0; Fat (g) = 0; Protein = 0

Water Bottled Non-Carbonated Calistoga ☞ serving size: 1 fl oz = 29.6 g; Calories = 0; Total Carb (g) = 0; Net Carb (g) = 0; Fat (g) = 0; Protein = 0

Water Bottled Non-Carbonated Crystal Geyser ☞ serving size: 1 fl oz = 29.6 g; Calories = 0; Total Carb (g) = 0; Net Carb (g) = 0; Fat (g) = 0; Protein = 0

Water Bottled Non-Carbonated Dannon ☞ serving size: 1 fl oz = 29.6 g; Calories = 0; Total Carb (g) = 0; Net Carb (g) = 0; Fat (g) = 0; Protein = 0

Water Bottled Non-Carbonated Dannon Fluoride To Go ☞ serving size: 1 fl oz = 29.6 g; Calories = 0; Total Carb (g) = 0; Net Carb (g) = 0; Fat (g) = 0; Protein = 0

Water Bottled Non-Carbonated Evian ☞ serving size: 1 fl oz = 29.6 g; Calories = 0; Total Carb (g) = 0; Net Carb (g) = 0; Fat (g) = 0; Protein = 0

Water Bottled Non-Carbonated Naya ☞ serving size: 1 fl oz = 29.6 g; Calories = 0; Total Carb (g) = 0; Net Carb (g) = 0; Fat (g) = 0; Protein = 0

Water Bottled Non-Carbonated Pepsi Aquafina ☞ serving size: 1 fl oz = 29.6 g; Calories = 0; Total Carb (g) = 0; Net Carb (g) = 0; Fat (g) = 0; Protein = 0

Water Bottled Perrier ☞ serving size: 1 fl oz = 29.6 g; Calories = 0; Total Carb (g) = 0; Net Carb (g) = 0; Fat (g) = 0; Protein = 0

Water Bottled Poland Spring ☞ serving size: 1 fl oz = 29.6 g; Calories = 0; Total Carb (g) = 0; Net Carb (g) = 0; Fat (g) = 0; Protein = 0

Water Non-Carbonated Bottles Natural Fruit Flavors Sweetened With Low Calorie Sweetener ☞ serving size: 1 fl oz = 29.6 g; Calories = 0.3; Total Carb (g) = 0; Net Carb (g) = 0; Fat (g) = 0; Protein = 0

Water Tap Municipal ☞ serving size: 1 fl oz = 29.6 g; Calories = 0; Total Carb (g) = 0; Net Carb (g) = 0; Fat (g) = 0; Protein = 0

Water With Added Vitamins And Minerals Bottles Sweetened Assorted Fruit Flavors ☞ serving size: 8 fl oz (1 nlea serving) = 237 g; Calories = 52.1; Total Carb (g) = 13; Net Carb (g) = 13; Fat (g) = 0; Protein = 0

Water With Corn Syrup And/or Sugar And Low Calorie Sweetener Fruit Flavored ☞ serving size: 1 pouch = 200 g; Calories = 36; Total Carb (g) = 9; Net Carb (g) = 9; Fat (g) = 0; Protein = 0

Well Water ☞ serving size: 1 fl oz = 29.6 g; Calories = 0; Total Carb (g) = 0; Net Carb (g) = 0; Fat (g) = 0; Protein = 0

Wendys Tea Ready-To-Drink Unsweetened ☞ serving size: 1 fl oz = 29.6 g; Calories = 0.3; Total Carb (g) = 0; Net Carb (g) = 0; Fat (g) = 0; Protein = 0.1

Whey Protein Powder Isolate ☞ serving size: 3 scoop = 86 g; Calories = 308.7; Total Carb (g) = 25; Net Carb (g) = 25; Fat (g) = 1; Protein = 50

Whiskey ☞ serving size: 1 fl oz = 27.8 g; Calories = 69.5; Total Carb (g) = 0; Net Carb (g) = 0; Fat (g) = 0; Protein = 0

Whiskey And Cola ☞ serving size: 1 fl oz = 30 g; Calories = 26.7; Total Carb (g) = 2.3; Net Carb (g) = 2.3; Fat (g) = 0.1; Protein = 0

Whiskey And Diet Cola ☞ serving size: 1 fl oz = 30 g; Calories = 18; Total Carb (g) = 0.1; Net Carb (g) = 0.1; Fat (g) = 0; Protein = 0

Whiskey And Ginger Ale ☞ serving size: 1 fl oz = 30 g; Calories = 24.9; Total Carb (g) = 2; Net Carb (g) = 2; Fat (g) = 0; Protein = 0

Whiskey And Water ☞ serving size: 1 fl oz = 30 g; Calories = 17.7; Total Carb (g) = 0; Net Carb (g) = 0; Fat (g) = 0; Protein = 0

Whiskey Sour Mix ☞ serving size: 1 packet = 17 g; Calories = 65.1; Total Carb (g) = 16.5; Net Carb (g) = 16.5; Fat (g) = 0; Protein = 0.1

Whiskey Sour Mix Bottled ☞ serving size: 1 fl oz = 32.3 g; Calories = 28.1; Total Carb (g) = 6.9; Net Carb (g) = 6.9; Fat (g) = 0; Protein = 0

Whiskey Sour Mix Bottled With Added Potassium And Sodium ☞ serving size: 1 fl oz = 32.3 g; Calories = 27.1; Total Carb (g) = 6.9; Net Carb (g) = 6.9; Fat (g) = 0; Protein = 0

White Wine ☞ serving size: 1 fl oz = 29.4 g; Calories = 24.1; Total Carb (g) = 0.8; Net Carb (g) = 0.8; Fat (g) = 0; Protein = 0

Wine Non-Alcoholic ☞ serving size: 1 fl oz = 29 g; Calories = 1.7; Total Carb (g) = 0.3; Net Carb (g) = 0.3; Fat (g) = 0; Protein = 0.2

Yellow Green Colored Citrus Soft Drink With Caffeine ☞ serving size: 16 fl oz = 473 g; Calories = 231.8; Total Carb (g) = 60.7; Net Carb (g) = 60.7; Fat (g) = 0; Protein = 0

Zevia Cola ☞ serving size: 1 can = 355 g; Calories = 0; Total Carb (g) = 4; Net Carb (g) = 4; Fat (g) = 0; Protein = 0

Zevia Cola Caffeine Free ☞ serving size: 1 can = 355 g; Calories = 0; Total Carb (g) = 4; Net Carb (g) = 4; Fat (g) = 0; Protein = 0

Zinfandel ☞ serving size: 1 fl oz = 29.4 g; Calories = 25.9; Total Carb (g) = 0.8; Net Carb (g) = 0.8; Fat (g) = 0; Protein = 0

14

BREAKFAST CEREALS

👅 Alpen ☞ serving size: 2/3 cup (1 nlea serving) = 55 g; Calories = 193.6; Total Carb (g) = 41.6; Net Carb (g) = 36.6; Fat (g) = 1.8; Protein = 6.2

👅 Barbaras Puffins Original ☞ serving size: 3/4 cup (1 nlea serving) = 27 g; Calories = 89.9; Total Carb (g) = 22.7; Net Carb (g) = 17.7; Fat (g) = 1; Protein = 2

👅 Cereal (General Mills 25% Less Sugar Cocoa Puffs) ☞ serving size: 1 cup = 32 g; Calories = 121.6; Total Carb (g) = 26.5; Net Carb (g) = 24.3; Fat (g) = 1.7; Protein = 2.1

👅 Cereal (General Mills 25% Less Sugar Trix) ☞ serving size: 1 cup = 30 g; Calories = 114.9; Total Carb (g) = 25.7; Net Carb (g) = 24.4; Fat (g) = 1.2; Protein = 1.6

👅 Cereal (General Mills Basic 4) ☞ serving size: 1 cup = 55 g; Calories = 196.9; Total Carb (g) = 43.5; Net Carb (g) = 38.5; Fat (g) = 2.2; Protein = 3.7

👅 Cereal (General Mills Boo Berry) ☞ serving size: 1 cup = 33 g;

Calories = 127.4; Total Carb (g) = 28.2; Net Carb (g) = 26.8; Fat (g) = 1.4; Protein = 1.8

🥣 Cereal (General Mills Cheerios Apple Cinnamon) ☞ serving size: 1 cup = 40 g; Calories = 154.4; Total Carb (g) = 32; Net Carb (g) = 29; Fat (g) = 2.4; Protein = 3.3

🥣 Cereal (General Mills Cheerios Banana Nut) ☞ serving size: 1 cup = 37 g; Calories = 138.8; Total Carb (g) = 31.3; Net Carb (g) = 29.1; Fat (g) = 1.5; Protein = 2

🥣 Cereal (General Mills Cheerios Berry Burst) ☞ serving size: 1 cup = 36 g; Calories = 136.1; Total Carb (g) = 29; Net Carb (g) = 26.2; Fat (g) = 1.6; Protein = 3.2

🥣 Cereal (General Mills Cheerios Chocolate) ☞ serving size: 1 cup = 36 g; Calories = 136.8; Total Carb (g) = 30.1; Net Carb (g) = 27.8; Fat (g) = 1.8; Protein = 2.1

🥣 Cereal (General Mills Cheerios Frosted) ☞ serving size: 1 cup = 37 g; Calories = 139.1; Total Carb (g) = 29.5; Net Carb (g) = 26.8; Fat (g) = 1.7; Protein = 3.3

🥣 Cereal (General Mills Cheerios Fruity) ☞ serving size: 1 cup = 36 g; Calories = 137.2; Total Carb (g) = 30.3; Net Carb (g) = 28.2; Fat (g) = 1.7; Protein = 2.1

🥣 Cereal (General Mills Cheerios Honey Nut) ☞ serving size: 1 cup = 37 g; Calories = 139.1; Total Carb (g) = 29.5; Net Carb (g) = 26.9; Fat (g) = 1.9; Protein = 3.3

🥣 Cereal (General Mills Cheerios Multigrain) ☞ serving size: 1 cup = 30 g; Calories = 111; Total Carb (g) = 24.4; Net Carb (g) = 21.8; Fat (g) = 1.2; Protein = 2.5

🥣 Cereal (General Mills Cheerios Oat Cluster Crunch) ☞ serving size: 1 cup = 36 g; Calories = 136.1; Total Carb (g) = 29.1; Net Carb (g) = 26.5; Fat (g) = 1.7; Protein = 3.1

🥣 Cereal (General Mills Cheerios Protein) ☞ serving size: 1 cup =

28 g; Calories = 105.8; Total Carb (g) = 21.3; Net Carb (g) = 19.4; Fat (g) = 1.4; Protein = 3.4

☙ Cereal (General Mills Cheerios Yogurt Burst) ☞ serving size: 1 cup = 40 g; Calories = 160; Total Carb (g) = 32.7; Net Carb (g) = 30; Fat (g) = 2.1; Protein = 2.7

☙ Cereal (General Mills Cheerios) ☞ serving size: 10 cheerios = 1 g; Calories = 3.8; Total Carb (g) = 0.7; Net Carb (g) = 0.6; Fat (g) = 0.1; Protein = 0.1

☙ Cereal (General Mills Chex Chocolate) ☞ serving size: 1 cup = 43 g; Calories = 177.2; Total Carb (g) = 34.9; Net Carb (g) = 34; Fat (g) = 3.6; Protein = 2.1

☙ Cereal (General Mills Chex Cinnamon) ☞ serving size: 1 cup = 39 g; Calories = 157.2; Total Carb (g) = 32.1; Net Carb (g) = 31.2; Fat (g) = 2.6; Protein = 2

☙ Cereal (General Mills Chex Corn) ☞ serving size: 1 piece = 0 g; Calories = 0; Total Carb (g) = 0; Net Carb (g) = 0; Fat (g) = 0; Protein = 0

☙ Cereal (General Mills Chex Honey Nut) ☞ serving size: 1 piece = 0 g; Calories = 0; Total Carb (g) = 0; Net Carb (g) = 0; Fat (g) = 0; Protein = 0

☙ Cereal (General Mills Chex Rice) ☞ serving size: 1 cup = 27 g; Calories = 101.3; Total Carb (g) = 23; Net Carb (g) = 22.4; Fat (g) = 0.5; Protein = 1.7

☙ Cereal (General Mills Cinnamon Toast Crunch) ☞ serving size: 1 cup = 40 g; Calories = 164; Total Carb (g) = 31.2; Net Carb (g) = 28.5; Fat (g) = 4.1; Protein = 2.2

☙ Cereal (General Mills Cocoa Puffs) ☞ serving size: 1 cup = 36 g; Calories = 137.9; Total Carb (g) = 30.1; Net Carb (g) = 28.1; Fat (g) = 1.9; Protein = 2

☙ Cereal (General Mills Cookie Crisp) ☞ serving size: 1 cup = 35 g;

Calories = 133; Total Carb (g) = 29.6; Net Carb (g) = 27.8; Fat (g) = 1.5; Protein = 1.8

🥣 Cereal (General Mills Count Chocula) ☞ serving size: 1 cup = 36 g; Calories = 137.9; Total Carb (g) = 30.4; Net Carb (g) = 28.6; Fat (g) = 1.7; Protein = 1.9

🥣 Cereal (General Mills Frankenberry) ☞ serving size: 1 cup = 33 g; Calories = 127.4; Total Carb (g) = 28.2; Net Carb (g) = 26.8; Fat (g) = 1.4; Protein = 1.8

🥣 Cereal (General Mills Golden Grahams) ☞ serving size: 1 cup = 40 g; Calories = 149.6; Total Carb (g) = 34; Net Carb (g) = 31.8; Fat (g) = 1.3; Protein = 2.1

🥣 Cereal (General Mills Honey Nut Clusters) ☞ serving size: 1 cup = 55 g; Calories = 205.7; Total Carb (g) = 46.9; Net Carb (g) = 43.4; Fat (g) = 1.1; Protein = 4.2

🥣 Cereal (General Mills Kix Berry Berry) ☞ serving size: 1 cup = 33 g; Calories = 124.1; Total Carb (g) = 27.7; Net Carb (g) = 25.8; Fat (g) = 1.4; Protein = 2

🥣 Cereal (General Mills Lucky Charms Chocolate) ☞ serving size: 1 cup = 37 g; Calories = 141; Total Carb (g) = 31.2; Net Carb (g) = 29.3; Fat (g) = 1.6; Protein = 2.1

🥣 Cereal (General Mills Lucky Charms) ☞ serving size: 1 cup = 36 g; Calories = 136.8; Total Carb (g) = 29.1; Net Carb (g) = 27.3; Fat (g) = 1.8; Protein = 2.8

🥣 Cereal (General Mills Oatmeal Crisp With Almonds) ☞ serving size: 1 cup = 60 g; Calories = 234; Total Carb (g) = 46.9; Net Carb (g) = 41.9; Fat (g) = 4; Protein = 5.9

🥣 Cereal (General Mills Oatmeal Crisp With Raisins) ☞ serving size: 1 cup = 62 g; Calories = 230.6; Total Carb (g) = 50.1; Net Carb (g) = 45.5; Fat (g) = 2.4; Protein = 5.3

🥣 Cereal (General Mills Reese's Puffs) ☞ serving size: 1 cup = 40 g;

Calories = 165.2; Total Carb (g) = 30.2; Net Carb (g) = 28.4; Fat (g) = 4.4; Protein = 2.7

🥣 Cereal (General Mills Trix) ☞ serving size: 1 cup = 32 g; Calories = 122.9; Total Carb (g) = 27.6; Net Carb (g) = 26.3; Fat (g) = 1.2; Protein = 1.6

🥣 Cereal (Kashi Heart To Heart Oat Flakes And Blueberry Clusters) ☞ serving size: 1 cup = 55 g; Calories = 206.8; Total Carb (g) = 44.2; Net Carb (g) = 40.1; Fat (g) = 2.1; Protein = 5.7

🥣 Cereal (Kellogg's Cinnabon) ☞ serving size: 1 cup = 30 g; Calories = 123; Total Carb (g) = 25; Net Carb (g) = 23.8; Fat (g) = 2.2; Protein = 1.7

🥣 Cereal (Kellogg's Cocoa Krispies) ☞ serving size: 1 cup = 41 g; Calories = 159.5; Total Carb (g) = 36; Net Carb (g) = 35.5; Fat (g) = 1.1; Protein = 1.9

🥣 Cereal (Kellogg's Corn Flakes) ☞ serving size: 1 cup = 28 g; Calories = 100; Total Carb (g) = 23.6; Net Carb (g) = 22.6; Fat (g) = 0.1; Protein = 2.1

🥣 Cereal (Kellogg's Corn Pops) ☞ serving size: 1 cup = 29 g; Calories = 112.2; Total Carb (g) = 26; Net Carb (g) = 23.6; Fat (g) = 0.4; Protein = 1.4

🥣 Cereal (Kellogg's Crispix) ☞ serving size: 1 cup = 29 g; Calories = 109.6; Total Carb (g) = 25.3; Net Carb (g) = 25; Fat (g) = 0.2; Protein = 1.9

🥣 Cereal (Kellogg's Froot Loops Marshmallow) ☞ serving size: 1 cup = 29 g; Calories = 109; Total Carb (g) = 25.9; Net Carb (g) = 23.8; Fat (g) = 0.8; Protein = 1.3

🥣 Cereal (Kellogg's Frosted Flakes Reduced Sugar) ☞ serving size: 1 cup = 31 g; Calories = 110.7; Total Carb (g) = 27.1; Net Carb (g) = 23.9; Fat (g) = 0.1; Protein = 1.7

🥣 Cereal (Kellogg's Frosted Flakes) ☞ serving size: 1 cup = 41 g;

Calories = 151.3; Total Carb (g) = 36.6; Net Carb (g) = 35.7; Fat (g) = 0.7; Protein = 1.6

👆 Cereal (Kellogg's Frosted Krispies) ☞ serving size: 1 cup = 40 g; Calories = 153.6; Total Carb (g) = 36.5; Net Carb (g) = 36.3; Fat (g) = 0.2; Protein = 1.7

👆 Cereal (Kellogg's Honey Crunch Corn Flakes) ☞ serving size: 1 cup = 40 g; Calories = 154; Total Carb (g) = 34.8; Net Carb (g) = 33.4; Fat (g) = 0.8; Protein = 2.7

👆 Cereal (Kellogg's Honey Smacks) ☞ serving size: 1 cup = 36 g; Calories = 136.8; Total Carb (g) = 31.9; Net Carb (g) = 30.1; Fat (g) = 0.8; Protein = 2.1

👆 Cereal (Kellogg's Low Fat Granola With Raisins) ☞ serving size: 1 cup = 90 g; Calories = 342.9; Total Carb (g) = 72.1; Net Carb (g) = 65.4; Fat (g) = 4.7; Protein = 8.1

👆 Cereal (Kellogg's Low Fat Granola) ☞ serving size: 1 cup = 98 g; Calories = 381.2; Total Carb (g) = 79.3; Net Carb (g) = 72.4; Fat (g) = 5.6; Protein = 8.5

👆 Cereal (Kellogg's Product 19) ☞ serving size: 1 cup = 30 g; Calories = 112.2; Total Carb (g) = 25.3; Net Carb (g) = 24.5; Fat (g) = 0.4; Protein = 2.6

👆 Cereal (Kellogg's Rice Krispies Treats Cereal) ☞ serving size: 1 cup = 40 g; Calories = 158; Total Carb (g) = 34.2; Net Carb (g) = 34.1; Fat (g) = 1.7; Protein = 1.7

👆 Cereal (Kellogg's Rice Krispies) ☞ serving size: 1 cup = 26 g; Calories = 99.1; Total Carb (g) = 22.1; Net Carb (g) = 22; Fat (g) = 0.5; Protein = 1.8

👆 Cereal (Kellogg's Smart Start Strong) ☞ serving size: 1 cup = 50 g; Calories = 185.5; Total Carb (g) = 43.4; Net Carb (g) = 40.7; Fat (g) = 0.8; Protein = 3.8

👆 Cereal (Kellogg's Special K Blueberry) ☞ serving size: 1 cup = 40

g; Calories = 145.2; Total Carb (g) = 34.5; Net Carb (g) = 31.1; Fat (g) = 0.6; Protein = 2.8

🥣 Cereal (Kellogg's Special K Low Fat Granola) ☞ serving size: 1 cup = 104 g; Calories = 404.6; Total Carb (g) = 84.1; Net Carb (g) = 76.9; Fat (g) = 5.9; Protein = 9.1

🥣 Cereal (Kellogg's Special K) ☞ serving size: 1 cup = 31 g; Calories = 116.9; Total Carb (g) = 22.8; Net Carb (g) = 22.3; Fat (g) = 0.6; Protein = 5.5

🥣 Cereal (Malt-O-Meal Blueberry Muffin Tops) ☞ serving size: 1 cup = 40 g; Calories = 149.6; Total Carb (g) = 34; Net Carb (g) = 31.8; Fat (g) = 1.3; Protein = 2.1

🥣 Cereal (Malt-O-Meal Crispy Rice) ☞ serving size: 1 cup = 28 g; Calories = 106.7; Total Carb (g) = 23.8; Net Carb (g) = 23.7; Fat (g) = 0.6; Protein = 1.9

🥣 Cereal (Malt-O-Meal Golden Puffs) ☞ serving size: 1 cup = 32 g; Calories = 121.6; Total Carb (g) = 28.3; Net Carb (g) = 26.7; Fat (g) = 0.7; Protein = 1.8

🥣 Cereal (Malt-O-Meal Honey Graham Squares) ☞ serving size: 1 cup = 40 g; Calories = 149.6; Total Carb (g) = 34; Net Carb (g) = 31.8; Fat (g) = 1.3; Protein = 2.1

🥣 Cereal (Malt-O-Meal Honey Nut Toasty O's) ☞ serving size: 1 cup = 38 g; Calories = 142.9; Total Carb (g) = 30.3; Net Carb (g) = 27.6; Fat (g) = 1.9; Protein = 3.4

🥣 Cereal (Malt-O-Meal Toasted Oat Cereal) ☞ serving size: 1 cup = 22 g; Calories = 82.7; Total Carb (g) = 16.1; Net Carb (g) = 14; Fat (g) = 1.5; Protein = 2.7

🥣 Cereal (Nature Valley Granola) ☞ serving size: 1 cup = 82 g; Calories = 312.4; Total Carb (g) = 65.1; Net Carb (g) = 61; Fat (g) = 3.9; Protein = 6.5

🥣 Cereal Cooked Nfs ☞ serving size: 1 cup, cooked = 240 g; Calo-

ries = 153.6; Total Carb (g) = 27.3; Net Carb (g) = 23.2; Fat (g) = 2.6; Protein = 5.3

☛ Cereal Corn Flakes ☞ serving size: 1 cup = 25 g; Calories = 89.3; Total Carb (g) = 21; Net Carb (g) = 20.2; Fat (g) = 0.1; Protein = 1.9

☛ Cereal Crispy Brown Rice ☞ serving size: 1 cup = 32 g; Calories = 126.1; Total Carb (g) = 27.6; Net Carb (g) = 27.4; Fat (g) = 0.4; Protein = 2.1

☛ Cereal Frosted Corn Flakes ☞ serving size: 1 cup = 40 g; Calories = 147.6; Total Carb (g) = 35.7; Net Carb (g) = 34.8; Fat (g) = 0.7; Protein = 1.6

☛ Cereal Frosted Rice ☞ serving size: 1 cup = 45 g; Calories = 172.8; Total Carb (g) = 41.1; Net Carb (g) = 40.9; Fat (g) = 0.2; Protein = 1.9

☛ Cereal Granola ☞ serving size: 1 cup = 111 g; Calories = 422.9; Total Carb (g) = 88.9; Net Carb (g) = 80.7; Fat (g) = 5.8; Protein = 10

☛ Cereal Muesli ☞ serving size: 1 cup = 85 g; Calories = 301.8; Total Carb (g) = 63.7; Net Carb (g) = 57.1; Fat (g) = 4.6; Protein = 7.3

☛ Cereal Oat Nfs ☞ serving size: 1 cup, nfs = 33 g; Calories = 124.1; Total Carb (g) = 24.2; Net Carb (g) = 21.1; Fat (g) = 2.2; Protein = 4

☛ Cereal Puffed Wheat Sweetened ☞ serving size: 1 cup = 38 g; Calories = 144.4; Total Carb (g) = 33.6; Net Carb (g) = 31.7; Fat (g) = 0.8; Protein = 2.2

☛ Cereal Ready-To-Eat Nfs ☞ serving size: 1 cup = 40 g; Calories = 149.6; Total Carb (g) = 31.8; Net Carb (g) = 29.1; Fat (g) = 1.9; Protein = 3.6

☛ Cereal Rice Flakes ☞ serving size: 1 cup = 27 g; Calories = 106.4; Total Carb (g) = 23.3; Net Carb (g) = 23.1; Fat (g) = 0.3; Protein = 1.8

☛ Chocolate-Flavored Frosted Puffed Corn ☞ serving size: 1 cup = 30 g; Calories = 121.5; Total Carb (g) = 26.2; Net Carb (g) = 25; Fat (g) = 1.1; Protein = 1

🥣 Corn Grits White Regular And Quick Enriched Cooked With Water With Salt ☞ serving size: 1 cup = 257 g; Calories = 182.5; Total Carb (g) = 37.9; Net Carb (g) = 35.9; Fat (g) = 1.2; Protein = 4.4

🥣 Corn Grits White Regular And Quick Enriched Dry ☞ serving size: 1 tbsp = 9.7 g; Calories = 35.9; Total Carb (g) = 7.7; Net Carb (g) = 7.2; Fat (g) = 0.2; Protein = 0.7

🥣 Corn Grits Yellow Regular And Quick Unenriched Dry ☞ serving size: 1 tbsp = 9.7 g; Calories = 36; Total Carb (g) = 7.7; Net Carb (g) = 7.6; Fat (g) = 0.1; Protein = 0.9

🥣 Corn Grits Yellow Regular Quick Enriched Cooked With Water With Salt ☞ serving size: 1 cup = 233 g; Calories = 151.5; Total Carb (g) = 32.3; Net Carb (g) = 30.7; Fat (g) = 0.9; Protein = 2.9

🥣 Cornmeal Mush Fat Added In Cooking ☞ serving size: 1 cup, cooked = 240 g; Calories = 168; Total Carb (g) = 29.4; Net Carb (g) = 28; Fat (g) = 4.3; Protein = 2.7

🥣 Cornmeal Mush Fat Not Added In Cooking ☞ serving size: 1 cup, cooked = 240 g; Calories = 139.2; Total Carb (g) = 29.9; Net Carb (g) = 28.5; Fat (g) = 0.7; Protein = 2.7

🥣 Cornmeal Mush Ns As To Fat Added In Cooking ☞ serving size: 1 cup, cooked = 240 g; Calories = 168; Total Carb (g) = 29.4; Net Carb (g) = 28; Fat (g) = 4.3; Protein = 2.7

🥣 Cornmeal Puerto Rican Style ☞ serving size: 1 cup, cooked = 240 g; Calories = 355.2; Total Carb (g) = 67.6; Net Carb (g) = 66.4; Fat (g) = 5.2; Protein = 9.7

🥣 Cream Of Rice Cooked With Water With Salt ☞ serving size: 1 cup = 244 g; Calories = 126.9; Total Carb (g) = 28.1; Net Carb (g) = 27.8; Fat (g) = 0.2; Protein = 2.2

🥣 Cream Of Rice Dry ☞ serving size: 1/4 cup (1 nlea serving) = 45 g; Calories = 166.5; Total Carb (g) = 37.1; Net Carb (g) = 36.8; Fat (g) = 0.2; Protein = 2.8

☙ Cream Of Rye ☞ serving size: 1 cup, cooked = 240 g; Calories = 98.4; Total Carb (g) = 21.3; Net Carb (g) = 17.9; Fat (g) = 0.4; Protein = 3.1

☙ Cream Of Wheat 1 Minute Cook Time Cooked With Water Microwaved Without Salt ☞ serving size: 1 cup = 237 g; Calories = 130.4; Total Carb (g) = 25.3; Net Carb (g) = 21.7; Fat (g) = 0.9; Protein = 4.6

☙ Cream Of Wheat 1 Minute Cook Time Cooked With Water Stove-Top Without Salt ☞ serving size: 1 cup = 245 g; Calories = 137.2; Total Carb (g) = 27.3; Net Carb (g) = 26.4; Fat (g) = 1; Protein = 4

☙ Cream Of Wheat 1 Minute Cook Time Dry ☞ serving size: 3 tablespoon (1 serving) = 33 g; Calories = 118.5; Total Carb (g) = 24; Net Carb (g) = 22.5; Fat (g) = 0.5; Protein = 3.9

☙ Cream Of Wheat 2 1/2 Minute Cook Time Cooked With Water Microwaved Without Salt ☞ serving size: 1 cup = 231 g; Calories = 120.1; Total Carb (g) = 23.3; Net Carb (g) = 21.7; Fat (g) = 0.9; Protein = 4.3

☙ Cream Of Wheat 2 1/2 Minute Cook Time Cooked With Water Stove-Top Without Salt ☞ serving size: 1 cup = 244 g; Calories = 136.6; Total Carb (g) = 28.7; Net Carb (g) = 26.9; Fat (g) = 0.5; Protein = 3.5

☙ Cream Of Wheat 2 1/2 Minute Cook Time Dry ☞ serving size: 3 tablespoon (1 nlea serving) = 33 g; Calories = 117.2; Total Carb (g) = 23.7; Net Carb (g) = 22.2; Fat (g) = 0.5; Protein = 3.8

☙ Cream Of Wheat Instant Dry ☞ serving size: 1 tbsp = 11.5 g; Calories = 42.1; Total Carb (g) = 8.7; Net Carb (g) = 8.3; Fat (g) = 0.2; Protein = 1.2

☙ Cream Of Wheat Instant Made With Milk Fat Added In Cooking ☞ serving size: 1 cup, cooked = 240 g; Calories = 290.4; Total Carb (g) = 43.1; Net Carb (g) = 41.9; Fat (g) = 8.8; Protein = 9.9

🥣 Cream Of Wheat Instant Made With Milk Fat Not Added In Cooking ☞ serving size: 1 cup, cooked = 240 g; Calories = 259.2; Total Carb (g) = 44.2; Net Carb (g) = 43; Fat (g) = 4.5; Protein = 10.1

🥣 Cream Of Wheat Instant Made With Milk Ns As To Fat Added In Cooking ☞ serving size: 1 cup, cooked = 240 g; Calories = 290.4; Total Carb (g) = 43.1; Net Carb (g) = 41.9; Fat (g) = 8.8; Protein = 9.9

🥣 Cream Of Wheat Instant Made With Non-Dairy Milk Fat Added In Cooking ☞ serving size: 1 cup, cooked = 240 g; Calories = 254.4; Total Carb (g) = 41.4; Net Carb (g) = 39.9; Fat (g) = 7.2; Protein = 5.7

🥣 Cream Of Wheat Instant Made With Non-Dairy Milk Fat Not Added In Cooking ☞ serving size: 1 cup, cooked = 240 g; Calories = 220.8; Total Carb (g) = 42.4; Net Carb (g) = 41; Fat (g) = 3; Protein = 5.9

🥣 Cream Of Wheat Instant Made With Non-Dairy Milk Ns As To Fat Added In Cooking ☞ serving size: 1 cup, cooked = 240 g; Calories = 254.4; Total Carb (g) = 41.4; Net Carb (g) = 39.9; Fat (g) = 7.2; Protein = 5.7

🥣 Cream Of Wheat Instant Made With Water Fat Added In Cooking ☞ serving size: 1 cup, cooked = 240 g; Calories = 194.4; Total Carb (g) = 33.8; Net Carb (g) = 32.6; Fat (g) = 4.8; Protein = 3.6

🥣 Cream Of Wheat Instant Made With Water Fat Not Added In Cooking ☞ serving size: 1 cup, cooked = 240 g; Calories = 158.4; Total Carb (g) = 34.6; Net Carb (g) = 33.4; Fat (g) = 0.5; Protein = 3.7

🥣 Cream Of Wheat Instant Made With Water Ns As To Fat Added In Cooking ☞ serving size: 1 cup, cooked = 240 g; Calories = 194.4; Total Carb (g) = 33.8; Net Carb (g) = 32.6; Fat (g) = 4.8; Protein = 3.6

🥣 Cream Of Wheat Instant Prepared With Water Without Salt ☞ serving size: 1 cup = 241 g; Calories = 149.4; Total Carb (g) = 31.5; Net Carb (g) = 30.1; Fat (g) = 0.6; Protein = 4.4

🥣 Cream Of Wheat Ns As To Regular Quick Or Instant Fat Added

In Cooking ☞ serving size: 1 cup, cooked = 240 g; Calories = 153.6; Total Carb (g) = 24.9; Net Carb (g) = 23.7; Fat (g) = 4.2; Protein = 3.5

🥣 Cream Of Wheat Ns As To Regular Quick Or Instant Fat Not Added In Cooking ☞ serving size: 1 cup, cooked = 240 g; Calories = 122.4; Total Carb (g) = 25.4; Net Carb (g) = 24.2; Fat (g) = 0.5; Protein = 3.5

🥣 Cream Of Wheat Ns As To Regular Quick Or Instant Ns As To Fat Added In Cooking ☞ serving size: 1 cup, cooked = 240 g; Calories = 153.6; Total Carb (g) = 24.9; Net Carb (g) = 23.7; Fat (g) = 4.2; Protein = 3.5

🥣 Cream Of Wheat Regular (10 Minute) Cooked With Water With Salt ☞ serving size: 1 cup (1 serving) = 251 g; Calories = 125.5; Total Carb (g) = 26.8; Net Carb (g) = 25.5; Fat (g) = 0.5; Protein = 3.7

🥣 Cream Of Wheat Regular (10 Minute) Cooked With Water Without Salt ☞ serving size: 1 cup (1 serving) = 251 g; Calories = 125.5; Total Carb (g) = 26.4; Net Carb (g) = 25.2; Fat (g) = 0.5; Protein = 3.6

🥣 Cream Of Wheat Regular 10 Minute Cooking Dry ☞ serving size: 1 tbsp = 10.6 g; Calories = 39.2; Total Carb (g) = 8.1; Net Carb (g) = 7.7; Fat (g) = 0.2; Protein = 1.1

🥣 Cream Of Wheat Regular Or Quick Made With Milk Fat Added In Cooking ☞ serving size: 1 cup, cooked = 240 g; Calories = 276; Total Carb (g) = 36.8; Net Carb (g) = 35.6; Fat (g) = 9.2; Protein = 11.4

🥣 Cream Of Wheat Regular Or Quick Made With Milk Fat Not Added In Cooking ☞ serving size: 1 cup, cooked = 240 g; Calories = 249.6; Total Carb (g) = 37.4; Net Carb (g) = 36.2; Fat (g) = 5.6; Protein = 11.6

🥣 Cream Of Wheat Regular Or Quick Made With Milk Ns As To Fat Added In Cooking ☞ serving size: 1 cup, cooked = 240 g; Calories = 276; Total Carb (g) = 36.8; Net Carb (g) = 35.6; Fat (g) = 9.2; Protein = 11.4

🥣 Cream Of Wheat Regular Or Quick Made With Non-Dairy Milk Fat Added In Cooking ☞ serving size: 1 cup, cooked = 240 g; Calories = 230.4; Total Carb (g) = 34.6; Net Carb (g) = 32.9; Fat (g) = 7.3; Protein = 6.2

🥣 Cream Of Wheat Regular Or Quick Made With Non-Dairy Milk Fat Not Added In Cooking ☞ serving size: 1 cup, cooked = 240 g; Calories = 201.6; Total Carb (g) = 35.2; Net Carb (g) = 33.5; Fat (g) = 3.6; Protein = 6.3

🥣 Cream Of Wheat Regular Or Quick Made With Non-Dairy Milk Ns As To Fat Added In Cooking ☞ serving size: 1 cup, cooked = 240 g; Calories = 230.4; Total Carb (g) = 34.6; Net Carb (g) = 32.9; Fat (g) = 7.3; Protein = 6.2

🥣 Cream Of Wheat Regular Or Quick Made With Water Fat Added In Cooking ☞ serving size: 1 cup, cooked = 240 g; Calories = 153.6; Total Carb (g) = 24.9; Net Carb (g) = 23.7; Fat (g) = 4.2; Protein = 3.5

🥣 Cream Of Wheat Regular Or Quick Made With Water Fat Not Added In Cooking ☞ serving size: 1 cup, cooked = 240 g; Calories = 122.4; Total Carb (g) = 25.4; Net Carb (g) = 24.2; Fat (g) = 0.5; Protein = 3.5

🥣 Cream Of Wheat Regular Or Quick Made With Water Ns As To Fat Added In Cooking ☞ serving size: 1 cup, cooked = 240 g; Calories = 153.6; Total Carb (g) = 24.9; Net Carb (g) = 23.7; Fat (g) = 4.2; Protein = 3.5

🥣 Familia ☞ serving size: 1 cup = 122 g; Calories = 473.4; Total Carb (g) = 90; Net Carb (g) = 79.7; Fat (g) = 7.7; Protein = 11.6

🥣 Farina Enriched Assorted Brands Including Cream Of Wheat Quick (1-3 Minutes) Cooked With Wat ☞ serving size: 1 cup = 240 g; Calories = 132; Total Carb (g) = 26.2; Net Carb (g) = 24.3; Fat (g) = 0.8; Protein = 4.4

🥣 Farina Enriched Assorted Brands Including Cream Of Wheat

Quick (1-3 Minutes) Dry ☞ serving size: 1 tbsp = 11 g; Calories = 39.6; Total Carb (g) = 8.1; Net Carb (g) = 7.6; Fat (g) = 0.2; Protein = 1.3

🥣 Farina Enriched Cooked With Water With Salt ☞ serving size: 1 cup = 233 g; Calories = 123.5; Total Carb (g) = 25.4; Net Carb (g) = 23.6; Fat (g) = 0.8; Protein = 4.2

🥣 Farina Unenriched Dry ☞ serving size: 1 tbsp = 10.9 g; Calories = 40.2; Total Carb (g) = 8.5; Net Carb (g) = 8.3; Fat (g) = 0.1; Protein = 1.2

🥣 Frosted Oat Cereal With Marshmallows ☞ serving size: 3/4 cup (1 nlea serving) = 30 g; Calories = 120; Total Carb (g) = 25.4; Net Carb (g) = 24.1; Fat (g) = 1; Protein = 2.1

🥣 General Mills Cheerios ☞ serving size: 1 cup (1 nlea serving) = 28 g; Calories = 104.2; Total Carb (g) = 20.5; Net Carb (g) = 17.7; Fat (g) = 1.9; Protein = 3.5

🥣 Granola Homemade ☞ serving size: 1 cup = 122 g; Calories = 596.6; Total Carb (g) = 65.7; Net Carb (g) = 54.9; Fat (g) = 29.7; Protein = 16.7

🥣 Grits Instant Made With Milk Fat Added In Cooking ☞ serving size: 1 cup, cooked = 240 g; Calories = 297.6; Total Carb (g) = 43.6; Net Carb (g) = 41.7; Fat (g) = 10.5; Protein = 9.4

🥣 Grits Instant Made With Milk Fat Not Added In Cooking ☞ serving size: 1 cup, cooked = 240 g; Calories = 254.4; Total Carb (g) = 45.1; Net Carb (g) = 43.1; Fat (g) = 4.9; Protein = 9.7

🥣 Grits Instant Made With Milk Ns As To Fat Added In Cooking ☞ serving size: 1 cup, cooked = 240 g; Calories = 297.6; Total Carb (g) = 43.6; Net Carb (g) = 41.7; Fat (g) = 10.5; Protein = 9.4

🥣 Grits Instant Made With Non-Dairy Milk Fat Added In Cooking ☞ serving size: 1 cup, cooked = 240 g; Calories = 261.6; Total Carb (g) = 41.9; Net Carb (g) = 39.7; Fat (g) = 9; Protein = 5.4

🥣 Grits Instant Made With Non-Dairy Milk Ns As To Fat Added In

Cooking ☞ serving size: 1 cup, cooked = 240 g; Calories = 261.6; Total Carb (g) = 41.9; Net Carb (g) = 39.7; Fat (g) = 9; Protein = 5.4

🥄 Grits Instant Made With Water Fat Added In Cooking ☞ serving size: 1 cup, cooked = 240 g; Calories = 201.6; Total Carb (g) = 34.5; Net Carb (g) = 32.5; Fat (g) = 6.6; Protein = 3.3

🥄 Grits Instant Made With Water Fat Not Added In Cooking ☞ serving size: 1 cup, cooked = 240 g; Calories = 156; Total Carb (g) = 35.6; Net Carb (g) = 33.7; Fat (g) = 1; Protein = 3.3

🥄 Grits Instant Made With Water Ns As To Fat Added In Cooking ☞ serving size: 1 cup, cooked = 240 g; Calories = 201.6; Total Carb (g) = 34.5; Net Carb (g) = 32.5; Fat (g) = 6.6; Protein = 3.3

🥄 Grits Ns As To Regular Quick Or Instant Fat Added In Cooking ☞ serving size: 1 cup, cooked = 240 g; Calories = 168; Total Carb (g) = 29.3; Net Carb (g) = 27.6; Fat (g) = 4.3; Protein = 2.9

🥄 Grits Ns As To Regular Quick Or Instant Fat Not Added In Cooking ☞ serving size: 1 cup, cooked = 240 g; Calories = 139.2; Total Carb (g) = 29.8; Net Carb (g) = 28.1; Fat (g) = 0.7; Protein = 2.9

🥄 Grits Ns As To Regular Quick Or Instant Ns As To Fat Added In Cooking ☞ serving size: 1 cup, cooked = 240 g; Calories = 168; Total Carb (g) = 29.3; Net Carb (g) = 27.6; Fat (g) = 4.3; Protein = 2.9

🥄 Grits Regular Or Quick Made With Milk Fat Added In Cooking ☞ serving size: 1 cup, cooked = 240 g; Calories = 290.4; Total Carb (g) = 40.9; Net Carb (g) = 39.2; Fat (g) = 9.2; Protein = 10.7

🥄 Grits Regular Or Quick Made With Milk Fat Not Added In Cooking ☞ serving size: 1 cup, cooked = 240 g; Calories = 264; Total Carb (g) = 41.6; Net Carb (g) = 40; Fat (g) = 5.7; Protein = 10.9

🥄 Grits Regular Or Quick Made With Milk Ns As To Fat Added In Cooking ☞ serving size: 1 cup, cooked = 240 g; Calories = 290.4; Total Carb (g) = 40.9; Net Carb (g) = 39.2; Fat (g) = 9.2; Protein = 10.7

🥄 Grits Regular Or Quick Made With Non-Dairy Milk Fat

Added In Cooking ☞ serving size: 1 cup, cooked = 240 g; Calories = 244.8; Total Carb (g) = 38.7; Net Carb (g) = 36.6; Fat (g) = 7.3; Protein = 5.5

🥣 Grits Regular Or Quick Made With Non-Dairy Milk Fat Not Added In Cooking ☞ serving size: 1 cup, cooked = 240 g; Calories = 216; Total Carb (g) = 39.4; Net Carb (g) = 37.3; Fat (g) = 3.7; Protein = 5.6

🥣 Grits Regular Or Quick Made With Non-Dairy Milk Ns As To Fat Added In Cooking ☞ serving size: 1 cup, cooked = 240 g; Calories = 244.8; Total Carb (g) = 38.7; Net Carb (g) = 36.6; Fat (g) = 7.3; Protein = 5.5

🥣 Grits Regular Or Quick Made With Water Fat Added In Cooking ☞ serving size: 1 cup, cooked = 240 g; Calories = 168; Total Carb (g) = 29.3; Net Carb (g) = 27.6; Fat (g) = 4.3; Protein = 2.9

🥣 Grits Regular Or Quick Made With Water Fat Not Added In Cooking ☞ serving size: 1 cup, cooked = 240 g; Calories = 139.2; Total Carb (g) = 29.8; Net Carb (g) = 28.1; Fat (g) = 0.7; Protein = 2.9

🥣 Grits Regular Or Quick Made With Water Ns As To Fat Added In Cooking ☞ serving size: 1 cup, cooked = 240 g; Calories = 168; Total Carb (g) = 29.3; Net Carb (g) = 27.6; Fat (g) = 4.3; Protein = 2.9

🥣 Grits With Cheese Fat Added In Cooking ☞ serving size: 1 cup, cooked = 240 g; Calories = 256.8; Total Carb (g) = 27.4; Net Carb (g) = 26; Fat (g) = 12.4; Protein = 8.4

🥣 Grits With Cheese Fat Not Added In Cooking ☞ serving size: 1 cup, cooked = 240 g; Calories = 230.4; Total Carb (g) = 27.9; Net Carb (g) = 26.2; Fat (g) = 9.2; Protein = 8.5

🥣 Grits With Cheese Ns As To Fat Added In Cooking ☞ serving size: 1 cup, cooked = 240 g; Calories = 256.8; Total Carb (g) = 27.4; Net Carb (g) = 26; Fat (g) = 12.4; Protein = 8.4

🥣 Health Valley Fiber 7 Flakes ☞ serving size: 3/4 cup (1 nlea serv-

ing) = 31 g; Calories = 109.4; Total Carb (g) = 24.2; Net Carb (g) = 19.9; Fat (g) = 0.4; Protein = 4.5

🥄 Hominy Cooked Fat Added In Cooking ☞ serving size: 1 cup = 170 g; Calories = 147.9; Total Carb (g) = 23.4; Net Carb (g) = 19.4; Fat (g) = 4.9; Protein = 2.5

🥄 Hominy Cooked Fat Not Added In Cooking ☞ serving size: 1 cup = 165 g; Calories = 118.8; Total Carb (g) = 23.4; Net Carb (g) = 19.3; Fat (g) = 1.5; Protein = 2.4

🥄 Hominy Cooked Ns As To Fat Added In Cooking ☞ serving size: 1 cup = 170 g; Calories = 147.9; Total Carb (g) = 23.4; Net Carb (g) = 19.4; Fat (g) = 4.9; Protein = 2.5

🥄 Incaparina Dry Mix (Corn And Soy Flours) Unprepared ☞ serving size: 1 tbsp = 8.9 g; Calories = 33.7; Total Carb (g) = 5.4; Net Carb (g) = 4.5; Fat (g) = 0.5; Protein = 1.9

🥄 Instant Grits (Made with Vegetable Fat) ☞ serving size: 1 cup, cooked = 240 g; Calories = 218.4; Total Carb (g) = 43.3; Net Carb (g) = 41.1; Fat (g) = 3.4; Protein = 5.5

🥄 Malt-O-Meal Apple Zings ☞ serving size: 1 cup (1 nlea serving) = 33 g; Calories = 128.7; Total Carb (g) = 28.8; Net Carb (g) = 28.1; Fat (g) = 0.9; Protein = 1.5

🥄 Malt-O-Meal Berry Colossal Crunch ☞ serving size: 3/4 cup (1 nlea serving) = 30 g; Calories = 118.8; Total Carb (g) = 26; Net Carb (g) = 25.4; Fat (g) = 1.3; Protein = 1.3

🥄 Malt-O-Meal Blueberry Mini Spooners ☞ serving size: 1 cup (1 nlea serving) = 55 g; Calories = 192.5; Total Carb (g) = 43.7; Net Carb (g) = 38; Fat (g) = 1.1; Protein = 4.9

🥄 Malt-O-Meal Blueberry Muffin Tops Cereal ☞ serving size: 3/4 cup (1 nlea serving) = 30 g; Calories = 132.9; Total Carb (g) = 24; Net Carb (g) = 22.6; Fat (g) = 3.4; Protein = 1.5

🥄 Malt-O-Meal Chocolate Dry ☞ serving size: 3 tbsp (1 nlea serv-

ing) = 35 g; Calories = 127.1; Total Carb (g) = 27.8; Net Carb (g) = 26.9; Fat (g) = 0.3; Protein = 3.7

🥄 Malt-O-Meal Chocolate Marshmallow Mateys ☞ serving size: 3/4 cup (1 nlea serving) = 30 g; Calories = 117.6; Total Carb (g) = 26.5; Net Carb (g) = 25.7; Fat (g) = 1.1; Protein = 1.1

🥄 Malt-O-Meal Chocolate Prepared With Water Without Salt ☞ serving size: 1 serving (3 t dry cereal plus 1 cup water) = 268 g; Calories = 126; Total Carb (g) = 24.7; Net Carb (g) = 23.6; Fat (g) = 0.3; Protein = 3.7

🥄 Malt-O-Meal Cinnamon Toasters ☞ serving size: 3/4 cup (1 nlea serving) = 30 g; Calories = 127.5; Total Carb (g) = 23.5; Net Carb (g) = 22; Fat (g) = 3.6; Protein = 1

🥄 Malt-O-Meal Coco-Roos ☞ serving size: 3/4 cup (1 nlea serving) = 30 g; Calories = 116.7; Total Carb (g) = 26; Net Carb (g) = 25; Fat (g) = 1.4; Protein = 1

🥄 Malt-O-Meal Cocoa Dyno-Bites ☞ serving size: 3/4 cup (1 nlea serving) = 29 g; Calories = 115.1; Total Carb (g) = 25.5; Net Carb (g) = 25.2; Fat (g) = 1; Protein = 1.2

🥄 Malt-O-Meal Colossal Crunch ☞ serving size: 3/4 cup (1 nlea serving) = 30 g; Calories = 120.3; Total Carb (g) = 24.5; Net Carb (g) = 24; Fat (g) = 1.6; Protein = 1.1

🥄 Malt-O-Meal Corn Bursts ☞ serving size: 1 cup (1 nlea serving) = 31 g; Calories = 119.4; Total Carb (g) = 28.1; Net Carb (g) = 27.5; Fat (g) = 0.1; Protein = 1

🥄 Malt-O-Meal Crispy Rice ☞ serving size: 1 (1/4) cup (1 nlea serving) = 33 g; Calories = 114.2; Total Carb (g) = 28.5; Net Carb (g) = 28.4; Fat (g) = 0.4; Protein = 2

🥄 Malt-O-Meal Farina Hot Wheat Cereal Dry ☞ serving size: 3 tbsp (1 nlea serving) = 35 g; Calories = 127.8; Total Carb (g) = 27; Net Carb (g) = 26; Fat (g) = 0.2; Protein = 3.7

🥣 Malt-O-Meal Frosted Flakes ☞ serving size: 3/4 cup (1 nlea serving) = 31 g; Calories = 120.6; Total Carb (g) = 28; Net Carb (g) = 27.6; Fat (g) = 0.3; Protein = 1.3

🥣 Malt-O-Meal Frosted Mini Spooners ☞ serving size: 1 cup (1 nlea serving) = 55 g; Calories = 194.7; Total Carb (g) = 45; Net Carb (g) = 39; Fat (g) = 1.1; Protein = 5

🥣 Malt-O-Meal Fruity Dyno-Bites ☞ serving size: 3/4 cup = 27 g; Calories = 109.1; Total Carb (g) = 24.3; Net Carb (g) = 24.1; Fat (g) = 0.9; Protein = 1.1

🥣 Malt-O-Meal Golden Puffs ☞ serving size: 3/4 cup (1 nlea serving) = 27 g; Calories = 99.9; Total Carb (g) = 24.2; Net Carb (g) = 23.5; Fat (g) = 0.2; Protein = 1.6

🥣 Malt-O-Meal Honey Buzzers ☞ serving size: 1 (1/3) cup = 29 g; Calories = 109.9; Total Carb (g) = 26; Net Carb (g) = 25; Fat (g) = 0.5; Protein = 1

🥣 Malt-O-Meal Honey Graham Squares ☞ serving size: 3/4 cup (1 nlea serving) = 30 g; Calories = 119.4; Total Carb (g) = 22.4; Net Carb (g) = 21.1; Fat (g) = 3; Protein = 1.3

🥣 Malt-O-Meal Honey Nut Scooters ☞ serving size: 1 cup (1 nlea serving) = 30 g; Calories = 116.1; Total Carb (g) = 23.9; Net Carb (g) = 22; Fat (g) = 1.4; Protein = 2.6

🥣 Malt-O-Meal Maple & Brown Sugar Hot Wheat Cereal Dry ☞ serving size: 1/4 cup (1 nlea serving) = 45 g; Calories = 165.6; Total Carb (g) = 36.2; Net Carb (g) = 35.4; Fat (g) = 0.2; Protein = 4

🥣 Malt-O-Meal Marshmallow Mateys ☞ serving size: 1 cup = 30 g; Calories = 116.1; Total Carb (g) = 24.8; Net Carb (g) = 23.4; Fat (g) = 1.1; Protein = 2.1

🥣 Malt-O-Meal Oat Blenders With Honey ☞ serving size: 3/4 cup (1 nlea serving) = 30 g; Calories = 118.8; Total Carb (g) = 25.5; Net Carb (g) = 24; Fat (g) = 1.3; Protein = 2

🥣 Malt-O-Meal Oat Blenders With Honey & Almonds ☞ serving size: 3/4 cup (1 nlea serving) = 30 g; Calories = 113.7; Total Carb (g) = 23.2; Net Carb (g) = 21.4; Fat (g) = 1.5; Protein = 2.3

🥣 Malt-O-Meal Original Plain Dry ☞ serving size: 3 tbsp (1 nlea serving) = 35 g; Calories = 127.8; Total Carb (g) = 27; Net Carb (g) = 26.3; Fat (g) = 0.3; Protein = 4.1

🥣 Malt-O-Meal Original Plain Prepared With Water Without Salt ☞ serving size: 1 serving (3 t dry cereal plus 1 cup water) = 268 g; Calories = 128.6; Total Carb (g) = 27; Net Carb (g) = 26.2; Fat (g) = 0.2; Protein = 4.5

🥣 Malt-O-Meal Raisin Bran Cereal ☞ serving size: 1 cup (1 nlea serving) = 59 g; Calories = 201.8; Total Carb (g) = 47.4; Net Carb (g) = 41.4; Fat (g) = 1.1; Protein = 4.5

🥣 Malt-O-Meal Tootie Fruities ☞ serving size: 1 cup (1 nlea serving) = 32 g; Calories = 125.1; Total Carb (g) = 27.5; Net Carb (g) = 26.8; Fat (g) = 1; Protein = 1.5

🥣 Masa Harina Cooked ☞ serving size: 1 cup, cooked = 240 g; Calories = 232.8; Total Carb (g) = 49.2; Net Carb (g) = 45.1; Fat (g) = 2.4; Protein = 5.4

🥣 Millet Puffed ☞ serving size: 1 cup = 21 g; Calories = 74.3; Total Carb (g) = 16.8; Net Carb (g) = 16.2; Fat (g) = 0.7; Protein = 2.7

🥣 Moms Best Honey Nut Toasty Os ☞ serving size: 1 cup (1 nlea serving) = 30 g; Calories = 116.4; Total Carb (g) = 24; Net Carb (g) = 22.1; Fat (g) = 1.4; Protein = 2.6

🥣 Moms Best Sweetened Wheat-Fuls ☞ serving size: 1 cup (1 nlea serving) = 55 g; Calories = 205.2; Total Carb (g) = 44.5; Net Carb (g) = 39; Fat (g) = 1; Protein = 4.5

🥣 Natures Path Organic Flax Plus Flakes ☞ serving size: 3/4 cup (1 nlea serving) = 30 g; Calories = 105; Total Carb (g) = 22.6; Net Carb (g) = 17.6; Fat (g) = 1.6; Protein = 3.6

🥄 Natures Path Organic Flax Plus Pumpkin Granola ☞ serving size: 3/4 cup (1 nlea serving) = 55 g; Calories = 256.9; Total Carb (g) = 36.4; Net Carb (g) = 31.7; Fat (g) = 10.1; Protein = 6.2

🥄 Oat Bran Flakes Health Valley ☞ serving size: 1 cup (1 nlea serving) = 50 g; Calories = 190; Total Carb (g) = 39; Net Carb (g) = 35; Fat (g) = 1.5; Protein = 5

🥄 Oatmeal Instant Plain Made With Milk Fat Added In Cooking ☞ serving size: 1 cup, cooked = 240 g; Calories = 304.8; Total Carb (g) = 39.7; Net Carb (g) = 35.4; Fat (g) = 12.6; Protein = 11.4

🥄 Oatmeal From Fast Food Fruit Flavored ☞ serving size: 1 cup, cooked = 240 g; Calories = 292.8; Total Carb (g) = 59.1; Net Carb (g) = 54.7; Fat (g) = 4.9; Protein = 5.5

🥄 Oatmeal From Fast Food Maple Flavored ☞ serving size: 1 cup, cooked = 240 g; Calories = 261.6; Total Carb (g) = 48.9; Net Carb (g) = 45.1; Fat (g) = 5.3; Protein = 5.8

🥄 Oatmeal From Fast Food Other Flavors ☞ serving size: 1 cup, cooked = 240 g; Calories = 261.6; Total Carb (g) = 48.9; Net Carb (g) = 45.1; Fat (g) = 5.3; Protein = 5.8

🥄 Oatmeal From Fast Food Plain ☞ serving size: 1 cup, cooked = 240 g; Calories = 189.6; Total Carb (g) = 28.7; Net Carb (g) = 24.6; Fat (g) = 5.8; Protein = 6.2

🥄 Oatmeal Instant Fruit Flavored Fat Added In Cooking ☞ serving size: 1 cup, cooked = 240 g; Calories = 268.8; Total Carb (g) = 46.8; Net Carb (g) = 42.3; Fat (g) = 8; Protein = 5.5

🥄 Oatmeal Instant Fruit Flavored Fat Not Added In Cooking ☞ serving size: 1 cup, cooked = 240 g; Calories = 230.4; Total Carb (g) = 48.2; Net Carb (g) = 43.7; Fat (g) = 2.9; Protein = 5.6

🥄 Oatmeal Instant Fruit Flavored Ns As To Fat Added In Cooking ☞ serving size: 1 cup, cooked = 240 g; Calories = 268.8; Total Carb (g) = 46.8; Net Carb (g) = 42.3; Fat (g) = 8; Protein = 5.5

🥣 Oatmeal Instant Maple Flavored Fat Added In Cooking ☞
serving size: 1 cup, cooked = 240 g; Calories = 271.2; Total Carb (g) =
47.1; Net Carb (g) = 42.8; Fat (g) = 8.1; Protein = 5.7

🥣 Oatmeal Instant Maple Flavored Fat Not Added In Cooking ☞
serving size: 1 cup, cooked = 240 g; Calories = 232.8; Total Carb (g) =
48.6; Net Carb (g) = 44; Fat (g) = 3; Protein = 5.9

🥣 Oatmeal Instant Maple Flavored Ns As To Fat Added In
Cooking ☞ serving size: 1 cup, cooked = 240 g; Calories = 271.2; Total
Carb (g) = 47.1; Net Carb (g) = 42.8; Fat (g) = 8.1; Protein = 5.7

🥣 Oatmeal Instant Other Flavors Fat Added In Cooking ☞ serving
size: 1 cup, cooked = 240 g; Calories = 271.2; Total Carb (g) = 47.1; Net
Carb (g) = 42.8; Fat (g) = 8.1; Protein = 5.7

🥣 Oatmeal Instant Other Flavors Fat Not Added In Cooking ☞
serving size: 1 cup, cooked = 240 g; Calories = 232.8; Total Carb (g) =
48.6; Net Carb (g) = 44; Fat (g) = 3; Protein = 5.9

🥣 Oatmeal Instant Other Flavors Ns As To Fat Added In Cooking
☞ serving size: 1 cup, cooked = 240 g; Calories = 271.2; Total Carb (g)
= 47.1; Net Carb (g) = 42.8; Fat (g) = 8.1; Protein = 5.7

🥣 Oatmeal Instant Plain Made With Milk Fat Not Added In
Cooking ☞ serving size: 1 cup, cooked = 240 g; Calories = 264; Total
Carb (g) = 41; Net Carb (g) = 36.4; Fat (g) = 7.1; Protein = 11.8

🥣 Oatmeal Instant Plain Made With Milk Ns As To Fat Added In
Cooking ☞ serving size: 1 cup, cooked = 240 g; Calories = 304.8;
Total Carb (g) = 39.7; Net Carb (g) = 35.4; Fat (g) = 12.6; Protein = 11.4

🥣 Oatmeal Instant Plain Made With Non-Dairy Milk Fat Added
In Cooking ☞ serving size: 1 cup, cooked = 240 g; Calories =
268.8; Total Carb (g) = 38; Net Carb (g) = 33.2; Fat (g) = 11.1; Protein
= 7.4

🥣 Oatmeal Instant Plain Made With Non-Dairy Milk Fat Not
Added In Cooking ☞ serving size: 1 cup, cooked = 240 g; Calories =

225.6; Total Carb (g) = 39.2; Net Carb (g) = 34.4; Fat (g) = 5.6; Protein = 7.6

🥣 Oatmeal Instant Plain Made With Non-Dairy Milk Ns As To Fat Added In Cooking ☞ serving size: 1 cup, cooked = 240 g; Calories = 268.8; Total Carb (g) = 38; Net Carb (g) = 33.2; Fat (g) = 11.1; Protein = 7.4

🥣 Oatmeal Instant Plain Made With Water Fat Added In Cooking ☞ serving size: 1 cup, cooked = 240 g; Calories = 208.8; Total Carb (g) = 30.6; Net Carb (g) = 26.3; Fat (g) = 8.7; Protein = 5.3

🥣 Oatmeal Instant Plain Made With Water Fat Not Added In Cooking ☞ serving size: 1 cup, cooked = 240 g; Calories = 163.2; Total Carb (g) = 31.6; Net Carb (g) = 27; Fat (g) = 3.1; Protein = 5.4

🥣 Oatmeal Instant Plain Made With Water Ns As To Fat Added In Cooking ☞ serving size: 1 cup, cooked = 240 g; Calories = 208.8; Total Carb (g) = 30.6; Net Carb (g) = 26.3; Fat (g) = 8.7; Protein = 5.3

🥣 Oatmeal Made With Milk And Sugar Puerto Rican Style ☞ serving size: 1 cup, cooked = 240 g; Calories = 348; Total Carb (g) = 63.3; Net Carb (g) = 59.9; Fat (g) = 6.3; Protein = 11

🥣 Oatmeal Multigrain Fat Added In Cooking ☞ serving size: 1 cup, cooked = 240 g; Calories = 163.2; Total Carb (g) = 28.8; Net Carb (g) = 24; Fat (g) = 4.7; Protein = 5

🥣 Oatmeal Multigrain Fat Not Added In Cooking ☞ serving size: 1 cup, cooked = 240 g; Calories = 134.4; Total Carb (g) = 29.3; Net Carb (g) = 24.5; Fat (g) = 1.1; Protein = 5.1

🥣 Oatmeal Multigrain Ns As To Fat Added In Cooking ☞ serving size: 1 cup, cooked = 240 g; Calories = 163.2; Total Carb (g) = 28.8; Net Carb (g) = 24; Fat (g) = 4.7; Protein = 5

🥣 Oatmeal Ns As To Regular Quick Or Instant Fat Added In Cooking ☞ serving size: 1 cup, cooked = 240 g; Calories = 182.4; Total Carb (g) = 26.8; Net Carb (g) = 22.7; Fat (g) = 6.2; Protein = 5.2

Oatmeal Ns As To Regular Quick Or Instant Fat Not Added In Cooking ☞ serving size: 1 cup, cooked = 240 g; Calories = 153.6; Total Carb (g) = 27.3; Net Carb (g) = 23.2; Fat (g) = 2.6; Protein = 5.3

Oatmeal Ns As To Regular Quick Or Instant Ns As To Fat Added In Cooking ☞ serving size: 1 cup, cooked = 240 g; Calories = 182.4; Total Carb (g) = 26.8; Net Carb (g) = 22.7; Fat (g) = 6.2; Protein = 5.2

Oatmeal Reduced Sugar Flavored Fat Added In Cooking ☞ serving size: 1 cup, cooked = 240 g; Calories = 240; Total Carb (g) = 38.7; Net Carb (g) = 34.3; Fat (g) = 8.4; Protein = 5.5

Oatmeal Reduced Sugar Flavored Fat Not Added In Cooking ☞ serving size: 1 cup, cooked = 240 g; Calories = 199.2; Total Carb (g) = 39.9; Net Carb (g) = 35.3; Fat (g) = 3.1; Protein = 5.6

Oatmeal Reduced Sugar Flavored Ns As To Fat Added In Cooking ☞ serving size: 1 cup, cooked = 240 g; Calories = 240; Total Carb (g) = 38.7; Net Carb (g) = 34.3; Fat (g) = 8.4; Protein = 5.5

Oatmeal Reduced Sugar Plain Fat Added In Cooking ☞ serving size: 1 cup, cooked = 240 g; Calories = 240; Total Carb (g) = 38.7; Net Carb (g) = 34.3; Fat (g) = 8.4; Protein = 5.5

Oatmeal Reduced Sugar Plain Fat Not Added In Cooking ☞ serving size: 1 cup, cooked = 240 g; Calories = 199.2; Total Carb (g) = 39.9; Net Carb (g) = 35.3; Fat (g) = 3.1; Protein = 5.6

Oatmeal Reduced Sugar Plain Ns As To Fat Added In Cooking ☞ serving size: 1 cup, cooked = 240 g; Calories = 240; Total Carb (g) = 38.7; Net Carb (g) = 34.3; Fat (g) = 8.4; Protein = 5.5

Oatmeal Regular Or Quick Made With Milk Fat Added In Cooking ☞ serving size: 1 cup, cooked = 240 g; Calories = 302.4; Total Carb (g) = 38.3; Net Carb (g) = 34.3; Fat (g) = 11; Protein = 13

Oatmeal Regular Or Quick Made With Milk Fat Not Added In Cooking ☞ serving size: 1 cup, cooked = 240 g; Calories = 276; Total Carb (g) = 39; Net Carb (g) = 34.9; Fat (g) = 7.6; Protein = 13.2

🥣 Oatmeal Regular Or Quick Made With Milk Ns As To Fat Added In Cooking ☞ serving size: 1 cup, cooked = 240 g; Calories = 302.4; Total Carb (g) = 38.3; Net Carb (g) = 34.3; Fat (g) = 11; Protein = 13

🥣 Oatmeal Regular Or Quick Made With Non-Dairy Milk Fat Added In Cooking ☞ serving size: 1 cup, cooked = 240 g; Calories = 256.8; Total Carb (g) = 36.2; Net Carb (g) = 31.6; Fat (g) = 9.1; Protein = 7.9

🥣 Oatmeal Regular Or Quick Made With Non-Dairy Milk Fat Not Added In Cooking ☞ serving size: 1 cup, cooked = 240 g; Calories = 230.4; Total Carb (g) = 36.8; Net Carb (g) = 32.3; Fat (g) = 5.6; Protein = 8

🥣 Oatmeal Regular Or Quick Made With Non-Dairy Milk Ns As To Fat Added In Cooking ☞ serving size: 1 cup, cooked = 240 g; Calories = 256.8; Total Carb (g) = 36.2; Net Carb (g) = 31.6; Fat (g) = 9.1; Protein = 7.9

🥣 Oatmeal Regular Or Quick Made With Water Fat Added In Cooking ☞ serving size: 1 cup, cooked = 240 g; Calories = 182.4; Total Carb (g) = 26.8; Net Carb (g) = 22.7; Fat (g) = 6.2; Protein = 5.2

🥣 Oatmeal Regular Or Quick Made With Water Fat Not Added In Cooking ☞ serving size: 1 cup, cooked = 240 g; Calories = 153.6; Total Carb (g) = 27.3; Net Carb (g) = 23.2; Fat (g) = 2.6; Protein = 5.3

🥣 Oatmeal Regular Or Quick Made With Water Ns As To Fat Added In Cooking ☞ serving size: 1 cup, cooked = 240 g; Calories = 182.4; Total Carb (g) = 26.8; Net Carb (g) = 22.7; Fat (g) = 6.2; Protein = 5.2

🥣 Oats Instant Fortified Maple And Brown Sugar Dry ☞ serving size: 1 packet = 43 g; Calories = 166; Total Carb (g) = 33; Net Carb (g) = 29.9; Fat (g) = 2; Protein = 4

🥣 Oats Instant Fortified Plain Dry ☞ serving size: 1 packet = 28 g; Calories = 101.4; Total Carb (g) = 19.5; Net Carb (g) = 16.7; Fat (g) = 1.9; Protein = 3.3

🥣 Oats Instant Fortified Plain Prepared With Water (Boiling Water Added Or Microwaved) ☞ serving size: 1 cup, cooked = 234 g; Calories = 159.1; Total Carb (g) = 27.3; Net Carb (g) = 23.3; Fat (g) = 3.2; Protein = 5.6

🥣 Oats Instant Fortified With Cinnamon And Spice Dry ☞ serving size: 1 packet = 45 g; Calories = 166.1; Total Carb (g) = 34.2; Net Carb (g) = 30.6; Fat (g) = 2.2; Protein = 4.3

🥣 Oats Instant Fortified With Cinnamon And Spice Prepared With Water ☞ serving size: 1 cup = 240 g; Calories = 230.4; Total Carb (g) = 45.5; Net Carb (g) = 40.7; Fat (g) = 2.9; Protein = 5.7

🥣 Oats Instant Fortified With Raisins And Spice Prepared With Water ☞ serving size: 1 cup = 240 g; Calories = 211.2; Total Carb (g) = 43; Net Carb (g) = 39.9; Fat (g) = 2.3; Protein = 4.8

🥣 Oats Regular And Quick And Instant Unenriched Cooked With Water (Includes Boiling And Microw ☞ serving size: 1 cup = 234 g; Calories = 166.1; Total Carb (g) = 28.1; Net Carb (g) = 24.1; Fat (g) = 3.6; Protein = 5.9

🥣 Oats Regular And Quick Not Fortified Dry ☞ serving size: 1 cup = 81 g; Calories = 307; Total Carb (g) = 54.8; Net Carb (g) = 46.7; Fat (g) = 5.3; Protein = 10.7

🥣 Post Alpha-Bits ☞ serving size: 1 cup (1 nlea serving for adults) = 30 g; Calories = 116.7; Total Carb (g) = 24.1; Net Carb (g) = 22; Fat (g) = 1.4; Protein = 3

🥣 Post Bran Flakes ☞ serving size: 3/4 cup (1 nlea serving) = 30 g; Calories = 98.4; Total Carb (g) = 24.2; Net Carb (g) = 18.7; Fat (g) = 0.6; Protein = 3

🥣 Post Cocoa Pebbles ☞ serving size: 3/4 cup (1 nlea serving) = 29 g; Calories = 115.1; Total Carb (g) = 24.9; Net Carb (g) = 24.4; Fat (g) = 1.2; Protein = 1.4

🥣 Post Fruity Pebbles ☞ serving size: 3/4 cup (1 nlea serving) = 27 g;

Calories = 108.5; Total Carb (g) = 23.3; Net Carb (g) = 23; Fat (g) = 1.1; Protein = 1.3

🥣 Post Golden Crisp ☞ serving size: 3/4 cup (1 nlea serving) = 27 g; Calories = 102.6; Total Carb (g) = 24.3; Net Carb (g) = 23; Fat (g) = 0.5; Protein = 1.5

🥣 Post Grape-Nuts Cereal ☞ serving size: 1/2 cup (1 nlea serving) = 58 g; Calories = 209.4; Total Carb (g) = 46.7; Net Carb (g) = 39.1; Fat (g) = 1.1; Protein = 6.5

🥣 Post Grape-Nuts Flakes ☞ serving size: 3/4 cup (1 nlea serving) = 29 g; Calories = 109; Total Carb (g) = 23.8; Net Carb (g) = 20.8; Fat (g) = 1.1; Protein = 2.7

🥣 Post Great Grains Banana Nut Crunch ☞ serving size: 1 cup (1 nlea serving) = 59 g; Calories = 230.1; Total Carb (g) = 41.8; Net Carb (g) = 35.2; Fat (g) = 5.2; Protein = 5.8

🥣 Post Great Grains Cranberry Almond Crunch ☞ serving size: 3/4 cup (1 nlea serving) = 48 g; Calories = 184.3; Total Carb (g) = 36.8; Net Carb (g) = 31.4; Fat (g) = 2.8; Protein = 4.3

🥣 Post Great Grains Crunchy Pecan Cereal ☞ serving size: 3/4 cup (1 nlea serving) = 52 g; Calories = 209.6; Total Carb (g) = 38; Net Carb (g) = 32.9; Fat (g) = 5.5; Protein = 4.7

🥣 Post Great Grains Raisin Date & Pecan ☞ serving size: 3/4 cup (1 nlea serving) = 55 g; Calories = 207.9; Total Carb (g) = 40.9; Net Carb (g) = 35.8; Fat (g) = 3.9; Protein = 4.4

🥣 Post Honey Bunches Of Oats Honey Roasted ☞ serving size: 3/4 cup (1 nlea serving) = 30 g; Calories = 120.3; Total Carb (g) = 24.4; Net Carb (g) = 23.1; Fat (g) = 1.6; Protein = 2.1

🥣 Post Honey Bunches Of Oats Pecan Bunches ☞ serving size: 3/4 cup (1 nlea serving) = 29 g; Calories = 115.7; Total Carb (g) = 23.8; Net Carb (g) = 22.3; Fat (g) = 1.6; Protein = 2

🥣 Post Honey Bunches Of Oats With Almonds ☞ serving size: 3/4 cup (1 nlea serving) = 32 g; Calories = 130.9; Total Carb (g) = 25.5; Net Carb (g) = 23.7; Fat (g) = 2.3; Protein = 2.5

👌 Post Honey Bunches Of Oats With Cinnamon Bunches 👉 serving size: 3/4 cup (1 nlea serving) = 30 g; Calories = 120; Total Carb (g) = 24.8; Net Carb (g) = 23.1; Fat (g) = 1.5; Protein = 2.1

👌 Post Honey Bunches Of Oats With Real Strawberries 👉 serving size: 3/4 cup (1 nlea serving) = 31 g; Calories = 123.7; Total Carb (g) = 25.8; Net Carb (g) = 24.2; Fat (g) = 1.5; Protein = 2.1

👌 Post Honey Bunches Of Oats With Vanilla Bunches 👉 serving size: 1 cup (1 nlea serving) = 56 g; Calories = 220.6; Total Carb (g) = 45.8; Net Carb (g) = 41.4; Fat (g) = 2.9; Protein = 4.4

👌 Post Honey Nut Shredded Wheat 👉 serving size: 1 cup (1 nlea serving) = 59 g; Calories = 220.1; Total Carb (g) = 49.3; Net Carb (g) = 43; Fat (g) = 1.7; Protein = 5

👌 Post Honeycomb Cereal 👉 serving size: 1 (1/2) cup (1 nlea serving) = 32 g; Calories = 126.1; Total Carb (g) = 27.7; Net Carb (g) = 26.7; Fat (g) = 0.9; Protein = 1.9

👌 Post Raisin Bran Cereal 👉 serving size: 1 cup (1 nlea serving) = 59 g; Calories = 191.2; Total Carb (g) = 46.6; Net Carb (g) = 38.5; Fat (g) = 0.9; Protein = 4.5

👌 Post Selects Blueberry Morning 👉 serving size: 1 (1/4) cup (1 nlea serving) = 55 g; Calories = 217.3; Total Carb (g) = 44.9; Net Carb (g) = 42.3; Fat (g) = 2.9; Protein = 3.6

👌 Post Selects Maple Pecan Crunch 👉 serving size: 3/4 cup (1 nlea serving) = 52 g; Calories = 214.8; Total Carb (g) = 40.3; Net Carb (g) = 36.4; Fat (g) = 4.5; Protein = 4.4

👌 Post Shredded Wheat Lightly Frosted Spoon-Size 👉 serving size: 1 cup (1 nlea serving) = 52 g; Calories = 183; Total Carb (g) = 43.6; Net Carb (g) = 38.6; Fat (g) = 1; Protein = 4.1

👌 Post Shredded Wheat N Bran Spoon-Size 👉 serving size: 1 (1/4) cup (1 nlea serving) = 59 g; Calories = 200; Total Carb (g) = 47.6; Net Carb (g) = 38.9; Fat (g) = 1.2; Protein = 6.5

🥣 Post Shredded Wheat Original Big Biscuit ☞ serving size: 2 biscuits (1 nlea serving) = 47 g; Calories = 158.4; Total Carb (g) = 37.1; Net Carb (g) = 31.3; Fat (g) = 0.9; Protein = 5.3

🥣 Post Shredded Wheat Original Spoon-Size ☞ serving size: 1 cup (1 nlea serving) = 49 g; Calories = 172; Total Carb (g) = 39.9; Net Carb (g) = 33.8; Fat (g) = 1; Protein = 5.8

🥣 Post Waffle Crisp ☞ serving size: 1 cup (1 nlea serving) = 30 g; Calories = 117; Total Carb (g) = 24.9; Net Carb (g) = 23.6; Fat (g) = 1.5; Protein = 2

🥣 Quaker 100% Natural Granola Oats Wheat And Honey ☞ serving size: 1/2 cup (1 nlea serving) = 48 g; Calories = 202.1; Total Carb (g) = 35.4; Net Carb (g) = 30.5; Fat (g) = 5.6; Protein = 5.1

🥣 Quaker Capn Crunch ☞ serving size: 3/4 cup (1 nlea serving) = 27 g; Calories = 107.5; Total Carb (g) = 23.1; Net Carb (g) = 22.4; Fat (g) = 1.4; Protein = 1.2

🥣 Quaker Capn Crunch With Crunchberries ☞ serving size: 3/4 cup (1 nlea serving) = 26 g; Calories = 103.2; Total Carb (g) = 22.3; Net Carb (g) = 21.7; Fat (g) = 1.3; Protein = 1.2

🥣 Quaker Capn Crunchs Halloween Crunch ☞ serving size: 3/4 cup (1 nlea serving) = 26 g; Calories = 104.5; Total Carb (g) = 22.1; Net Carb (g) = 21.5; Fat (g) = 1.5; Protein = 1.2

🥣 Quaker Capn Crunchs Oops! All Berries Cereal ☞ serving size: 1 cup (1 nlea serving) = 32 g; Calories = 126.4; Total Carb (g) = 27.9; Net Carb (g) = 27; Fat (g) = 1.3; Protein = 1.5

🥣 Quaker Capn Crunchs Peanut Butter Crunch ☞ serving size: 3/4 cup (1 nlea serving) = 27 g; Calories = 112.6; Total Carb (g) = 21.2; Net Carb (g) = 20.5; Fat (g) = 2.5; Protein = 1.9

🥣 Quaker Christmas Crunch ☞ serving size: 3/4 cup (1 nlea serv-

ing) = 26 g; Calories = 103.2; Total Carb (g) = 22.3; Net Carb (g) = 21.7; Fat (g) = 1.3; Protein = 1.2

🥄 Quaker Corn Grits Instant Cheddar Cheese Flavor Dry ☞ serving size: 1 packet (1 nlea serving) = 28 g; Calories = 101.6; Total Carb (g) = 20.4; Net Carb (g) = 19.3; Fat (g) = 1.5; Protein = 2.5

🥄 Quaker Corn Grits Instant Plain Dry ☞ serving size: 1 packet = 29 g; Calories = 99.5; Total Carb (g) = 22.7; Net Carb (g) = 21.5; Fat (g) = 0.6; Protein = 2.1

🥄 Quaker Corn Grits Instant Plain Prepared (Microwaved Or Boiling Water Added) Without Salt ☞ serving size: 1 cup = 219 g; Calories = 162.1; Total Carb (g) = 34.9; Net Carb (g) = 32.5; Fat (g) = 1.1; Protein = 3.5

🥄 Quaker Hominy Grits White Quick Dry ☞ serving size: 1/4 cup = 37 g; Calories = 128.8; Total Carb (g) = 29.5; Net Carb (g) = 27.7; Fat (g) = 0.4; Protein = 3.3

🥄 Quaker Hominy Grits White Regular Dry ☞ serving size: 1/4 cup (1 nlea serving) = 41 g; Calories = 148; Total Carb (g) = 32.5; Net Carb (g) = 31.8; Fat (g) = 0.7; Protein = 3.6

🥄 Quaker Honey Graham Oh!s ☞ serving size: 3/4 cup (1 nlea serving) = 27 g; Calories = 111.2; Total Carb (g) = 22.6; Net Carb (g) = 22; Fat (g) = 2.1; Protein = 1.1

🥄 Quaker Instant Grits Butter Flavor Dry ☞ serving size: 1 packet (1 nlea serving) = 28 g; Calories = 103.3; Total Carb (g) = 21; Net Carb (g) = 19.6; Fat (g) = 1.6; Protein = 2.3

🥄 Quaker Instant Grits Country Bacon Flavor Dry ☞ serving size: 1 packet (1 nlea serving) = 28 g; Calories = 95.2; Total Carb (g) = 21.1; Net Carb (g) = 19.7; Fat (g) = 0.5; Protein = 2.8

🥄 Quaker Instant Grits Ham N Cheese Flavor Dry ☞ serving size: 1 packet (1 nlea serving) = 28 g; Calories = 99.4; Total Carb (g) = 19.9; Net Carb (g) = 18.7; Fat (g) = 1.3; Protein = 3

🥣 Quaker Instant Grits Product With American Cheese Flavor Dry ☞ serving size: 1 packet (1 nlea serving) = 28 g; Calories = 100.8; Total Carb (g) = 20.8; Net Carb (g) = 19.6; Fat (g) = 1.3; Protein = 2.5

🥣 Quaker Instant Grits Redeye Gravy & Country Ham Flavor Dry ☞ serving size: 1 packet (1 nlea serving) = 28 g; Calories = 95.8; Total Carb (g) = 21.2; Net Carb (g) = 20; Fat (g) = 0.4; Protein = 2.8

🥣 Quaker Instant Oatmeal Apple And Cinnamon Reduced Sugar ☞ serving size: 1 packet (1 nlea serving) = 31 g; Calories = 111; Total Carb (g) = 22.4; Net Carb (g) = 19.4; Fat (g) = 1.8; Protein = 3.2

🥣 Quaker Instant Oatmeal Apples And Cinnamon Dry ☞ serving size: 1 packet (1 nlea serving) = 43 g; Calories = 157.4; Total Carb (g) = 33; Net Carb (g) = 29.4; Fat (g) = 2; Protein = 3.7

🥣 Quaker Instant Oatmeal Banana Bread Dry ☞ serving size: 1 packet (1 nlea serving) = 41 g; Calories = 150.9; Total Carb (g) = 31; Net Carb (g) = 28.3; Fat (g) = 2; Protein = 3.7

🥣 Quaker Instant Oatmeal Cinnamon Spice Reduced Sugar ☞ serving size: 1 packet (1 nlea serving) = 34 g; Calories = 121.7; Total Carb (g) = 23.6; Net Carb (g) = 20.6; Fat (g) = 2.1; Protein = 3.8

🥣 Quaker Instant Oatmeal Cinnamon Swirl High Fiber ☞ serving size: 1 packet (1 nlea serving) = 45 g; Calories = 164.7; Total Carb (g) = 34.1; Net Carb (g) = 24; Fat (g) = 2.2; Protein = 4

🥣 Quaker Instant Oatmeal Cinnamon-Spice Dry ☞ serving size: 1 packet (1 nlea serving) = 43 g; Calories = 158.7; Total Carb (g) = 32; Net Carb (g) = 28.5; Fat (g) = 2.2; Protein = 4.5

🥣 Quaker Instant Oatmeal Dinosaur Eggs Brown Sugar Dry ☞ serving size: 1 packet (1 nlea serving) = 50 g; Calories = 192; Total Carb (g) = 36.8; Net Carb (g) = 33.6; Fat (g) = 3.8; Protein = 4.4

🥣 Quaker Instant Oatmeal Fruit And Cream Variety Dry ☞ serving size: 1 packet = 35 g; Calories = 132.7; Total Carb (g) = 26.4; Net Carb (g) = 24.3; Fat (g) = 2.2; Protein = 2.9

🥣 Quaker Instant Oatmeal Fruit And Cream Variety Of Flavors Reduced Sugar ☞ serving size: 1 packet = 33 g; Calories = 124.1; Total Carb (g) = 23.6; Net Carb (g) = 20.9; Fat (g) = 2.5; Protein = 3.4

🥣 Quaker Instant Oatmeal Maple And Brown Sugar Dry ☞ serving size: 1 packet = 43 g; Calories = 158.2; Total Carb (g) = 33.1; Net Carb (g) = 30; Fat (g) = 2; Protein = 4

🥣 Quaker Instant Oatmeal Organic Regular ☞ serving size: 1 packet = 41 g; Calories = 150.5; Total Carb (g) = 27.5; Net Carb (g) = 23.5; Fat (g) = 2.6; Protein = 6.6

🥣 Quaker Instant Oatmeal Raisin And Spice Dry ☞ serving size: 1 packet (1 nlea serving) = 43 g; Calories = 154.8; Total Carb (g) = 32.5; Net Carb (g) = 30.1; Fat (g) = 1.7; Protein = 3.9

🥣 Quaker Instant Oatmeal Raisins Dates And Walnuts Dry ☞ serving size: 1 packet = 37 g; Calories = 137.3; Total Carb (g) = 26.8; Net Carb (g) = 24.2; Fat (g) = 2.6; Protein = 3.3

🥣 Quaker Instant Oatmeal Weight Control Cinnamon ☞ serving size: 1 packet (1 nlea serving) = 45 g; Calories = 162.5; Total Carb (g) = 28.9; Net Carb (g) = 23; Fat (g) = 2.8; Protein = 7.4

🥣 Quaker King Vitaman ☞ serving size: 1 (1/2) cup (1 nlea serving) = 31 g; Calories = 118.1; Total Carb (g) = 26; Net Carb (g) = 24.9; Fat (g) = 1.1; Protein = 2

🥣 Quaker Low Fat 100% Natural Granola With Raisins ☞ serving size: 2/3 cup (1 nlea serving) = 55 g; Calories = 213.4; Total Carb (g) = 44.3; Net Carb (g) = 39; Fat (g) = 3; Protein = 4.6

🥣 Quaker Maple Brown Sugar Life Cereal ☞ serving size: 3/4 cup (1 nlea serving) = 32 g; Calories = 119.4; Total Carb (g) = 25.2; Net Carb (g) = 23.2; Fat (g) = 1.3; Protein = 2.9

🥣 Quaker Mothers Cinnamon Oat Crunch ☞ serving size: 1 cup (1 nlea serving) = 60 g; Calories = 229.2; Total Carb (g) = 47.9; Net Carb (g) = 43; Fat (g) = 2.7; Protein = 6.4

🥣 Quaker Mothers Cocoa Bumpers ☞ serving size: 1 cup (1 nlea serving) = 33 g; Calories = 126.1; Total Carb (g) = 29.7; Net Carb (g) = 28.8; Fat (g) = 0.5; Protein = 1.4

🥣 Quaker Mothers Graham Bumpers ☞ serving size: 3/4 cup (1 nlea serving) = 28 g; Calories = 106.1; Total Carb (g) = 24.9; Net Carb (g) = 24.2; Fat (g) = 0.4; Protein = 1.3

🥣 Quaker Mothers Peanut Butter Bumpers Cereal ☞ serving size: 1 cup (1 nlea serving) = 33 g; Calories = 134.3; Total Carb (g) = 26.3; Net Carb (g) = 25.5; Fat (g) = 2.4; Protein = 2.5

🥣 Quaker Mothers Toasted Oat Bran Cereal ☞ serving size: 3/4 cup (1 nlea serving) = 32 g; Calories = 119; Total Carb (g) = 24.1; Net Carb (g) = 21.4; Fat (g) = 1.6; Protein = 3.7

🥣 Quaker Natural Granola Apple Cranberry Almond ☞ serving size: 1/2 cup (1 nlea serving) = 49 g; Calories = 204.8; Total Carb (g) = 36.6; Net Carb (g) = 31.8; Fat (g) = 5.4; Protein = 4.5

🥣 Quaker Oat Bran Quaker/mothers Oat Bran Dry ☞ serving size: 1/2 cup (1 nlea serving) = 40 g; Calories = 145.6; Total Carb (g) = 25.2; Net Carb (g) = 19.5; Fat (g) = 3.2; Protein = 6.8

🥣 Quaker Oatmeal Real Medleys Apple Walnut Dry ☞ serving size: 1 package (1 nlea serving) = 75 g; Calories = 292.5; Total Carb (g) = 52.9; Net Carb (g) = 47.7; Fat (g) = 7.8; Protein = 6.1

🥣 Quaker Oatmeal Real Medleys Blueberry Hazelnut Dry ☞ serving size: 1 package (1 nlea serving) = 70 g; Calories = 270.2; Total Carb (g) = 48.6; Net Carb (g) = 43.2; Fat (g) = 6.9; Protein = 6.9

🥣 Quaker Oatmeal Real Medleys Cherry Pistachio Dry ☞ serving size: 1 package (1 nlea serving) = 73 g; Calories = 287.6; Total Carb (g) = 48.7; Net Carb (g) = 43.5; Fat (g) = 8; Protein = 8.8

🥣 Quaker Oatmeal Real Medleys Peach Almond Dry ☞ serving size: 1 package (1 nlea serving) = 75 g; Calories = 290.3; Total Carb (g) = 51.5; Net Carb (g) = 45.9; Fat (g) = 7.4; Protein = 7.6

👝 Quaker Oatmeal Real Medleys Summer Berry Dry ☞ serving size: 1 package (1 nlea serving) = 70 g; Calories = 247.1; Total Carb (g) = 50.8; Net Carb (g) = 44.9; Fat (g) = 3.1; Protein = 7.9

👝 Quaker Oatmeal Squares ☞ serving size: 1 cup (1 nlea serving) = 56 g; Calories = 212.2; Total Carb (g) = 43.6; Net Carb (g) = 38.9; Fat (g) = 2.7; Protein = 6.4

👝 Quaker Oatmeal Squares Cinnamon ☞ serving size: 1 cup (1 nlea serving) = 56 g; Calories = 212.2; Total Carb (g) = 43.7; Net Carb (g) = 38.9; Fat (g) = 2.7; Protein = 6.3

👝 Quaker Oatmeal Squares Golden Maple ☞ serving size: 1 cup (1 nlea serving) = 56 g; Calories = 212.8; Total Carb (g) = 43.7; Net Carb (g) = 39.1; Fat (g) = 2.7; Protein = 6.3

👝 Quaker Quaker 100% Natural Granola With Oats Wheat Honey And Raisins ☞ serving size: 1/2 cup (1 nlea serving) = 51 g; Calories = 210.1; Total Carb (g) = 38.1; Net Carb (g) = 33.3; Fat (g) = 5.3; Protein = 4.9

👝 Quaker Quaker Crunchy Bran ☞ serving size: 3/4 cup (1 nlea serving) = 27 g; Calories = 89.4; Total Carb (g) = 22.6; Net Carb (g) = 18.5; Fat (g) = 1.1; Protein = 1.7

👝 Quaker Quaker Honey Graham Life Cereal ☞ serving size: 3/4 cup (1 nlea serving) = 32 g; Calories = 119.4; Total Carb (g) = 25.1; Net Carb (g) = 23.1; Fat (g) = 1.3; Protein = 3

👝 Quaker Quaker Multigrain Oatmeal Dry ☞ serving size: 1/2 cup (1 nlea serving) = 40 g; Calories = 133.6; Total Carb (g) = 29.1; Net Carb (g) = 24.3; Fat (g) = 1.1; Protein = 5.1

👝 Quaker Quaker Oat Cinnamon Life ☞ serving size: 3/4 cup (1 nlea serving) = 32 g; Calories = 119.7; Total Carb (g) = 25.3; Net Carb (g) = 23.3; Fat (g) = 1.3; Protein = 2.9

👝 Quaker Quaker Oat Life Plain ☞ serving size: 3/4 cup (1 nlea serving) = 32 g; Calories = 119.7; Total Carb (g) = 24.9; Net Carb (g) = 22.8; Fat (g) = 1.4; Protein = 3.2

🍪 Quaker Quaker Puffed Rice ☞ serving size: 3/4 cup (1 nlea serving) = 14 g; Calories = 53.6; Total Carb (g) = 12.3; Net Carb (g) = 12.1; Fat (g) = 0.1; Protein = 1

🍪 Quaker Quaker Puffed Wheat ☞ serving size: 1 cup (1 nlea serving) = 15 g; Calories = 54.9; Total Carb (g) = 11.5; Net Carb (g) = 10.1; Fat (g) = 0.3; Protein = 2.4

🍪 Quaker Quick Oats Dry ☞ serving size: 1/2 cup = 40 g; Calories = 148.4; Total Carb (g) = 27.3; Net Carb (g) = 23.5; Fat (g) = 2.8; Protein = 5.5

🍪 Quaker Quick Oats With Iron Dry ☞ serving size: 1/2 cup = 40 g; Calories = 148.4; Total Carb (g) = 27.3; Net Carb (g) = 23.5; Fat (g) = 2.8; Protein = 5.5

🍪 Quaker Shredded Wheat Bagged Cereal ☞ serving size: 3 biscuits (1 nlea serving) = 63 g; Calories = 219.2; Total Carb (g) = 51; Net Carb (g) = 43.6; Fat (g) = 1.3; Protein = 7.1

🍪 Quaker Sweet Crunch/quisp ☞ serving size: 1 cup (1 nlea serving) = 27 g; Calories = 109.6; Total Carb (g) = 23; Net Carb (g) = 22.3; Fat (g) = 1.6; Protein = 1.2

🍪 Quaker Toasted Multigrain Crisps ☞ serving size: 1 (1/4) cup (1 nlea serving) = 57 g; Calories = 212; Total Carb (g) = 42.7; Net Carb (g) = 36.9; Fat (g) = 2.9; Protein = 7.1

🍪 Quaker Weight Control Instant Oatmeal Banana Bread ☞ serving size: 1 packet (1 nlea serving) = 45 g; Calories = 162.5; Total Carb (g) = 29; Net Carb (g) = 23.3; Fat (g) = 2.8; Protein = 7.4

🍪 Quaker Weight Control Instant Oatmeal Maple And Brown Sugar ☞ serving size: 1 packet (1 nlea serving) = 45 g; Calories = 162.5; Total Carb (g) = 28.9; Net Carb (g) = 23.1; Fat (g) = 2.8; Protein = 7.4

🥣 Quaker Whole Hearts Oat Cereal ☞ serving size: 3/4 cup (1 nlea serving) = 28 g; Calories = 105.3; Total Carb (g) = 22.4; Net Carb (g) = 19.9; Fat (g) = 1.6; Protein = 2.1

🥣 Quaker Whole Wheat Natural Cereal Dry ☞ serving size: 1/2 cup = 40 g; Calories = 133.2; Total Carb (g) = 29.9; Net Carb (g) = 26; Fat (g) = 0.8; Protein = 4.7

🥣 Ralston Corn Biscuits ☞ serving size: 1 cup (nlea serving) = 30 g; Calories = 112.8; Total Carb (g) = 25.7; Net Carb (g) = 25; Fat (g) = 0.3; Protein = 1.8

🥣 Ralston Corn Flakes ☞ serving size: 1 cup (1 nlea serving) = 28 g; Calories = 107.5; Total Carb (g) = 24.6; Net Carb (g) = 23.9; Fat (g) = 0.3; Protein = 1.7

🥣 Ralston Crisp Rice ☞ serving size: 1 (1/4) cup (1 nlea serving) = 33 g; Calories = 126.4; Total Carb (g) = 28.5; Net Carb (g) = 28.2; Fat (g) = 0.4; Protein = 2.2

🥣 Ralston Crispy Hexagons ☞ serving size: 1 cup (1 nlea serving) = 29 g; Calories = 109.9; Total Carb (g) = 25.2; Net Carb (g) = 24.7; Fat (g) = 0.3; Protein = 1.7

🥣 Ralston Enriched Bran Flakes ☞ serving size: 1 serving (nlea serving size = 0.75 cup) = 29 g; Calories = 113.1; Total Carb (g) = 23.1; Net Carb (g) = 18.2; Fat (g) = 1; Protein = 3

🥣 Ralston Tasteeos ☞ serving size: 1 cup (1 nlea serving) = 28 g; Calories = 110.6; Total Carb (g) = 21.3; Net Carb (g) = 18.3; Fat (g) = 1.5; Protein = 3

🥣 Rice Cream Of Cooked Fat Added In Cooking ☞ serving size: 1 cup, cooked = 240 g; Calories = 192; Total Carb (g) = 36.1; Net Carb (g) = 35.8; Fat (g) = 3.7; Protein = 2.8

🥣 Rice Cream Of Cooked Fat Not Added In Cooking ☞ serving size: 1 cup, cooked = 240 g; Calories = 165.6; Total Carb (g) = 36.7; Net Carb (g) = 36.4; Fat (g) = 0.2; Protein = 2.8

🥣 Rice Cream Of Cooked Made With Milk ☞ serving size: 1 cup, cooked = 240 g; Calories = 312; Total Carb (g) = 47.4; Net Carb (g) = 47.1; Fat (g) = 8.5; Protein = 10.4

🥣 Rice Cream Of Cooked Ns As To Fat Added In Cooking ☞ serving size: 1 cup, cooked = 240 g; Calories = 192; Total Carb (g) = 36.1; Net Carb (g) = 35.8; Fat (g) = 3.7; Protein = 2.8

🥣 Rice Creamed Made With Milk And Sugar Puerto Rican Style ☞ serving size: 1 cup, cooked = 245 g; Calories = 215.6; Total Carb (g) = 42.8; Net Carb (g) = 42.6; Fat (g) = 2.4; Protein = 5.4

🥣 Rice Puffed Fortified ☞ serving size: 1 cup = 14 g; Calories = 56.3; Total Carb (g) = 12.6; Net Carb (g) = 12.3; Fat (g) = 0.1; Protein = 0.9

🥣 Sun Country Kretschmer Honey Crunch Wheat Germ ☞ serving size: 2 tbsp (1 nlea serving) = 14 g; Calories = 52.1; Total Carb (g) = 8.1; Net Carb (g) = 6.7; Fat (g) = 1.1; Protein = 3.7

🥣 Sun Country Kretschmer Toasted Wheat Bran ☞ serving size: 1/4 cup (1 nlea serving) = 16 g; Calories = 32; Total Carb (g) = 9.5; Net Carb (g) = 2.9; Fat (g) = 0.8; Protein = 2.8

🥣 Sun Country Kretschmer Wheat Germ Regular ☞ serving size: 2 tbsp (1 nlea serving) = 14 g; Calories = 51.2; Total Carb (g) = 6.9; Net Carb (g) = 5.3; Fat (g) = 1.3; Protein = 4.4

🥣 Toasted Wheat Germ ☞ serving size: 1 oz = 28.4 g; Calories = 108.5; Total Carb (g) = 14.1; Net Carb (g) = 9.8; Fat (g) = 3; Protein = 8.3

🥣 Uncle Sam Cereal ☞ serving size: 3/4 cup (1 nlea serving) = 55 g; Calories = 190.3; Total Carb (g) = 36.2; Net Carb (g) = 25; Fat (g) = 6.4; Protein = 8.8

🥣 Upma Indian Breakfast Dish ☞ serving size: 1 cup, cooked = 170 g; Calories = 147.9; Total Carb (g) = 23.9; Net Carb (g) = 21.8; Fat (g) = 4.4; Protein = 3.5

🥣 Weetabix Whole Grain Cereal ☞ serving size: 2 biscuits (1 nlea serving) = 35 g; Calories = 129.9; Total Carb (g) = 28.5; Net Carb (g) = 24.5; Fat (g) = 1; Protein = 4

☙ Wheat And Bran Presweetened With Nuts And Fruits ☞ serving size: 1 cup (1 nlea serving) = 55 g; Calories = 211.8; Total Carb (g) = 41.9; Net Carb (g) = 36.6; Fat (g) = 3.1; Protein = 3.9

☙ Wheat Cereal Chocolate Flavored Cooked ☞ serving size: 1 cup, cooked = 240 g; Calories = 117.6; Total Carb (g) = 26.5; Net Carb (g) = 22.4; Fat (g) = 1.1; Protein = 4.3

☙ Wheat Cream Of Cooked Made With Milk And Sugar Puerto Rican Style ☞ serving size: 1 cup, cooked = 245 g; Calories = 267.1; Total Carb (g) = 46.2; Net Carb (g) = 45.2; Fat (g) = 4.8; Protein = 9.7

☙ Wheat Puffed Fortified ☞ serving size: 1 cup = 12 g; Calories = 43.7; Total Carb (g) = 9.6; Net Carb (g) = 9; Fat (g) = 0.1; Protein = 1.8

☙ Wheatena Cooked With Water ☞ serving size: 1 cup = 243 g; Calories = 136.1; Total Carb (g) = 28.7; Net Carb (g) = 22.1; Fat (g) = 1.2; Protein = 4.9

☙ Wheatena Cooked With Water With Salt ☞ serving size: 1 cup = 243 g; Calories = 143.4; Total Carb (g) = 28.5; Net Carb (g) = 23.7; Fat (g) = 1.1; Protein = 4.9

☙ Wheatena Dry ☞ serving size: 1/3 cup (1 nlea serving) = 40 g; Calories = 142.8; Total Carb (g) = 30.2; Net Carb (g) = 25.1; Fat (g) = 1.2; Protein = 5.2

☙ White Cornmeal (Grits) ☞ serving size: 1 cup = 257 g; Calories = 182.5; Total Carb (g) = 37.9; Net Carb (g) = 35.9; Fat (g) = 1.2; Protein = 4.4

☙ Whole Wheat Cereal Cooked Fat Added In Cooking ☞ serving size: 1 cup, cooked = 240 g; Calories = 144; Total Carb (g) = 24.5; Net Carb (g) = 21.4; Fat (g) = 4.3; Protein = 3.7

☙ Whole Wheat Cereal Cooked Fat Not Added In Cooking ☞

serving size: 1 cup, cooked = 240 g; Calories = 112.8; Total Carb (g) = 24.9; Net Carb (g) = 21.8; Fat (g) = 0.7; Protein = 3.7

🥣 Whole Wheat Cereal Cooked Ns As To Fat Added In Cooking ☞ serving size: 1 cup, cooked = 240 g; Calories = 144; Total Carb (g) = 24.5; Net Carb (g) = 21.4; Fat (g) = 4.3; Protein = 3.7

🥣 Whole Wheat Hot Natural Cereal Cooked With Water With Salt ☞ serving size: 1 cup = 242 g; Calories = 150; Total Carb (g) = 33.2; Net Carb (g) = 29.3; Fat (g) = 1; Protein = 4.8

🥣 Whole Wheat Hot Natural Cereal Cooked With Water Without Salt ☞ serving size: 1 cup = 242 g; Calories = 150; Total Carb (g) = 33.2; Net Carb (g) = 29.3; Fat (g) = 1; Protein = 4.8

🥣 Whole Wheat Hot Natural Cereal Dry ☞ serving size: 1 cup = 94 g; Calories = 321.5; Total Carb (g) = 70.7; Net Carb (g) = 61.8; Fat (g) = 1.9; Protein = 10.5

15

DAIRY AND EGG PRODUCTS

🥛 Almond Milk Unsweetened ☞ serving size: 1 cup = 244 g; Calories = 36.6; Total Carb (g) = 1.4; Net Carb (g) = 1.4; Fat (g) = 2.7; Protein = 1.4

🥛 American Cheese ☞ serving size: 1 cup = 113 g; Calories = 372.9; Total Carb (g) = 9.7; Net Carb (g) = 9.7; Fat (g) = 29; Protein = 19.1

🥛 American Cheese Spread ☞ serving size: 1 cup, diced = 140 g; Calories = 406; Total Carb (g) = 12.2; Net Carb (g) = 12.2; Fat (g) = 29.7; Protein = 23

🥛 Baked Alaska ☞ serving size: 1 baked alaska = 820 g; Calories = 2033.6; Total Carb (g) = 290.6; Net Carb (g) = 285.7; Fat (g) = 80.3; Protein = 40.9

🥛 Beverage Instant Breakfast Powder Chocolate Not Reconstituted ☞ serving size: 1 tbsp = 7.4 g; Calories = 26.1; Total Carb (g) = 4.9; Net Carb (g) = 4.9; Fat (g) = 0.1; Protein = 1.5

🥛 Beverage Instant Breakfast Powder Chocolate Sugar-Free Not Reconstituted ☞ serving size: 1 tbsp = 5.6 g; Calories = 20; Total Carb (g) = 2.3; Net Carb (g) = 2.2; Fat (g) = 0.3; Protein = 2

Blue Cheese ☞ serving size: 1 oz = 28.4 g; Calories = 100.3; Total Carb (g) = 0.7; Net Carb (g) = 0.7; Fat (g) = 8.2; Protein = 6.1

Breast Milk (Human) ☞ serving size: 1 fl oz = 30.8 g; Calories = 21.6; Total Carb (g) = 2.1; Net Carb (g) = 2.1; Fat (g) = 1.4; Protein = 0.3

Brick Cheese ☞ serving size: 1 cup, diced = 132 g; Calories = 489.7; Total Carb (g) = 3.7; Net Carb (g) = 3.7; Fat (g) = 39.2; Protein = 30.7

Brie Cheese ☞ serving size: 1 oz = 28.4 g; Calories = 94.9; Total Carb (g) = 0.1; Net Carb (g) = 0.1; Fat (g) = 7.9; Protein = 5.9

Buttermilk ☞ serving size: 1 cup = 245 g; Calories = 151.9; Total Carb (g) = 12; Net Carb (g) = 12; Fat (g) = 8.1; Protein = 7.9

Buttermilk Fat Free (Skim) ☞ serving size: 1 cup = 244 g; Calories = 97.6; Total Carb (g) = 11.7; Net Carb (g) = 11.7; Fat (g) = 2.2; Protein = 8.1

Buttermilk Low Fat (1%) ☞ serving size: 1 cup = 244 g; Calories = 97.6; Total Carb (g) = 11.7; Net Carb (g) = 11.7; Fat (g) = 2.2; Protein = 8.1

Camambert ☞ serving size: 1 oz = 28.4 g; Calories = 85.2; Total Carb (g) = 0.1; Net Carb (g) = 0.1; Fat (g) = 6.9; Protein = 5.6

Caraway Cheese ☞ serving size: 1 oz = 28.4 g; Calories = 106.8; Total Carb (g) = 0.9; Net Carb (g) = 0.9; Fat (g) = 8.3; Protein = 7.2

Cheddar Cheese ☞ serving size: 1 cup, diced = 132 g; Calories = 532; Total Carb (g) = 4.5; Net Carb (g) = 4.5; Fat (g) = 44; Protein = 30.2

Cheddar Cheese (Non-Fat Or Fat Free) ☞ serving size: 1 serving = 28 g; Calories = 44; Total Carb (g) = 2; Net Carb (g) = 2; Fat (g) = 0; Protein = 9

Cheese American Cheddar Imitation ☞ serving size: 1 slice = 21 g; Calories = 50.2; Total Carb (g) = 2.4; Net Carb (g) = 2.4; Fat (g) = 2.9; Protein = 3.5

Cheese Cheddar ☞ serving size: 1 cracker-size slice = 9 g; Calo-

ries = 36.4; Total Carb (g) = 0.3; Net Carb (g) = 0.3; Fat (g) = 3; Protein = 2.1

🥛 Cheese Cheddar Reduced Fat ☞ serving size: 1 slice = 21 g; Calories = 66.4; Total Carb (g) = 0.6; Net Carb (g) = 0.6; Fat (g) = 4.3; Protein = 5.7

🥛 Cheese Colby Jack ☞ serving size: 1 cracker-size slice = 9 g; Calories = 34.6; Total Carb (g) = 0.2; Net Carb (g) = 0.2; Fat (g) = 2.8; Protein = 2.2

🥛 Cheese Cottage Cheese With Gelatin Dessert ☞ serving size: 1 cup = 240 g; Calories = 194.4; Total Carb (g) = 20.1; Net Carb (g) = 20.1; Fat (g) = 5.6; Protein = 15.7

🥛 Cheese Cottage Cheese With Gelatin Dessert And Fruit ☞ serving size: 1 cup = 240 g; Calories = 211.2; Total Carb (g) = 31.6; Net Carb (g) = 30.7; Fat (g) = 4.3; Protein = 12.2

🥛 Cheese Cottage Cheese With Gelatin Dessert And Vegetables ☞ serving size: 1 cup = 240 g; Calories = 196.8; Total Carb (g) = 15.1; Net Carb (g) = 14.6; Fat (g) = 6.8; Protein = 18.5

🥛 Cheese Cottage Lowfat 1% Milkfat Lactose Reduced ☞ serving size: 4 oz = 113 g; Calories = 83.6; Total Carb (g) = 3.6; Net Carb (g) = 2.9; Fat (g) = 1.1; Protein = 14

🥛 Cheese Cottage Lowfat 1% Milkfat No Sodium Added ☞ serving size: 4 oz = 113 g; Calories = 81.4; Total Carb (g) = 3.1; Net Carb (g) = 3.1; Fat (g) = 1.1; Protein = 14

🥛 Cheese Cottage Lowfat 1% Milkfat With Vegetables ☞ serving size: 4 oz = 113 g; Calories = 75.7; Total Carb (g) = 3.4; Net Carb (g) = 3.4; Fat (g) = 1.1; Protein = 12.3

🥛 Cheese Cottage Lowfat With Fruit ☞ serving size: 1 cup = 226 g; Calories = 160.5; Total Carb (g) = 18.7; Net Carb (g) = 17.5; Fat (g) = 3.3; Protein = 15.6

🥛 Cheese Cottage With Vegetables ☞ serving size: 4 oz = 113 g;

Calories = 107.4; Total Carb (g) = 3.4; Net Carb (g) = 3.3; Fat (g) = 4.8; Protein = 12.3

🥛 Cheese Cream Low Fat ☞ serving size: 1 tbsp = 15 g; Calories = 31.2; Total Carb (g) = 1; Net Carb (g) = 1; Fat (g) = 2.5; Protein = 1.2

🥛 Cheese Dry White Queso Seco ☞ serving size: 1 cup grated = 97 g; Calories = 315.3; Total Carb (g) = 2; Net Carb (g) = 2; Fat (g) = 23.6; Protein = 23.8

🥛 Cheese Food Pasteurized Process American Without Added Vitamin D ☞ serving size: 1 cup = 113 g; Calories = 372.9; Total Carb (g) = 9.7; Net Carb (g) = 9.7; Fat (g) = 29; Protein = 19.1

🥛 Cheese Food Pasteurized Process Swiss ☞ serving size: 1 oz = 28.4 g; Calories = 91.7; Total Carb (g) = 1.3; Net Carb (g) = 1.3; Fat (g) = 6.9; Protein = 6.2

🥛 Cheese Goat ☞ serving size: 1 cup, crumbled = 140 g; Calories = 504; Total Carb (g) = 1.1; Net Carb (g) = 1.1; Fat (g) = 40.4; Protein = 32.9

🥛 Cheese Goat Semisoft Type ☞ serving size: 1 oz = 28.4 g; Calories = 103.4; Total Carb (g) = 0; Net Carb (g) = 0; Fat (g) = 8.5; Protein = 6.1

🥛 Cheese Gouda Or Edam ☞ serving size: 1 cracker-size slice = 9 g; Calories = 32.1; Total Carb (g) = 0.2; Net Carb (g) = 0.2; Fat (g) = 2.5; Protein = 2.3

🥛 Cheese Mexican Blend Reduced Fat ☞ serving size: 1 oz = 28.4 g; Calories = 80.1; Total Carb (g) = 1; Net Carb (g) = 1; Fat (g) = 5.5; Protein = 7

🥛 Cheese Mexican Queso Anejo ☞ serving size: 1 cup, crumbled = 132 g; Calories = 492.4; Total Carb (g) = 6.1; Net Carb (g) = 6.1; Fat (g) = 39.6; Protein = 28.3

🥛 Cheese Mexican Queso Asadero ☞ serving size: 1 cup, diced =

132 g; Calories = 469.9; Total Carb (g) = 5.5; Net Carb (g) = 5.5; Fat (g) = 33; Protein = 29.8

🥛 Cheese Monterey Low Fat ☞ serving size: 1 cup, diced = 132 g; Calories = 413.2; Total Carb (g) = 0.9; Net Carb (g) = 0.9; Fat (g) = 28.5; Protein = 37.2

🥛 Cheese Mozzarella Low Moisture Part-Skim Shredded ☞ serving size: 1 cup = 86 g; Calories = 261.4; Total Carb (g) = 6.9; Net Carb (g) = 6.9; Fat (g) = 17; Protein = 20.3

🥛 Cheese Mozzarella Low Sodium ☞ serving size: 1 cup, diced = 132 g; Calories = 369.6; Total Carb (g) = 4.1; Net Carb (g) = 4.1; Fat (g) = 22.6; Protein = 36.3

🥛 Cheese Muenster Low Fat ☞ serving size: 1 cup, shredded = 113 g; Calories = 306.2; Total Carb (g) = 4; Net Carb (g) = 4; Fat (g) = 19.9; Protein = 27.9

🥛 Cheese Nfs ☞ serving size: 1 cracker-size slice = 9 g; Calories = 32.9; Total Carb (g) = 0.5; Net Carb (g) = 0.5; Fat (g) = 2.6; Protein = 1.8

🥛 Cheese Parmesan Dry Grated Reduced Fat ☞ serving size: 1 cup = 100 g; Calories = 265; Total Carb (g) = 1.4; Net Carb (g) = 1.4; Fat (g) = 20; Protein = 20

🥛 Cheese Pasteurized Process American Low Fat ☞ serving size: 1 cup, diced = 140 g; Calories = 252; Total Carb (g) = 4.9; Net Carb (g) = 4.9; Fat (g) = 9.8; Protein = 34.4

🥛 Cheese Pasteurized Process American Without Added Vitamin D ☞ serving size: 1 oz = 28.4 g; Calories = 105.4; Total Carb (g) = 1.1; Net Carb (g) = 1.1; Fat (g) = 9; Protein = 5.2

🥛 Cheese Pasteurized Process Cheddar Or American Low Sodium ☞ serving size: 1 cup, diced = 140 g; Calories = 526.4; Total Carb (g) = 2.2; Net Carb (g) = 2.2; Fat (g) = 43.7; Protein = 31.1

🥛 Cheese Product Pasteurized Process American Reduced Fat Fortified With Vitamin D ☞ serving size: 1 slice 3/4 oz = 21 g; Calo-

ries = 50.4; Total Carb (g) = 2.2; Net Carb (g) = 2.2; Fat (g) = 3; Protein = 3.7

🥛 Cheese Product Pasteurized Process American Vitamin D Fortified ☞ serving size: 1 slice (2/3 oz) = 19 g; Calories = 58.3; Total Carb (g) = 1.7; Net Carb (g) = 1.7; Fat (g) = 4.4; Protein = 3.1

🥛 Cheese Ricotta ☞ serving size: 1 cup = 246 g; Calories = 383.8; Total Carb (g) = 10.1; Net Carb (g) = 10.1; Fat (g) = 25.7; Protein = 27.9

🥛 Cheese Sauce Prepared From Recipe ☞ serving size: 2 tbsp = 30 g; Calories = 59.1; Total Carb (g) = 1.6; Net Carb (g) = 1.6; Fat (g) = 4.5; Protein = 3.1

🥛 Cheese Souffle ☞ serving size: 1 cup = 95 g; Calories = 193.8; Total Carb (g) = 6.1; Net Carb (g) = 6; Fat (g) = 14.9; Protein = 8.9

🥛 Cheese Spread American Or Cheddar Cheese Base Reduced Fat ☞ serving size: 1 piece = 21 g; Calories = 37; Total Carb (g) = 2.3; Net Carb (g) = 2.3; Fat (g) = 1.9; Protein = 2.8

🥛 Cheese Spread Cream Cheese Base ☞ serving size: 1 oz = 28.4 g; Calories = 83.8; Total Carb (g) = 1; Net Carb (g) = 1; Fat (g) = 8.1; Protein = 2

🥛 Cheese Substitute Mozzarella ☞ serving size: 1 cup, shredded = 113 g; Calories = 280.2; Total Carb (g) = 26.8; Net Carb (g) = 26.8; Fat (g) = 13.8; Protein = 13

🥛 Cheese Swiss Low Fat ☞ serving size: 1 slice (1 oz) = 28 g; Calories = 50.1; Total Carb (g) = 1; Net Carb (g) = 1; Fat (g) = 1.4; Protein = 8

🥛 Cheese Swiss Low Sodium ☞ serving size: 1 slice = 28 g; Calories = 104.7; Total Carb (g) = 1; Net Carb (g) = 1; Fat (g) = 7.7; Protein = 8

🥛 Cheese With Nuts ☞ serving size: 1 tablespoon = 15 g; Calories = 63.6; Total Carb (g) = 0.9; Net Carb (g) = 0.7; Fat (g) = 5.7; Protein = 2.7

🥛 Chesire Cheese ☞ serving size: 1 oz = 28.4 g; Calories = 109.9; Total Carb (g) = 1.4; Net Carb (g) = 1.4; Fat (g) = 8.7; Protein = 6.6

🥛 Chicken Or Turkey Souffle ☞ serving size: 1 cup = 159 g; Calories = 268.7; Total Carb (g) = 8.7; Net Carb (g) = 8.6; Fat (g) = 17.7; Protein = 18.6

🥛 Chocolate Milk Made From Dry Mix Ns As To Type Of Milk ☞ serving size: 1 cup = 248 g; Calories = 178.6; Total Carb (g) = 25.1; Net Carb (g) = 24.3; Fat (g) = 5.1; Protein = 8.3

🥛 Chocolate Milk Made From Dry Mix Ns As To Type Of Milk (Nesquik) ☞ serving size: 1 cup = 248 g; Calories = 178.6; Total Carb (g) = 25.1; Net Carb (g) = 24.3; Fat (g) = 5.1; Protein = 8.3

🥛 Chocolate Milk Made From Dry Mix With Fat Free Milk ☞ serving size: 1 cup = 248 g; Calories = 141.4; Total Carb (g) = 25.3; Net Carb (g) = 24.6; Fat (g) = 0.6; Protein = 8.5

🥛 Chocolate Milk Made From Dry Mix With Fat Free Milk (Nesquik) ☞ serving size: 1 cup = 248 g; Calories = 141.4; Total Carb (g) = 25.3; Net Carb (g) = 24.6; Fat (g) = 0.6; Protein = 8.5

🥛 Chocolate Milk Made From Dry Mix With Low Fat Milk ☞ serving size: 1 cup = 248 g; Calories = 158.7; Total Carb (g) = 25.4; Net Carb (g) = 24.7; Fat (g) = 2.6; Protein = 8.5

🥛 Chocolate Milk Made From Dry Mix With Low Fat Milk (Nesquik) ☞ serving size: 1 cup = 248 g; Calories = 158.7; Total Carb (g) = 25.4; Net Carb (g) = 24.7; Fat (g) = 2.6; Protein = 8.5

🥛 Chocolate Milk Made From Dry Mix With Non-Dairy Milk ☞ serving size: 1 cup = 248 g; Calories = 156.2; Total Carb (g) = 27.2; Net Carb (g) = 25.7; Fat (g) = 3.3; Protein = 4.2

🥛 Chocolate Milk Made From Dry Mix With Non-Dairy Milk (Nesquik) ☞ serving size: 1 cup = 248 g; Calories = 156.2; Total Carb (g) = 27.2; Net Carb (g) = 25.7; Fat (g) = 3.3; Protein = 4.2

🥛 Chocolate Milk Made From Dry Mix With Reduced Fat Milk ☞ serving size: 1 cup = 248 g; Calories = 178.6; Total Carb (g) = 25; Net Carb (g) = 24.2; Fat (g) = 5; Protein = 8.4

Chocolate Milk Made From Dry Mix With Reduced Fat Milk (Nesquik) ☞ serving size: 1 cup = 248 g; Calories = 178.6; Total Carb (g) = 25; Net Carb (g) = 24.2; Fat (g) = 5; Protein = 8.4

Chocolate Milk Made From Dry Mix With Whole Milk ☞ serving size: 1 cup = 248 g; Calories = 203.4; Total Carb (g) = 25; Net Carb (g) = 24.2; Fat (g) = 7.9; Protein = 8

Chocolate Milk Made From Dry Mix With Whole Milk (Nesquik) ☞ serving size: 1 cup = 248 g; Calories = 203.4; Total Carb (g) = 25; Net Carb (g) = 24.2; Fat (g) = 7.9; Protein = 8

Chocolate Milk Made From Light Syrup Ns As To Type Of Milk ☞ serving size: 1 cup = 248 g; Calories = 158.7; Total Carb (g) = 21.3; Net Carb (g) = 21.3; Fat (g) = 4.7; Protein = 7.5

Chocolate Milk Made From Light Syrup With Fat Free Milk ☞ serving size: 1 cup = 248 g; Calories = 121.5; Total Carb (g) = 21.5; Net Carb (g) = 21.5; Fat (g) = 0.5; Protein = 7.7

Chocolate Milk Made From Light Syrup With Low Fat Milk ☞ serving size: 1 cup = 248 g; Calories = 138.9; Total Carb (g) = 21.6; Net Carb (g) = 21.6; Fat (g) = 2.4; Protein = 7.7

Chocolate Milk Made From Light Syrup With Non-Dairy Milk ☞ serving size: 1 cup = 248 g; Calories = 136.4; Total Carb (g) = 23.2; Net Carb (g) = 22.5; Fat (g) = 3; Protein = 3.7

Chocolate Milk Made From Light Syrup With Reduced Fat Milk ☞ serving size: 1 cup = 248 g; Calories = 156.2; Total Carb (g) = 21.2; Net Carb (g) = 21.2; Fat (g) = 4.6; Protein = 7.6

Chocolate Milk Made From Light Syrup With Whole Milk ☞ serving size: 1 cup = 248 g; Calories = 181; Total Carb (g) = 21.2; Net Carb (g) = 21.2; Fat (g) = 7.3; Protein = 7.3

Chocolate Milk Made From No Sugar Added Dry Mix Ns As To Type Of Milk (Nesquik) ☞ serving size: 1 cup = 248 g; Calories =

161.2; Total Carb (g) = 18.3; Net Carb (g) = 17.3; Fat (g) = 5.8; Protein = 8.7

🥛 Chocolate Milk Made From No Sugar Added Dry Mix With Fat Free Milk (Nesquik) ☞ serving size: 1 cup = 248 g; Calories = 121.5; Total Carb (g) = 18.6; Net Carb (g) = 17.6; Fat (g) = 1.2; Protein = 9

🥛 Chocolate Milk Made From No Sugar Added Dry Mix With Low Fat Milk (Nesquik) ☞ serving size: 1 cup = 248 g; Calories = 138.9; Total Carb (g) = 18.7; Net Carb (g) = 17.7; Fat (g) = 3.3; Protein = 9

🥛 Chocolate Milk Made From No Sugar Added Dry Mix With Non-Dairy Milk (Nesquik) ☞ serving size: 1 cup = 248 g; Calories = 136.4; Total Carb (g) = 20.5; Net Carb (g) = 18.7; Fat (g) = 3.9; Protein = 4.6

🥛 Chocolate Milk Made From No Sugar Added Dry Mix With Reduced Fat Milk (Nesquik) ☞ serving size: 1 cup = 248 g; Calories = 158.7; Total Carb (g) = 18.2; Net Carb (g) = 17.2; Fat (g) = 5.7; Protein = 8.8

🥛 Chocolate Milk Made From No Sugar Added Dry Mix With Whole Milk (Nesquik) ☞ serving size: 1 cup = 248 g; Calories = 183.5; Total Carb (g) = 18.2; Net Carb (g) = 17.2; Fat (g) = 8.7; Protein = 8.5

🥛 Chocolate Milk Made From Reduced Sugar Mix Ns As To Type Of Milk ☞ serving size: 1 cup = 248 g; Calories = 161.2; Total Carb (g) = 18.3; Net Carb (g) = 17.3; Fat (g) = 5.8; Protein = 8.7

🥛 Chocolate Milk Made From Reduced Sugar Mix With Fat Free Milk ☞ serving size: 1 cup = 248 g; Calories = 121.5; Total Carb (g) = 18.6; Net Carb (g) = 17.6; Fat (g) = 1.2; Protein = 9

🥛 Chocolate Milk Made From Reduced Sugar Mix With Low Fat Milk ☞ serving size: 1 cup = 248 g; Calories = 138.9; Total Carb (g) = 18.7; Net Carb (g) = 17.7; Fat (g) = 3.3; Protein = 9

🥛 Chocolate Milk Made From Reduced Sugar Mix With Non-

Dairy Milk ☞ serving size: 1 cup = 248 g; Calories = 136.4; Total Carb (g) = 20.5; Net Carb (g) = 18.7; Fat (g) = 3.9; Protein = 4.6

🥛 Chocolate Milk Made From Reduced Sugar Mix With Reduced Fat Milk ☞ serving size: 1 cup = 248 g; Calories = 158.7; Total Carb (g) = 18.2; Net Carb (g) = 17.2; Fat (g) = 5.7; Protein = 8.8

🥛 Chocolate Milk Made From Reduced Sugar Mix With Whole Milk ☞ serving size: 1 cup = 248 g; Calories = 183.5; Total Carb (g) = 18.2; Net Carb (g) = 17.2; Fat (g) = 8.7; Protein = 8.5

🥛 Chocolate Milk Made From Sugar Free Syrup Ns As To Type Of Milk ☞ serving size: 1 cup = 248 g; Calories = 124; Total Carb (g) = 14.9; Net Carb (g) = 13.9; Fat (g) = 5.1; Protein = 8

🥛 Chocolate Milk Made From Sugar Free Syrup With Fat Free Milk ☞ serving size: 1 cup = 248 g; Calories = 86.8; Total Carb (g) = 15.2; Net Carb (g) = 14.2; Fat (g) = 0.8; Protein = 8.2

🥛 Chocolate Milk Made From Sugar Free Syrup With Low Fat Milk ☞ serving size: 1 cup = 248 g; Calories = 104.2; Total Carb (g) = 15.2; Net Carb (g) = 14.2; Fat (g) = 2.7; Protein = 8.2

🥛 Chocolate Milk Made From Sugar Free Syrup With Non-Dairy Milk ☞ serving size: 1 cup = 248 g; Calories = 101.7; Total Carb (g) = 16.9; Net Carb (g) = 15.4; Fat (g) = 3.4; Protein = 4.2

🥛 Chocolate Milk Made From Sugar Free Syrup With Reduced Fat Milk ☞ serving size: 1 cup = 248 g; Calories = 121.5; Total Carb (g) = 14.8; Net Carb (g) = 13.8; Fat (g) = 4.9; Protein = 8.1

🥛 Chocolate Milk Made From Sugar Free Syrup With Whole Milk ☞ serving size: 1 cup = 248 g; Calories = 146.3; Total Carb (g) = 14.8; Net Carb (g) = 13.8; Fat (g) = 7.7; Protein = 7.7

🥛 Chocolate Milk Made From Syrup Ns As To Type Of Milk ☞ serving size: 1 cup = 248 g; Calories = 198.4; Total Carb (g) = 32.6; Net Carb (g) = 32.6; Fat (g) = 4.4; Protein = 7

🥛 Chocolate Milk Made From Syrup With Fat Free Milk ☞

serving size: 1 cup = 248 g; Calories = 161.2; Total Carb (g) = 32.9; Net Carb (g) = 32.9; Fat (g) = 0.2; Protein = 7.2

🥛 Chocolate Milk Made From Syrup With Low Fat Milk ☞ serving size: 1 cup = 248 g; Calories = 178.6; Total Carb (g) = 32.9; Net Carb (g) = 32.9; Fat (g) = 2.1; Protein = 7.2

🥛 Chocolate Milk Made From Syrup With Non-Dairy Milk ☞ serving size: 1 cup = 248 g; Calories = 176.1; Total Carb (g) = 34.6; Net Carb (g) = 33.8; Fat (g) = 2.7; Protein = 3.3

🥛 Chocolate Milk Made From Syrup With Reduced Fat Milk ☞ serving size: 1 cup = 248 g; Calories = 195.9; Total Carb (g) = 32.5; Net Carb (g) = 32.5; Fat (g) = 4.3; Protein = 7.1

🥛 Chocolate Milk Made From Syrup With Whole Milk ☞ serving size: 1 cup = 248 g; Calories = 220.7; Total Carb (g) = 32.5; Net Carb (g) = 32.5; Fat (g) = 7; Protein = 6.8

🥛 Chocolate Milk Ready To Drink Low Fat ☞ serving size: 1 fl oz = 31 g; Calories = 19.2; Total Carb (g) = 3.1; Net Carb (g) = 3; Fat (g) = 0.3; Protein = 1.1

🥛 Chocolate Milk Ready To Drink Low Fat (Nesquik) ☞ serving size: 1 cup = 248 g; Calories = 153.8; Total Carb (g) = 24.5; Net Carb (g) = 24.2; Fat (g) = 2.5; Protein = 8.6

🥛 Chocolate Milk Ready To Drink Low Fat No Sugar Added (Nesquik) ☞ serving size: 1 cup = 248 g; Calories = 153.8; Total Carb (g) = 24.5; Net Carb (g) = 24.2; Fat (g) = 2.5; Protein = 8.6

🥛 Chocolate Milk Ready To Drink Reduced Sugar Ns As To Milk ☞ serving size: 1 cup = 248 g; Calories = 133.9; Total Carb (g) = 19.1; Net Carb (g) = 19.1; Fat (g) = 2.6; Protein = 8.5

🥛 Colby Cheese ☞ serving size: 1 cup, diced = 132 g; Calories = 520.1; Total Carb (g) = 3.4; Net Carb (g) = 3.4; Fat (g) = 42.4; Protein = 31.4

🥛 Cold Pack American Cheese ☞ serving size: 1 oz = 28.4 g; Calories = 94; Total Carb (g) = 2.4; Net Carb (g) = 2.4; Fat (g) = 7; Protein = 5.6

Cottage Cheese (Blended With Fruit) ☞ serving size: 4 oz = 113 g; Calories = 109.6; Total Carb (g) = 5.2; Net Carb (g) = 5; Fat (g) = 4.4; Protein = 12.1

Cottage Cheese (Blended) ☞ serving size: 4 oz = 113 g; Calories = 110.7; Total Carb (g) = 3.8; Net Carb (g) = 3.8; Fat (g) = 4.9; Protein = 12.6

Cottage Cheese Farmer's ☞ serving size: 1 cup = 210 g; Calories = 300.3; Total Carb (g) = 6.7; Net Carb (g) = 6.7; Fat (g) = 20.6; Protein = 22

Cream Cheese ☞ serving size: 1 tbsp = 14.5 g; Calories = 50.8; Total Carb (g) = 0.8; Net Carb (g) = 0.8; Fat (g) = 5; Protein = 0.9

Cream Half And Half Fat Free ☞ serving size: 2 tbsp = 29 g; Calories = 17.1; Total Carb (g) = 2.6; Net Carb (g) = 2.6; Fat (g) = 0.4; Protein = 0.8

Cream Substitute Flavored Liquid ☞ serving size: 1 tbsp = 15 g; Calories = 37.7; Total Carb (g) = 5.3; Net Carb (g) = 5.1; Fat (g) = 2; Protein = 0.1

Cream Substitute Flavored Powdered ☞ serving size: 4 tsp = 12 g; Calories = 57.8; Total Carb (g) = 9.1; Net Carb (g) = 8.9; Fat (g) = 2.6; Protein = 0.1

Cream Substitute Liquid Light ☞ serving size: 1 fl oz = 30 g; Calories = 21.3; Total Carb (g) = 2.7; Net Carb (g) = 2.7; Fat (g) = 1.1; Protein = 0.2

Cream Substitute Liquid With Hydrogenated Vegetable Oil And Soy Protein ☞ serving size: 1 container, individual = 15 g; Calories = 20.4; Total Carb (g) = 1.7; Net Carb (g) = 1.7; Fat (g) = 1.5; Protein = 0.2

Cream Substitute Liquid With Lauric Acid Oil And Sodium Caseinate ☞ serving size: 1 container, individual = 15 g; Calories =

20.4; Total Carb (g) = 1.7; Net Carb (g) = 1.7; Fat (g) = 1.5; Protein = 0.2

🥛 Cream Substitute Powdered ☞ serving size: 1 cup = 94 g; Calories = 497.3; Total Carb (g) = 55.7; Net Carb (g) = 55.7; Fat (g) = 30.9; Protein = 2.3

🥛 Cream Substitute Powdered Light ☞ serving size: 1 cup = 94 g; Calories = 405.1; Total Carb (g) = 69; Net Carb (g) = 69; Fat (g) = 14.8; Protein = 1.8

🥛 Cultured Sour Cream ☞ serving size: 1 tbsp = 12 g; Calories = 23.8; Total Carb (g) = 0.6; Net Carb (g) = 0.6; Fat (g) = 2.3; Protein = 0.3

🥛 Dehydrated Milk ☞ serving size: 1/4 cup = 32 g; Calories = 158.7; Total Carb (g) = 12.3; Net Carb (g) = 12.3; Fat (g) = 8.6; Protein = 8.4

🥛 Dessert Topping Powdered ☞ serving size: 1 (1/2) oz = 43 g; Calories = 248.1; Total Carb (g) = 22.6; Net Carb (g) = 22.6; Fat (g) = 17.2; Protein = 2.1

🥛 Dessert Topping Powdered 1.5 Ounce Prepared With 1/2 Cup Milk ☞ serving size: 1 cup = 80 g; Calories = 155.2; Total Carb (g) = 13.7; Net Carb (g) = 13.7; Fat (g) = 10.2; Protein = 2.9

🥛 Dessert Topping Pressurized ☞ serving size: 1 cup = 70 g; Calories = 184.8; Total Carb (g) = 11.3; Net Carb (g) = 11.3; Fat (g) = 15.6; Protein = 0.7

🥛 Dessert Topping Semi Solid Frozen ☞ serving size: 1 cup = 75 g; Calories = 238.5; Total Carb (g) = 17.3; Net Carb (g) = 17.3; Fat (g) = 19; Protein = 0.9

🥛 Dried Eggs ☞ serving size: 1 cup, sifted = 85 g; Calories = 503.2; Total Carb (g) = 1; Net Carb (g) = 1; Fat (g) = 37.3; Protein = 40.8

🥛 Dried Sweet Whey Powder ☞ serving size: 1 cup = 145 g; Calories = 511.9; Total Carb (g) = 108; Net Carb (g) = 108; Fat (g) = 1.6; Protein = 18.8

🍸 Dried Whey Powder (Acid) ☞ serving size: 1 cup = 57 g; Calories = 193.2; Total Carb (g) = 41.9; Net Carb (g) = 41.9; Fat (g) = 0.3; Protein = 6.7

🍸 Duck Egg Cooked ☞ serving size: 1 egg = 70 g; Calories = 146.3; Total Carb (g) = 1.2; Net Carb (g) = 1.2; Fat (g) = 10.9; Protein = 10.1

🍸 Dulce De Leche ☞ serving size: 1 tbsp = 19 g; Calories = 59.9; Total Carb (g) = 10.5; Net Carb (g) = 10.5; Fat (g) = 1.4; Protein = 1.3

🍸 Edam Cheese ☞ serving size: 1 oz = 28.4 g; Calories = 101.4; Total Carb (g) = 0.4; Net Carb (g) = 0.4; Fat (g) = 8.1; Protein = 7.1

🍸 Egg Benedict ☞ serving size: 1 medium egg = 149 g; Calories = 427.6; Total Carb (g) = 12.3; Net Carb (g) = 11.4; Fat (g) = 33.6; Protein = 18.9

🍸 Egg Creamed ☞ serving size: 1 medium egg = 139 g; Calories = 208.5; Total Carb (g) = 7.7; Net Carb (g) = 7.6; Fat (g) = 14.7; Protein = 10.7

🍸 Egg Deviled ☞ serving size: 1/2 small egg = 24 g; Calories = 47.5; Total Carb (g) = 0.3; Net Carb (g) = 0.3; Fat (g) = 3.8; Protein = 2.8

🍸 Egg Duck Whole Fresh Raw ☞ serving size: 1 egg = 70 g; Calories = 129.5; Total Carb (g) = 1; Net Carb (g) = 1; Fat (g) = 9.6; Protein = 9

🍸 Egg Goose Whole Fresh Raw ☞ serving size: 1 egg = 144 g; Calories = 266.4; Total Carb (g) = 1.9; Net Carb (g) = 1.9; Fat (g) = 19.1; Protein = 20

🍸 Egg Omelet ☞ serving size: 1 tbsp = 15 g; Calories = 23.1; Total Carb (g) = 0.1; Net Carb (g) = 0.1; Fat (g) = 1.8; Protein = 1.6

🍸 Egg Quail Whole Fresh Raw ☞ serving size: 1 egg = 9 g; Calories = 14.2; Total Carb (g) = 0; Net Carb (g) = 0; Fat (g) = 1; Protein = 1.2

🍸 Egg Turkey Whole Fresh Raw ☞ serving size: 1 egg = 79 g; Calo-

ries = 135.1; Total Carb (g) = 0.9; Net Carb (g) = 0.9; Fat (g) = 9.4; Protein = 10.8

🥛 Egg White Cooked Fat Added In Cooking ☞ serving size: 1 small egg white = 24 g; Calories = 26.6; Total Carb (g) = 0.2; Net Carb (g) = 0.2; Fat (g) = 1.6; Protein = 2.8

🥛 Egg White Cooked Fat Not Added In Cooking ☞ serving size: 1 small egg white = 24 g; Calories = 14.2; Total Carb (g) = 0.2; Net Carb (g) = 0.2; Fat (g) = 0.1; Protein = 3

🥛 Egg White Cooked Ns As To Fat Added In Cooking ☞ serving size: 1 small egg white = 24 g; Calories = 26.6; Total Carb (g) = 0.2; Net Carb (g) = 0.2; Fat (g) = 1.6; Protein = 2.8

🥛 Egg White Dried ☞ serving size: 1 oz = 28 g; Calories = 107; Total Carb (g) = 2.2; Net Carb (g) = 2.2; Fat (g) = 0; Protein = 22.7

🥛 Egg White Powder ☞ serving size: 1 cup, sifted = 107 g; Calories = 382; Total Carb (g) = 4.8; Net Carb (g) = 4.8; Fat (g) = 0.3; Protein = 90

🥛 Egg Whites (Raw) ☞ serving size: 1 large = 33 g; Calories = 17.2; Total Carb (g) = 0.2; Net Carb (g) = 0.2; Fat (g) = 0.1; Protein = 3.6

🥛 Egg Whole Boiled Or Poached ☞ serving size: 1 small = 37 g; Calories = 52.5; Total Carb (g) = 0.3; Net Carb (g) = 0.3; Fat (g) = 3.5; Protein = 4.6

🥛 Egg Whole Cooked Ns As To Cooking Method ☞ serving size: 1 small = 37 g; Calories = 66.2; Total Carb (g) = 0.4; Net Carb (g) = 0.4; Fat (g) = 5; Protein = 4.6

🥛 Egg Whole Pickled ☞ serving size: 1 large egg = 47 g; Calories = 72.4; Total Carb (g) = 0.5; Net Carb (g) = 0.5; Fat (g) = 5; Protein = 5.9

🥛 Egg Yolks (Raw) ☞ serving size: 1 large = 17 g; Calories = 54.7; Total Carb (g) = 0.6; Net Carb (g) = 0.6; Fat (g) = 4.5; Protein = 2.7

🥛 Eggnog ☞ serving size: 1 cup = 254 g; Calories = 223.5; Total Carb (g) = 20.5; Net Carb (g) = 20.5; Fat (g) = 10.6; Protein = 11.6

Eggnog Lowfat / Light ☞ serving size: 1 cup = 256 g; Calories = 189.4; Total Carb (g) = 16.7; Net Carb (g) = 16.7; Fat (g) = 8.1; Protein = 12.1

Eggs (Raw) ☞ serving size: 1 large = 50 g; Calories = 71.5; Total Carb (g) = 0.4; Net Carb (g) = 0.4; Fat (g) = 4.8; Protein = 6.3

Evaporated Milk ☞ serving size: 1 fl oz = 31.9 g; Calories = 24.9; Total Carb (g) = 3.6; Net Carb (g) = 3.6; Fat (g) = 0.1; Protein = 2.4

Fat Free Cream Cheese ☞ serving size: 1 tbsp = 18 g; Calories = 18.9; Total Carb (g) = 1.4; Net Carb (g) = 1.4; Fat (g) = 0.2; Protein = 2.8

Fat Free Ice Cream No Sugar Added Flavors Other Than Chocolate ☞ serving size: 1/2 cup = 68 g; Calories = 90.4; Total Carb (g) = 19.6; Net Carb (g) = 14.6; Fat (g) = 0; Protein = 3

Fat Free Sour Cream ☞ serving size: 1 tablespoon = 12 g; Calories = 8.9; Total Carb (g) = 1.9; Net Carb (g) = 1.9; Fat (g) = 0; Protein = 0.4

Fatfree Swiss Cheese ☞ serving size: 1 serving = 28 g; Calories = 35.6; Total Carb (g) = 1; Net Carb (g) = 1; Fat (g) = 0; Protein = 8

Feta Cheese ☞ serving size: 1 cup, crumbled = 150 g; Calories = 397.5; Total Carb (g) = 5.8; Net Carb (g) = 5.8; Fat (g) = 32.2; Protein = 21.3

Fontina Cheese ☞ serving size: 1 cup, diced = 132 g; Calories = 513.5; Total Carb (g) = 2.1; Net Carb (g) = 2.1; Fat (g) = 41.1; Protein = 33.8

Ghee (Clarified Butter) ☞ serving size: 1 tbsp = 12.8 g; Calories = 112.1; Total Carb (g) = 0; Net Carb (g) = 0; Fat (g) = 12.7; Protein = 0

Gjetost Cheese ☞ serving size: 1 oz = 28.4 g; Calories = 132.3; Total Carb (g) = 12.1; Net Carb (g) = 12.1; Fat (g) = 8.4; Protein = 2.7

Goat Milk ☞ serving size: 1 fl oz = 30.5 g; Calories = 21; Total Carb (g) = 1.4; Net Carb (g) = 1.4; Fat (g) = 1.3; Protein = 1.1

🥛 Goose Egg Cooked ☞ serving size: 1 egg = 144 g; Calories = 301; Total Carb (g) = 2.2; Net Carb (g) = 2.2; Fat (g) = 21.6; Protein = 22.5

🥛 Gouda Cheese ☞ serving size: 1 oz = 28.4 g; Calories = 101.1; Total Carb (g) = 0.6; Net Carb (g) = 0.6; Fat (g) = 7.8; Protein = 7.1

🥛 Grated Parmesan ☞ serving size: 1 cup = 100 g; Calories = 420; Total Carb (g) = 13.9; Net Carb (g) = 13.9; Fat (g) = 27.8; Protein = 28.4

🥛 Grated Parmesan (Hard) ☞ serving size: 1 oz = 28.4 g; Calories = 111.3; Total Carb (g) = 0.9; Net Carb (g) = 0.9; Fat (g) = 7.1; Protein = 10.2

🥛 Grated Parmesan Cheese (Low-Sodium) ☞ serving size: 1 cup, grated = 100 g; Calories = 451; Total Carb (g) = 3.7; Net Carb (g) = 3.7; Fat (g) = 30; Protein = 41.6

🥛 Gruyere Cheese ☞ serving size: 1 oz = 28.4 g; Calories = 117.3; Total Carb (g) = 0.1; Net Carb (g) = 0.1; Fat (g) = 9.2; Protein = 8.5

🥛 Half And Half Cream ☞ serving size: 1 fl oz = 30.2 g; Calories = 39.6; Total Carb (g) = 1.3; Net Carb (g) = 1.3; Fat (g) = 3.5; Protein = 1

🥛 Hard Goat Cheese ☞ serving size: 1 oz = 28.4 g; Calories = 128.4; Total Carb (g) = 0.6; Net Carb (g) = 0.6; Fat (g) = 10.1; Protein = 8.7

🥛 Heavy Whipping Cream ☞ serving size: 1 cup, whipped = 120 g; Calories = 408; Total Carb (g) = 3.4; Net Carb (g) = 3.4; Fat (g) = 43.3; Protein = 3.4

🥛 High Fat Milk (3.7% Fat) ☞ serving size: 1 cup = 244 g; Calories = 156.2; Total Carb (g) = 11.4; Net Carb (g) = 11.4; Fat (g) = 8.9; Protein = 8

🥛 Hot Chocolate / Cocoa Made With Dry Mix And Fat Free Milk ☞ serving size: 1 cup = 248 g; Calories = 203.4; Total Carb (g) = 38.2; Net Carb (g) = 37; Fat (g) = 1.5; Protein = 9.5

🥛 Hot Chocolate / Cocoa Made With Dry Mix And Low Fat Milk

☞ serving size: 1 cup = 248 g; Calories = 220.7; Total Carb (g) = 38.3; Net Carb (g) = 37.1; Fat (g) = 3.4; Protein = 9.5

🥛 Hot Cocoa ☞ serving size: 1 cup = 250 g; Calories = 192.5; Total Carb (g) = 26.9; Net Carb (g) = 24.4; Fat (g) = 5.9; Protein = 8.8

🥛 Huevos Rancheros ☞ serving size: 1 egg, ns as to size = 118 g; Calories = 139.2; Total Carb (g) = 10.3; Net Carb (g) = 8.3; Fat (g) = 7.7; Protein = 8.1

🥛 Ice Cream Bar Cake Covered ☞ serving size: 1 bar = 59 g; Calories = 164; Total Carb (g) = 21.7; Net Carb (g) = 21.1; Fat (g) = 8; Protein = 2.6

🥛 Ice Cream Bar Or Stick Chocolate Covered ☞ serving size: 1 bar = 50 g; Calories = 165.5; Total Carb (g) = 12.3; Net Carb (g) = 11.9; Fat (g) = 12.1; Protein = 2.1

🥛 Ice Cream Bar Or Stick Chocolate Ice Cream Chocolate Covered ☞ serving size: 1 bar = 49 g; Calories = 139.2; Total Carb (g) = 17.1; Net Carb (g) = 16.3; Fat (g) = 7.4; Protein = 2.3

🥛 Kefir Ns As To Fat Content ☞ serving size: 1 cup = 244 g; Calories = 126.9; Total Carb (g) = 17.9; Net Carb (g) = 17.9; Fat (g) = 2.2; Protein = 8.8

🥛 Kraft Breakstones Free Fat Free Sour Cream ☞ serving size: 2 tbsp = 32 g; Calories = 29.1; Total Carb (g) = 4.8; Net Carb (g) = 4.8; Fat (g) = 0.4; Protein = 1.5

🥛 Kraft Breakstones Reduced Fat Sour Cream ☞ serving size: 2 tbsp = 31 g; Calories = 47.1; Total Carb (g) = 2; Net Carb (g) = 2; Fat (g) = 3.7; Protein = 1.4

🥛 Kraft Cheez Whiz Light Pasteurized Process Cheese Product ☞ serving size: 2 tbsp = 35 g; Calories = 75.3; Total Carb (g) = 5.7; Net Carb (g) = 5.6; Fat (g) = 3.3; Protein = 5.7

🥛 Kraft Cheez Whiz Pasteurized Process Cheese Sauce ☞ serving size: 2 tbsp = 33 g; Calories = 91.1; Total Carb (g) = 3; Net Carb (g) = 2.9; Fat (g) = 6.9; Protein = 4

🥛 Kraft Free Singles American Nonfat Pasteurized Process Cheese Product ☞ serving size: 1 slice = 21 g; Calories = 31.1; Total Carb (g) = 2.5; Net Carb (g) = 2.4; Fat (g) = 0.2; Protein = 4.8

🥛 Kraft Velveeta Light Reduced Fat Pasteurized Process Cheese Product ☞ serving size: 1 oz = 28 g; Calories = 62.2; Total Carb (g) = 3.3; Net Carb (g) = 3.3; Fat (g) = 3; Protein = 5.5

🥛 Kraft Velveeta Pasteurized Process Cheese Spread ☞ serving size: 1 oz = 28 g; Calories = 84.8; Total Carb (g) = 2.7; Net Carb (g) = 2.7; Fat (g) = 6.2; Protein = 4.6

🥛 Light Cream (Coffe Cream) ☞ serving size: 1 fl oz = 30 g; Calories = 58.5; Total Carb (g) = 1.1; Net Carb (g) = 1.1; Fat (g) = 5.7; Protein = 0.9

🥛 Light Ice Cream Bar Or Stick Chocolate Coated ☞ serving size: 1 bar (3 fl oz) = 56 g; Calories = 161.8; Total Carb (g) = 17; Net Carb (g) = 16.6; Fat (g) = 9.8; Protein = 2.2

🥛 Light Ice Cream Bar Or Stick Chocolate Covered With Nuts ☞ serving size: 1 bar = 149 g; Calories = 490.2; Total Carb (g) = 42.2; Net Carb (g) = 39.7; Fat (g) = 32.8; Protein = 10.6

🥛 Light Ice Cream Cone Chocolate ☞ serving size: 1 cone and single dip (or 1 small cone) = 78 g; Calories = 131; Total Carb (g) = 23.4; Net Carb (g) = 23; Fat (g) = 2.7; Protein = 3.6

🥛 Light Ice Cream Cone Flavors Other Than Chocolate ☞ serving size: 1 cone and single dip (or 1 small cone) = 78 g; Calories = 115.4; Total Carb (g) = 20.4; Net Carb (g) = 20.3; Fat (g) = 2.3; Protein = 4

🥛 Light Ice Cream Cone Nfs ☞ serving size: 1 cone and single dip (or 1 small cone) = 78 g; Calories = 115.4; Total Carb (g) = 20.4; Net Carb (g) = 20.3; Fat (g) = 2.3; Protein = 4

🥛 Light Ice Cream Creamsicle Or Dreamsicle No Sugar Added ☞

serving size: 1 sicle = 40 g; Calories = 20; Total Carb (g) = 4.6; Net Carb (g) = 3.9; Fat (g) = 0; Protein = 0.4

Light Ice Cream Fudgesicle ☞ serving size: 1 sicle (2.5 fl oz) = 73 g; Calories = 132.9; Total Carb (g) = 22.4; Net Carb (g) = 21.3; Fat (g) = 3.8; Protein = 3.9

Light Whipping Cream ☞ serving size: 1 cup, whipped = 120 g; Calories = 350.4; Total Carb (g) = 3.6; Net Carb (g) = 3.6; Fat (g) = 37.1; Protein = 2.6

Limburger Cheese ☞ serving size: 1 cup = 134 g; Calories = 438.2; Total Carb (g) = 0.7; Net Carb (g) = 0.7; Fat (g) = 36.5; Protein = 26.9

Low Fat Fruit Yogurt (With Vitamin D) ☞ serving size: 1 container (6 oz) = 170 g; Calories = 173.4; Total Carb (g) = 32.4; Net Carb (g) = 32.4; Fat (g) = 1.8; Protein = 7.4

Low Fat Provolone ☞ serving size: 1 cup, diced = 132 g; Calories = 361.7; Total Carb (g) = 4.6; Net Carb (g) = 4.6; Fat (g) = 23.2; Protein = 32.6

Low Fat Sour Cream ☞ serving size: 1 tablespoon = 12 g; Calories = 21.7; Total Carb (g) = 0.8; Net Carb (g) = 0.8; Fat (g) = 1.7; Protein = 0.8

Low-Fat Milk 1% ☞ serving size: 1 cup = 244 g; Calories = 102.5; Total Carb (g) = 12.2; Net Carb (g) = 12.2; Fat (g) = 2.4; Protein = 8.2

Low-Fat Milk 2% ☞ serving size: 1 cup = 244 g; Calories = 122; Total Carb (g) = 11.7; Net Carb (g) = 11.7; Fat (g) = 4.8; Protein = 8.1

Low-Fat Yogurt ☞ serving size: 1 container (6 oz) = 170 g; Calories = 107.1; Total Carb (g) = 12; Net Carb (g) = 12; Fat (g) = 2.6; Protein = 8.9

Low-Sodium Cheddar Cheese ☞ serving size: 1 cup, diced = 132 g; Calories = 525.4; Total Carb (g) = 2.5; Net Carb (g) = 2.5; Fat (g) = 43.1; Protein = 32.1

🥛 Lowfat Buttermilk ☞ serving size: 1 cup = 245 g; Calories = 98; Total Carb (g) = 11.7; Net Carb (g) = 11.7; Fat (g) = 2.6; Protein = 8.1

🥛 Lowfat Cheddar Cheese ☞ serving size: 1 cup, diced = 132 g; Calories = 228.4; Total Carb (g) = 2.5; Net Carb (g) = 2.5; Fat (g) = 9.2; Protein = 32.1

🥛 Lowfat Chocolate Milk ☞ serving size: 1 cup = 250 g; Calories = 190; Total Carb (g) = 30.3; Net Carb (g) = 28.6; Fat (g) = 4.8; Protein = 7.5

🥛 Lowfat Cottage Cheese (1%) ☞ serving size: 4 oz = 113 g; Calories = 81.4; Total Carb (g) = 3.1; Net Carb (g) = 3.1; Fat (g) = 1.2; Protein = 14

🥛 Lowfat Cottage Cheese (2%) ☞ serving size: 4 oz = 113 g; Calories = 91.5; Total Carb (g) = 5.4; Net Carb (g) = 5.4; Fat (g) = 2.6; Protein = 11.8

🥛 Lowfat Greek Strawberry Yogurt ☞ serving size: 1 container (5.3 oz) = 150 g; Calories = 157.5; Total Carb (g) = 18.4; Net Carb (g) = 16.9; Fat (g) = 3.9; Protein = 12.3

🥛 Lowfat Greek Yogurt ☞ serving size: 1 container (7 oz) = 200 g; Calories = 146; Total Carb (g) = 7.9; Net Carb (g) = 7.9; Fat (g) = 3.8; Protein = 19.9

🥛 Lowfat Ricotta ☞ serving size: 1/2 cup = 124 g; Calories = 171.1; Total Carb (g) = 6.4; Net Carb (g) = 6.4; Fat (g) = 9.8; Protein = 14.1

🥛 Lowfat Sour Cream ☞ serving size: 1 tbsp = 15 g; Calories = 20.3; Total Carb (g) = 0.6; Net Carb (g) = 0.6; Fat (g) = 1.8; Protein = 0.4

🥛 Mexican Blend Cheese ☞ serving size: 1/4 cup shredded = 28 g; Calories = 107.5; Total Carb (g) = 0; Net Carb (g) = 0; Fat (g) = 9; Protein = 6.6

🥛 Milk Buttermilk Dried ☞ serving size: 1/4 cup = 30 g; Calories = 116.1; Total Carb (g) = 14.7; Net Carb (g) = 14.7; Fat (g) = 1.7; Protein = 10.3

🥛 Milk Buttermilk Fluid Cultured Reduced Fat ☞ serving size: 1 cup = 245 g; Calories = 137.2; Total Carb (g) = 13; Net Carb (g) = 13; Fat (g) = 4.9; Protein = 10.1

🥛 Milk Canned Evaporated With Added Vitamin A ☞ serving size: 1 fl oz = 31.5 g; Calories = 42.2; Total Carb (g) = 3.2; Net Carb (g) = 3.2; Fat (g) = 2.4; Protein = 2.2

🥛 Milk Canned Evaporated With Added Vitamin D And Without Added Vitamin A ☞ serving size: 1 fl oz = 31.5 g; Calories = 42.2; Total Carb (g) = 3.2; Net Carb (g) = 3.2; Fat (g) = 2.4; Protein = 2.2

🥛 Milk Chocolate Fluid Commercial Reduced Fat With Added Calcium ☞ serving size: 1 cup = 250 g; Calories = 195; Total Carb (g) = 30.3; Net Carb (g) = 28.6; Fat (g) = 4.8; Protein = 7.5

🥛 Milk Chocolate Fluid Commercial Whole With Added Vitamin A And Vitamin D ☞ serving size: 1 cup = 250 g; Calories = 207.5; Total Carb (g) = 25.9; Net Carb (g) = 23.9; Fat (g) = 8.5; Protein = 7.9

🥛 Milk Chocolate Lowfat With Added Vitamin A And Vitamin D ☞ serving size: 1 cup = 250 g; Calories = 160; Total Carb (g) = 25.4; Net Carb (g) = 25.1; Fat (g) = 2.8; Protein = 8.7

🥛 Milk Dessert Bar Frozen Made From Lowfat Milk ☞ serving size: 1 bar = 68 g; Calories = 100; Total Carb (g) = 21.8; Net Carb (g) = 17.3; Fat (g) = 1; Protein = 3

🥛 Milk Dessert Bar Or Stick Frozen With Coconut ☞ serving size: 1 frut stix bar (4 fl oz) = 129 g; Calories = 202.5; Total Carb (g) = 27.4; Net Carb (g) = 25.4; Fat (g) = 7.6; Protein = 6.9

🥛 Milk Dessert Sandwich Bar Frozen Made From Lowfat Milk ☞ serving size: 1 weight watchers sandwich bar (2.75 fl oz plus 2 wafers) = 64 g; Calories = 121; Total Carb (g) = 22.8; Net Carb (g) = 22.2; Fat (g) = 2; Protein = 3.5

🥛 Milk Dessert Sandwich Bar Frozen With Low-Calorie Sweetener Made From Lowfat Milk ☞ serving size: 1 eskimo pie sandwich (3.2 fl oz) = 59 g; Calories = 186.4; Total Carb (g) = 31.5; Net Carb (g) = 30.2; Fat (g) = 5.8; Protein = 3.5

🥛 Milk Dry Nonfat Calcium Reduced ☞ serving size: 1 oz = 28.4 g; Calories = 100.5; Total Carb (g) = 14.7; Net Carb (g) = 14.7; Fat (g) = 0.1; Protein = 10.1

🥛 Milk Dry Nonfat Instant With Added Vitamin A And Vitamin D ☞ serving size: 1 cup = 68 g; Calories = 243.4; Total Carb (g) = 35.5; Net Carb (g) = 35.5; Fat (g) = 0.5; Protein = 23.9

🥛 Milk Dry Nonfat Instant Without Added Vitamin A And Vitamin D ☞ serving size: 1 cup = 68 g; Calories = 243.4; Total Carb (g) = 35.5; Net Carb (g) = 35.5; Fat (g) = 0.5; Protein = 23.9

🥛 Milk Dry Nonfat Regular With Added Vitamin A And Vitamin D ☞ serving size: 1/4 cup = 30 g; Calories = 108.6; Total Carb (g) = 15.6; Net Carb (g) = 15.6; Fat (g) = 0.2; Protein = 10.9

🥛 Milk Dry Nonfat Regular Without Added Vitamin A And Vitamin D ☞ serving size: 1/4 cup = 30 g; Calories = 108.6; Total Carb (g) = 15.6; Net Carb (g) = 15.6; Fat (g) = 0.2; Protein = 10.9

🥛 Milk Dry Reconstituted Fat Free (Skim) ☞ serving size: 1 cup = 244 g; Calories = 78.1; Total Carb (g) = 11.3; Net Carb (g) = 11.3; Fat (g) = 0.2; Protein = 7.6

🥛 Milk Dry Reconstituted Low Fat (1%) ☞ serving size: 1 cup = 244 g; Calories = 97.6; Total Carb (g) = 11.2; Net Carb (g) = 11.2; Fat (g) = 2.5; Protein = 7.5

🥛 Milk Dry Reconstituted Ns As To Fat Content ☞ serving size: 1 cup = 244 g; Calories = 78.1; Total Carb (g) = 11.3; Net Carb (g) = 11.3; Fat (g) = 0.2; Protein = 7.6

🥛 Milk Dry Reconstituted Whole ☞ serving size: 1 cup = 244 g; Calories = 185.4; Total Carb (g) = 14.3; Net Carb (g) = 14.3; Fat (g) = 10; Protein = 9.8

🥛 Milk Dry Whole Without Added Vitamin D ☞ serving size: 1

cup = 128 g; Calories = 634.9; Total Carb (g) = 49.2; Net Carb (g) = 49.2; Fat (g) = 34.2; Protein = 33.7

🥛 Milk Evaporated 2% Fat With Added Vitamin A And Vitamin D ☞ serving size: 1 cup = 252 g; Calories = 269.6; Total Carb (g) = 39.7; Net Carb (g) = 39.7; Fat (g) = 5; Protein = 16.8

🥛 Milk Evaporated Reduced Fat (2%) ☞ serving size: 1 cup = 252 g; Calories = 231.8; Total Carb (g) = 28.1; Net Carb (g) = 28.1; Fat (g) = 4.9; Protein = 18.7

🥛 Milk Filled Fluid With Blend Of Hydrogenated Vegetable Oils ☞ serving size: 1 cup = 244 g; Calories = 153.7; Total Carb (g) = 11.6; Net Carb (g) = 11.6; Fat (g) = 8.4; Protein = 8.1

🥛 Milk Filled Fluid With Lauric Acid Oil ☞ serving size: 1 cup = 244 g; Calories = 153.7; Total Carb (g) = 11.6; Net Carb (g) = 11.6; Fat (g) = 8.3; Protein = 8.1

🥛 Milk Fluid 1% Fat Without Added Vitamin A And Vitamin D ☞ serving size: 1 cup = 244 g; Calories = 102.5; Total Carb (g) = 12.2; Net Carb (g) = 12.2; Fat (g) = 2.4; Protein = 8.2

🥛 Milk Fluid Nonfat Calcium Fortified (Fat Free Or Skim) ☞ serving size: 1 cup = 247 g; Calories = 86.5; Total Carb (g) = 12; Net Carb (g) = 12; Fat (g) = 0.4; Protein = 8.4

🥛 Milk Imitation Non-Soy ☞ serving size: 1 cup = 244 g; Calories = 112.2; Total Carb (g) = 12.9; Net Carb (g) = 12.9; Fat (g) = 4.9; Protein = 3.9

🥛 Milk Indian Buffalo Fluid ☞ serving size: 1 cup = 244 g; Calories = 236.7; Total Carb (g) = 12.6; Net Carb (g) = 12.6; Fat (g) = 16.8; Protein = 9.2

🥛 Milk Low Sodium Fluid ☞ serving size: 1 cup = 244 g; Calories = 148.8; Total Carb (g) = 10.9; Net Carb (g) = 10.9; Fat (g) = 8.4; Protein = 7.6

🥛 Milk Lowfat Fluid 1% Milkfat Protein Fortified With Added

Vitamin A And Vitamin D ☞ serving size: 1 cup = 246 g; Calories = 118.1; Total Carb (g) = 13.6; Net Carb (g) = 13.6; Fat (g) = 2.9; Protein = 9.7

🥛 Milk Lowfat Fluid 1% Milkfat With Added Nonfat Milk Solids Vitamin A And Vitamin D ☞ serving size: 1 cup = 245 g; Calories = 105.4; Total Carb (g) = 12.2; Net Carb (g) = 12.2; Fat (g) = 2.4; Protein = 8.5

🥛 Milk Malted ☞ serving size: 1 cup = 256 g; Calories = 166.4; Total Carb (g) = 22.1; Net Carb (g) = 22.1; Fat (g) = 5; Protein = 8

🥛 Milk Nfs ☞ serving size: 1 cup = 244 g; Calories = 124.4; Total Carb (g) = 11.8; Net Carb (g) = 11.8; Fat (g) = 5; Protein = 8

🥛 Milk Nonfat Fluid Protein Fortified With Added Vitamin A And Vitamin D (Fat Free And Skim) ☞ serving size: 1 cup = 246 g; Calories = 100.9; Total Carb (g) = 13.7; Net Carb (g) = 13.7; Fat (g) = 0.6; Protein = 9.7

🥛 Milk Nonfat Fluid With Added Nonfat Milk Solids Vitamin A And Vitamin D (Fat Free Or Skim) ☞ serving size: 1 cup = 245 g; Calories = 90.7; Total Carb (g) = 12.3; Net Carb (g) = 12.3; Fat (g) = 0.6; Protein = 8.8

🥛 Milk Nonfat Fluid Without Added Vitamin A And Vitamin D (Fat Free Or Skim) ☞ serving size: 1 cup = 245 g; Calories = 85.8; Total Carb (g) = 11.9; Net Carb (g) = 11.9; Fat (g) = 0.4; Protein = 8.3

🥛 Milk Reduced Fat Fluid 2% Milkfat Protein Fortified With Added Vitamin A And Vitamin D ☞ serving size: 1 cup = 246 g; Calories = 137.8; Total Carb (g) = 13.5; Net Carb (g) = 13.5; Fat (g) = 4.9; Protein = 9.7

🥛 Milk Reduced Fat Fluid 2% Milkfat With Added Nonfat Milk Solids And Vitamin A And Vitamin D ☞ serving size: 1 cup = 245 g; Calories = 125; Total Carb (g) = 12.2; Net Carb (g) = 12.2; Fat (g) = 4.7; Protein = 8.5

🥛 Milk Reduced Fat Fluid 2% Milkfat With Added Nonfat Milk Solids Without Added Vitamin A ☞ serving size: 1 cup = 245 g; Calories = 137.2; Total Carb (g) = 13.5; Net Carb (g) = 13.5; Fat (g) = 4.9; Protein = 9.7

🥛 Milk Reduced Fat Fluid 2% Milkfat Without Added Vitamin A And Vitamin D ☞ serving size: 1 cup = 246 g; Calories = 123; Total Carb (g) = 11.8; Net Carb (g) = 11.8; Fat (g) = 4.9; Protein = 8.1

🥛 Milk Shake Bottled Chocolate ☞ serving size: 1 fl oz = 31 g; Calories = 46.5; Total Carb (g) = 6.3; Net Carb (g) = 5.8; Fat (g) = 2.1; Protein = 1.2

🥛 Milk Shake Home Recipe Chocolate ☞ serving size: 1 fl oz = 28 g; Calories = 33.6; Total Carb (g) = 3.8; Net Carb (g) = 3.7; Fat (g) = 1.7; Protein = 1

🥛 Milk Shake Home Recipe Chocolate Light ☞ serving size: 1 fl oz = 28 g; Calories = 27.2; Total Carb (g) = 3.6; Net Carb (g) = 3.5; Fat (g) = 0.9; Protein = 1.1

🥛 Milk Shake Home Recipe Flavors Other Than Chocolate ☞ serving size: 1 fl oz = 28 g; Calories = 32.5; Total Carb (g) = 3.3; Net Carb (g) = 3.3; Fat (g) = 1.7; Protein = 0.9

🥛 Milk Shake Home Recipe Flavors Other Than Chocolate Light ☞ serving size: 1 fl oz = 28 g; Calories = 26.3; Total Carb (g) = 4; Net Carb (g) = 4; Fat (g) = 0.7; Protein = 1.1

🥛 Milk Shake With Malt ☞ serving size: 1 fl oz = 28 g; Calories = 35.6; Total Carb (g) = 3.9; Net Carb (g) = 3.9; Fat (g) = 1.8; Protein = 1

🥛 Milk Shakes Thick Chocolate ☞ serving size: 1 fl oz = 28.4 g; Calories = 33.8; Total Carb (g) = 6; Net Carb (g) = 5.9; Fat (g) = 0.8; Protein = 0.9

🥛 Milk Shakes Thick Vanilla ☞ serving size: 1 fl oz = 28.4 g; Calories = 31.8; Total Carb (g) = 5; Net Carb (g) = 5; Fat (g) = 0.9; Protein = 1.1

🥛 Milk Sheep Fluid ☞ serving size: 1 cup = 245 g; Calories = 264.6; Total Carb (g) = 13.1; Net Carb (g) = 13.1; Fat (g) = 17.2; Protein = 14.7

🥛 Milk Substitutes Fluid With Lauric Acid Oil ☞ serving size: 1 cup = 244 g; Calories = 148.8; Total Carb (g) = 15; Net Carb (g) = 15; Fat (g) = 8.3; Protein = 4.3

🥛 Milk Whole 3.25% Milkfat Without Added Vitamin A And Vitamin D ☞ serving size: 1 cup = 244 g; Calories = 148.8; Total Carb (g) = 11.7; Net Carb (g) = 11.7; Fat (g) = 8; Protein = 7.7

🥛 Monterey Cheese ☞ serving size: 1 cup, diced = 132 g; Calories = 492.4; Total Carb (g) = 0.9; Net Carb (g) = 0.9; Fat (g) = 40; Protein = 32.3

🥛 Mozzarella ☞ serving size: 1 cup, shredded = 112 g; Calories = 334.9; Total Carb (g) = 2.7; Net Carb (g) = 2.7; Fat (g) = 24.8; Protein = 24.8

🥛 Mozzarella (Hard And Lowfat) ☞ serving size: 1 cup, diced = 132 g; Calories = 389.4; Total Carb (g) = 7.4; Net Carb (g) = 7.4; Fat (g) = 26.1; Protein = 31.4

🥛 Mozzarella (Hard) ☞ serving size: 1 oz = 28.4 g; Calories = 90.3; Total Carb (g) = 0.7; Net Carb (g) = 0.7; Fat (g) = 7; Protein = 6.1

🥛 Mozzarella (Lowfat) ☞ serving size: 1 oz = 28.4 g; Calories = 72.1; Total Carb (g) = 0.8; Net Carb (g) = 0.8; Fat (g) = 4.5; Protein = 6.9

🥛 Mozzarella Cheese (Non-Fat Or Fat Free) ☞ serving size: 1 cup, shredded = 113 g; Calories = 159.3; Total Carb (g) = 4; Net Carb (g) = 1.9; Fat (g) = 0; Protein = 35.8

🥛 Muenster Cheese ☞ serving size: 1 cup, diced = 132 g; Calories = 485.8; Total Carb (g) = 1.5; Net Carb (g) = 1.5; Fat (g) = 39.7; Protein = 30.9

🥛 Neufchatel Cheese ☞ serving size: 1 oz = 28.4 g; Calories = 71.9; Total Carb (g) = 1; Net Carb (g) = 1; Fat (g) = 6.5; Protein = 2.6

🥛 Non-Dairy Milk Nfs ☞ serving size: 1 cup = 244 g; Calories = 78.1; Total Carb (g) = 9.6; Net Carb (g) = 9.2; Fat (g) = 3.1; Protein = 2.7

🥛 Non-Fat Yogurt ☞ serving size: 1 container (6 oz) = 170 g; Calories = 95.2; Total Carb (g) = 13.1; Net Carb (g) = 13.1; Fat (g) = 0.3; Protein = 9.7

🥛 Nonfat American Cheese ☞ serving size: 1 serving = 19 g; Calories = 23.9; Total Carb (g) = 2; Net Carb (g) = 2; Fat (g) = 0; Protein = 4

🥛 Nonfat Chocolate Yogurt ☞ serving size: 1 container (6 oz) = 170 g; Calories = 190.4; Total Carb (g) = 40; Net Carb (g) = 38; Fat (g) = 0; Protein = 6

🥛 Nonfat Cottage Cheese ☞ serving size: 1 cup (not packed) = 145 g; Calories = 104.4; Total Carb (g) = 9.7; Net Carb (g) = 9.7; Fat (g) = 0.4; Protein = 15

🥛 Nonfat Greek Strawberry Yogurt ☞ serving size: 1 container (5.3 oz) = 150 g; Calories = 123; Total Carb (g) = 18.1; Net Carb (g) = 17.2; Fat (g) = 0.2; Protein = 12.1

🥛 Nonfat Greek Vanilla Yogurt ☞ serving size: 1 container (5.3 oz) = 150 g; Calories = 117; Total Carb (g) = 15.6; Net Carb (g) = 14.8; Fat (g) = 0.3; Protein = 13

🥛 Nonfat Greek Yogurt ☞ serving size: 1 container = 170 g; Calories = 100.3; Total Carb (g) = 6.1; Net Carb (g) = 6.1; Fat (g) = 0.7; Protein = 17.3

🥛 Nonfat Strawberry Yogurt ☞ serving size: 5oz serving = 150 g; Calories = 126; Total Carb (g) = 18.8; Net Carb (g) = 18.2; Fat (g) = 0.3; Protein = 12.1

🥛 Nonfat Vanilla Yogurt ☞ serving size: 1 cup (8 fl oz) = 245 g; Calories = 191.1; Total Carb (g) = 41.8; Net Carb (g) = 41.8; Fat (g) = 0; Protein = 7.2

🥛 Nutritional Supplement For People With Diabetes Liquid ☞

serving size: 1 can = 227 g; Calories = 199.8; Total Carb (g) = 27; Net Carb (g) = 22; Fat (g) = 7; Protein = 10

🥛 Parmesan Cheese Topping Fat Free ☞ serving size: 1 tablespoon = 5 g; Calories = 18.5; Total Carb (g) = 2; Net Carb (g) = 2; Fat (g) = 0.3; Protein = 2

🥛 Plain Yogurt ☞ serving size: 1 container (6 oz) = 170 g; Calories = 103.7; Total Carb (g) = 7.9; Net Carb (g) = 7.9; Fat (g) = 5.5; Protein = 5.9

🥛 Poached Eggs ☞ serving size: 1 large = 50 g; Calories = 71.5; Total Carb (g) = 0.4; Net Carb (g) = 0.4; Fat (g) = 4.7; Protein = 6.3

🥛 Port De Salut Cheese ☞ serving size: 1 cup, diced = 132 g; Calories = 464.6; Total Carb (g) = 0.8; Net Carb (g) = 0.8; Fat (g) = 37.2; Protein = 31.4

🥛 Processed American Cheese (With Vitamin D) ☞ serving size: 1 oz = 28.4 g; Calories = 103.9; Total Carb (g) = 1.4; Net Carb (g) = 1.4; Fat (g) = 8.7; Protein = 5.2

🥛 Processed Pimento Cheese ☞ serving size: 1 cup, diced = 140 g; Calories = 525; Total Carb (g) = 2.4; Net Carb (g) = 2.3; Fat (g) = 43.7; Protein = 31

🥛 Processed Swiss Cheese ☞ serving size: 1 cup, diced = 140 g; Calories = 467.6; Total Carb (g) = 2.9; Net Carb (g) = 2.9; Fat (g) = 35; Protein = 34.6

🥛 Protein Supplement Milk Based Muscle Milk Light Powder ☞ serving size: 2 scoop = 50 g; Calories = 198; Total Carb (g) = 11; Net Carb (g) = 10; Fat (g) = 6; Protein = 25

🥛 Protein Supplement Milk Based Muscle Milk Powder ☞ serving size: 1 tbsp = 11 g; Calories = 45.2; Total Carb (g) = 2; Net Carb (g) = 1.3; Fat (g) = 1.9; Protein = 5

🥛 Provolone Cheese ☞ serving size: 1 cup, diced = 132 g; Calories = 463.3; Total Carb (g) = 2.8; Net Carb (g) = 2.8; Fat (g) = 35.1; Protein = 33.8

🥛 Puerto Rican White Cheese ☞ serving size: 1 cup = 128 g; Calories = 222.7; Total Carb (g) = 3.9; Net Carb (g) = 3.9; Fat (g) = 16.6; Protein = 14.4

🥛 Quail Egg Canned ☞ serving size: 1 egg = 9 g; Calories = 16; Total Carb (g) = 0; Net Carb (g) = 0; Fat (g) = 1.1; Protein = 1.3

🥛 Queso Asadero ☞ serving size: 1 cracker-size slice = 9 g; Calories = 32; Total Carb (g) = 0.3; Net Carb (g) = 0.3; Fat (g) = 2.5; Protein = 2

🥛 Queso Blanco ☞ serving size: 1 cup, crumbled = 118 g; Calories = 365.8; Total Carb (g) = 3; Net Carb (g) = 3; Fat (g) = 28.7; Protein = 24.1

🥛 Queso Chihuahua ☞ serving size: 1 cup, diced = 132 g; Calories = 493.7; Total Carb (g) = 7.3; Net Carb (g) = 7.3; Fat (g) = 39.2; Protein = 28.5

🥛 Queso Cotija ☞ serving size: 2 tsp = 5 g; Calories = 18.3; Total Carb (g) = 0.2; Net Carb (g) = 0.2; Fat (g) = 1.5; Protein = 1

🥛 Queso Fresco ☞ serving size: 1 cup, crumbled = 122 g; Calories = 364.8; Total Carb (g) = 3.6; Net Carb (g) = 3.6; Fat (g) = 29.1; Protein = 22.1

🥛 Reddi Wip Fat Free Whipped Topping ☞ serving size: 1 tablespoon = 4 g; Calories = 6; Total Carb (g) = 1; Net Carb (g) = 1; Fat (g) = 0.2; Protein = 0.1

🥛 Rice Dessert Bar Frozen Chocolate Nondairy Chocolate Covered ☞ serving size: 1 bar (4 oz) = 113 g; Calories = 267.8; Total Carb (g) = 28.3; Net Carb (g) = 23.8; Fat (g) = 16.8; Protein = 4.6

🥛 Rice Dessert Bar Frozen Flavors Other Than Chocolate Nondairy Carob Covered ☞ serving size: 1 bar (4 oz) = 113 g; Calories = 248.6; Total Carb (g) = 27.9; Net Carb (g) = 23.8; Fat (g) = 15.5; Protein = 2.6

🥛 Rice Frozen Dessert Nondairy Flavors Other Than Chocolate ☞ serving size: 1 cup = 172 g; Calories = 259.7; Total Carb (g) = 39.7; Net Carb (g) = 37.6; Fat (g) = 10.4; Protein = 3.1

🥛 Ricotta Cheese ☞ serving size: 1/2 cup = 124 g; Calories = 186; Total Carb (g) = 9; Net Carb (g) = 9; Fat (g) = 12.6; Protein = 9.4

🥛 Ripe Plantain Omelet Puerto Rican Style ☞ serving size: 1 medium egg = 79 g; Calories = 177; Total Carb (g) = 14.3; Net Carb (g) = 13.3; Fat (g) = 11.7; Protein = 5.2

🥛 Romano Cheese ☞ serving size: 1 oz = 28.4 g; Calories = 109.9; Total Carb (g) = 1; Net Carb (g) = 1; Fat (g) = 7.7; Protein = 9

🥛 Roquefort ☞ serving size: 1 oz = 28.4 g; Calories = 104.8; Total Carb (g) = 0.6; Net Carb (g) = 0.6; Fat (g) = 8.7; Protein = 6.1

🥛 Salted Butter ☞ serving size: 1 pat (1 inch sq, 1/3 inch high) = 5 g; Calories = 35.9; Total Carb (g) = 0; Net Carb (g) = 0; Fat (g) = 4.1; Protein = 0

🥛 Scrambled Eggs ☞ serving size: 1 large = 61 g; Calories = 90.9; Total Carb (g) = 1; Net Carb (g) = 1; Fat (g) = 6.7; Protein = 6.1

🥛 Scrambled Eggs With Jerked Beef Puerto Rican Style ☞ serving size: 1 cup = 140 g; Calories = 364; Total Carb (g) = 4.2; Net Carb (g) = 3.9; Fat (g) = 24.9; Protein = 30

🥛 Seafood Souffle ☞ serving size: 1 cup = 159 g; Calories = 240.1; Total Carb (g) = 8.7; Net Carb (g) = 8.5; Fat (g) = 15.6; Protein = 15.8

🥛 Sharp Cheddar Cheese ☞ serving size: 1 slice (2/3 oz) = 19 g; Calories = 77.9; Total Carb (g) = 0.4; Net Carb (g) = 0.4; Fat (g) = 6.4; Protein = 4.6

🥛 Shredded Parmesan ☞ serving size: 1 tbsp = 5 g; Calories = 20.8; Total Carb (g) = 0.2; Net Carb (g) = 0.2; Fat (g) = 1.4; Protein = 1.9

🥛 Shrimp-Egg Patty ☞ serving size: 1 patty (about 2" dia) = 18 g; Calories = 87.7; Total Carb (g) = 2.1; Net Carb (g) = 2; Fat (g) = 6.4; Protein = 5.1

🥛 Skim Milk ☞ serving size: 1 cup = 245 g; Calories = 83.3; Total Carb (g) = 12.2; Net Carb (g) = 12.2; Fat (g) = 0.2; Protein = 8.3

🥛 Soft Goat Cheese ☞ serving size: 1 oz = 28.4 g; Calories = 75; Total Carb (g) = 0; Net Carb (g) = 0; Fat (g) = 6; Protein = 5.3

🥛 Soft Serve Chocolate Ice Cream ☞ serving size: 1/2 cup = 86 g; Calories = 190.9; Total Carb (g) = 19.1; Net Carb (g) = 18.5; Fat (g) = 11.2; Protein = 3.5

🥛 Sour Cream Light ☞ serving size: 1 tablespoon = 12 g; Calories = 16.3; Total Carb (g) = 0.9; Net Carb (g) = 0.9; Fat (g) = 1.3; Protein = 0.4

🥛 Sour Dressing Non-Butterfat Cultured Filled Cream-Type ☞ serving size: 1 tbsp = 12 g; Calories = 21.4; Total Carb (g) = 0.6; Net Carb (g) = 0.6; Fat (g) = 2; Protein = 0.4

🥛 Squash Summer Souffle ☞ serving size: 1 cup = 136 g; Calories = 165.9; Total Carb (g) = 9.4; Net Carb (g) = 8.3; Fat (g) = 11.9; Protein = 6

🥛 Squash Winter Souffle ☞ serving size: 1 cup = 157 g; Calories = 122.5; Total Carb (g) = 19.1; Net Carb (g) = 15.8; Fat (g) = 3.4; Protein = 5.3

🥛 Strawberry Milk Fat Free ☞ serving size: 1 fl oz = 31 g; Calories = 17.4; Total Carb (g) = 3.3; Net Carb (g) = 3.3; Fat (g) = 0; Protein = 1

🥛 Strawberry Milk Low Fat ☞ serving size: 1 cup = 248 g; Calories = 156.2; Total Carb (g) = 26.7; Net Carb (g) = 26.7; Fat (g) = 2.3; Protein = 7.9

🥛 Strawberry Milk Nfs ☞ serving size: 1 fl oz = 31 g; Calories = 16.1; Total Carb (g) = 1.6; Net Carb (g) = 1.6; Fat (g) = 0.6; Protein = 1

🥛 Strawberry Milk Non-Dairy ☞ serving size: 1 cup = 248 g; Calories = 153.8; Total Carb (g) = 28.5; Net Carb (g) = 27.8; Fat (g) = 3; Protein = 3.5

🥛 Strawberry Milk Reduced Fat ☞ serving size: 1 cup = 248 g; Calories = 176.1; Total Carb (g) = 26.3; Net Carb (g) = 26.3; Fat (g) = 4.6; Protein = 7.7

🥛 Strawberry Milk Whole ☞ serving size: 1 cup = 248 g; Calories =

200.9; Total Carb (g) = 26.3; Net Carb (g) = 26.3; Fat (g) = 7.6; Protein = 7.3

Sweet Whey Fluid ☞ serving size: 1 cup = 246 g; Calories = 66.4; Total Carb (g) = 12.6; Net Carb (g) = 12.6; Fat (g) = 0.9; Protein = 2.1

Sweetened Condensed Milk ☞ serving size: 1 fl oz = 38.2 g; Calories = 122.6; Total Carb (g) = 20.8; Net Carb (g) = 20.8; Fat (g) = 3.3; Protein = 3

Swiss Cheese ☞ serving size: 1 cup, diced = 132 g; Calories = 518.8; Total Carb (g) = 1.9; Net Carb (g) = 1.9; Fat (g) = 40.9; Protein = 35.6

Tilsit Cheese ☞ serving size: 1 oz = 28.4 g; Calories = 96.6; Total Carb (g) = 0.5; Net Carb (g) = 0.5; Fat (g) = 7.4; Protein = 6.9

Tofu Frozen Dessert Chocolate ☞ serving size: 1 cup = 164 g; Calories = 388.7; Total Carb (g) = 41; Net Carb (g) = 35.3; Fat (g) = 24.2; Protein = 5.5

Tofu Frozen Dessert Flavors Other Than Chocolate ☞ serving size: 1 cup = 164 g; Calories = 428; Total Carb (g) = 36.7; Net Carb (g) = 35.6; Fat (g) = 30.6; Protein = 7.9

Unsalted Butter ☞ serving size: 1 pat (1 inch sq, 1/3 inch high) = 5 g; Calories = 35.9; Total Carb (g) = 0; Net Carb (g) = 0; Fat (g) = 4.1; Protein = 0

Whey Acid Fluid ☞ serving size: 1 cup = 246 g; Calories = 59; Total Carb (g) = 12.6; Net Carb (g) = 12.6; Fat (g) = 0.2; Protein = 1.9

Whipped Butter (Salted) ☞ serving size: 1 pat (1 inch sq, 1/3 inch high) = 3.8 g; Calories = 27.8; Total Carb (g) = 0; Net Carb (g) = 0; Fat (g) = 3; Protein = 0

Whipped Cream ☞ serving size: 1 cup = 60 g; Calories = 154.2; Total Carb (g) = 7.5; Net Carb (g) = 7.5; Fat (g) = 13.3; Protein = 1.9

Whipped Cream Substitute Dietetic Made From Powdered Mix

☞ serving size: 1 cup = 80 g; Calories = 80; Total Carb (g) = 8.5; Net Carb (g) = 8.5; Fat (g) = 4.8; Protein = 0.7

🥛 Whipped Topping Frozen Low Fat ☞ serving size: 1 cup = 75 g; Calories = 168; Total Carb (g) = 17.7; Net Carb (g) = 17.7; Fat (g) = 9.8; Protein = 2.3

🥛 Whole Milk ☞ serving size: 1 cup = 244 g; Calories = 148.8; Total Carb (g) = 11.7; Net Carb (g) = 11.7; Fat (g) = 7.9; Protein = 7.7

🥛 Yogurt Chocolate Nonfat Milk ☞ serving size: 1 container (6 oz) = 170 g; Calories = 190.4; Total Carb (g) = 40; Net Carb (g) = 38; Fat (g) = 0; Protein = 6

🥛 Yogurt Coconut Milk ☞ serving size: 1 6 oz container = 170 g; Calories = 108.8; Total Carb (g) = 13.5; Net Carb (g) = 13.5; Fat (g) = 6; Protein = 0.5

🥛 Yogurt Frozen Chocolate Lowfat Milk ☞ serving size: 1 cup = 200 g; Calories = 226; Total Carb (g) = 43.6; Net Carb (g) = 40.4; Fat (g) = 3.9; Protein = 10.5

🥛 Yogurt Frozen Chocolate-Coated ☞ serving size: 1 bar = 41 g; Calories = 110.7; Total Carb (g) = 11.9; Net Carb (g) = 11.8; Fat (g) = 6.7; Protein = 1.3

🥛 Yogurt Frozen Cone Chocolate ☞ serving size: 1 small cone = 78 g; Calories = 175.5; Total Carb (g) = 24.4; Net Carb (g) = 23.2; Fat (g) = 7.1; Protein = 4.1

🥛 Yogurt Frozen Cone Chocolate Lowfat Milk ☞ serving size: 1 small cone = 78 g; Calories = 102.2; Total Carb (g) = 19.6; Net Carb (g) = 18.4; Fat (g) = 1.8; Protein = 4.2

🥛 Yogurt Frozen Cone Flavors Other Than Chocolate ☞ serving size: 1 small cone = 78 g; Calories = 147.4; Total Carb (g) = 24.6; Net Carb (g) = 24.4; Fat (g) = 4.2; Protein = 3.5

🥛 Yogurt Frozen Cone Flavors Other Than Chocolate Lowfat Milk

☞ serving size: 1 small cone = 78 g; Calories = 65.5; Total Carb (g) = 8.8; Net Carb (g) = 8.6; Fat (g) = 1.5; Protein = 4.2

🥛 Yogurt Frozen Flavors Not Chocolate Nonfat Milk With Low-Calorie Sweetener ☞ serving size: 1/2 cup = 68 g; Calories = 70.7; Total Carb (g) = 13.4; Net Carb (g) = 12; Fat (g) = 0.5; Protein = 3

🥛 Yogurt Frozen Flavors Other Than Chocolate With Sorbet Or Sorbet-Coated ☞ serving size: 1 haagen-dazs bar (2.3 fl oz) = 75 g; Calories = 114; Total Carb (g) = 20; Net Carb (g) = 19.6; Fat (g) = 2.6; Protein = 2.8

🥛 Yogurt Frozen Ns As To Flavor Nonfat Milk ☞ serving size: 1 cup = 159 g; Calories = 192.4; Total Carb (g) = 39.4; Net Carb (g) = 38; Fat (g) = 0.7; Protein = 7

🥛 Yogurt Frozen Sandwich ☞ serving size: 1 sandwich = 85 g; Calories = 180.2; Total Carb (g) = 32; Net Carb (g) = 31.7; Fat (g) = 4.4; Protein = 3.9

🥛 Yogurt Fruit Low Fat 10 Grams Protein Per 8 Ounce ☞ serving size: 1 container (6 oz) = 170 g; Calories = 173.4; Total Carb (g) = 32.4; Net Carb (g) = 32.4; Fat (g) = 1.8; Protein = 7.4

🥛 Yogurt Fruit Low Fat 11 Grams Protein Per 8 Ounce ☞ serving size: 1 container (6 oz) = 170 g; Calories = 178.5; Total Carb (g) = 31.6; Net Carb (g) = 31.6; Fat (g) = 2.4; Protein = 8.3

🥛 Yogurt Fruit Low Fat 9 Grams Protein Per 8 Ounce ☞ serving size: 1 container (6 oz) = 170 g; Calories = 168.3; Total Carb (g) = 31.7; Net Carb (g) = 31.7; Fat (g) = 2; Protein = 6.8

🥛 Yogurt Fruit Low Fat 9 Grams Protein Per 8 Ounce Fortified With Vitamin D ☞ serving size: 1 container (6 oz) = 170 g; Calories = 168.3; Total Carb (g) = 31.7; Net Carb (g) = 31.7; Fat (g) = 2; Protein = 6.8

🥛 Yogurt Fruit Lowfat With Low Calorie Sweetener ☞ serving

size: 1 container (6 oz) = 170 g; Calories = 178.5; Total Carb (g) = 31.6; Net Carb (g) = 31.6; Fat (g) = 2.4; Protein = 8.3

🥛 Yogurt Fruit Lowfat With Low Calorie Sweetener Fortified With Vitamin D ☞ serving size: 1 container (6 oz) = 170 g; Calories = 178.5; Total Carb (g) = 31.6; Net Carb (g) = 31.6; Fat (g) = 2.4; Protein = 8.3

🥛 Yogurt Fruit Variety Nonfat ☞ serving size: 1 container (6 oz) = 170 g; Calories = 161.5; Total Carb (g) = 32.3; Net Carb (g) = 32.3; Fat (g) = 0.3; Protein = 7.5

🥛 Yogurt Fruit Variety Nonfat Fortified With Vitamin D ☞ serving size: 1 container (6 oz) = 170 g; Calories = 161.5; Total Carb (g) = 32.3; Net Carb (g) = 32.3; Fat (g) = 0.3; Protein = 7.5

🥛 Yogurt Greek Low Fat Milk Fruit ☞ serving size: 1 tube = 57 g; Calories = 58.7; Total Carb (g) = 6.8; Net Carb (g) = 6.2; Fat (g) = 1.5; Protein = 4.7

🥛 Yogurt Greek Nonfat Vanilla Chobani ☞ serving size: oz = 150 g; Calories = 106.5; Total Carb (g) = 12.1; Net Carb (g) = 11.7; Fat (g) = 0.3; Protein = 13.6

🥛 Yogurt Greek Nonfat Vanilla Dannon Oikos ☞ serving size: 5oz serving = 150 g; Calories = 127.5; Total Carb (g) = 19.1; Net Carb (g) = 18.3; Fat (g) = 0.2; Protein = 12.2

🥛 Yogurt Greek Ns As To Type Of Milk Fruit ☞ serving size: 1 5.3 oz container = 150 g; Calories = 154.5; Total Carb (g) = 17.8; Net Carb (g) = 16.3; Fat (g) = 3.9; Protein = 12.3

🥛 Yogurt Greek Strawberry Dannon Oikos ☞ serving size: 5oz serving = 150 g; Calories = 159; Total Carb (g) = 17.5; Net Carb (g) = 16; Fat (g) = 4.4; Protein = 12.4

🥛 Yogurt Greek Whole Milk Flavors Other Than Fruit ☞ serving size: 1 5.3 oz container = 150 g; Calories = 166.5; Total Carb (g) = 14; Net Carb (g) = 14; Fat (g) = 6.7; Protein = 12.7

Yogurt Liquid ☞ serving size: 1 bottle = 93 g; Calories = 67; Total Carb (g) = 11; Net Carb (g) = 10.9; Fat (g) = 1; Protein = 3.5

Yogurt Low Fat Milk Flavors Other Than Fruit ☞ serving size: 1 tube = 64 g; Calories = 46.7; Total Carb (g) = 6.3; Net Carb (g) = 6.3; Fat (g) = 1; Protein = 3.3

Yogurt Low Fat Milk Fruit ☞ serving size: 1 tube = 64 g; Calories = 57; Total Carb (g) = 9.3; Net Carb (g) = 9.2; Fat (g) = 0.9; Protein = 3

Yogurt Nonfat Milk Flavors Other Than Fruit ☞ serving size: 1 4 oz container = 113 g; Calories = 74.6; Total Carb (g) = 11.8; Net Carb (g) = 11.8; Fat (g) = 0.2; Protein = 6.3

Yogurt Nonfat Milk Fruit ☞ serving size: 1 4 oz container = 113 g; Calories = 93.8; Total Carb (g) = 17; Net Carb (g) = 16.9; Fat (g) = 0.2; Protein = 5.8

Yogurt Ns As To Type Of Milk Flavors Other Than Fruit ☞ serving size: 1 4 oz container = 113 g; Calories = 82.5; Total Carb (g) = 11.1; Net Carb (g) = 11.1; Fat (g) = 1.7; Protein = 5.8

Yogurt Ns As To Type Of Milk Fruit ☞ serving size: 1 4 oz container = 113 g; Calories = 100.6; Total Carb (g) = 16.3; Net Carb (g) = 16.2; Fat (g) = 1.6; Protein = 5.3

Yogurt Vanilla Flavor Lowfat Milk Sweetened With Low Calorie Sweetener ☞ serving size: 1 container = 170 g; Calories = 146.2; Total Carb (g) = 23.5; Net Carb (g) = 23.5; Fat (g) = 2.1; Protein = 8.4

Yogurt Vanilla Low Fat 11 Grams Protein Per 8 Ounce ☞ serving size: 1 container (6 oz) = 170 g; Calories = 144.5; Total Carb (g) = 23.5; Net Carb (g) = 23.5; Fat (g) = 2.1; Protein = 8.4

Yogurt Vanilla Low Fat 11 Grams Protein Per 8 Ounce Fortified With Vitamin D ☞ serving size: 1 container (6 oz) = 170 g; Calories = 144.5; Total Carb (g) = 23.5; Net Carb (g) = 23.5; Fat (g) = 2.1; Protein = 8.4

Yogurt Vanilla Or Lemon Flavor Nonfat Milk Sweetened With

Low-Calorie Sweetener ☞ serving size: 1 container (6 oz) = 170 g; Calories = 73.1; Total Carb (g) = 12.8; Net Carb (g) = 12.8; Fat (g) = 0.3; Protein = 6.6

◙ Yogurt Vanilla Or Lemon Flavor Nonfat Milk Sweetened With Low-Calorie Sweetener Fortified With Vitamin D ☞ serving size: 1 container (6 oz) = 170 g; Calories = 73.1; Total Carb (g) = 12.8; Net Carb (g) = 12.8; Fat (g) = 0.3; Protein = 6.6

◙ Yogurt Whole Milk Flavors Other Than Fruit ☞ serving size: 1 4 oz container = 113 g; Calories = 87; Total Carb (g) = 10.7; Net Carb (g) = 10.7; Fat (g) = 3.5; Protein = 3.7

FAST FOODS

🍔 Arbys Roast Beef Sandwich Classic ☞ serving size: 1 sandwich = 149 g; Calories = 360.6; Total Carb (g) = 33.1; Net Carb (g) = 31.2; Fat (g) = 15.4; Protein = 22.6

🍔 Bacon And Cheese Sandwich With Spread ☞ serving size: 1 sandwich = 121 g; Calories = 378.7; Total Carb (g) = 31.7; Net Carb (g) = 30.3; Fat (g) = 20.5; Protein = 16.3

🍔 Bacon And Egg Sandwich ☞ serving size: 1 sandwich = 177 g; Calories = 419.5; Total Carb (g) = 38.5; Net Carb (g) = 36.6; Fat (g) = 18.9; Protein = 21.9

🍔 Bacon Breaded Fried Chicken Fillet And Tomato Club With Lettuce And Spread ☞ serving size: 1 sandwich = 227 g; Calories = 583.4; Total Carb (g) = 47.3; Net Carb (g) = 43.5; Fat (g) = 31.4; Protein = 28.2

🍔 Bacon Cheeseburger 1 Large Patty With Condiments On Bun From Fast Food / Restaurant ☞ serving size: 1 (1/3 lb) cheeseburger = 335 g; Calories = 794; Total Carb (g) = 39.6; Net Carb (g) = 37.3; Fat (g) = 49.7; Protein = 45.6

🍔 Bacon Cheeseburger 1 Medium Patty Plain On Bun From Fast Food / Restaurant ☞ serving size: 1 (1/4 lb) bacon cheeseburger = 170 g; Calories = 552.5; Total Carb (g) = 37.3; Net Carb (g) = 34.7; Fat (g) = 30.3; Protein = 32.1

🍔 Bacon Cheeseburger 1 Medium Patty Plain On White Bun ☞ serving size: 1 (1/4 lb) bacon cheeseburger = 180 g; Calories = 543.6; Total Carb (g) = 31; Net Carb (g) = 29.9; Fat (g) = 29.1; Protein = 36.9

🍔 Bacon Cheeseburger 1 Medium Patty With Condiments On Bun From Fast Food / Restaurant ☞ serving size: 1 (1/4 lb) bacon cheeseburger = 240 g; Calories = 676.8; Total Carb (g) = 44.4; Net Carb (g) = 41.8; Fat (g) = 37.9; Protein = 39.6

🍔 Bacon Cheeseburger 1 Medium Patty With Condiments On Wheat Bun ☞ serving size: 1 (1/4 lb) bacon cheeseburger = 240 g; Calories = 585.6; Total Carb (g) = 32.4; Net Carb (g) = 28.5; Fat (g) = 33; Protein = 38.8

🍔 Bacon Cheeseburger 1 Medium Patty With Condiments On White Bun ☞ serving size: 1 (1/4 lb) bacon cheeseburger = 240 g; Calories = 595.2; Total Carb (g) = 35.3; Net Carb (g) = 33.6; Fat (g) = 33; Protein = 37.8

🍔 Bacon Cheeseburger 1 Medium Patty With Condiments On Whole Wheat Bun ☞ serving size: 1 (1/4 lb) bacon cheeseburger = 240 g; Calories = 585.6; Total Carb (g) = 32.4; Net Carb (g) = 28.5; Fat (g) = 33; Protein = 38.8

🍔 Bacon Cheeseburger 1 Small Patty With Condiments On Bun From Fast Food / Restaurant ☞ serving size: 1 bacon cheeseburger = 160 g; Calories = 459.2; Total Carb (g) = 37.6; Net Carb (g) = 34.8; Fat (g) = 23.6; Protein = 24.3

🍔 Bacon Cheeseburger 1 Small Patty With Condiments On Bun From Fast Food / Restaurant (Wendy's Jr. Bacon Cheeseburger) ☞ serving size: 1 wendy's jr. bacon cheeseburger = 150 g; Calories =

408; Total Carb (g) = 34.5; Net Carb (g) = 32.6; Fat (g) = 20.2; Protein = 22.2

🍪 Bacon Chicken And Tomato Club Sandwich On Multigrain Roll With Lettuce And Spread ☞ serving size: 1 sandwich = 194 g; Calories = 432.6; Total Carb (g) = 23.6; Net Carb (g) = 21.3; Fat (g) = 21.7; Protein = 35.1

🍪 Bacon Lettuce And Tomato Sandwich With Spread ☞ serving size: 1 sandwich = 164 g; Calories = 339.5; Total Carb (g) = 34.8; Net Carb (g) = 32.1; Fat (g) = 16.9; Protein = 12.2

🍪 Bacon Lettuce Tomato And Cheese Submarine Sandwich With Spread ☞ serving size: 1 submarine = 260 g; Calories = 605.8; Total Carb (g) = 40.8; Net Carb (g) = 37.4; Fat (g) = 36.3; Protein = 28.5

🍪 Bacon On Biscuit ☞ serving size: 1 sandwich = 93 g; Calories = 330.2; Total Carb (g) = 43.9; Net Carb (g) = 42.9; Fat (g) = 13.1; Protein = 9.1

🍪 Bacon Sandwich With Spread ☞ serving size: 1 sandwich = 91 g; Calories = 324; Total Carb (g) = 27.8; Net Carb (g) = 26.3; Fat (g) = 16.2; Protein = 15.6

🍪 Bagel With Breakfast Steak Egg Cheese And Condiments ☞ serving size: 1 item = 254 g; Calories = 716.3; Total Carb (g) = 58.4; Net Carb (g) = 57.9; Fat (g) = 35.7; Protein = 40.5

🍪 Bagel With Egg Sausage Patty Cheese And Condiments ☞ serving size: 1 item = 219 g; Calories = 646.1; Total Carb (g) = 49.6; Net Carb (g) = 49.1; Fat (g) = 37.2; Protein = 28.4

🍪 Beef Barbecue Sandwich Or Sloppy Joe On Bun ☞ serving size: 1 barbecue sandwich = 186 g; Calories = 433.4; Total Carb (g) = 61.3; Net Carb (g) = 59.6; Fat (g) = 11.6; Protein = 19.1

🍪 Beef Barbecue Submarine Sandwich On Bun ☞ serving size: 1 sandwich = 192 g; Calories = 424.3; Total Carb (g) = 50; Net Carb (g) = 48.5; Fat (g) = 10.3; Protein = 32.1

🍔 Beef Sandwich Nfs ☞ serving size: 1 sandwich = 133 g; Calories = 252.7; Total Carb (g) = 24.8; Net Carb (g) = 24.1; Fat (g) = 9.8; Protein = 15.9

🍔 Biscuit With Crispy Chicken Fillet ☞ serving size: 1 item = 132 g; Calories = 396; Total Carb (g) = 40.3; Net Carb (g) = 38.5; Fat (g) = 19.7; Protein = 15.8

🍔 Biscuit With Egg And Bacon ☞ serving size: 1 biscuit = 150 g; Calories = 457.5; Total Carb (g) = 28.6; Net Carb (g) = 27.8; Fat (g) = 31.1; Protein = 17

🍔 Biscuit With Egg And Ham ☞ serving size: 1 biscuit = 182 g; Calories = 424.1; Total Carb (g) = 29.8; Net Carb (g) = 29.1; Fat (g) = 25.6; Protein = 19.4

🍔 Biscuit With Egg Cheese And Bacon ☞ serving size: 1 item = 145 g; Calories = 436.5; Total Carb (g) = 35.4; Net Carb (g) = 35.2; Fat (g) = 25.4; Protein = 17.4

🍔 Biscuit With Gravy ☞ serving size: 1 biscuit with gravy = 221 g; Calories = 475.2; Total Carb (g) = 44.9; Net Carb (g) = 44.1; Fat (g) = 27.2; Protein = 13

🍔 Biscuit With Ham ☞ serving size: 1 biscuit = 162 g; Calories = 554; Total Carb (g) = 62.8; Net Carb (g) = 61.6; Fat (g) = 26.4; Protein = 19.2

🍔 Biscuit With Sausage ☞ serving size: 1 item = 111 g; Calories = 411.8; Total Carb (g) = 33.3; Net Carb (g) = 32.8; Fat (g) = 27.1; Protein = 10.7

🍔 Blended Soft Serve Ice Cream With Cookies ☞ serving size: 12 fl oz cup = 337 g; Calories = 569.5; Total Carb (g) = 86.1; Net Carb (g) = 85.8; Fat (g) = 19.1; Protein = 13.4

🍔 Blintz Cheese-Filled ☞ serving size: 1 blintz = 70 g; Calories = 130.2; Total Carb (g) = 14.1; Net Carb (g) = 13.8; Fat (g) = 5.3; Protein = 6.3

🍶 Blintz Fruit-Filled ☞ serving size: 1 blintz = 70 g; Calories = 122.5; Total Carb (g) = 17.4; Net Carb (g) = 16.9; Fat (g) = 4.3; Protein = 3.9

🍶 Bologna And Cheese Sandwich With Spread ☞ serving size: 1 sandwich = 111 g; Calories = 335.2; Total Carb (g) = 30.1; Net Carb (g) = 28.6; Fat (g) = 17.8; Protein = 13.1

🍶 Bologna Sandwich With Spread ☞ serving size: 1 sandwich = 83 g; Calories = 249.8; Total Carb (g) = 27.3; Net Carb (g) = 25.9; Fat (g) = 11.5; Protein = 8.7

🍶 Breadstick Soft Prepared With Garlic And Parmesan Cheese ☞ serving size: 1 breadstick = 43 g; Calories = 147.5; Total Carb (g) = 19.1; Net Carb (g) = 18.1; Fat (g) = 5.5; Protein = 5.3

🍶 Breakfast Burrito With Egg Cheese And Sausage ☞ serving size: 1 burrito = 109 g; Calories = 301.9; Total Carb (g) = 25; Net Carb (g) = 23.7; Fat (g) = 17; Protein = 12.1

🍶 Breakfast Pizza With Egg ☞ serving size: 1 piece, nfs = 144 g; Calories = 427.7; Total Carb (g) = 37.7; Net Carb (g) = 35.4; Fat (g) = 21.9; Protein = 19

🍶 Bruschetta ☞ serving size: 1 slice = 43 g; Calories = 74.4; Total Carb (g) = 9.5; Net Carb (g) = 8.7; Fat (g) = 3.3; Protein = 1.7

🍶 Buffalo Chicken Submarine Sandwich ☞ serving size: 1 submarine = 240 g; Calories = 446.4; Total Carb (g) = 45.9; Net Carb (g) = 43.3; Fat (g) = 18.7; Protein = 23.5

🍶 Buffalo Chicken Submarine Sandwich With Cheese ☞ serving size: 1 submarine = 260 g; Calories = 527.8; Total Carb (g) = 45.1; Net Carb (g) = 42.5; Fat (g) = 25.4; Protein = 29.7

🍶 Burger King Cheeseburger ☞ serving size: 1 item = 133 g; Calories = 380.4; Total Carb (g) = 31.5; Net Carb (g) = 30.2; Fat (g) = 19.7; Protein = 19.4

🍶 Burger King Chicken Strips ☞ serving size: 1 strip = 36 g; Calo-

ries = 105.1; Total Carb (g) = 7.4; Net Carb (g) = 6.9; Fat (g) = 5.5; Protein = 6.6

⬤ Burger King Croissanwich With Egg And Cheese ☞ serving size: 1 item = 110 g; Calories = 311.3; Total Carb (g) = 27.3; Net Carb (g) = 26.5; Fat (g) = 17.4; Protein = 11.4

⬤ Burger King Croissanwich With Sausage And Cheese ☞ serving size: 1 item = 131 g; Calories = 492.6; Total Carb (g) = 30.1; Net Carb (g) = 29.2; Fat (g) = 33.3; Protein = 18

⬤ Burger King Croissanwich With Sausage Egg And Cheese ☞ serving size: 1 sandwich = 171 g; Calories = 526.7; Total Carb (g) = 27.2; Net Carb (g) = 24.1; Fat (g) = 37.2; Protein = 20.7

⬤ Burger King Double Cheeseburger ☞ serving size: 1 sandwich = 162 g; Calories = 456.8; Total Carb (g) = 28.2; Net Carb (g) = 28.2; Fat (g) = 26.1; Protein = 27.3

⬤ Burger King Double Whopper No Cheese ☞ serving size: 1 item = 374 g; Calories = 942.5; Total Carb (g) = 51.4; Net Carb (g) = 46.2; Fat (g) = 58.6; Protein = 52.1

⬤ Burger King Double Whopper With Cheese ☞ serving size: 1 item = 399 g; Calories = 1061.3; Total Carb (g) = 53.9; Net Carb (g) = 47.6; Fat (g) = 68.1; Protein = 57.7

⬤ Burger King French Fries ☞ serving size: 1 small serving = 74 g; Calories = 207.2; Total Carb (g) = 28.6; Net Carb (g) = 26.5; Fat (g) = 9.2; Protein = 2.4

⬤ Burger King French Toast Sticks ☞ serving size: 1 stick = 21 g; Calories = 73.3; Total Carb (g) = 8.7; Net Carb (g) = 8.4; Fat (g) = 3.7; Protein = 1.3

⬤ Burger King Hamburger ☞ serving size: 1 sandwich = 99 g; Calories = 258.4; Total Carb (g) = 26.5; Net Carb (g) = 25.5; Fat (g) = 10.4; Protein = 14.7

⬤ Burger King Hash Brown Rounds ☞ serving size: 1 piece = 5.6 g;

Calories = 16.9; Total Carb (g) = 1.6; Net Carb (g) = 1.5; Fat (g) = 1.1; Protein = 0.2

Burger King Onion Rings ☞ serving size: 1 small = 91 g; Calories = 379.5; Total Carb (g) = 39.7; Net Carb (g) = 37.2; Fat (g) = 23; Protein = 3.5

Burger King Original Chicken Sandwich ☞ serving size: 1 sandwich = 199 g; Calories = 569.1; Total Carb (g) = 52.2; Net Carb (g) = 47.4; Fat (g) = 29.2; Protein = 24.2

Burger King Premium Fish Sandwich ☞ serving size: 1 sandwich = 220 g; Calories = 572; Total Carb (g) = 58.7; Net Carb (g) = 56.7; Fat (g) = 27.4; Protein = 22.6

Burger King Vanilla Shake ☞ serving size: 1 fl oz = 24.8 g; Calories = 41.7; Total Carb (g) = 4.7; Net Carb (g) = 4.7; Fat (g) = 2.2; Protein = 0.8

Burger King Whopper No Cheese ☞ serving size: 1 item = 291 g; Calories = 678; Total Carb (g) = 54; Net Carb (g) = 48.7; Fat (g) = 37.4; Protein = 31.3

Burger King Whopper With Cheese ☞ serving size: 1 item = 316 g; Calories = 790; Total Carb (g) = 52.8; Net Carb (g) = 49.6; Fat (g) = 48.4; Protein = 35.4

Burrito Taco Or Quesadilla With Egg ☞ serving size: 1 small = 110 g; Calories = 251.9; Total Carb (g) = 21.7; Net Carb (g) = 20.1; Fat (g) = 13; Protein = 11.3

Burrito Taco Or Quesadilla With Egg And Breakfast Meat ☞ serving size: 1 small = 123 g; Calories = 297.7; Total Carb (g) = 21.2; Net Carb (g) = 19.6; Fat (g) = 17.1; Protein = 14

Burrito Taco Or Quesadilla With Egg And Potato ☞ serving size: 1 small = 127 g; Calories = 298.5; Total Carb (g) = 26.9; Net Carb (g) = 24.8; Fat (g) = 16.1; Protein = 11.5

Burrito Taco Or Quesadilla With Egg Beans And Breakfast Meat

☞ serving size: 1 small = 150 g; Calories = 336; Total Carb (g) = 26; Net Carb (g) = 23; Fat (g) = 18.7; Protein = 15.7

🥟 Burrito Taco Or Quesadilla With Egg Potato And Breakfast Meat ☞ serving size: 1 small = 144 g; Calories = 354.2; Total Carb (g) = 27.2; Net Carb (g) = 25; Fat (g) = 20.7; Protein = 14.6

🥟 Burrito Taco Or Quesadilla With Egg Potato And Breakfast Meat From Fast Food ☞ serving size: 1 small = 144 g; Calories = 348.5; Total Carb (g) = 25.6; Net Carb (g) = 23.7; Fat (g) = 20.1; Protein = 16.1

🥟 Burrito With Beans ☞ serving size: 2 pieces = 217 g; Calories = 447; Total Carb (g) = 71.4; Net Carb (g) = 71.4; Fat (g) = 13.5; Protein = 14.1

🥟 Burrito With Beans And Beef ☞ serving size: 1 item = 241 g; Calories = 460.3; Total Carb (g) = 47; Net Carb (g) = 39.8; Fat (g) = 18; Protein = 27.8

🥟 Burrito With Beans And Cheese ☞ serving size: 1 each burrito = 185 g; Calories = 379.3; Total Carb (g) = 57.8; Net Carb (g) = 50; Fat (g) = 11.2; Protein = 13.6

🥟 Burrito With Beans Cheese And Beef ☞ serving size: 1 burrito = 241 g; Calories = 433.8; Total Carb (g) = 56.3; Net Carb (g) = 47.4; Fat (g) = 16.4; Protein = 16.9

🥟 Cheese Pizza ☞ serving size: 1 slice = 107 g; Calories = 284.6; Total Carb (g) = 35.7; Net Carb (g) = 33.2; Fat (g) = 10.4; Protein = 12.2

🥟 Cheeseburger 1 Large Patty Plain On Bun From Fast Food / Restaurant ☞ serving size: 1 (1/3 lb) cheeseburger = 200 g; Calories = 600; Total Carb (g) = 32; Net Carb (g) = 31; Fat (g) = 35; Protein = 37.2

🥟 Cheeseburger 1 Large Patty With Condiments On Bun From Fast Food / Restaurant ☞ serving size: 1 (1/3 lb) cheeseburger = 315 g; Calories = 689.9; Total Carb (g) = 39.7; Net Carb (g) = 37.5; Fat (g) = 41.8; Protein = 38

Cheeseburger 1 Medium Patty Plain On Wheat Bun ☞ serving size: 1 (1/4 lb) cheeseburger = 165 g; Calories = 462; Total Carb (g) = 28; Net Carb (g) = 24.8; Fat (g) = 23.7; Protein = 32.6

Cheeseburger 1 Medium Patty Plain On White Bun ☞ serving size: 1 (1/4 lb) cheeseburger = 165 g; Calories = 471.9; Total Carb (g) = 30.8; Net Carb (g) = 29.7; Fat (g) = 23.7; Protein = 31.7

Cheeseburger 1 Medium Patty Plain On Whole Wheat Bun ☞ serving size: 1 cheeseburger = 165 g; Calories = 462; Total Carb (g) = 28; Net Carb (g) = 24.8; Fat (g) = 23.7; Protein = 32.6

Cheeseburger 1 Medium Patty With Condiments On Wheat Bun ☞ serving size: 1 (1/4 lb) cheeseburger = 225 g; Calories = 513; Total Carb (g) = 32.2; Net Carb (g) = 28.4; Fat (g) = 27.5; Protein = 33.5

Cheeseburger 1 Medium Patty With Condiments On White Bun ☞ serving size: 1 (1/4 lb) cheeseburger = 225 g; Calories = 524.3; Total Carb (g) = 35.2; Net Carb (g) = 33.6; Fat (g) = 27.5; Protein = 32.5

Cheeseburger 1 Medium Patty With Condiments On Whole Wheat Bun ☞ serving size: 1 (1/4 lb) cheeseburger = 225 g; Calories = 513; Total Carb (g) = 32.2; Net Carb (g) = 28.4; Fat (g) = 27.5; Protein = 33.5

Cheeseburger 1 Miniature Patty On Miniature Bun From School ☞ serving size: 1 miniature = 60 g; Calories = 150; Total Carb (g) = 12.8; Net Carb (g) = 11.1; Fat (g) = 5.6; Protein = 11.8

Cheeseburger 1 Miniature Patty Plain On Miniature Bun From Fast Food / Restaurant ☞ serving size: 1 miniature = 60 g; Calories = 178.8; Total Carb (g) = 15; Net Carb (g) = 14.5; Fat (g) = 8.6; Protein = 9.7

Cheeseburger 1 Miniature Patty With Condiments On Miniature Bun From Fast Food / Restaurant ☞ serving size: 1 miniature = 75 g; Calories = 198; Total Carb (g) = 16.3; Net Carb (g) = 15.6; Fat (g) = 10.3; Protein = 9.7

🍔 Cheeseburger 1 Small Patty Plain On Wheat Bun ☞ serving size: 1 cheeseburger = 140 g; Calories = 394.8; Total Carb (g) = 24.9; Net Carb (g) = 22.1; Fat (g) = 20.2; Protein = 27.2

🍔 Cheeseburger 1 Small Patty Plain On White Bun ☞ serving size: 1 cheeseburger = 140 g; Calories = 403.2; Total Carb (g) = 27.4; Net Carb (g) = 26.4; Fat (g) = 20.2; Protein = 26.3

🍔 Cheeseburger 1 Small Patty With Condiments On Bun From Fast Food / Restaurant (Burger King Whopper Jr. With Cheese) ☞ serving size: 1 burger king whopper jr = 170 g; Calories = 382.5; Total Carb (g) = 30.8; Net Carb (g) = 29.3; Fat (g) = 20.2; Protein = 19

🍔 Cheeseburger 1 Small Patty With Condiments On Bun From Fast Food / Restaurant (Wendy's Jr. Cheeseburger Deluxe) ☞ serving size: 1 wendy's jr. cheeseburger deluxe = 160 g; Calories = 360; Total Carb (g) = 29; Net Carb (g) = 27.5; Fat (g) = 19; Protein = 17.9

🍔 Cheeseburger 1 Small Patty With Condiments On Wheat Bun ☞ serving size: 1 cheeseburger = 195 g; Calories = 434.9; Total Carb (g) = 28.3; Net Carb (g) = 25; Fat (g) = 23.3; Protein = 27.2

🍔 Cheeseburger 1 Small Patty With Condiments On White Bun ☞ serving size: 1 cheeseburger = 195 g; Calories = 442.7; Total Carb (g) = 30.8; Net Carb (g) = 29.3; Fat (g) = 23.3; Protein = 26.3

🍔 Cheeseburger 1 Small Patty With Condiments On Whole Wheat Bun ☞ serving size: 1 cheeseburger = 195 g; Calories = 434.9; Total Carb (g) = 28.3; Net Carb (g) = 25; Fat (g) = 23.3; Protein = 27.2

🍔 Cheeseburger Double Regular Patty And Bun With Condiments ☞ serving size: 1 sandwich = 155 g; Calories = 437.1; Total Carb (g) = 27.9; Net Carb (g) = 26.3; Fat (g) = 25.1; Protein = 25.2

🍔 Cheeseburger Nfs ☞ serving size: 1 cheeseburger = 225 g; Calories = 524.3; Total Carb (g) = 35.2; Net Carb (g) = 33.6; Fat (g) = 27.5; Protein = 32.5

🍔 Cheeseburger On Bun From School ☞ serving size: 1 cheeseburger = 115 g; Calories = 280.6; Total Carb (g) = 25.5; Net Carb (g) = 21.9; Fat (g) = 9.7; Protein = 22.2

Cheeseburger; Double Large Patty; With Condiments ☞ serving size: 1 item = 280 g; Calories = 761.6; Total Carb (g) = 40.4; Net Carb (g) = 37.6; Fat (g) = 45.4; Protein = 47.5

Cheeseburger; Double Regular Patty; Double Decker Bun With Condiments And Special Sauce ☞ serving size: 1 item = 219 g; Calories = 571.6; Total Carb (g) = 47.2; Net Carb (g) = 44.1; Fat (g) = 30.9; Protein = 26.2

Cheeseburger; Double Regular Patty; With Condiments ☞ serving size: 1 sandwich = 155 g; Calories = 437.1; Total Carb (g) = 27.9; Net Carb (g) = 26.5; Fat (g) = 25.1; Protein = 25.2

Cheeseburger; Single Large Patty; Plain ☞ serving size: 1 sandwich = 182 g; Calories = 564.2; Total Carb (g) = 43.8; Net Carb (g) = 40.7; Fat (g) = 29.1; Protein = 31.5

Cheeseburger; Single Large Patty; With Condiments ☞ serving size: 1 item = 199 g; Calories = 535.3; Total Carb (g) = 39.2; Net Carb (g) = 36.9; Fat (g) = 28.7; Protein = 30.3

Cheeseburger; Single Large Patty; With Condiments Vegetables And Mayonnaise ☞ serving size: 1 sandwich = 215 g; Calories = 576.2; Total Carb (g) = 38.1; Net Carb (g) = 35.8; Fat (g) = 34; Protein = 29.4

Cheeseburger; Single Regular Patty With Condiments ☞ serving size: 1 item = 127 g; Calories = 342.9; Total Carb (g) = 32.3; Net Carb (g) = 29.9; Fat (g) = 16.4; Protein = 17.1

Cheeseburger; Single Regular Patty With Condiments And Vegetables ☞ serving size: 1 sandwich = 115 g; Calories = 292.1; Total Carb (g) = 28.7; Net Carb (g) = 27.1; Fat (g) = 13.2; Protein = 15

Cheeseburger; Single Regular Patty; Plain ☞ serving size: 1

sandwich = 91 g; Calories = 280.3; Total Carb (g) = 25.5; Net Carb (g) = 23.7; Fat (g) = 13.4; Protein = 15

● Chick-Fil-A Chick-N-Strips ☞ serving size: 1 strip = 50 g; Calories = 114; Total Carb (g) = 5.2; Net Carb (g) = 4.8; Fat (g) = 5.6; Protein = 10.7

● Chick-Fil-A Chicken Sandwich ☞ serving size: 1 sandwich = 187 g; Calories = 465.6; Total Carb (g) = 39.1; Net Carb (g) = 36.5; Fat (g) = 20.9; Protein = 30.4

● Chick-Fil-A Hash Browns ☞ serving size: 1 piece = 5.5 g; Calories = 16.6; Total Carb (g) = 1.7; Net Carb (g) = 1.5; Fat (g) = 1; Protein = 0.2

● Chicken Barbecue Sandwich ☞ serving size: 1 sandwich = 239 g; Calories = 530.6; Total Carb (g) = 62.5; Net Carb (g) = 59.4; Fat (g) = 11.7; Protein = 41

● Chicken Breaded And Fried Boneless Pieces Plain ☞ serving size: 6 pieces = 96 g; Calories = 294.7; Total Carb (g) = 14.3; Net Carb (g) = 13.5; Fat (g) = 19.6; Protein = 15.3

● Chicken Fillet Breaded Fried Sandwich With Cheese Lettuce Tomato And Spread ☞ serving size: 1 sandwich = 241 g; Calories = 689.3; Total Carb (g) = 60.3; Net Carb (g) = 57.2; Fat (g) = 37.1; Protein = 28.1

● Chicken Fillet Broiled Sandwich On Oat Bran Bun With Lettuce Tomato Spread ☞ serving size: 1 burger king sandwich = 155 g; Calories = 311.6; Total Carb (g) = 26.2; Net Carb (g) = 23.8; Fat (g) = 10.9; Protein = 25.5

● Chicken Fillet Broiled Sandwich On Whole Wheat Roll With Lettuce Tomato And Spread ☞ serving size: 1 sandwich = 173 g; Calories = 352.9; Total Carb (g) = 34; Net Carb (g) = 28.8; Fat (g) = 12.1; Protein = 28

● Chicken Fillet Broiled Sandwich With Cheese On Whole Wheat Roll With Lettuce Tomato And Non-Mayonnaise Type

Spread ☞ serving size: 1 wendy's sandwich = 242 g; Calories = 479.2; Total Carb (g) = 47.1; Net Carb (g) = 40.6; Fat (g) = 15.6; Protein = 39

🥟 Chicken Fillet Sandwich Plain With Pickles ☞ serving size: 1 sandwich = 187 g; Calories = 467.5; Total Carb (g) = 39.1; Net Carb (g) = 36.5; Fat (g) = 20.9; Protein = 30.4

🥟 Chicken Patty Sandwich Miniature With Spread ☞ serving size: 1 miniature sandwich = 31 g; Calories = 93.6; Total Carb (g) = 9.3; Net Carb (g) = 8.9; Fat (g) = 4.3; Protein = 4.3

🥟 Chicken Patty Sandwich Or Biscuit ☞ serving size: 1 sandwich = 173 g; Calories = 532.8; Total Carb (g) = 65; Net Carb (g) = 62.8; Fat (g) = 21.3; Protein = 20.7

🥟 Chicken Patty Sandwich With Cheese On Wheat Bun With Lettuce Tomato And Spread ☞ serving size: 1 sandwich = 227 g; Calories = 576.6; Total Carb (g) = 55.8; Net Carb (g) = 48.7; Fat (g) = 28.8; Protein = 27

🥟 Chicken Salad Or Chicken Spread Sandwich ☞ serving size: 1 sandwich = 141 g; Calories = 324.3; Total Carb (g) = 28; Net Carb (g) = 26.2; Fat (g) = 15.2; Protein = 18.5

🥟 Chicken Sandwich With Cheese And Spread ☞ serving size: 1 sandwich = 136 g; Calories = 321; Total Carb (g) = 29; Net Carb (g) = 27.5; Fat (g) = 11.9; Protein = 23.9

🥟 Chicken Sandwich With Spread ☞ serving size: 1 sandwich = 112 g; Calories = 249.8; Total Carb (g) = 26.4; Net Carb (g) = 25; Fat (g) = 7; Protein = 19.9

🥟 Chicken Tenders ☞ serving size: 1 strip = 30 g; Calories = 81.3; Total Carb (g) = 5.2; Net Carb (g) = 4.8; Fat (g) = 4.2; Protein = 5.8

🥟 Chiliburger With Or Without Cheese On Bun ☞ serving size: 1 chiliburger = 160 g; Calories = 403.2; Total Carb (g) = 29.6; Net Carb (g) = 27.7; Fat (g) = 20.2; Protein = 24.9

🥟 Chinese Pancake ☞ serving size: 1 pancake = 28 g; Calories = 58;

Total Carb (g) = 12.7; Net Carb (g) = 12.5; Fat (g) = 0.1; Protein = 1.1

🍔 Coleslaw (Fast Food) ☞ serving size: 1 cup = 191 g; Calories = 292.2; Total Carb (g) = 28.4; Net Carb (g) = 24.8; Fat (g) = 18.9; Protein = 1.8

🍔 Corned Beef Sandwich ☞ serving size: 1 sandwich = 130 g; Calories = 267.8; Total Carb (g) = 25.8; Net Carb (g) = 24.1; Fat (g) = 9.5; Protein = 18.6

🍔 Crab Cake Sandwich On Bun ☞ serving size: 1 sandwich = 140 g; Calories = 327.6; Total Carb (g) = 30.2; Net Carb (g) = 29.1; Fat (g) = 14.6; Protein = 17.7

🍔 Crepe Chocolate Filled ☞ serving size: 1 crepe with filling, any size = 80 g; Calories = 124.8; Total Carb (g) = 16.7; Net Carb (g) = 16.1; Fat (g) = 4.4; Protein = 4.4

🍔 Crepe Fruit Filled ☞ serving size: 1 crepe with filling, any size = 80 g; Calories = 147.2; Total Carb (g) = 21.2; Net Carb (g) = 20.2; Fat (g) = 5.6; Protein = 3.6

🍔 Crepe Nfs ☞ serving size: 1 crepe, any size = 80 g; Calories = 178.4; Total Carb (g) = 17.4; Net Carb (g) = 16.9; Fat (g) = 8.8; Protein = 7

🍔 Crepe Ns As To Filling ☞ serving size: 1 crepe with filling, any size = 80 g; Calories = 147.2; Total Carb (g) = 21.2; Net Carb (g) = 20.2; Fat (g) = 5.6; Protein = 3.6

🍔 Crepe Plain ☞ serving size: 1 crepe, any size = 65 g; Calories = 145; Total Carb (g) = 14.1; Net Carb (g) = 13.7; Fat (g) = 7.1; Protein = 5.7

🍔 Crispy Chicken Bacon And Tomato Club Sandwich With Cheese Lettuce And Mayonnaise ☞ serving size: 1 sandwich = 271 g; Calories = 696.5; Total Carb (g) = 61.3; Net Carb (g) = 58; Fat (g) = 31.9; Protein = 41.7

🍔 Crispy Chicken In Tortilla With Lettuce Cheese And Ranch

Sauce ☞ serving size: 1 item = 133 g; Calories = 365.8; Total Carb (g) = 30.9; Net Carb (g) = 29.2; Fat (g) = 20.1; Protein = 15.3

🥐 Croissant Sandwich Filled With Broccoli And Cheese ☞ serving size: 1 croissant = 113 g; Calories = 302.8; Total Carb (g) = 29.4; Net Carb (g) = 28.1; Fat (g) = 17.2; Protein = 8

🥐 Croissant Sandwich Filled With Chicken Broccoli And Cheese Sauce ☞ serving size: 1 croissant = 128 g; Calories = 346.9; Total Carb (g) = 28.2; Net Carb (g) = 27.1; Fat (g) = 18.8; Protein = 15.7

🥐 Croissant Sandwich Filled With Ham And Cheese ☞ serving size: 1 croissant = 113 g; Calories = 337.9; Total Carb (g) = 25.5; Net Carb (g) = 24.7; Fat (g) = 19.6; Protein = 14.5

🥐 Croissant Sandwich With Bacon And Egg ☞ serving size: 1 croissant = 113 g; Calories = 371.8; Total Carb (g) = 25; Net Carb (g) = 23.6; Fat (g) = 23.1; Protein = 15.2

🥐 Croissant Sandwich With Bacon Egg And Cheese ☞ serving size: 1 croissant = 131 g; Calories = 408.7; Total Carb (g) = 27.2; Net Carb (g) = 25.9; Fat (g) = 26.2; Protein = 16.5

🥐 Croissant Sandwich With Sausage And Egg ☞ serving size: 1 croissant = 142 g; Calories = 497; Total Carb (g) = 30.7; Net Carb (g) = 29; Fat (g) = 34; Protein = 16.1

🥐 Croissant With Egg Cheese And Bacon ☞ serving size: 1 item = 128 g; Calories = 369.9; Total Carb (g) = 28.8; Net Carb (g) = 27.5; Fat (g) = 21; Protein = 16.5

🥐 Croissant With Egg Cheese And Ham ☞ serving size: 1 item = 155 g; Calories = 404.6; Total Carb (g) = 29.4; Net Carb (g) = 28; Fat (g) = 23.2; Protein = 19.3

🥐 Croissant With Egg Cheese And Sausage ☞ serving size: 1 sandwich = 171 g; Calories = 526.7; Total Carb (g) = 27.2; Net Carb (g) = 24.1; Fat (g) = 37.2; Protein = 20.7

🥐 Cuban Sandwich With Spread ☞ serving size: 1 sandwich (6"

long) = 255 g; Calories = 698.7; Total Carb (g) = 57.8; Net Carb (g) = 55.7; Fat (g) = 30.6; Protein = 45.4

● Digiorno Pizza Cheese Topping Cheese Stuffed Crust Frozen Baked ☞ serving size: 1 slice 1/4 of pie = 164 g; Calories = 457.6; Total Carb (g) = 49; Net Carb (g) = 45.9; Fat (g) = 19.2; Protein = 22.1

● Digiorno Pizza Cheese Topping Rising Crust Frozen Baked ☞ serving size: 1 slice 1/4 of pie = 183 g; Calories = 468.5; Total Carb (g) = 58.2; Net Carb (g) = 53.8; Fat (g) = 15.7; Protein = 23.4

● Digiorno Pizza Cheese Topping Thin Crispy Crust Frozen Baked ☞ serving size: 1 slice 1/4 of pie = 161 g; Calories = 397.7; Total Carb (g) = 42.6; Net Carb (g) = 37.8; Fat (g) = 16; Protein = 20.9

● Digiorno Pizza Pepperoni Topping Cheese Stuffed Crust Frozen Baked ☞ serving size: 1 slice 1/4 of pie = 179 g; Calories = 499.4; Total Carb (g) = 52.7; Net Carb (g) = 49; Fat (g) = 21; Protein = 24.9

● Digiorno Pizza Pepperoni Topping Rising Crust Frozen Baked ☞ serving size: 1 slice 1/4 of pie = 207 g; Calories = 548.6; Total Carb (g) = 64.5; Net Carb (g) = 59.7; Fat (g) = 20.9; Protein = 25.8

● Digiorno Pizza Pepperoni Topping Thin Crispy Crust Frozen Baked ☞ serving size: 1 slice 1/4 of pie = 145 g; Calories = 410.4; Total Carb (g) = 41.6; Net Carb (g) = 37.5; Fat (g) = 18.7; Protein = 19.2

● Digiorno Pizza Supreme Topping Rising Crust Frozen Baked ☞ serving size: 1 slice 1/4 of pie = 227 g; Calories = 578.9; Total Carb (g) = 63.4; Net Carb (g) = 58.2; Fat (g) = 24.2; Protein = 26.7

● Digiorno Pizza Supreme Topping Thin Crispy Crust Frozen Baked ☞ serving size: 1 slice 1/4 of pie = 155 g; Calories = 395.3; Total Carb (g) = 43.5; Net Carb (g) = 39.1; Fat (g) = 16.7; Protein = 17.7

● Dominos 14 Inch Cheese Pizza Classic Hand-Tossed Crust ☞ serving size: 1 slice = 108 g; Calories = 277.6; Total Carb (g) = 35.9; Net Carb (g) = 33.5; Fat (g) = 9.7; Protein = 11.7

● Dominos 14 Inch Cheese Pizza Crunchy Thin Crust ☞ serving

size: 1 slice = 70 g; Calories = 208.6; Total Carb (g) = 19.7; Net Carb (g) = 18; Fat (g) = 10.6; Protein = 8.6

Dominos 14 Inch Cheese Pizza Ultimate Deep Dish Crust ☞ serving size: 1 slice = 118 g; Calories = 312.7; Total Carb (g) = 39.5; Net Carb (g) = 36.7; Fat (g) = 11.6; Protein = 12.7

Dominos 14 Inch Extravaganzza Feast Pizza Classic Hand-Tossed Crust ☞ serving size: 1 slice = 151 g; Calories = 368.4; Total Carb (g) = 38.8; Net Carb (g) = 35.8; Fat (g) = 16.8; Protein = 15.6

Dominos 14 Inch Pepperoni Pizza Classic Hand-Tossed Crust ☞ serving size: 1 slice = 113 g; Calories = 308.5; Total Carb (g) = 36; Net Carb (g) = 33.6; Fat (g) = 12.6; Protein = 12.7

Dominos 14 Inch Pepperoni Pizza Crunchy Thin Crust ☞ serving size: 1 slice = 79 g; Calories = 259.1; Total Carb (g) = 20; Net Carb (g) = 18; Fat (g) = 15.1; Protein = 11

Dominos 14 Inch Pepperoni Pizza Ultimate Deep Dish Crust ☞ serving size: 1 slice = 123 g; Calories = 348.1; Total Carb (g) = 39.2; Net Carb (g) = 36.3; Fat (g) = 14.9; Protein = 14.2

Dominos 14 Inch Sausage Pizza Classic Hand-Tossed Crust ☞ serving size: 1 slice = 114 g; Calories = 311.2; Total Carb (g) = 36.3; Net Carb (g) = 33.6; Fat (g) = 12.8; Protein = 12.6

Dominos 14 Inch Sausage Pizza Crunchy Thin Crust ☞ serving size: 1 slice = 78 g; Calories = 248.8; Total Carb (g) = 19.7; Net Carb (g) = 17.7; Fat (g) = 14.5; Protein = 10

Dominos 14 Inch Sausage Pizza Ultimate Deep Dish Crust ☞ serving size: 1 slice = 129 g; Calories = 357.3; Total Carb (g) = 40.2; Net Carb (g) = 36.9; Fat (g) = 15.5; Protein = 14.2

Dosa (Indian) Plain ☞ serving size: 1 small = 35 g; Calories = 73.2; Total Carb (g) = 13; Net Carb (g) = 12.4; Fat (g) = 1.4; Protein = 2

Double Bacon Cheeseburger 2 Large Patties With Condiments On Bun From Fast Food / Restaurant ☞ serving size: 1 sandwich =

400 g; Calories = 1172; Total Carb (g) = 68; Net Carb (g) = 64.8; Fat (g) = 69.3; Protein = 69.2

🍔 Double Bacon Cheeseburger 2 Medium Patties Plain On Bun From Fast Food / Restaurant ☞ serving size: 1 double bacon cheeseburger = 275 g; Calories = 855.3; Total Carb (g) = 31.9; Net Carb (g) = 30.8; Fat (g) = 54.4; Protein = 56.2

🍔 Double Bacon Cheeseburger 2 Medium Patties With Condiments On Bun From Fast Food / Restaurant ☞ serving size: 1 double bacon cheeseburger = 335 g; Calories = 907.9; Total Carb (g) = 36.1; Net Carb (g) = 34.4; Fat (g) = 58.3; Protein = 57.2

🍔 Double Bacon Cheeseburger 2 Medium Patties With Condiments On Bun From Fast Food / Restaurant (Wendy's Baconator) ☞ serving size: 1 wendy's baconator = 335 g; Calories = 907.9; Total Carb (g) = 36.1; Net Carb (g) = 34.4; Fat (g) = 58.3; Protein = 57.2

🍔 Double Bacon Cheeseburger 2 Small Patties With Condiments On Bun From Fast Food / Restaurant (Burger King Bacon Double Cheeseburger) ☞ serving size: 1 burger king double bacon cheeseburger = 200 g; Calories = 510; Total Carb (g) = 27.5; Net Carb (g) = 26.1; Fat (g) = 30.5; Protein = 29.8

🍔 Double Cheeseburger 2 Medium Patties Plain On Bun From Fast Food / Restaurant ☞ serving size: 1 double cheeseburger = 235 g; Calories = 716.8; Total Carb (g) = 37.3; Net Carb (g) = 34.7; Fat (g) = 42.2; Protein = 45.2

🍔 Double Cheeseburger 2 Small Patties Plain On Bun From Fast Food / Restaurant ☞ serving size: 1 double cheeseburger = 155 g; Calories = 472.8; Total Carb (g) = 32.2; Net Carb (g) = 29.9; Fat (g) = 25.7; Protein = 28.2

🍔 Double Hamburger 2 Medium Patties Plain On Bun From Fast Food / Restaurant ☞ serving size: 1 double hamburger = 220 g; Calories = 638; Total Carb (g) = 30; Net Carb (g) = 28.9; Fat (g) = 37.2; Protein = 42.6

⬛ Double Hamburger 2 Small Patties Plain On Bun From Fast Food / Restaurant ☞ serving size: 1 double hamburger = 135 g; Calories = 388.8; Total Carb (g) = 26.6; Net Carb (g) = 25.6; Fat (g) = 19.9; Protein = 24

⬛ Double Hamburger 2 Small Patties With Condiments On Bun From Fast Food / Restaurant ☞ serving size: 1 double hamburger = 190 g; Calories = 427.5; Total Carb (g) = 30; Net Carb (g) = 28.5; Fat (g) = 23; Protein = 24

⬛ Egg And Cheese On Biscuit ☞ serving size: 1 sandwich = 140 g; Calories = 378; Total Carb (g) = 30.4; Net Carb (g) = 29.7; Fat (g) = 22.8; Protein = 12.6

⬛ Egg And Steak On Biscuit ☞ serving size: 1 sandwich = 179 g; Calories = 508.4; Total Carb (g) = 55.6; Net Carb (g) = 54.4; Fat (g) = 23; Protein = 19.4

⬛ Egg Cheese And Bacon On Bagel ☞ serving size: 1 sandwich = 246 g; Calories = 590.4; Total Carb (g) = 53.6; Net Carb (g) = 52.1; Fat (g) = 26.9; Protein = 31.9

⬛ Egg Cheese And Beef On English Muffin ☞ serving size: 1 great starts sandwich (5.2 oz) = 147 g; Calories = 402.8; Total Carb (g) = 26.2; Net Carb (g) = 24.1; Fat (g) = 23.6; Protein = 21.1

⬛ Egg Cheese And Ham On Bagel ☞ serving size: 1 mcdonald's sandwich = 218 g; Calories = 569; Total Carb (g) = 42.4; Net Carb (g) = 40.3; Fat (g) = 31.4; Protein = 28

⬛ Egg Cheese And Ham On Biscuit ☞ serving size: 1 sandwich = 174 g; Calories = 440.2; Total Carb (g) = 25.8; Net Carb (g) = 25.1; Fat (g) = 28.3; Protein = 21

⬛ Egg Cheese And Sausage On Bun ☞ serving size: 1 sandwich = 148 g; Calories = 401.1; Total Carb (g) = 25.7; Net Carb (g) = 24.8; Fat (g) = 23.7; Protein = 20.2

⬛ Egg Cheese Ham And Bacon On Bun ☞ serving size: 1 jack-in-the-box sandwich = 226 g; Calories = 589.9; Total Carb (g) = 40.5; Net Carb (g) = 38.7; Fat (g) = 31.5; Protein = 33.9

🍔 Egg Extra Cheese And Extra Sausage On Bun ☞ serving size: 1 jack-in-the-box sandwich = 213 g; Calories = 583.6; Total Carb (g) = 29.9; Net Carb (g) = 29.1; Fat (g) = 37.7; Protein = 30.5

🍔 Egg Salad Sandwich ☞ serving size: 1 sandwich = 159 g; Calories = 470.6; Total Carb (g) = 27.9; Net Carb (g) = 26.5; Fat (g) = 33; Protein = 14.3

🍔 Egg Scrambled ☞ serving size: 2 eggs = 96 g; Calories = 203.5; Total Carb (g) = 2; Net Carb (g) = 2; Fat (g) = 15.5; Protein = 13.3

🍔 English Muffin With Cheese And Sausage ☞ serving size: 1 item = 108 g; Calories = 365; Total Carb (g) = 27.3; Net Carb (g) = 26.8; Fat (g) = 22.3; Protein = 14.3

🍔 English Muffin With Egg Cheese And Canadian Bacon ☞ serving size: 1 sandwich = 126 g; Calories = 287.3; Total Carb (g) = 27.3; Net Carb (g) = 26.8; Fat (g) = 12.2; Protein = 17.2

🍔 English Muffin With Egg Cheese And Sausage ☞ serving size: 1 item = 165 g; Calories = 471.9; Total Carb (g) = 28.8; Net Carb (g) = 28.5; Fat (g) = 29.9; Protein = 22.1

🍔 Fajita-Style Beef Sandwich With Cheese On Pita Bread With Lettuce And Tomato ☞ serving size: 1 pita sandwich = 175 g; Calories = 280; Total Carb (g) = 26.9; Net Carb (g) = 24.8; Fat (g) = 12.1; Protein = 15.9

🍔 Fajita-Style Chicken Sandwich With Cheese On Pita Bread With Lettuce And Tomato ☞ serving size: 1 pita sandwich = 207 g; Calories = 322.9; Total Carb (g) = 31.6; Net Carb (g) = 29.1; Fat (g) = 11.9; Protein = 21.8

🍔 Fast Food Biscuit ☞ serving size: 1 biscuit = 55 g; Calories = 203.5; Total Carb (g) = 23.6; Net Carb (g) = 22.2; Fat (g) = 10.4; Protein = 3.9

🍔 Fast Food Pizza Chain 14 Inch Pizza Cheese Topping Stuffed

Crust ☞ serving size: 1 slice 1/8 pizza = 117 g; Calories = 320.6; Total Carb (g) = 35.1; Net Carb (g) = 33.1; Fat (g) = 13.6; Protein = 14.3

Fast Food Pizza Chain 14 Inch Pizza Cheese Topping Thick Crust ☞ serving size: 1 slice = 115 g; Calories = 311.7; Total Carb (g) = 38.2; Net Carb (g) = 35.6; Fat (g) = 12.1; Protein = 12.4

Fast Food Pizza Chain 14 Inch Pizza Cheese Topping Thin Crust ☞ serving size: 1 slice = 76 g; Calories = 229.5; Total Carb (g) = 23.7; Net Carb (g) = 21.8; Fat (g) = 10.6; Protein = 9.8

Fast Food Pizza Chain 14 Inch Pizza Meat And Vegetable Topping Regular Crust ☞ serving size: 1 slice = 136 g; Calories = 331.8; Total Carb (g) = 34.5; Net Carb (g) = 31.5; Fat (g) = 14.8; Protein = 15

Fast Food Pizza Chain 14 Inch Pizza Pepperoni Topping Thick Crust ☞ serving size: 1 slice = 118 g; Calories = 338.7; Total Carb (g) = 37.6; Net Carb (g) = 35; Fat (g) = 14.8; Protein = 13.6

Fast Food Pizza Chain 14 Inch Pizza Pepperoni Topping Thin Crust ☞ serving size: 1 slice = 79 g; Calories = 261.5; Total Carb (g) = 22.9; Net Carb (g) = 21.1; Fat (g) = 13.9; Protein = 11.1

Fast Food Pizza Chain 14 Inch Pizza Sausage Topping Thick Crust ☞ serving size: 1 slice = 127 g; Calories = 358.1; Total Carb (g) = 38.6; Net Carb (g) = 35.6; Fat (g) = 16.4; Protein = 14.1

Fast Food Pizza Chain 14 Inch Pizza Sausage Topping Thin Crust ☞ serving size: 1 slice = 88 g; Calories = 282.5; Total Carb (g) = 23.8; Net Carb (g) = 21.6; Fat (g) = 15.6; Protein = 11.8

Fast Foods Biscuit With Egg And Sausage ☞ serving size: 1 item = 162 g; Calories = 505.4; Total Carb (g) = 34.1; Net Carb (g) = 33.8; Fat (g) = 33.7; Protein = 18

Fast Foods Cheeseburger; Double Large Patty; With Condiments Vegetables And Mayonnaise ☞ serving size: 1 item = 355 g;

Calories = 898.2; Total Carb (g) = 44.8; Net Carb (g) = 40.2; Fat (g) = 55.5; Protein = 55

🍔 Fast Foods Crispy Chicken Filet Sandwich With Lettuce And Mayonnaise ☞ serving size: 1 sandwich = 152 g; Calories = 419.5; Total Carb (g) = 41.7; Net Carb (g) = 39.5; Fat (g) = 20.7; Protein = 16.6

🍔 Fast Foods Fried Chicken Breast Meat And Skin And Breading ☞ serving size: 1 breast, with skin = 203 g; Calories = 466.9; Total Carb (g) = 12.2; Net Carb (g) = 12; Fat (g) = 25.3; Protein = 47.7

🍔 Fast Foods Fried Chicken Breast Meat Only Skin And Breading Removed ☞ serving size: 1 breast without skin = 142 g; Calories = 217.3; Total Carb (g) = 0; Net Carb (g) = 0; Fat (g) = 6.5; Protein = 39.7

🍔 Fast Foods Fried Chicken Drumstick Meat And Skin With Breading ☞ serving size: 1 drumstick, with skin = 75 g; Calories = 200.3; Total Carb (g) = 5.7; Net Carb (g) = 5.3; Fat (g) = 12.7; Protein = 15.9

🍔 Fast Foods Fried Chicken Drumstick Meat Only Skin And Breading Removed ☞ serving size: 1 drumstick, bone and skin removed = 40 g; Calories = 68.8; Total Carb (g) = 0; Net Carb (g) = 0; Fat (g) = 3; Protein = 10.5

🍔 Fast Foods Fried Chicken Thigh Meat And Skin And Breading ☞ serving size: 1 thigh with skin = 136 g; Calories = 372.6; Total Carb (g) = 11.8; Net Carb (g) = 11.7; Fat (g) = 24.6; Protein = 26.2

🍔 Fast Foods Fried Chicken Thigh Meat Only Skin And Breading Removed ☞ serving size: 1 thigh without skin = 84 g; Calories = 149.5; Total Carb (g) = 0.2; Net Carb (g) = 0.2; Fat (g) = 7.9; Protein = 19.5

🍔 Fast Foods Fried Chicken Wing Meat And Skin And Breading ☞ serving size: 1 wing, with skin = 58 g; Calories = 179.8; Total Carb (g) = 6.5; Net Carb (g) = 6.4; Fat (g) = 11.7; Protein = 12.3

🍔 Fast Foods Fried Chicken Wing Meat Only Skin And Breading

Removed ☞ serving size: 1 wing without skin = 37 g; Calories = 79.6; Total Carb (g) = 0.8; Net Carb (g) = 0.8; Fat (g) = 3.8; Protein = 10.6

🍪 Fast Foods Grilled Chicken Filet Sandwich With Lettuce Tomato And Spread ☞ serving size: 1 sandwich = 230 g; Calories = 418.6; Total Carb (g) = 38.6; Net Carb (g) = 36.5; Fat (g) = 10.5; Protein = 39.9

🍪 Fish Sandwich With Tartar Sauce ☞ serving size: 1 sandwich = 220 g; Calories = 565.4; Total Carb (g) = 58.7; Net Carb (g) = 56.5; Fat (g) = 27.4; Protein = 22.6

🍪 Fish Sandwich With Tartar Sauce And Cheese ☞ serving size: 1 sandwich = 134 g; Calories = 373.9; Total Carb (g) = 35.4; Net Carb (g) = 34.3; Fat (g) = 19.6; Protein = 15.1

🍪 Frankfurter Or Hot Dog Sandwich Beef And Pork Plain On Multigrain Bread ☞ serving size: 1 frankfurter on bread = 93 g; Calories = 266.9; Total Carb (g) = 19.4; Net Carb (g) = 16.7; Fat (g) = 16.1; Protein = 10.9

🍪 Frankfurter Or Hot Dog Sandwich Beef And Pork Plain On Multigrain Bun ☞ serving size: 1 frankfurter on bun = 102 g; Calories = 290.7; Total Carb (g) = 24.1; Net Carb (g) = 22.3; Fat (g) = 17.4; Protein = 10.4

🍪 Frankfurter Or Hot Dog Sandwich Beef And Pork Plain On Wheat Bread ☞ serving size: 1 frankfurter on bread = 85 g; Calories = 247.4; Total Carb (g) = 17; Net Carb (g) = 15.8; Fat (g) = 15.8; Protein = 9

🍪 Frankfurter Or Hot Dog Sandwich Beef And Pork Plain On Wheat Bun ☞ serving size: 1 frankfurter on bun = 102 g; Calories = 293.8; Total Carb (g) = 25.4; Net Carb (g) = 23.4; Fat (g) = 16.2; Protein = 11.4

🍪 Frankfurter Or Hot Dog Sandwich Beef And Pork Plain On White Bread ☞ serving size: 1 frankfurter on bread = 85 g; Calories

= 244.8; Total Carb (g) = 17.6; Net Carb (g) = 16.8; Fat (g) = 15.5; Protein = 8.4

🍔 Frankfurter Or Hot Dog Sandwich Beef And Pork Plain On White Bun ☞ serving size: 1 frankfurter on bun = 102 g; Calories = 298.9; Total Carb (g) = 26.8; Net Carb (g) = 25.9; Fat (g) = 16.4; Protein = 10.5

🍔 Frankfurter Or Hot Dog Sandwich Beef And Pork Plain On Whole Grain White Bread ☞ serving size: 1 frankfurter on bread = 93 g; Calories = 256.7; Total Carb (g) = 19.7; Net Carb (g) = 16.2; Fat (g) = 15.3; Protein = 9.9

🍔 Frankfurter Or Hot Dog Sandwich Beef And Pork Plain On Whole Grain White Bun ☞ serving size: 1 frankfurter on bun = 102 g; Calories = 286.6; Total Carb (g) = 25; Net Carb (g) = 23.9; Fat (g) = 16.2; Protein = 10.2

🍔 Frankfurter Or Hot Dog Sandwich Beef And Pork Plain On Whole Wheat Bread ☞ serving size: 1 frankfurter on bread = 93 g; Calories = 261.3; Total Carb (g) = 19.2; Net Carb (g) = 17; Fat (g) = 15.8; Protein = 10.6

🍔 Frankfurter Or Hot Dog Sandwich Beef And Pork Plain On Whole Wheat Bun ☞ serving size: 1 frankfurter on bun = 102 g; Calories = 293.8; Total Carb (g) = 24.3; Net Carb (g) = 21.4; Fat (g) = 16.6; Protein = 11.7

🍔 Frankfurter Or Hot Dog Sandwich Beef Plain On Multigrain Bread ☞ serving size: 1 frankfurter on bread = 93 g; Calories = 284.6; Total Carb (g) = 17.4; Net Carb (g) = 14.7; Fat (g) = 18.4; Protein = 11.8

🍔 Frankfurter Or Hot Dog Sandwich Beef Plain On Multigrain Bun ☞ serving size: 1 frankfurter on bun = 102 g; Calories = 307; Total Carb (g) = 21.9; Net Carb (g) = 20.1; Fat (g) = 19.6; Protein = 11.3

🍔 Frankfurter Or Hot Dog Sandwich Beef Plain On Wheat Bread ☞ serving size: 1 frankfurter on bread = 85 g; Calories = 266.1; Total Carb (g) = 15.1; Net Carb (g) = 14; Fat (g) = 18.1; Protein = 10

Frankfurter Or Hot Dog Sandwich Beef Plain On Wheat Bun ☞ serving size: 1 frankfurter on bun = 102 g; Calories = 310.1; Total Carb (g) = 23.1; Net Carb (g) = 21.1; Fat (g) = 18.5; Protein = 12.3

Frankfurter Or Hot Dog Sandwich Beef Plain On White Bread ☞ serving size: 1 frankfurter on bread = 85 g; Calories = 263.5; Total Carb (g) = 15.6; Net Carb (g) = 14.9; Fat (g) = 17.8; Protein = 9.5

Frankfurter Or Hot Dog Sandwich Beef Plain On White Bun ☞ serving size: 1 frankfurter on bun = 102 g; Calories = 314.2; Total Carb (g) = 24.3; Net Carb (g) = 23.5; Fat (g) = 18.6; Protein = 11.4

Frankfurter Or Hot Dog Sandwich Beef Plain On Whole Grain White Bread ☞ serving size: 1 frankfurter on bread = 93 g; Calories = 274.4; Total Carb (g) = 17.6; Net Carb (g) = 14.2; Fat (g) = 17.6; Protein = 10.9

Frankfurter Or Hot Dog Sandwich Beef Plain On Whole Grain White Bun ☞ serving size: 1 frankfurter on bun = 102 g; Calories = 304; Total Carb (g) = 22.7; Net Carb (g) = 21.7; Fat (g) = 18.4; Protein = 11.2

Frankfurter Or Hot Dog Sandwich Beef Plain On Whole Wheat Bread ☞ serving size: 1 frankfurter on bread = 93 g; Calories = 279.9; Total Carb (g) = 17.2; Net Carb (g) = 15; Fat (g) = 18.1; Protein = 11.5

Frankfurter Or Hot Dog Sandwich Beef Plain On Whole Wheat Bun ☞ serving size: 1 frankfurter on bun = 102 g; Calories = 310.1; Total Carb (g) = 22; Net Carb (g) = 19.3; Fat (g) = 18.8; Protein = 12.6

Frankfurter Or Hot Dog Sandwich Chicken And/or Turkey Plain On Multigrain Bread ☞ serving size: 1 frankfurter on bread = 93 g; Calories = 228.8; Total Carb (g) = 17.2; Net Carb (g) = 14.6; Fat (g) = 11.2; Protein = 14.1

Frankfurter Or Hot Dog Sandwich Chicken And/or Turkey Plain On Multigrain Bun ☞ serving size: 1 frankfurter on bun = 102 g; Calories = 251.9; Total Carb (g) = 21.7; Net Carb (g) = 20; Fat (g) = 12.4; Protein = 13.6

Frankfurter Or Hot Dog Sandwich Chicken And/or Turkey Plain On Wheat Bread ☞ serving size: 1 frankfurter on bread = 85 g; Calories = 210.8; Total Carb (g) = 15; Net Carb (g) = 13.9; Fat (g) = 11; Protein = 12.3

Frankfurter Or Hot Dog Sandwich Chicken And/or Turkey Plain On Wheat Bun ☞ serving size: 1 frankfurter on bun = 102 g; Calories = 255; Total Carb (g) = 22.9; Net Carb (g) = 21; Fat (g) = 11.3; Protein = 14.6

Frankfurter Or Hot Dog Sandwich Chicken And/or Turkey Plain On White Bread ☞ serving size: 1 frankfurter on bread = 85 g; Calories = 208.3; Total Carb (g) = 15.5; Net Carb (g) = 14.7; Fat (g) = 10.6; Protein = 11.8

Frankfurter Or Hot Dog Sandwich Chicken And/or Turkey Plain On White Bun ☞ serving size: 1 frankfurter on bun = 102 g; Calories = 259.1; Total Carb (g) = 24.2; Net Carb (g) = 23.4; Fat (g) = 11.5; Protein = 13.7

Frankfurter Or Hot Dog Sandwich Chicken And/or Turkey Plain On Whole Grain White Bread ☞ serving size: 1 frankfurter on bread = 93 g; Calories = 219.5; Total Carb (g) = 17.5; Net Carb (g) = 14.1; Fat (g) = 10.5; Protein = 13.1

Frankfurter Or Hot Dog Sandwich Chicken And/or Turkey Plain On Whole Grain White Bun ☞ serving size: 1 frankfurter on bun = 102 g; Calories = 248.9; Total Carb (g) = 22.6; Net Carb (g) = 21.6; Fat (g) = 11.3; Protein = 13.5

Frankfurter Or Hot Dog Sandwich Chicken And/or Turkey Plain On Whole Wheat Bread ☞ serving size: 1 frankfurter on bread = 93 g; Calories = 224.1; Total Carb (g) = 17; Net Carb (g) = 14.9; Fat (g) = 11; Protein = 13.8

Frankfurter Or Hot Dog Sandwich Chicken And/or Turkey Plain On Whole Wheat Bun ☞ serving size: 1 frankfurter on bun =

102 g; Calories = 255; Total Carb (g) = 21.9; Net Carb (g) = 19.1; Fat (g) = 11.7; Protein = 14.9

🍔 Frankfurter Or Hot Dog Sandwich Fat Free Plain On Multigrain Bread ☞ serving size: 1 frankfurter on bread = 93 g; Calories = 160.9; Total Carb (g) = 22.3; Net Carb (g) = 19.6; Fat (g) = 2.5; Protein = 12.3

🍔 Frankfurter Or Hot Dog Sandwich Fat Free Plain On Multigrain Bun ☞ serving size: 1 frankfurter on bun = 102 g; Calories = 183.6; Total Carb (g) = 26.8; Net Carb (g) = 25.1; Fat (g) = 3.7; Protein = 11.8

🍔 Frankfurter Or Hot Dog Sandwich Fat Free Plain On Wheat Bread ☞ serving size: 1 frankfurter on bread = 85 g; Calories = 142; Total Carb (g) = 20; Net Carb (g) = 18.9; Fat (g) = 2.2; Protein = 10.5

🍔 Frankfurter Or Hot Dog Sandwich Fat Free Plain On Wheat Bun ☞ serving size: 1 frankfurter on bun = 102 g; Calories = 186.7; Total Carb (g) = 28; Net Carb (g) = 26.1; Fat (g) = 2.6; Protein = 12.8

🍔 Frankfurter Or Hot Dog Sandwich Fat Free Plain On White Bread ☞ serving size: 1 frankfurter on bread = 85 g; Calories = 140.3; Total Carb (g) = 20.6; Net Carb (g) = 19.8; Fat (g) = 1.9; Protein = 10

🍔 Frankfurter Or Hot Dog Sandwich Fat Free Plain On White Bun ☞ serving size: 1 frankfurter on bun = 102 g; Calories = 190.7; Total Carb (g) = 29.3; Net Carb (g) = 28.5; Fat (g) = 2.7; Protein = 11.9

🍔 Frankfurter Or Hot Dog Sandwich Fat Free Plain On Whole Grain White Bread ☞ serving size: 1 frankfurter on bread = 93 g; Calories = 150.7; Total Carb (g) = 22.5; Net Carb (g) = 19.2; Fat (g) = 1.7; Protein = 11.3

🍔 Frankfurter Or Hot Dog Sandwich Fat Free Plain On Whole Grain White Bun ☞ serving size: 1 frankfurter on bun = 102 g; Calories = 180.5; Total Carb (g) = 27.7; Net Carb (g) = 26.6; Fat (g) = 2.5; Protein = 11.7

🍔 Frankfurter Or Hot Dog Sandwich Fat Free Plain On Whole Wheat Bread ☞ serving size: 1 frankfurter on bread = 93 g; Calories

= 156.2; Total Carb (g) = 22.1; Net Carb (g) = 20; Fat (g) = 2.2; Protein = 12

🍪 Frankfurter Or Hot Dog Sandwich Fat Free Plain On Whole Wheat Bun ☞ serving size: 1 frankfurter on bun = 102 g; Calories = 186.7; Total Carb (g) = 27; Net Carb (g) = 24.2; Fat (g) = 2.9; Protein = 13.1

🍪 Frankfurter Or Hot Dog Sandwich Meat And Poultry Plain On Multigrain Bread ☞ serving size: 1 frankfurter on bread = 93 g; Calories = 261.3; Total Carb (g) = 18.6; Net Carb (g) = 15.9; Fat (g) = 16; Protein = 10.6

🍪 Frankfurter Or Hot Dog Sandwich Meat And Poultry Plain On Multigrain Bun ☞ serving size: 1 frankfurter on bun = 102 g; Calories = 284.6; Total Carb (g) = 23.1; Net Carb (g) = 21.4; Fat (g) = 17.2; Protein = 10.2

🍪 Frankfurter Or Hot Dog Sandwich Meat And Poultry Plain On Wheat Bread ☞ serving size: 1 frankfurter on bread = 85 g; Calories = 243.1; Total Carb (g) = 16.3; Net Carb (g) = 15.2; Fat (g) = 15.8; Protein = 8.8

🍪 Frankfurter Or Hot Dog Sandwich Meat And Poultry Plain On Wheat Bun ☞ serving size: 1 frankfurter on bun = 102 g; Calories = 287.6; Total Carb (g) = 24.3; Net Carb (g) = 22.4; Fat (g) = 16.1; Protein = 11.1

🍪 Frankfurter Or Hot Dog Sandwich Meat And Poultry Plain On White Bread ☞ serving size: 1 frankfurter on bread = 85 g; Calories = 240.6; Total Carb (g) = 16.9; Net Carb (g) = 16.1; Fat (g) = 15.4; Protein = 8.3

🍪 Frankfurter Or Hot Dog Sandwich Meat And Poultry Plain On White Bun ☞ serving size: 1 frankfurter on bun = 102 g; Calories = 291.7; Total Carb (g) = 25.6; Net Carb (g) = 24.8; Fat (g) = 16.3; Protein = 10.2

🍪 Frankfurter Or Hot Dog Sandwich Meat And Poultry Plain On

Whole Grain White Bread ☞ serving size: 1 frankfurter on bread = 93 g; Calories = 252; Total Carb (g) = 18.8; Net Carb (g) = 15.5; Fat (g) = 15.3; Protein = 9.7

🥫 Frankfurter Or Hot Dog Sandwich Meat And Poultry Plain On Whole Grain White Bun ☞ serving size: 1 frankfurter on bun = 102 g; Calories = 280.5; Total Carb (g) = 23.9; Net Carb (g) = 22.9; Fat (g) = 16.1; Protein = 10

🥫 Frankfurter Or Hot Dog Sandwich Meat And Poultry Plain On Whole Wheat Bread ☞ serving size: 1 frankfurter on bread = 93 g; Calories = 256.7; Total Carb (g) = 18.4; Net Carb (g) = 16.3; Fat (g) = 15.8; Protein = 10.3

🥫 Frankfurter Or Hot Dog Sandwich Meat And Poultry Plain On Whole Wheat Bun ☞ serving size: 1 frankfurter on bun = 102 g; Calories = 287.6; Total Carb (g) = 23.2; Net Carb (g) = 20.5; Fat (g) = 16.5; Protein = 11.4

🥫 Frankfurter Or Hot Dog Sandwich Meatless On Bread With Meatless Chili ☞ serving size: 1 frankfurter on bread = 162 g; Calories = 302.9; Total Carb (g) = 27.7; Net Carb (g) = 22; Fat (g) = 12.9; Protein = 20.1

🥫 Frankfurter Or Hot Dog Sandwich Meatless On Bun With Meatless Chili ☞ serving size: 1 frankfurter on bun = 179 g; Calories = 354.4; Total Carb (g) = 36.4; Net Carb (g) = 30.7; Fat (g) = 13.8; Protein = 22

🥫 Frankfurter Or Hot Dog Sandwich Meatless Plain On Bread ☞ serving size: 1 frankfurter on bread = 98 g; Calories = 237.2; Total Carb (g) = 19.2; Net Carb (g) = 15.7; Fat (g) = 10.5; Protein = 16.2

🥫 Frankfurter Or Hot Dog Sandwich Meatless Plain On Bun ☞ serving size: 1 frankfurter on bun = 115 g; Calories = 288.7; Total Carb (g) = 28; Net Carb (g) = 24.4; Fat (g) = 11.4; Protein = 18.1

🥫 Frankfurter Or Hot Dog Sandwich NFS Plain On Multigrain

Bread ☞ serving size: 1 frankfurter on bread = 93 g; Calories = 284.6; Total Carb (g) = 17.4; Net Carb (g) = 14.7; Fat (g) = 18.4; Protein = 11.8

🍴 Frankfurter Or Hot Dog Sandwich NFS Plain On Multigrain Bun ☞ serving size: 1 frankfurter on bun = 102 g; Calories = 307; Total Carb (g) = 21.9; Net Carb (g) = 20.1; Fat (g) = 19.6; Protein = 11.3

🍴 Frankfurter Or Hot Dog Sandwich NFS Plain On Wheat Bread ☞ serving size: 1 frankfurter on bread = 85 g; Calories = 266.1; Total Carb (g) = 15.1; Net Carb (g) = 14; Fat (g) = 18.1; Protein = 10

🍴 Frankfurter Or Hot Dog Sandwich NFS Plain On Wheat Bun ☞ serving size: 1 frankfurter on bun = 102 g; Calories = 310.1; Total Carb (g) = 23.1; Net Carb (g) = 21.1; Fat (g) = 18.5; Protein = 12.3

🍴 Frankfurter Or Hot Dog Sandwich NFS Plain On White Bread ☞ serving size: 1 frankfurter on bread = 85 g; Calories = 263.5; Total Carb (g) = 15.6; Net Carb (g) = 14.9; Fat (g) = 17.8; Protein = 9.5

🍴 Frankfurter Or Hot Dog Sandwich NFS Plain On White Bun ☞ serving size: 1 frankfurter on bun = 102 g; Calories = 314.2; Total Carb (g) = 24.3; Net Carb (g) = 23.5; Fat (g) = 18.6; Protein = 11.4

🍴 Frankfurter Or Hot Dog Sandwich NFS Plain On Whole Grain White Bread ☞ serving size: 1 frankfurter on bread = 93 g; Calories = 274.4; Total Carb (g) = 17.6; Net Carb (g) = 14.2; Fat (g) = 17.6; Protein = 10.9

🍴 Frankfurter Or Hot Dog Sandwich NFS Plain On Whole Grain White Bun ☞ serving size: 1 frankfurter on bun = 102 g; Calories = 304; Total Carb (g) = 22.7; Net Carb (g) = 21.7; Fat (g) = 18.4; Protein = 11.2

🍴 Frankfurter Or Hot Dog Sandwich NFS Plain On Whole Wheat Bread ☞ serving size: 1 frankfurter on bread = 93 g; Calories = 279.9; Total Carb (g) = 17.2; Net Carb (g) = 15; Fat (g) = 18.1; Protein = 11.5

🍴 Frankfurter Or Hot Dog Sandwich NFS Plain On Whole Wheat

Bun ☞ serving size: 1 frankfurter on bun = 102 g; Calories = 310.1; Total Carb (g) = 22; Net Carb (g) = 19.3; Fat (g) = 18.8; Protein = 12.6

Frankfurter Or Hot Dog Sandwich Reduced Fat Or Light Plain On Multigrain Bread ☞ serving size: 1 frankfurter on bread = 93 g; Calories = 168.3; Total Carb (g) = 20.7; Net Carb (g) = 18; Fat (g) = 3.2; Protein = 14.1

Frankfurter Or Hot Dog Sandwich Reduced Fat Or Light Plain On Multigrain Bun ☞ serving size: 1 frankfurter on bun = 102 g; Calories = 190.7; Total Carb (g) = 25.1; Net Carb (g) = 23.4; Fat (g) = 4.4; Protein = 13.6

Frankfurter Or Hot Dog Sandwich Reduced Fat Or Light Plain On Wheat Bread ☞ serving size: 1 frankfurter on bread = 85 g; Calories = 149.6; Total Carb (g) = 18.4; Net Carb (g) = 17.2; Fat (g) = 3; Protein = 12.3

Frankfurter Or Hot Dog Sandwich Reduced Fat Or Light Plain On Wheat Bun ☞ serving size: 1 frankfurter on bun = 102 g; Calories = 193.8; Total Carb (g) = 26.3; Net Carb (g) = 24.4; Fat (g) = 3.3; Protein = 14.6

Frankfurter Or Hot Dog Sandwich Reduced Fat Or Light Plain On White Bread ☞ serving size: 1 frankfurter on bread = 85 g; Calories = 147.1; Total Carb (g) = 18.9; Net Carb (g) = 18; Fat (g) = 2.6; Protein = 11.8

Frankfurter Or Hot Dog Sandwich Reduced Fat Or Light Plain On White Bun ☞ serving size: 1 frankfurter on bun = 102 g; Calories = 197.9; Total Carb (g) = 27.6; Net Carb (g) = 26.7; Fat (g) = 3.4; Protein = 13.7

Frankfurter Or Hot Dog Sandwich Reduced Fat Or Light Plain On Whole Grain White Bread ☞ serving size: 1 frankfurter on bread = 93 g; Calories = 158.1; Total Carb (g) = 20.9; Net Carb (g) = 17.5; Fat (g) = 2.5; Protein = 13.1

Frankfurter Or Hot Dog Sandwich Reduced Fat Or Light Plain

On Whole Grain White Bun ☞ serving size: 1 frankfurter on bun = 102 g; Calories = 187.7; Total Carb (g) = 26; Net Carb (g) = 24.9; Fat (g) = 3.3; Protein = 13.5

🍲 Frankfurter Or Hot Dog Sandwich Reduced Fat Or Light Plain On Whole Wheat Bread ☞ serving size: 1 frankfurter on bread = 93 g; Calories = 163.7; Total Carb (g) = 20.4; Net Carb (g) = 18.2; Fat (g) = 2.9; Protein = 13.8

🍲 Frankfurter Or Hot Dog Sandwich Reduced Fat Or Light Plain On Whole Wheat Bun ☞ serving size: 1 frankfurter on bun = 102 g; Calories = 193.8; Total Carb (g) = 25.3; Net Carb (g) = 22.4; Fat (g) = 3.7; Protein = 14.9

🍲 Frankfurter Or Hot Dog Sandwich With Chili On Multigrain Bread ☞ serving size: 1 frankfurter on bread = 157 g; Calories = 353.3; Total Carb (g) = 25.8; Net Carb (g) = 21.1; Fat (g) = 20.6; Protein = 15.5

🍲 Frankfurter Or Hot Dog Sandwich With Chili On Multigrain Bun ☞ serving size: 1 frankfurter on bun = 166 g; Calories = 375.2; Total Carb (g) = 30.2; Net Carb (g) = 26.4; Fat (g) = 21.8; Protein = 15

🍲 Frankfurter Or Hot Dog Sandwich With Chili On Wheat Bread ☞ serving size: 1 frankfurter on bread = 149 g; Calories = 333.8; Total Carb (g) = 23.5; Net Carb (g) = 20.2; Fat (g) = 20.4; Protein = 13.7

🍲 Frankfurter Or Hot Dog Sandwich With Chili On Wheat Bun ☞ serving size: 1 frankfurter on bun = 166 g; Calories = 378.5; Total Carb (g) = 31.5; Net Carb (g) = 27.5; Fat (g) = 20.7; Protein = 16

🍲 Frankfurter Or Hot Dog Sandwich With Chili On White Bread ☞ serving size: 1 frankfurter on bread = 149 g; Calories = 332.3; Total Carb (g) = 24; Net Carb (g) = 21.2; Fat (g) = 20; Protein = 13.2

🍲 Frankfurter Or Hot Dog Sandwich With Chili On White Bun ☞ serving size: 1 frankfurter on bun = 166 g; Calories = 383.5; Total Carb (g) = 32.7; Net Carb (g) = 29.7; Fat (g) = 20.8; Protein = 15.1

🍲 Frankfurter Or Hot Dog Sandwich With Chili On Whole Grain

White Bread ☞ serving size: 1 frankfurter on bread = 157 g; Calories = 343.8; Total Carb (g) = 26; Net Carb (g) = 20.5; Fat (g) = 19.9; Protein = 14.6

🍔 Frankfurter Or Hot Dog Sandwich With Chili On Whole Grain White Bun ☞ serving size: 1 frankfurter on bun = 166 g; Calories = 371.8; Total Carb (g) = 31.1; Net Carb (g) = 27.9; Fat (g) = 20.7; Protein = 14.9

🍔 Frankfurter Or Hot Dog Sandwich With Chili On Whole Wheat Bread ☞ serving size: 1 frankfurter on bread = 157 g; Calories = 348.5; Total Carb (g) = 25.5; Net Carb (g) = 21.3; Fat (g) = 20.4; Protein = 15.2

🍔 Frankfurter Or Hot Dog Sandwich With Chili On Whole Wheat Bun ☞ serving size: 1 frankfurter on bun = 166 g; Calories = 378.5; Total Carb (g) = 31.5; Net Carb (g) = 27.5; Fat (g) = 20.7; Protein = 16

🍔 Frankfurter Or Hot Dog Sandwich With Meatless Chili On Multigrain Bread ☞ serving size: 1 frankfurter on bread = 157 g; Calories = 350.1; Total Carb (g) = 25.9; Net Carb (g) = 21.2; Fat (g) = 20.8; Protein = 15.8

🍔 Frankfurter Or Hot Dog Sandwich With Meatless Chili On Multigrain Bun ☞ serving size: 1 frankfurter on bun = 166 g; Calories = 373.5; Total Carb (g) = 30.3; Net Carb (g) = 26.5; Fat (g) = 22; Protein = 15.3

🍔 Frankfurter Or Hot Dog Sandwich With Meatless Chili On Wheat Bread ☞ serving size: 1 frankfurter on bread = 149 g; Calories = 332.3; Total Carb (g) = 23.6; Net Carb (g) = 20.3; Fat (g) = 20.5; Protein = 13.9

🍔 Frankfurter Or Hot Dog Sandwich With Meatless Chili On Wheat Bun ☞ serving size: 1 frankfurter on bun = 166 g; Calories = 375.2; Total Carb (g) = 31.5; Net Carb (g) = 27.6; Fat (g) = 20.9; Protein = 16.2

Frankfurter Or Hot Dog Sandwich With Meatless Chili On White Bread ☞ serving size: 1 frankfurter on bread = 149 g; Calories = 329.3; Total Carb (g) = 24.1; Net Carb (g) = 21.3; Fat (g) = 20.2; Protein = 13.4

Frankfurter Or Hot Dog Sandwich With Meatless Chili On White Bun ☞ serving size: 1 frankfurter on bun = 166 g; Calories = 380.1; Total Carb (g) = 32.8; Net Carb (g) = 29.8; Fat (g) = 21; Protein = 15.3

Frankfurter Or Hot Dog Sandwich With Meatless Chili On Whole Grain White Bread ☞ serving size: 1 frankfurter on bread = 157 g; Calories = 340.7; Total Carb (g) = 26.1; Net Carb (g) = 20.6; Fat (g) = 20; Protein = 14.8

Frankfurter Or Hot Dog Sandwich With Meatless Chili On Whole Grain White Bun ☞ serving size: 1 frankfurter on bun = 166 g; Calories = 370.2; Total Carb (g) = 31.2; Net Carb (g) = 28; Fat (g) = 20.8; Protein = 15.1

Frankfurter Or Hot Dog Sandwich With Meatless Chili On Whole Wheat Bread ☞ serving size: 1 frankfurter on bread = 157 g; Calories = 348.5; Total Carb (g) = 25.5; Net Carb (g) = 21.3; Fat (g) = 20.4; Protein = 15.2

Frankfurter Or Hot Dog Sandwich With Meatless Chili On Whole Wheat Bun ☞ serving size: 1 frankfurter on bun = 166 g; Calories = 375.2; Total Carb (g) = 30.5; Net Carb (g) = 25.7; Fat (g) = 21.2; Protein = 16.5

French Toast From School Nfs ☞ serving size: 1 bite size = 10 g; Calories = 16; Total Carb (g) = 2.2; Net Carb (g) = 2; Fat (g) = 0.4; Protein = 0.9

French Toast Gluten Free ☞ serving size: 1 slice, any size = 65 g; Calories = 169.7; Total Carb (g) = 19.9; Net Carb (g) = 18.4; Fat (g) = 7.7; Protein = 5.1

French Toast Gluten Free From Frozen ☞ serving size: 1 bite size

= 10 g; Calories = 17.3; Total Carb (g) = 2.8; Net Carb (g) = 2.6; Fat (g) = 0.5; Protein = 0.5

🝔 French Toast Nfs ☞ serving size: 1 slice, any size = 65 g; Calories = 175.5; Total Carb (g) = 21; Net Carb (g) = 20.1; Fat (g) = 7.1; Protein = 6.6

🝔 French Toast Plain ☞ serving size: 1 slice, any size = 65 g; Calories = 175.5; Total Carb (g) = 21; Net Carb (g) = 20.1; Fat (g) = 7.1; Protein = 6.6

🝔 French Toast Plain From Fast Food / Restaurant ☞ serving size: 1 slice, any size = 85 g; Calories = 260.1; Total Carb (g) = 30.4; Net Carb (g) = 29.1; Fat (g) = 11.7; Protein = 8.1

🝔 French Toast Plain From Frozen ☞ serving size: 1 bite size = 10 g; Calories = 18.1; Total Carb (g) = 3; Net Carb (g) = 2.9; Fat (g) = 0.4; Protein = 0.7

🝔 French Toast Plain Reduced Fat ☞ serving size: 1 slice, any size = 65 g; Calories = 154.1; Total Carb (g) = 22.1; Net Carb (g) = 21.2; Fat (g) = 4; Protein = 6.9

🝔 French Toast Sticks ☞ serving size: 3 pieces = 65 g; Calories = 221; Total Carb (g) = 26.8; Net Carb (g) = 25.9; Fat (g) = 11.5; Protein = 3.9

🝔 French Toast Sticks From School Nfs ☞ serving size: 1 stick = 25 g; Calories = 40; Total Carb (g) = 5.6; Net Carb (g) = 4.9; Fat (g) = 0.9; Protein = 2.3

🝔 French Toast Sticks Nfs ☞ serving size: 1 stick = 25 g; Calories = 70.8; Total Carb (g) = 10.5; Net Carb (g) = 10; Fat (g) = 2.4; Protein = 1.8

🝔 French Toast Sticks Plain From Fast Food / Restaurant ☞ serving size: 1 stick = 25 g; Calories = 100; Total Carb (g) = 12.1; Net Carb (g) = 11.7; Fat (g) = 5.2; Protein = 1.8

🝔 French Toast Sticks Plain From Frozen ☞ serving size: 1 stick = 45 g; Calories = 127.4; Total Carb (g) = 18.9; Net Carb (g) = 18; Fat (g) = 4.3; Protein = 3.2

🍔 French Toast Sticks Whole Grain ☞ serving size: 1 stick = 45 g; Calories = 121.1; Total Carb (g) = 13.6; Net Carb (g) = 12.4; Fat (g) = 5.1; Protein = 5.1

🍔 French Toast Whole Grain ☞ serving size: 1 slice, any size = 65 g; Calories = 174.9; Total Carb (g) = 19.7; Net Carb (g) = 17.9; Fat (g) = 7.3; Protein = 7.4

🍔 French Toast Whole Grain From Fast Food / Restaurant ☞ serving size: 1 slice, any size = 85 g; Calories = 258.4; Total Carb (g) = 28.4; Net Carb (g) = 25.8; Fat (g) = 12; Protein = 9.4

🍔 French Toast Whole Grain From Frozen ☞ serving size: 1 bite size = 10 g; Calories = 18; Total Carb (g) = 2.8; Net Carb (g) = 2.5; Fat (g) = 0.4; Protein = 0.8

🍔 French Toast Whole Grain Reduced Fat ☞ serving size: 1 slice, any size = 65 g; Calories = 153.4; Total Carb (g) = 20.7; Net Carb (g) = 18.9; Fat (g) = 4.3; Protein = 7.8

🍔 Fried Bread Puerto Rican Style ☞ serving size: 2 fritters with syrup (4" x 2-1/2" x 3-1/4") = 110 g; Calories = 282.7; Total Carb (g) = 46; Net Carb (g) = 45.5; Fat (g) = 9; Protein = 5.5

🍔 Fried Egg Sandwich ☞ serving size: 1 sandwich = 96 g; Calories = 224.6; Total Carb (g) = 26.4; Net Carb (g) = 25; Fat (g) = 8.2; Protein = 10.6

🍔 Griddle Cake Sandwich Egg Cheese And Bacon ☞ serving size: 1 item 6.1 oz = 174 g; Calories = 473.3; Total Carb (g) = 45.6; Net Carb (g) = 44.2; Fat (g) = 23; Protein = 20.9

🍔 Griddle Cake Sandwich Egg Cheese And Sausage ☞ serving size: 1 item = 199 g; Calories = 579.1; Total Carb (g) = 43.9; Net Carb (g) = 42.7; Fat (g) = 35.3; Protein = 21.4

🍔 Griddle Cake Sandwich Sausage ☞ serving size: 1 item = 135 g; Calories = 429.3; Total Carb (g) = 42.2; Net Carb (g) = 40.8; Fat (g) = 24; Protein = 11.4

⬤ Grilled Chicken Bacon And Tomato Club Sandwich With Cheese Lettuce And Mayonnaise ☞ serving size: 1 sandwich = 268 g; Calories = 589.6; Total Carb (g) = 53.3; Net Carb (g) = 50; Fat (g) = 21.6; Protein = 46.1

⬤ Grilled Chicken In Tortilla With Lettuce Cheese And Ranch Sauce ☞ serving size: 1 item = 123 g; Calories = 273.1; Total Carb (g) = 22.7; Net Carb (g) = 21.6; Fat (g) = 12.7; Protein = 16.9

⬤ Gyro Sandwich (Pita Bread Beef Lamb Onion Condiments) With Tomato And Spread ☞ serving size: 1 gyro = 390 g; Calories = 651.3; Total Carb (g) = 71.9; Net Carb (g) = 68; Fat (g) = 18.6; Protein = 46.5

⬤ Ham And Cheese On English Muffin ☞ serving size: 1 jimmy dean sandwich = 57 g; Calories = 144.8; Total Carb (g) = 10.8; Net Carb (g) = 10; Fat (g) = 6.9; Protein = 9.6

⬤ Ham And Cheese Sandwich On Bun With Lettuce And Spread ☞ serving size: 1 sandwich = 154 g; Calories = 328; Total Carb (g) = 26.2; Net Carb (g) = 24.5; Fat (g) = 16.4; Protein = 18.1

⬤ Ham And Cheese Sandwich With Lettuce And Spread ☞ serving size: 1 sandwich = 155 g; Calories = 359.6; Total Carb (g) = 32.6; Net Carb (g) = 30.2; Fat (g) = 16.7; Protein = 19

⬤ Ham And Cheese Sandwich With Spread Grilled ☞ serving size: 1 sandwich = 141 g; Calories = 359.6; Total Carb (g) = 32.3; Net Carb (g) = 30; Fat (g) = 17; Protein = 18.7

⬤ Ham And Egg Sandwich ☞ serving size: 1 sandwich = 124 g; Calories = 271.6; Total Carb (g) = 27.7; Net Carb (g) = 26; Fat (g) = 10.6; Protein = 15.2

⬤ Ham And Tomato Club Sandwich With Lettuce And Spread ☞ serving size: 1 sandwich = 254 g; Calories = 602; Total Carb (g) = 49.3; Net Carb (g) = 45.7; Fat (g) = 33; Protein = 27.5

⬤ Ham Salad Sandwich ☞ serving size: 1 sandwich = 141 g; Calo-

ries = 311.6; Total Carb (g) = 28.2; Net Carb (g) = 26.4; Fat (g) = 14.4; Protein = 16.2

🍔 Ham Sandwich With Lettuce And Spread ☞ serving size: 1 sandwich = 127 g; Calories = 273.1; Total Carb (g) = 30.1; Net Carb (g) = 27.7; Fat (g) = 10.2; Protein = 14.5

🍔 Ham Sandwich With Spread ☞ serving size: 1 sandwich = 112 g; Calories = 269.9; Total Carb (g) = 28; Net Carb (g) = 25.9; Fat (g) = 11.1; Protein = 13.5

🍔 Hamburger 1 Medium Patty Plain On Wheat Bun ☞ serving size: 1 hamburger = 145 g; Calories = 388.6; Total Carb (g) = 27.2; Net Carb (g) = 24; Fat (g) = 17.8; Protein = 28.5

🍔 Hamburger 1 Medium Patty Plain On White Bun ☞ serving size: 1 hamburger = 145 g; Calories = 398.8; Total Carb (g) = 30.1; Net Carb (g) = 29.1; Fat (g) = 17.8; Protein = 27.5

🍔 Hamburger 1 Medium Patty Plain On Whole Wheat Bun ☞ serving size: 1 hamburger = 145 g; Calories = 388.6; Total Carb (g) = 27.2; Net Carb (g) = 24; Fat (g) = 17.8; Protein = 28.5

🍔 Hamburger 1 Medium Patty With Condiments On Wheat Bun ☞ serving size: 1 hamburger = 200 g; Calories = 430; Total Carb (g) = 30.7; Net Carb (g) = 26.9; Fat (g) = 21; Protein = 28.6

🍔 Hamburger 1 Medium Patty With Condiments On White Bun ☞ serving size: 1 hamburger = 200 g; Calories = 440; Total Carb (g) = 33.5; Net Carb (g) = 31.9; Fat (g) = 21; Protein = 27.6

🍔 Hamburger 1 Medium Patty With Condiments On Whole Wheat Bun ☞ serving size: 1 hamburger = 200 g; Calories = 430; Total Carb (g) = 30.7; Net Carb (g) = 26.9; Fat (g) = 21; Protein = 28.6

🍔 Hamburger 1 Miniature Patty On Miniature Bun From School ☞ serving size: 1 miniature hamburger = 50 g; Calories = 118.5; Total Carb (g) = 12.5; Net Carb (g) = 10.7; Fat (g) = 3.5; Protein = 9.1

🍔 Hamburger 1 Miniature Patty Plain On Miniature Bun From Fast

Food / Restaurant ☞ serving size: 1 miniature hamburger = 50 g; Calories = 143; Total Carb (g) = 14.6; Net Carb (g) = 14.1; Fat (g) = 5.7; Protein = 7.7

🍔 Hamburger 1 Miniature Patty With Condiments On Miniature Bun From Fast Food / Restaurant ☞ serving size: 1 miniature hamburger = 65 g; Calories = 162.5; Total Carb (g) = 15.9; Net Carb (g) = 15.2; Fat (g) = 7.4; Protein = 7.6

🍔 Hamburger 1 Small Patty Plain On Wheat Bun ☞ serving size: 1 hamburger = 115 g; Calories = 308.2; Total Carb (g) = 23.2; Net Carb (g) = 20.4; Fat (g) = 13.6; Protein = 22.1

🍔 Hamburger 1 Small Patty Plain On White Bun ☞ serving size: 1 hamburger = 115 g; Calories = 316.3; Total Carb (g) = 25.6; Net Carb (g) = 24.7; Fat (g) = 13.6; Protein = 21.3

🍔 Hamburger 1 Small Patty Plain On Whole Wheat Bun ☞ serving size: 1 hamburger = 115 g; Calories = 308.2; Total Carb (g) = 23.2; Net Carb (g) = 20.4; Fat (g) = 13.6; Protein = 22.1

🍔 Hamburger 1 Small Patty With Condiments On Bun From Fast Food / Restaurant (Burger King Whopper Jr.) ☞ serving size: 1 burger king whopper jr = 150 g; Calories = 310.5; Total Carb (g) = 30; Net Carb (g) = 28.5; Fat (g) = 14.3; Protein = 14.8

🍔 Hamburger 1 Small Patty With Condiments On White Bun ☞ serving size: 1 hamburger = 175 g; Calories = 369.3; Total Carb (g) = 30; Net Carb (g) = 28.4; Fat (g) = 17.4; Protein = 22.1

🍔 Hamburger 1 Small Patty With Condiments On Whole Wheat Bun ☞ serving size: 1 hamburger = 175 g; Calories = 360.5; Total Carb (g) = 27.5; Net Carb (g) = 24.2; Fat (g) = 17.4; Protein = 23

🍔 Hamburger Large Single Patty With Condiments ☞ serving size: 1 item = 171 g; Calories = 437.8; Total Carb (g) = 37.9; Net Carb (g) = 36; Fat (g) = 19.8; Protein = 26.8

🍔 Hamburger Nfs ☞ serving size: 1 hamburger = 200 g; Calories =

440; Total Carb (g) = 33.5; Net Carb (g) = 31.9; Fat (g) = 21; Protein = 27.6

Hamburger On Bun From School ☞ serving size: 1 hamburger = 95 g; Calories = 225.2; Total Carb (g) = 22.9; Net Carb (g) = 19.7; Fat (g) = 6.7; Protein = 17.5

Hamburger; Double Large Patty; With Condiments Vegetables And Mayonnaise ☞ serving size: 1 item = 374 g; Calories = 942.5; Total Carb (g) = 51.4; Net Carb (g) = 46.2; Fat (g) = 58.6; Protein = 52.1

Hamburger; Single Large Patty; With Condiments Vegetables And Mayonnaise ☞ serving size: 1 item = 247 g; Calories = 558.2; Total Carb (g) = 42.8; Net Carb (g) = 39.1; Fat (g) = 30.6; Protein = 28

Hamburger; Single Regular Patty; Double Decker Bun With Condiments And Special Sauce ☞ serving size: 1 item = 205 g; Calories = 531; Total Carb (g) = 46.5; Net Carb (g) = 43.6; Fat (g) = 27.3; Protein = 25

Hamburger; Single Regular Patty; Plain ☞ serving size: 1 sandwich = 78 g; Calories = 231.7; Total Carb (g) = 24.6; Net Carb (g) = 23.2; Fat (g) = 9.4; Protein = 12.9

Hamburger; Single Regular Patty; With Condiments ☞ serving size: 1 sandwich = 97 g; Calories = 255.1; Total Carb (g) = 28.7; Net Carb (g) = 26.9; Fat (g) = 9.9; Protein = 12.9

Hors D'oeuvres With Spread ☞ serving size: 1 hors d'oeuvre = 23 g; Calories = 47.4; Total Carb (g) = 6.6; Net Carb (g) = 6.3; Fat (g) = 1.1; Protein = 2.6

Hot Ham And Cheese Sandwich On Bun ☞ serving size: 1 sandwich = 162 g; Calories = 345.1; Total Carb (g) = 26.2; Net Carb (g) = 24.3; Fat (g) = 18.6; Protein = 17.4

Hush Puppies ☞ serving size: 1 piece = 22 g; Calories = 65.1; Total Carb (g) = 8.9; Net Carb (g) = 8.2; Fat (g) = 2.9; Protein = 1.4

🍪 Kfc Biscuit ☞ serving size: 1 biscuit = 49 g; Calories = 175.4; Total Carb (g) = 21.3; Net Carb (g) = 20.4; Fat (g) = 8.4; Protein = 3.7

🍪 Kfc Coleslaw ☞ serving size: 1 package = 112 g; Calories = 161.3; Total Carb (g) = 17.5; Net Carb (g) = 15.3; Fat (g) = 9.7; Protein = 1

🍪 Kfc Crispy Chicken Strips ☞ serving size: 1 strip = 47 g; Calories = 128.8; Total Carb (g) = 6.4; Net Carb (g) = 5.8; Fat (g) = 7.3; Protein = 9.5

🍪 Kfc Fried Chicken Breast ☞ serving size: 1 breast, with skin = 212 g; Calories = 568.2; Total Carb (g) = 18; Net Carb (g) = 18; Fat (g) = 35.1; Protein = 45

🍪 Kfc Fried Chicken Extra Crispy Breast Meat Only Skin And Breading Removed ☞ serving size: 1 breast, without skin = 140 g; Calories = 214.2; Total Carb (g) = 0.4; Net Carb (g) = 0.4; Fat (g) = 6.8; Protein = 38.2

🍪 Kfc Fried Chicken Extra Crispy Drumstick Meat And Skin With Breading ☞ serving size: 1 drumstick, with skin = 81 g; Calories = 221.9; Total Carb (g) = 6.5; Net Carb (g) = 6.5; Fat (g) = 14.4; Protein = 16.7

🍪 Kfc Fried Chicken Extra Crispy Drumstick Meat Only Skin And Breading Removed ☞ serving size: 1 drumstick, bone and skin removed = 41 g; Calories = 69.7; Total Carb (g) = 0; Net Carb (g) = 0; Fat (g) = 3.1; Protein = 10.6

🍪 Kfc Fried Chicken Extra Crispy Thigh Meat And Skin With Breading ☞ serving size: 1 thigh, with skin = 152 g; Calories = 469.7; Total Carb (g) = 15.7; Net Carb (g) = 15.7; Fat (g) = 33.7; Protein = 26.1

🍪 Kfc Fried Chicken Extra Crispy Thigh Meat Only Skin And Breading Removed ☞ serving size: 1 thigh, without skin = 91 g; Calories = 162.9; Total Carb (g) = 0; Net Carb (g) = 0; Fat (g) = 9.1; Protein = 20.4

🍪 Kfc Fried Chicken Extra Crispy Wing Meat And Skin With

Breading ☞ serving size: 1 wing, with skin = 68 g; Calories = 229.2; Total Carb (g) = 7.9; Net Carb (g) = 7.9; Fat (g) = 15.6; Protein = 14.1

🍪 Kfc Fried Chicken Extra Crispy Wing Meat Only Skin And Breading Removed ☞ serving size: 1 wing, without skin = 44 g; Calories = 103.8; Total Carb (g) = 1.3; Net Carb (g) = 1.3; Fat (g) = 5.3; Protein = 12.6

🍪 Kfc Fried Chicken Original Recipe Breast Meat And Skin With Breading ☞ serving size: 1 breast, with skin = 212 g; Calories = 489.7; Total Carb (g) = 13.3; Net Carb (g) = 13.3; Fat (g) = 27.8; Protein = 46.5

🍪 Kfc Fried Chicken Original Recipe Breast Meat Only Skin And Breading Removed ☞ serving size: 1 breast without skin = 152 g; Calories = 226.5; Total Carb (g) = 0; Net Carb (g) = 0; Fat (g) = 6.9; Protein = 40.9

🍪 Kfc Fried Chicken Original Recipe Drumstick Meat And Skin With Breading ☞ serving size: 1 drumstick, with skin = 75 g; Calories = 179.3; Total Carb (g) = 4; Net Carb (g) = 4; Fat (g) = 10.7; Protein = 16.7

🍪 Kfc Fried Chicken Original Recipe Drumstick Meat Only Skin And Breading Removed ☞ serving size: 1 drumstick, bone and skin removed = 40 g; Calories = 70; Total Carb (g) = 0; Net Carb (g) = 0; Fat (g) = 3.1; Protein = 10.5

🍪 Kfc Fried Chicken Original Recipe Thigh Meat And Skin With Breading ☞ serving size: 1 thigh, with skin = 135 g; Calories = 363.2; Total Carb (g) = 11.4; Net Carb (g) = 11.4; Fat (g) = 23.9; Protein = 25.5

🍪 Kfc Fried Chicken Original Recipe Thigh Meat Only Skin And Breading Removed ☞ serving size: 1 thigh without skin = 86 g; Calories = 150.5; Total Carb (g) = 0; Net Carb (g) = 0; Fat (g) = 8; Protein = 19.6

🍪 Kfc Fried Chicken Original Recipe Wing Meat And Skin With Breading ☞ serving size: 1 wing, with skin = 60 g; Calories = 178.2; Total Carb (g) = 6; Net Carb (g) = 6; Fat (g) = 11.3; Protein = 13

🍔 Kfc Fried Chicken Original Recipe Wing Meat Only Skin And Breading Removed ☞ serving size: 1 wing wing without skin = 39 g; Calories = 84.2; Total Carb (g) = 0.7; Net Carb (g) = 0.7; Fat (g) = 4.1; Protein = 11.2

🍔 Kfc Popcorn Chicken ☞ serving size: 1 piece = 6.4 g; Calories = 22.5; Total Carb (g) = 1.4; Net Carb (g) = 1.3; Fat (g) = 1.4; Protein = 1.1

🍔 Little Caesars 14 Inch Cheese Pizza Large Deep Dish Crust ☞ serving size: 1 slice = 102 g; Calories = 268.3; Total Carb (g) = 30.7; Net Carb (g) = 29.4; Fat (g) = 10.4; Protein = 12.9

🍔 Little Caesars 14 Inch Cheese Pizza Thin Crust ☞ serving size: 1 slice = 48 g; Calories = 148.3; Total Carb (g) = 11; Net Carb (g) = 10.2; Fat (g) = 8.2; Protein = 7.8

🍔 Little Caesars 14 Inch Original Round Cheese Pizza Regular Crust ☞ serving size: 1 slice = 89 g; Calories = 235.9; Total Carb (g) = 28; Net Carb (g) = 26.5; Fat (g) = 8.5; Protein = 11.9

🍔 Little Caesars 14 Inch Original Round Meat And Vegetable Pizza Regular Crust ☞ serving size: 1 slice = 115 g; Calories = 279.5; Total Carb (g) = 26.6; Net Carb (g) = 24.2; Fat (g) = 13.1; Protein = 13.9

🍔 Little Caesars 14 Inch Original Round Pepperoni Pizza Regular Crust ☞ serving size: 1 slice = 90 g; Calories = 245.7; Total Carb (g) = 27.9; Net Carb (g) = 26.4; Fat (g) = 9.5; Protein = 12.2

🍔 Little Caesars 14 Inch Pepperoni Pizza Large Deep Dish Crust ☞ serving size: 1 slice = 104 g; Calories = 275.6; Total Carb (g) = 30.2; Net Carb (g) = 28.6; Fat (g) = 11.2; Protein = 13.5

🍔 McDonalds Bacon Egg & Cheese Biscuit ☞ serving size: 1 item 4.9 oz = 142 g; Calories = 431.7; Total Carb (g) = 31.6; Net Carb (g) = 30.3; Fat (g) = 26.7; Protein = 19.1

🍔 McDonalds Bacon Egg & Cheese Mcgriddles ☞ serving size: 1 item 5.8 oz = 165 g; Calories = 448.8; Total Carb (g) = 43.2; Net Carb (g) = 41.9; Fat (g) = 21.8; Protein = 19.9

McDonalds Bacon Ranch Salad With Crispy Chicken ☞ serving size: 1 item 11.3 oz = 319 g; Calories = 389.2; Total Carb (g) = 19.4; Net Carb (g) = 16.2; Fat (g) = 20.1; Protein = 28.1

McDonalds Bacon Ranch Salad With Grilled Chicken ☞ serving size: 1 item 10.8 oz = 305 g; Calories = 247.1; Total Carb (g) = 11.1; Net Carb (g) = 8.1; Fat (g) = 9.6; Protein = 31.4

McDonalds Bacon Ranch Salad Without Chicken ☞ serving size: 1 item 7.8 oz = 223 g; Calories = 136; Total Carb (g) = 9.4; Net Carb (g) = 6; Fat (g) = 8.1; Protein = 9.2

McDonalds Big Breakfast ☞ serving size: 1 item 9.5 oz = 269 g; Calories = 766.7; Total Carb (g) = 47.1; Net Carb (g) = 44.1; Fat (g) = 52.1; Protein = 27.3

McDonalds Big Mac ☞ serving size: 1 item 7.6 oz = 219 g; Calories = 562.8; Total Carb (g) = 44; Net Carb (g) = 40.5; Fat (g) = 32.8; Protein = 25.9

McDonalds Big Mac (Without Big Mac Sauce) ☞ serving size: 1 item = 200 g; Calories = 468; Total Carb (g) = 42; Net Carb (g) = 38.6; Fat (g) = 23.1; Protein = 25.6

McDonalds Cheeseburger ☞ serving size: 1 item 4 oz = 119 g; Calories = 313; Total Carb (g) = 33.1; Net Carb (g) = 31.8; Fat (g) = 14; Protein = 15.4

McDonalds Chicken Mcnuggets ☞ serving size: 4 pieces = 64 g; Calories = 193.3; Total Carb (g) = 9.7; Net Carb (g) = 9.7; Fat (g) = 12.7; Protein = 10.1

McDonalds Deluxe Breakfast With Syrup And Margarine ☞ serving size: 1 item 14.8 oz = 420 g; Calories = 1197; Total Carb (g) = 123.8; Net Carb (g) = 119.6; Fat (g) = 64; Protein = 31.8

McDonalds Double Cheeseburger ☞ serving size: 1 sandwich = 155 g; Calories = 437.1; Total Carb (g) = 29.1; Net Carb (g) = 27.9; Fat (g) = 24.9; Protein = 24

🍔 McDonalds Double Quarter Pounder With Cheese ☞ serving size: 1 item = 280 g; Calories = 733.6; Total Carb (g) = 40.4; Net Carb (g) = 37.6; Fat (g) = 45.4; Protein = 47.5

🍔 McDonalds Egg Mcmuffin ☞ serving size: 1 sandwich = 126 g; Calories = 287.3; Total Carb (g) = 27.3; Net Carb (g) = 25.9; Fat (g) = 12.2; Protein = 17.2

🍔 McDonalds Filet-O-Fish ☞ serving size: 1 sandwich = 134 g; Calories = 377.9; Total Carb (g) = 35.4; Net Carb (g) = 33.5; Fat (g) = 19.6; Protein = 15.1

🍔 McDonalds Filet-O-Fish (Without Tartar Sauce) ☞ serving size: 1 item = 124 g; Calories = 301.3; Total Carb (g) = 38.5; Net Carb (g) = 37.3; Fat (g) = 9.5; Protein = 15.5

🍔 McDonalds French Fries ☞ serving size: 1 small serving = 71 g; Calories = 229.3; Total Carb (g) = 30.2; Net Carb (g) = 27.5; Fat (g) = 11; Protein = 2.4

🍔 McDonalds Fruit N Yogurt Parfait ☞ serving size: 1 item 5.2 oz = 149 g; Calories = 156.5; Total Carb (g) = 30.9; Net Carb (g) = 29.4; Fat (g) = 1.9; Protein = 4.1

🍔 McDonalds Fruit N Yogurt Parfait (Without Granola) ☞ serving size: 1 item = 142 g; Calories = 127.8; Total Carb (g) = 25.1; Net Carb (g) = 23.8; Fat (g) = 1.6; Protein = 3.5

🍔 McDonalds Hamburger ☞ serving size: 1 sandwich = 95 g; Calories = 250.8; Total Carb (g) = 28.8; Net Carb (g) = 27.5; Fat (g) = 9.6; Protein = 12.3

🍔 McDonalds Hash Brown ☞ serving size: 1 serving 1 patty = 53 g; Calories = 143.6; Total Carb (g) = 15.1; Net Carb (g) = 13.7; Fat (g) = 8.6; Protein = 1.3

🍔 McDonalds Hot Caramel Sundae ☞ serving size: 1 item (6.4 oz) = 182 g; Calories = 342.2; Total Carb (g) = 60.7; Net Carb (g) = 60.7; Fat (g) = 8.9; Protein = 6.5

🍪 McDonalds Hot Fudge Sundae ☞ serving size: 1 item (6.3 oz) = 179 g; Calories = 332.9; Total Carb (g) = 53.8; Net Carb (g) = 53.1; Fat (g) = 10.6; Protein = 7.4

🍪 McDonalds Hotcakes (Plain) ☞ serving size: 3 hotcakes 5.3 oz = 149 g; Calories = 339.7; Total Carb (g) = 57; Net Carb (g) = 54.9; Fat (g) = 8.7; Protein = 8.9

🍪 McDonalds Hotcakes And Sausage ☞ serving size: 1 item = 192 g; Calories = 564.5; Total Carb (g) = 72.1; Net Carb (g) = 69; Fat (g) = 24; Protein = 15

🍪 McDonalds Mcchicken Sandwich ☞ serving size: 1 sandwich = 131 g; Calories = 357.6; Total Carb (g) = 36.6; Net Carb (g) = 34.9; Fat (g) = 17.3; Protein = 13.7

🍪 McDonalds Mcchicken Sandwich (Without Mayonnaise) ☞ serving size: 1 item = 138 g; Calories = 331.2; Total Carb (g) = 42.7; Net Carb (g) = 40.8; Fat (g) = 11.7; Protein = 15.3

🍪 McDonalds Mcflurry With M&Ms ☞ serving size: 1 regular (12 fl oz) = 348 g; Calories = 616; Total Carb (g) = 93.3; Net Carb (g) = 92.6; Fat (g) = 22.5; Protein = 14

🍪 McDonalds Mcflurry With Oreo Cookies ☞ serving size: 1 regular (12 fl oz) = 337 g; Calories = 556.1; Total Carb (g) = 86.1; Net Carb (g) = 85.8; Fat (g) = 19.1; Protein = 13.4

🍪 McDonalds Pancakes ☞ serving size: 1 item = 221 g; Calories = 601.1; Total Carb (g) = 101.8; Net Carb (g) = 99.9; Fat (g) = 17.8; Protein = 9

🍪 McDonalds Quarter Pounder ☞ serving size: 1 item = 171 g; Calories = 417.2; Total Carb (g) = 37.9; Net Carb (g) = 35.2; Fat (g) = 19.8; Protein = 24.1

🍪 McDonalds Quarter Pounder With Cheese ☞ serving size: 1 item 7.1 oz = 199 g; Calories = 513.4; Total Carb (g) = 39.7; Net Carb (g) = 36.9; Fat (g) = 28.3; Protein = 29

🍔 McDonalds Ranch Snack Wrap Crispy ☞ serving size: 1 wrap = 133 g; Calories = 365.8; Total Carb (g) = 30.9; Net Carb (g) = 29.2; Fat (g) = 20.1; Protein = 15.3

🍔 McDonalds Ranch Snack Wrap Grilled ☞ serving size: 1 wrap = 123 g; Calories = 273.1; Total Carb (g) = 22.7; Net Carb (g) = 21.6; Fat (g) = 12.7; Protein = 16.9

🍔 McDonalds Sausage Biscuit ☞ serving size: 1 item 4.1 oz = 117 g; Calories = 439.9; Total Carb (g) = 31.8; Net Carb (g) = 30.4; Fat (g) = 29.7; Protein = 11.3

🍔 McDonalds Sausage Biscuit With Egg ☞ serving size: 1 item 5.7 oz = 163 g; Calories = 506.9; Total Carb (g) = 31.4; Net Carb (g) = 30.1; Fat (g) = 36.3; Protein = 18.4

🍔 McDonalds Sausage Burrito ☞ serving size: 1 burrito = 109 g; Calories = 301.9; Total Carb (g) = 25; Net Carb (g) = 23.7; Fat (g) = 17; Protein = 12.1

🍔 McDonalds Sausage Egg & Cheese Mcgriddles ☞ serving size: 1 item 7 oz = 199 g; Calories = 563.2; Total Carb (g) = 43.9; Net Carb (g) = 42.7; Fat (g) = 35.3; Protein = 21.4

🍔 McDonalds Sausage Mcgriddles ☞ serving size: 1 item = 135 g; Calories = 421.2; Total Carb (g) = 42.2; Net Carb (g) = 40.8; Fat (g) = 24; Protein = 11.4

🍔 McDonalds Sausage Mcmuffin ☞ serving size: 1 item 4 oz = 115 g; Calories = 383; Total Carb (g) = 28.2; Net Carb (g) = 26.6; Fat (g) = 24.2; Protein = 14.6

🍔 McDonalds Sausage Mcmuffin With Egg ☞ serving size: 1 item 5.8 oz = 165 g; Calories = 452.1; Total Carb (g) = 28.5; Net Carb (g) = 27; Fat (g) = 29.4; Protein = 20.8

🍔 McDonalds Side Salad ☞ serving size: 1 item 3.1 oz = 87 g; Calories = 17.4; Total Carb (g) = 3.7; Net Carb (g) = 2.4; Fat (g) = 0.2; Protein = 0.9

🍔 McDonalds Southern Style Chicken Biscuit ☞ serving size: 1 biscuit regular size biscuit = 132 g; Calories = 401.3; Total Carb (g) = 40.3; Net Carb (g) = 38.5; Fat (g) = 19.7; Protein = 15.8

🍔 McDonalds Strawberry Sundae ☞ serving size: 1 item (6.3 oz) = 178 g; Calories = 281.2; Total Carb (g) = 50; Net Carb (g) = 50; Fat (g) = 7; Protein = 5.7

🍔 McDonalds Vanilla Reduced Fat Ice Cream Cone ☞ serving size: 1 item (3.2 oz) = 90 g; Calories = 145.8; Total Carb (g) = 23.7; Net Carb (g) = 23.6; Fat (g) = 4.4; Protein = 3.8

🍔 Meat Sandwich Nfs ☞ serving size: 1 sandwich = 83 g; Calories = 249.8; Total Carb (g) = 27.3; Net Carb (g) = 25.9; Fat (g) = 11.5; Protein = 8.7

🍔 Meat Spread Or Potted Meat Sandwich ☞ serving size: 1 sandwich = 107 g; Calories = 267.5; Total Carb (g) = 32.7; Net Carb (g) = 31.2; Fat (g) = 11.1; Protein = 8.8

🍔 Midnight Sandwich With Spread ☞ serving size: 1 sandwich = 201 g; Calories = 472.4; Total Carb (g) = 40.5; Net Carb (g) = 39.1; Fat (g) = 18.1; Protein = 34.7

🍔 Miniature Cinnamon Rolls ☞ serving size: 1 each = 25 g; Calories = 100.8; Total Carb (g) = 13.4; Net Carb (g) = 12.8; Fat (g) = 4.5; Protein = 1.8

🍔 Nachos With Cheese ☞ serving size: 1 serving = 80 g; Calories = 274.4; Total Carb (g) = 27.9; Net Carb (g) = 25.4; Fat (g) = 17.2; Protein = 3.5

🍔 Nachos With Cheese Beans Ground Beef And Tomatoes ☞ serving size: 1 serving = 222 g; Calories = 486.2; Total Carb (g) = 47.5; Net Carb (g) = 39.3; Fat (g) = 27.7; Protein = 13.8

🍔 Onion Rings Breaded And Fried ☞ serving size: 1 package (18 onion rings) = 117 g; Calories = 480.9; Total Carb (g) = 51; Net Carb (g) = 47.8; Fat (g) = 29.5; Protein = 4.5

Pancakes Buckwheat ☞ serving size: 1 miniature/bite size pancake = 10 g; Calories = 26.7; Total Carb (g) = 3.2; Net Carb (g) = 2.8; Fat (g) = 1.3; Protein = 0.8

Pancakes Cornmeal ☞ serving size: 1 miniature/bite size pancake = 10 g; Calories = 20.2; Total Carb (g) = 3.2; Net Carb (g) = 3.1; Fat (g) = 0.6; Protein = 0.5

Pancakes From School Nfs ☞ serving size: 1 miniature/bite size pancake = 10 g; Calories = 23.1; Total Carb (g) = 4; Net Carb (g) = 3.5; Fat (g) = 0.7; Protein = 0.6

Pancakes Nfs ☞ serving size: 1 miniature/bite size pancake = 10 g; Calories = 27.8; Total Carb (g) = 3.5; Net Carb (g) = 3.3; Fat (g) = 1.2; Protein = 0.7

Pancakes Plain ☞ serving size: 1 miniature/bite size pancake = 10 g; Calories = 27.8; Total Carb (g) = 3.5; Net Carb (g) = 3.3; Fat (g) = 1.2; Protein = 0.7

Pancakes Plain From Fast Food / Restaurant ☞ serving size: 1 miniature/bite size pancake = 10 g; Calories = 30.3; Total Carb (g) = 3.4; Net Carb (g) = 3.2; Fat (g) = 1.5; Protein = 0.7

Pancakes Plain Reduced Fat From Fozen ☞ serving size: 1 miniature/bite size pancake = 10 g; Calories = 26.2; Total Carb (g) = 3.6; Net Carb (g) = 3.4; Fat (g) = 1; Protein = 0.8

Pancakes Pumpkin ☞ serving size: 1 miniature/bite size pancake = 10 g; Calories = 23.8; Total Carb (g) = 3.1; Net Carb (g) = 2.9; Fat (g) = 1; Protein = 0.6

Pancakes Whole Grain ☞ serving size: 1 miniature/bite size pancake = 10 g; Calories = 27.1; Total Carb (g) = 3.3; Net Carb (g) = 3; Fat (g) = 1.2; Protein = 0.8

Pancakes Whole Grain And Nuts From Fast Food / Restaurant ☞ serving size: 1 miniature/bite size pancake = 10 g; Calories = 35.1; Total Carb (g) = 3; Net Carb (g) = 2.6; Fat (g) = 2.3; Protein = 0.8

🥞 Pancakes Whole Grain From Fast Food / Restaurant ☞ serving size: 1 miniature/bite size pancake = 10 g; Calories = 29.6; Total Carb (g) = 3.2; Net Carb (g) = 2.9; Fat (g) = 1.6; Protein = 0.8

🥞 Pancakes Whole Grain From Frozen ☞ serving size: 1 miniature/bite size pancake = 10 g; Calories = 23.2; Total Carb (g) = 3.9; Net Carb (g) = 3.6; Fat (g) = 0.7; Protein = 0.6

🥞 Pancakes Whole Grain Reduced Fat ☞ serving size: 1 miniature/bite size pancake = 10 g; Calories = 25.3; Total Carb (g) = 3.4; Net Carb (g) = 3; Fat (g) = 1; Protein = 0.8

🥞 Pancakes Whole Grain Reduced Fat From Frozen ☞ serving size: 1 miniature/bite size pancake = 10 g; Calories = 23.2; Total Carb (g) = 3.9; Net Carb (g) = 3.6; Fat (g) = 0.7; Protein = 0.6

🥞 Pancakes With Chocolate ☞ serving size: 1 miniature/bite size pancake = 10 g; Calories = 33.8; Total Carb (g) = 4.1; Net Carb (g) = 3.9; Fat (g) = 1.6; Protein = 0.8

🥞 Pancakes With Chocolate From Fast Food / Restaurant ☞ serving size: 1 miniature/bite size pancake = 10 g; Calories = 35.7; Total Carb (g) = 4; Net Carb (g) = 3.8; Fat (g) = 1.9; Protein = 0.8

🥞 Pancakes With Chocolate From Frozen ☞ serving size: 1 miniature/bite size pancake = 10 g; Calories = 24.8; Total Carb (g) = 3.9; Net Carb (g) = 3.8; Fat (g) = 0.8; Protein = 0.5

🥞 Pancakes With Fruit ☞ serving size: 1 miniature/bite size pancake = 10 g; Calories = 23; Total Carb (g) = 3.1; Net Carb (g) = 2.8; Fat (g) = 0.9; Protein = 0.6

🥞 Pancakes With Fruit From Fast Food / Restaurant ☞ serving size: 1 miniature/bite size pancake = 10 g; Calories = 25; Total Carb (g) = 3; Net Carb (g) = 2.8; Fat (g) = 1.2; Protein = 0.6

🥞 Pancakes With Fruit From Frozen ☞ serving size: 1 miniature/bite size pancake = 10 g; Calories = 22.4; Total Carb (g) = 3.7; Net Carb (g) = 3.5; Fat (g) = 0.7; Protein = 0.5

Papa Johns 14 Inch Cheese Pizza Original Crust ☞ serving size: 1 slice = 117 g; Calories = 304.2; Total Carb (g) = 38.3; Net Carb (g) = 36.1; Fat (g) = 10.8; Protein = 13.5

Papa Johns 14 Inch Cheese Pizza Thin Crust ☞ serving size: 1 slice = 87 g; Calories = 256.7; Total Carb (g) = 22.9; Net Carb (g) = 20.9; Fat (g) = 13.6; Protein = 10.7

Papa Johns 14 Inch Pepperoni Pizza Original Crust ☞ serving size: 1 slice = 123 g; Calories = 338.3; Total Carb (g) = 37; Net Carb (g) = 35.5; Fat (g) = 14.6; Protein = 14.7

Papa Johns 14 Inch The Works Pizza Original Crust ☞ serving size: 1 slice = 153 g; Calories = 367.2; Total Carb (g) = 40.8; Net Carb (g) = 37; Fat (g) = 15.6; Protein = 15.7

Pastrami Sandwich ☞ serving size: 1 sandwich = 134 g; Calories = 221.1; Total Carb (g) = 26.8; Net Carb (g) = 25.1; Fat (g) = 4.9; Protein = 16.4

Pepperoni And Salami Submarine Sandwich With Lettuce Tomato And Spread ☞ serving size: 1 submarine = 240 g; Calories = 540; Total Carb (g) = 46.8; Net Carb (g) = 44.1; Fat (g) = 30.8; Protein = 17.9

Pepperoni Pizza ☞ serving size: 1 slice = 111 g; Calories = 313; Total Carb (g) = 35.5; Net Carb (g) = 32.9; Fat (g) = 13.2; Protein = 13

Pig In A Blanket Frankfurter Or Hot Dog Wrapped In Dough ☞ serving size: 1 pig in blanket = 85 g; Calories = 275.4; Total Carb (g) = 16.5; Net Carb (g) = 15.9; Fat (g) = 18.6; Protein = 10.1

Pizza Cheese Topping Regular Crust Frozen Cooked ☞ serving size: 1 serving 9 servings per 24 oz package = 81 g; Calories = 217.1; Total Carb (g) = 23.5; Net Carb (g) = 21.7; Fat (g) = 10; Protein = 8.4

Pizza Cheese Topping Rising Crust Frozen Cooked ☞ serving size: 1 serving 6 servings per 29.25 oz package = 139 g; Calories =

361.4; Total Carb (g) = 45.7; Net Carb (g) = 42.3; Fat (g) = 12.2; Protein = 17.2

Pizza Cheese Topping Thin Crust Frozen Cooked ☞ serving size: 1 slice = 69 g; Calories = 181.5; Total Carb (g) = 19.9; Net Carb (g) = 17.8; Fat (g) = 7.6; Protein = 8.2

Pizza Hut 12 Inch Cheese Pizza Hand-Tossed Crust ☞ serving size: 1 slice = 96 g; Calories = 260.2; Total Carb (g) = 30; Net Carb (g) = 28.2; Fat (g) = 10.5; Protein = 11.5

Pizza Hut 12 Inch Cheese Pizza Pan Crust ☞ serving size: 1 slice = 100 g; Calories = 280; Total Carb (g) = 29.9; Net Carb (g) = 28.2; Fat (g) = 12.6; Protein = 11.7

Pizza Hut 12 Inch Cheese Pizza Thin N Crispy Crust ☞ serving size: 1 slice = 69 g; Calories = 209.1; Total Carb (g) = 19.8; Net Carb (g) = 18.7; Fat (g) = 9.7; Protein = 10.6

Pizza Hut 12 Inch Pepperoni Pizza Hand-Tossed Crust ☞ serving size: 1 slice = 96 g; Calories = 268.8; Total Carb (g) = 30.3; Net Carb (g) = 28.7; Fat (g) = 10.9; Protein = 12.4

Pizza Hut 12 Inch Pepperoni Pizza Pan Crust ☞ serving size: 1 slice = 96 g; Calories = 286.1; Total Carb (g) = 29.3; Net Carb (g) = 27.5; Fat (g) = 13.6; Protein = 11.5

Pizza Hut 12 Inch Super Supreme Pizza Hand-Tossed Crust ☞ serving size: 1 slice = 127 g; Calories = 308.6; Total Carb (g) = 32.5; Net Carb (g) = 30; Fat (g) = 13.6; Protein = 13.8

Pizza Hut 14 Inch Cheese Pizza Hand-Tossed Crust ☞ serving size: 1 slice = 105 g; Calories = 288.8; Total Carb (g) = 35.1; Net Carb (g) = 32.6; Fat (g) = 10.9; Protein = 12.6

Pizza Hut 14 Inch Cheese Pizza Pan Crust' ☞ serving size: 1 slice = 112 g; Calories = 309.1; Total Carb (g) = 36.8; Net Carb (g) = 34.4; Fat (g) = 12.6; Protein = 12.2

Pizza Hut 14 Inch Cheese Pizza Stuffed Crust ☞ serving size: 1

slice = 117 g; Calories = 320.6; Total Carb (g) = 35.1; Net Carb (g) = 33.1; Fat (g) = 13.6; Protein = 14.3

🍽 Pizza Hut 14 Inch Cheese Pizza Thin N Crispy Crust ☞ serving size: 1 slice = 79 g; Calories = 241.7; Total Carb (g) = 27; Net Carb (g) = 25.1; Fat (g) = 10.1; Protein = 10.6

🍽 Pizza Hut 14 Inch Pepperoni Pizza Hand-Tossed Crust ☞ serving size: 1 slice = 110 g; Calories = 320.1; Total Carb (g) = 35.3; Net Carb (g) = 32.5; Fat (g) = 13.9; Protein = 13.5

🍽 Pizza Hut 14 Inch Pepperoni Pizza Pan Crust ☞ serving size: 1 slice = 113 g; Calories = 328.8; Total Carb (g) = 35.9; Net Carb (g) = 33.7; Fat (g) = 14.8; Protein = 13

🍽 Pizza Hut 14 Inch Pepperoni Pizza Thin N Crispy Crust ☞ serving size: 1 slice = 80 g; Calories = 266.4; Total Carb (g) = 26.1; Net Carb (g) = 24.5; Fat (g) = 12.9; Protein = 11.3

🍽 Pizza Hut 14 Inch Sausage Pizza Hand-Tossed Crust ☞ serving size: 1 slice = 119 g; Calories = 341.5; Total Carb (g) = 35; Net Carb (g) = 32.2; Fat (g) = 16.1; Protein = 14.2

🍽 Pizza Hut 14 Inch Sausage Pizza Pan Crust ☞ serving size: 1 slice = 125 g; Calories = 358.8; Total Carb (g) = 37; Net Carb (g) = 34.5; Fat (g) = 17.3; Protein = 13.9

🍽 Pizza Hut 14 Inch Sausage Pizza Thin N Crispy Crust ☞ serving size: 1 slice = 92 g; Calories = 297.2; Total Carb (g) = 26.4; Net Carb (g) = 24.2; Fat (g) = 15.6; Protein = 12.8

🍽 Pizza Hut 14 Inch Super Supreme Pizza Hand-Tossed Crust ☞ serving size: 1 slice = 123 g; Calories = 305; Total Carb (g) = 32; Net Carb (g) = 29.2; Fat (g) = 13.5; Protein = 14

🍽 Pizza Hut Breadstick Parmesan Garlic ☞ serving size: 1 breadstick = 43 g; Calories = 147.5; Total Carb (g) = 19.1; Net Carb (g) = 18.1; Fat (g) = 5.5; Protein = 5.3

🍽 Pizza Meat And Vegetable Topping Regular Crust Frozen

Cooked ☞ serving size: 1 serving 5 servings per 24.2 oz package = 143 g; Calories = 394.7; Total Carb (g) = 36; Net Carb (g) = 32.8; Fat (g) = 20.6; Protein = 16.1

● Pizza Meat And Vegetable Topping Rising Crust Frozen Cooked ☞ serving size: 1 serving 6 servings per 34.98 oz package = 170 g; Calories = 460.7; Total Carb (g) = 48.9; Net Carb (g) = 45; Fat (g) = 20; Protein = 21.5

● Pizza Meat Topping Thick Crust Frozen Cooked ☞ serving size: 1 slice 1/8 of 12 inch pizza = 103 g; Calories = 282.2; Total Carb (g) = 31.7; Net Carb (g) = 29.3; Fat (g) = 11.9; Protein = 12.1

● Pizza Pepperoni Topping Regular Crust Frozen Cooked ☞ serving size: 1/4 pizza 12 inch diameter = 127 g; Calories = 348; Total Carb (g) = 31.4; Net Carb (g) = 28.8; Fat (g) = 16.7; Protein = 18.3

● Popeyes Biscuit ☞ serving size: 1 biscuit = 60 g; Calories = 240.6; Total Carb (g) = 24.6; Net Carb (g) = 22.3; Fat (g) = 14.2; Protein = 3.6

● Popeyes Coleslaw ☞ serving size: 1 package = 120 g; Calories = 193.2; Total Carb (g) = 16.9; Net Carb (g) = 14.9; Fat (g) = 13.4; Protein = 1.2

● Popeyes Fried Chicken Mild Breast Meat And Skin With Breading ☞ serving size: 1 breast, with skin = 194 g; Calories = 531.6; Total Carb (g) = 19.1; Net Carb (g) = 18.3; Fat (g) = 32; Protein = 42

● Popeyes Fried Chicken Mild Breast Meat Only Skin And Breading Removed ☞ serving size: 1 breast without skin = 132 g; Calories = 207.2; Total Carb (g) = 0; Net Carb (g) = 0; Fat (g) = 6; Protein = 38.3

● Popeyes Fried Chicken Mild Drumstick Meat And Skin With Breading ☞ serving size: 1 drumstick, with skin = 76 g; Calories = 222.7; Total Carb (g) = 7.5; Net Carb (g) = 7.5; Fat (g) = 14.6; Protein = 15.5

● Popeyes Fried Chicken Mild Drumstick Meat Only Skin And

Breading Removed ☞ serving size: 1 drumstick, bone and skin removed = 44 g; Calories = 74.8; Total Carb (g) = 0; Net Carb (g) = 0; Fat (g) = 3.1; Protein = 11.7

🍲 Popeyes Fried Chicken Mild Thigh Meat And Skin With Breading ☞ serving size: 1 thigh with skin = 138 g; Calories = 427.8; Total Carb (g) = 15.5; Net Carb (g) = 14.8; Fat (g) = 29; Protein = 26.4

🍲 Popeyes Fried Chicken Mild Thigh Meat Only Skin And Breading Removed ☞ serving size: 1 thigh thigh without skin = 83 g; Calories = 156; Total Carb (g) = 0.7; Net Carb (g) = 0.7; Fat (g) = 8; Protein = 20.2

🍲 Popeyes Fried Chicken Mild Wing Meat And Skin With Breading ☞ serving size: 1 wing, with skin = 57 g; Calories = 192.7; Total Carb (g) = 7.7; Net Carb (g) = 7.4; Fat (g) = 12.8; Protein = 11.6

🍲 Popeyes Fried Chicken Mild Wing Meat Only Skin And Breading Removed ☞ serving size: 1 wing without skin, bone and breading = 16 g; Calories = 33.9; Total Carb (g) = 0.5; Net Carb (g) = 0.5; Fat (g) = 1.5; Protein = 4.6

🍲 Popeyes Mild Chicken Strips Analyzed 2006 ☞ serving size: 1 strip = 54 g; Calories = 146.3; Total Carb (g) = 10.4; Net Carb (g) = 10; Fat (g) = 7; Protein = 10.4

🍲 Popeyes Spicy Chicken Strips Analyzed 2006 ☞ serving size: 1 strip = 53 g; Calories = 134.1; Total Carb (g) = 9.8; Net Carb (g) = 9.2; Fat (g) = 5.9; Protein = 10.4

🍲 Pork Barbecue Sandwich Or Sloppy Joe On Bun ☞ serving size: 1 barbecue sandwich = 186 g; Calories = 388.7; Total Carb (g) = 56.1; Net Carb (g) = 54.6; Fat (g) = 7.8; Protein = 21.6

🍲 Pork Sandwich ☞ serving size: 1 sandwich = 136 g; Calories = 315.5; Total Carb (g) = 33.3; Net Carb (g) = 31.5; Fat (g) = 8.5; Protein = 24.7

🍲 Pork Sandwich On White Roll With Onions Dill Pickles And

Barbecue Sauce ☞ serving size: 1 sandwich = 189 g; Calories = 421.5; Total Carb (g) = 50.1; Net Carb (g) = 48.4; Fat (g) = 12.2; Protein = 25.8

Pork Sandwich With Gravy ☞ serving size: 1 sandwich = 218 g; Calories = 324.8; Total Carb (g) = 36; Net Carb (g) = 34; Fat (g) = 8.6; Protein = 23.8

Potato French Fried In Vegetable Oil ☞ serving size: 1 serving small = 71 g; Calories = 221.5; Total Carb (g) = 29.4; Net Carb (g) = 26.7; Fat (g) = 10.5; Protein = 2.4

Potato French Fries From Fresh Baked ☞ serving size: 1 shoestring = 2 g; Calories = 3.3; Total Carb (g) = 0.4; Net Carb (g) = 0.4; Fat (g) = 0.2; Protein = 0

Potato French Fries From Fresh Fried ☞ serving size: 1 shoestring = 2 g; Calories = 3.9; Total Carb (g) = 0.4; Net Carb (g) = 0.3; Fat (g) = 0.3; Protein = 0

Potato French Fries From Frozen Fried ☞ serving size: 1 shoestring = 2 g; Calories = 4.5; Total Carb (g) = 0.5; Net Carb (g) = 0.4; Fat (g) = 0.3; Protein = 0.1

Potato French Fries Nfs ☞ serving size: 1 shoestring = 2 g; Calories = 4.5; Total Carb (g) = 0.5; Net Carb (g) = 0.4; Fat (g) = 0.3; Protein = 0.1

Potato French Fries Ns As To Fresh Or Frozen ☞ serving size: 1 shoestring = 2 g; Calories = 4.5; Total Carb (g) = 0.5; Net Carb (g) = 0.4; Fat (g) = 0.3; Protein = 0.1

Potato French Fries School ☞ serving size: 1 shoestring = 2 g; Calories = 3.3; Total Carb (g) = 0.4; Net Carb (g) = 0.4; Fat (g) = 0.2; Protein = 0

Potato French Fries With Cheese ☞ serving size: 1 fry, any cut = 8 g; Calories = 20.7; Total Carb (g) = 2.4; Net Carb (g) = 2.2; Fat (g) = 1.1; Protein = 0.3

Potato French Fries With Cheese Fast Food / Restaurant ☞

serving size: 1 kids meal order = 107 g; Calories = 277.1; Total Carb (g) = 31.8; Net Carb (g) = 29; Fat (g) = 15.1; Protein = 3.6

🍔 Potato French Fries With Cheese School ☞ serving size: 1 fry, any cut = 11 g; Calories = 19.7; Total Carb (g) = 2; Net Carb (g) = 1.8; Fat (g) = 1.1; Protein = 0.5

🍔 Potato French Fries With Chili ☞ serving size: 1 fry, any cut = 8 g; Calories = 19.3; Total Carb (g) = 2.5; Net Carb (g) = 2.2; Fat (g) = 0.9; Protein = 0.3

🍔 Potato French Fries With Chili And Cheese ☞ serving size: 1 fry, any cut = 10 g; Calories = 22; Total Carb (g) = 2.5; Net Carb (g) = 2.3; Fat (g) = 1.1; Protein = 0.4

🍔 Potato French Fries With Chili And Cheese Fast Food / Restaurant ☞ serving size: 1 fry, any cut = 10 g; Calories = 22; Total Carb (g) = 2.5; Net Carb (g) = 2.3; Fat (g) = 1.1; Protein = 0.4

🍔 Potato French Fries With Chili Fast Food / Restaurant ☞ serving size: 1 fry, any cut = 8 g; Calories = 19.3; Total Carb (g) = 2.5; Net Carb (g) = 2.2; Fat (g) = 0.9; Protein = 0.3

🍔 Potato Hash Brown From Dry Mix ☞ serving size: 1 cup = 160 g; Calories = 347.2; Total Carb (g) = 45.2; Net Carb (g) = 40.1; Fat (g) = 18.4; Protein = 4.2

🍔 Potato Hash Brown From Fast Food With Cheese ☞ serving size: 1 patty = 55 g; Calories = 161.7; Total Carb (g) = 13.5; Net Carb (g) = 12.3; Fat (g) = 10.9; Protein = 3.3

🍔 Potato Hash Brown From Fresh ☞ serving size: 1 cup = 160 g; Calories = 302.4; Total Carb (g) = 29.7; Net Carb (g) = 27.2; Fat (g) = 19.6; Protein = 3.1

🍔 Potato Hash Brown From Fresh With Cheese ☞ serving size: 1 cup = 160 g; Calories = 353.6; Total Carb (g) = 26; Net Carb (g) = 23.8; Fat (g) = 24.6; Protein = 8.1

🍔 Potato Hash Brown From Restaurant With Cheese ☞ serving

size: 1 patty = 55 g; Calories = 161.7; Total Carb (g) = 13.5; Net Carb (g) = 12.3; Fat (g) = 10.9; Protein = 3.3

🟤 Potato Hash Brown From School Lunch ☞ serving size: 1 patty = 55 g; Calories = 119.9; Total Carb (g) = 15.6; Net Carb (g) = 13.9; Fat (g) = 6.4; Protein = 1.5

🟤 Potato Hash Brown Nfs ☞ serving size: 1 patty = 55 g; Calories = 119.4; Total Carb (g) = 15.5; Net Carb (g) = 13.8; Fat (g) = 6.3; Protein = 1.4

🟤 Potato Hash Brown Ready-To-Heat ☞ serving size: 1 patty = 55 g; Calories = 119.4; Total Carb (g) = 15.5; Net Carb (g) = 13.8; Fat (g) = 6.3; Protein = 1.4

🟤 Potato Hash Brown Ready-To-Heat With Cheese ☞ serving size: 1 patty = 55 g; Calories = 136.4; Total Carb (g) = 13.2; Net Carb (g) = 11.8; Fat (g) = 8.3; Protein = 3.3

🟤 Potato Home Fries From Fresh ☞ serving size: 1 cup = 200 g; Calories = 366; Total Carb (g) = 37.5; Net Carb (g) = 34.3; Fat (g) = 23; Protein = 3.9

🟤 Potato Home Fries From Restaurant / Fast Food ☞ serving size: 1 cup = 200 g; Calories = 426; Total Carb (g) = 35.8; Net Carb (g) = 32.6; Fat (g) = 30.4; Protein = 3.7

🟤 Potato Home Fries Nfs ☞ serving size: 1 cup = 200 g; Calories = 390; Total Carb (g) = 36.8; Net Carb (g) = 33.6; Fat (g) = 26.1; Protein = 3.8

🟤 Potato Home Fries Ready-To-Heat ☞ serving size: 1 cup = 200 g; Calories = 390; Total Carb (g) = 36.8; Net Carb (g) = 33.6; Fat (g) = 26.1; Protein = 3.8

🟤 Potato Home Fries With Vegetables ☞ serving size: 1 cup = 200 g; Calories = 342; Total Carb (g) = 31.2; Net Carb (g) = 28; Fat (g) = 23.5; Protein = 3.5

🟤 Potato Mashed ☞ serving size: 1 cup = 242 g; Calories = 215.4;

Total Carb (g) = 35.5; Net Carb (g) = 32.3; Fat (g) = 6.8; Protein = 4

🥔 Potato Patty ☞ serving size: 1 patty = 55 g; Calories = 93.5; Total Carb (g) = 7.4; Net Carb (g) = 6.6; Fat (g) = 6.2; Protein = 2.1

🥔 Potato Skins Nfs ☞ serving size: skin from 1 small = 25 g; Calories = 49.5; Total Carb (g) = 4.1; Net Carb (g) = 3.7; Fat (g) = 3.1; Protein = 1.5

🥔 Potato Skins With Cheese ☞ serving size: skin from 1 small = 35 g; Calories = 69.3; Total Carb (g) = 5.8; Net Carb (g) = 5.2; Fat (g) = 4.3; Protein = 2.1

🥔 Potato Skins With Cheese And Bacon ☞ serving size: skin from 1 small = 35 g; Calories = 74.6; Total Carb (g) = 5.5; Net Carb (g) = 5; Fat (g) = 4.8; Protein = 2.7

🥔 Potato Skins Without Topping ☞ serving size: skin from 1 small = 25 g; Calories = 37.5; Total Carb (g) = 4.9; Net Carb (g) = 4.4; Fat (g) = 1.9; Protein = 0.5

🥔 Potato Tots Fast Food / Restaurant ☞ serving size: 1 cup = 130 g; Calories = 306.8; Total Carb (g) = 31.6; Net Carb (g) = 28.6; Fat (g) = 20; Protein = 2.5

🥔 Potato Tots From Fresh Fried Or Baked ☞ serving size: 1 cup = 130 g; Calories = 306.8; Total Carb (g) = 31.7; Net Carb (g) = 28.7; Fat (g) = 20.1; Protein = 2.5

🥔 Potato Tots Frozen Baked ☞ serving size: 1 cup = 130 g; Calories = 243.1; Total Carb (g) = 33.9; Net Carb (g) = 30.8; Fat (g) = 11.9; Protein = 2.6

🥔 Potato Tots Frozen Fried ☞ serving size: 1 cup = 130 g; Calories = 306.8; Total Carb (g) = 31.7; Net Carb (g) = 28.7; Fat (g) = 20.1; Protein = 2.5

🥔 Potato Tots Frozen Ns As To Fried Or Baked ☞ serving size: 1 cup = 130 g; Calories = 306.8; Total Carb (g) = 31.7; Net Carb (g) = 28.7; Fat (g) = 20.1; Protein = 2.5

🍲 Potato Tots Nfs ☞ serving size: 1 cup = 130 g; Calories = 306.8; Total Carb (g) = 31.7; Net Carb (g) = 28.7; Fat (g) = 20.1; Protein = 2.5

🍲 Potato Tots School ☞ serving size: 1 cup = 130 g; Calories = 213.2; Total Carb (g) = 25.1; Net Carb (g) = 22.9; Fat (g) = 11.9; Protein = 2.6

🍲 Potatoes Hash Browns Round Pieces Or Patty ☞ serving size: 1 round piece = 5.5 g; Calories = 15; Total Carb (g) = 1.6; Net Carb (g) = 1.4; Fat (g) = 0.9; Protein = 0.1

🍲 Puerto Rican Sandwich ☞ serving size: 1 sandwich = 160 g; Calories = 534.4; Total Carb (g) = 51; Net Carb (g) = 49.2; Fat (g) = 28.8; Protein = 17.1

🍲 Quesadilla With Chicken ☞ serving size: 1 each quesadilla = 180 g; Calories = 529.2; Total Carb (g) = 43.3; Net Carb (g) = 40.2; Fat (g) = 27.5; Protein = 27.1

🍲 Reuben Sandwich Corned Beef Sandwich With Sauerkraut And Cheese With Spread ☞ serving size: 1 sandwich = 181 g; Calories = 515.9; Total Carb (g) = 35; Net Carb (g) = 31; Fat (g) = 31.2; Protein = 22.8

🍲 Roast Beef Sandwich Plain ☞ serving size: 1 sandwich = 149 g; Calories = 363.6; Total Carb (g) = 33.1; Net Carb (g) = 31.2; Fat (g) = 15.4; Protein = 22.6

🍲 Roast Beef Sandwich With Bacon And Cheese Sauce ☞ serving size: 1 sandwich = 218 g; Calories = 754.3; Total Carb (g) = 42.9; Net Carb (g) = 41.4; Fat (g) = 45.3; Protein = 41

🍲 Roast Beef Sandwich With Cheese ☞ serving size: 1 sandwich = 190 g; Calories = 619.4; Total Carb (g) = 32.9; Net Carb (g) = 31.2; Fat (g) = 37.9; Protein = 34.3

🍲 Roast Beef Sandwich With Gravy ☞ serving size: 1 sandwich = 222 g; Calories = 490.6; Total Carb (g) = 30.9; Net Carb (g) = 29.1; Fat (g) = 28.4; Protein = 26.6

🍲 Roast Beef Submarine Sandwich On Roll Au Jus ☞ serving size:

1 sandwich = 193 g; Calories = 461.3; Total Carb (g) = 33.9; Net Carb (g) = 32.7; Fat (g) = 24.7; Protein = 23.8

🍔 Roast Beef Submarine Sandwich With Cheese Lettuce Tomato And Spread ☞ serving size: 1 submarine = 260 g; Calories = 494; Total Carb (g) = 48.6; Net Carb (g) = 47; Fat (g) = 19.1; Protein = 31

🍔 Roast Beef Submarine Sandwich With Lettuce Tomato And Spread ☞ serving size: 1 submarine = 240 g; Calories = 434.4; Total Carb (g) = 46.6; Net Carb (g) = 44.9; Fat (g) = 14.8; Protein = 27.9

🍔 Salami Sandwich With Spread ☞ serving size: 1 sandwich = 82 g; Calories = 254.2; Total Carb (g) = 26.3; Net Carb (g) = 24.9; Fat (g) = 11.6; Protein = 10.3

🍔 Sandwich Nfs ☞ serving size: 1 sandwich = 83 g; Calories = 249.8; Total Carb (g) = 27.3; Net Carb (g) = 25.9; Fat (g) = 11.5; Protein = 8.7

🍔 Sardine Sandwich With Lettuce And Spread ☞ serving size: 1 sandwich = 214 g; Calories = 483.6; Total Carb (g) = 31.5; Net Carb (g) = 29.3; Fat (g) = 27.2; Protein = 26.7

🍔 Sausage And Spaghetti Sauce Sandwich ☞ serving size: 1 sandwich = 189 g; Calories = 480.1; Total Carb (g) = 37.2; Net Carb (g) = 35.3; Fat (g) = 26; Protein = 22.6

🍔 Sausage Pizza ☞ serving size: 1 slice = 116 g; Calories = 324.8; Total Carb (g) = 35.5; Net Carb (g) = 32.9; Fat (g) = 14.3; Protein = 13.3

🍔 Sausage Sandwich ☞ serving size: 1 sandwich = 107 g; Calories = 316.7; Total Carb (g) = 27; Net Carb (g) = 25.7; Fat (g) = 16.4; Protein = 14.7

🍔 School Lunch Chicken Nuggets Whole Grain Breaded ☞ serving size: 5 pieces = 88 g; Calories = 237.6; Total Carb (g) = 20.1; Net Carb (g) = 18.2; Fat (g) = 11.4; Protein = 13.8

🍔 School Lunch Chicken Patty Whole Grain Breaded ☞ serving size: 1 patty = 86 g; Calories = 211.6; Total Carb (g) = 10.8; Net Carb (g) = 8.8; Fat (g) = 12; Protein = 15.2

🍪 School Lunch Pizza Big Daddys Ls 16 Inch 51% Whole Grain Rolled Edge Cheese Pizza Frozen ☞ serving size: 1 slice 1/8 per pizza = 155 g; Calories = 376.7; Total Carb (g) = 42; Net Carb (g) = 37.8; Fat (g) = 13.7; Protein = 21.5

🍪 School Lunch Pizza Big Daddys Ls 16 Inch 51% Whole Grain Rolled Edge Turkey Pepperoni Pizza Frozen ☞ serving size: 1 slice 1/8 per pizza = 156 g; Calories = 386.9; Total Carb (g) = 42.7; Net Carb (g) = 36.3; Fat (g) = 14.6; Protein = 21.3

🍪 School Lunch Pizza Cheese Topping Thick Crust Whole Grain Frozen Cooked ☞ serving size: 1 slice per 1/10 pizza = 124 g; Calories = 315; Total Carb (g) = 34.8; Net Carb (g) = 31.2; Fat (g) = 11.5; Protein = 18.1

🍪 School Lunch Pizza Cheese Topping Thin Crust Whole Grain Frozen Cooked ☞ serving size: 1 piece 4 inchx6 inch = 130 g; Calories = 321.1; Total Carb (g) = 40.7; Net Carb (g) = 35.5; Fat (g) = 10.3; Protein = 16.5

🍪 School Lunch Pizza Pepperoni Topping Thick Crust Whole Grain Frozen Cooked ☞ serving size: 1 slice per 1/10 pizza = 124 g; Calories = 321.2; Total Carb (g) = 35.1; Net Carb (g) = 29.8; Fat (g) = 12.2; Protein = 17.8

🍪 School Lunch Pizza Pepperoni Topping Thin Crust Whole Grain Frozen Cooked ☞ serving size: 1 piece 4 inchx6 inch = 127 g; Calories = 322.6; Total Carb (g) = 39.7; Net Carb (g) = 34.2; Fat (g) = 11; Protein = 16.2

🍪 School Lunch Pizza Sausage Topping Thick Crust Whole Grain Frozen Cooked ☞ serving size: 1 slice per 1/10 pizza = 129 g; Calories = 331.5; Total Carb (g) = 39.5; Net Carb (g) = 34.3; Fat (g) = 11.7; Protein = 17.1

🍪 School Lunch Pizza Sausage Topping Thin Crust Whole Grain Frozen Cooked ☞ serving size: 1 piece 4 inch x 6 inch = 133 g; Calo-

ries = 332.5; Total Carb (g) = 42.9; Net Carb (g) = 37.7; Fat (g) = 10.4; Protein = 16.8

🍪 School Lunch Pizza Tonys Breakfast Pizza Sausage Frozen ☞ serving size: 1 piece 3.2 oz = 91 g; Calories = 218.4; Total Carb (g) = 24.6; Net Carb (g) = 22.7; Fat (g) = 9.1; Protein = 9.5

🍪 School Lunch Pizza Tonys Smartpizza Whole Grain 4x6 Cheese Pizza 50/50 Cheese Frozen ☞ serving size: 1 piece 4 inch x 6 inch = 130 g; Calories = 302.9; Total Carb (g) = 38.1; Net Carb (g) = 33.1; Fat (g) = 9.8; Protein = 15.7

🍪 School Lunch Pizza Tonys Smartpizza Whole Grain 4x6 Pepperoni Pizza 50/50 Cheese Frozen ☞ serving size: 1 piece 4 inchx6 inch = 127 g; Calories = 302.3; Total Carb (g) = 36.6; Net Carb (g) = 31.4; Fat (g) = 10.4; Protein = 15.4

🍪 Scrambled Egg Sandwich ☞ serving size: 1 sandwich = 112 g; Calories = 229.6; Total Carb (g) = 27.4; Net Carb (g) = 26; Fat (g) = 8.2; Protein = 10.6

🍪 Shrimp Breaded And Fried ☞ serving size: 3 pieces shrimp = 39 g; Calories = 120.1; Total Carb (g) = 10.9; Net Carb (g) = 10.6; Fat (g) = 7.4; Protein = 3.1

🍪 Soft Serve Blended With Chocolate Candy ☞ serving size: 12 fl oz cup = 348 g; Calories = 633.4; Total Carb (g) = 93.3; Net Carb (g) = 92.6; Fat (g) = 22.5; Protein = 14

🍪 Steak And Cheese Sandwich Plain On Roll ☞ serving size: 1 sandwich = 170 g; Calories = 421.6; Total Carb (g) = 30.8; Net Carb (g) = 29.8; Fat (g) = 17.4; Protein = 33.5

🍪 Steak And Cheese Submarine Sandwich Plain On Roll ☞ serving size: 1 submarine = 197 g; Calories = 496.4; Total Carb (g) = 42.7; Net Carb (g) = 41.3; Fat (g) = 18.8; Protein = 36.6

🍪 Steak And Cheese Submarine Sandwich With Fried Peppers And Onions On Roll ☞ serving size: 1 submarine = 260 g; Calories =

603.2; Total Carb (g) = 47.4; Net Carb (g) = 45; Fat (g) = 26.2; Protein = 42.3

Steak Sandwich Plain On Biscuit ☞ serving size: 1 sandwich = 142 g; Calories = 407.5; Total Carb (g) = 52; Net Carb (g) = 50.7; Fat (g) = 13.3; Protein = 19.4

Steak Sandwich Plain On Roll ☞ serving size: 1 sandwich = 142 g; Calories = 329.4; Total Carb (g) = 23.4; Net Carb (g) = 22.6; Fat (g) = 11.5; Protein = 30.7

Steak Submarine Sandwich With Lettuce And Tomato ☞ serving size: 1 sandwich = 186 g; Calories = 375.7; Total Carb (g) = 37.8; Net Carb (g) = 36.1; Fat (g) = 11.1; Protein = 29.4

Strawberry Banana Smoothie Made With Ice And Low-Fat Yogurt ☞ serving size: 12 fl oz = 347 g; Calories = 225.6; Total Carb (g) = 52.2; Net Carb (g) = 49.1; Fat (g) = 0.5; Protein = 3

Submarine Sandwich Bacon Lettuce And Tomato On White Bread ☞ serving size: 6 inch sub = 148 g; Calories = 303.4; Total Carb (g) = 39.5; Net Carb (g) = 37.1; Fat (g) = 9.5; Protein = 14.9

Submarine Sandwich Cold Cut On White Bread With Lettuce And Tomato ☞ serving size: 6 inch sub = 196 g; Calories = 417.5; Total Carb (g) = 40; Net Carb (g) = 37.7; Fat (g) = 19.7; Protein = 20.6

Submarine Sandwich Ham On White Bread With Lettuce And Tomato ☞ serving size: 6 inch sub = 184 g; Calories = 277.8; Total Carb (g) = 42.2; Net Carb (g) = 39.8; Fat (g) = 4.7; Protein = 16.8

Submarine Sandwich Meatball Marinara On White Bread ☞ serving size: 6 inch sub = 209 g; Calories = 457.7; Total Carb (g) = 54.4; Net Carb (g) = 50; Fat (g) = 17.7; Protein = 20.4

Submarine Sandwich Oven Roasted Chicken On White Bread With Lettuce And Tomato ☞ serving size: 6 inch sub = 198 g; Calories = 310.9; Total Carb (g) = 42.3; Net Carb (g) = 39.9; Fat (g) = 6.2; Protein = 21.5

⬛ Submarine Sandwich Roast Beef On White Bread With Lettuce And Tomato ☞ serving size: 6 inch sub = 190 g; Calories = 296.4; Total Carb (g) = 38.7; Net Carb (g) = 37.3; Fat (g) = 5.2; Protein = 23.1

⬛ Submarine Sandwich Steak And Cheese On White Bread With Cheese Lettuce And Tomato ☞ serving size: 6 inch sub = 201 g; Calories = 367.8; Total Carb (g) = 43.2; Net Carb (g) = 40.8; Fat (g) = 10.7; Protein = 24.7

⬛ Submarine Sandwich Sweet Onion Chicken Teriyaki On White Bread With Lettuce Tomato And Sweet Onion Sauce ☞ serving size: 6 inch sub = 228 g; Calories = 353.4; Total Carb (g) = 51.4; Net Carb (g) = 48.7; Fat (g) = 5.4; Protein = 24.9

⬛ Submarine Sandwich Tuna On White Bread With Lettuce And Tomato ☞ serving size: 6 inch sub = 237 g; Calories = 516.7; Total Carb (g) = 37.8; Net Carb (g) = 36.1; Fat (g) = 28.5; Protein = 29.2

⬛ Submarine Sandwich Turkey Breast On White Bread With Lettuce And Tomato ☞ serving size: 6 inch sub = 184 g; Calories = 270.5; Total Carb (g) = 41.3; Net Carb (g) = 38.9; Fat (g) = 4.3; Protein = 16.8

⬛ Submarine Sandwich Turkey Roast Beef And Ham On White Bread With Lettuce And Tomato ☞ serving size: 12 inch sub = 413 g; Calories = 603; Total Carb (g) = 84.1; Net Carb (g) = 78.3; Fat (g) = 10; Protein = 44

⬛ Subway B.l.t. Sub On White Bread With Bacon Lettuce And Tomato ☞ serving size: 6 inch sub = 148 g; Calories = 303.4; Total Carb (g) = 39.5; Net Carb (g) = 37.1; Fat (g) = 9.5; Protein = 14.9

⬛ Subway Black Forest Ham Sub On White Bread With Lettuce And Tomato ☞ serving size: 6 inch sub = 184 g; Calories = 277.8; Total Carb (g) = 42.2; Net Carb (g) = 39.8; Fat (g) = 4.7; Protein = 16.8

⬛ Subway Cold Cut Sub On White Bread With Lettuce And Tomato ☞ serving size: 6 inch sub = 196 g; Calories = 419.4; Total Carb (g) = 40; Net Carb (g) = 37.7; Fat (g) = 19.7; Protein = 20.6

Subway Meatball Marinara Sub On White Bread (No Toppings) ☞ serving size: 6 inch sub = 209 g; Calories = 457.7; Total Carb (g) = 54.4; Net Carb (g) = 50; Fat (g) = 17.7; Protein = 20.4

Subway Oven Roasted Chicken Sub On White Bread With Lettuce And Tomato ☞ serving size: 6 inch sub = 198 g; Calories = 310.9; Total Carb (g) = 42.3; Net Carb (g) = 39.9; Fat (g) = 6.2; Protein = 21.5

Subway Roast Beef Sub On White Bread With Lettuce And Tomato ☞ serving size: 6 inch sub = 190 g; Calories = 294.5; Total Carb (g) = 38.7; Net Carb (g) = 37.3; Fat (g) = 5.2; Protein = 23.1

Subway Steak & Cheese Sub On White Bread With American Cheese Lettuce And Tomato ☞ serving size: 6 inch sub = 201 g; Calories = 367.8; Total Carb (g) = 43.2; Net Carb (g) = 40.8; Fat (g) = 10.7; Protein = 24.7

Subway Subway Club Sub On White Bread With Lettuce And Tomato ☞ serving size: 6 inch sub = 207 g; Calories = 302.2; Total Carb (g) = 42.2; Net Carb (g) = 39.3; Fat (g) = 5; Protein = 22.1

Subway Sweet Onion Chicken Teriyaki Sub On White Bread With Lettuce Tomato And Sweet Onion Sauce ☞ serving size: 6 inch sub = 228 g; Calories = 353.4; Total Carb (g) = 51.4; Net Carb (g) = 48.7; Fat (g) = 5.4; Protein = 24.9

Subway Tuna Sub ☞ serving size: 6 inch sub = 237 g; Calories = 523.8; Total Carb (g) = 37.8; Net Carb (g) = 36.1; Fat (g) = 28.5; Protein = 29.2

Subway Turkey Breast Sub On White Bread With Lettuce And Tomato ☞ serving size: 6 inch sub = 184 g; Calories = 270.5; Total Carb (g) = 41.3; Net Carb (g) = 38.9; Fat (g) = 4.3; Protein = 16.8

Sundae Caramel ☞ serving size: 1 sundae = 155 g; Calories = 303.8; Total Carb (g) = 49.3; Net Carb (g) = 49.3; Fat (g) = 9.3; Protein = 7.3

🍪 Sundae Hot Fudge ☞ serving size: 1 sundae = 158 g; Calories = 284.4; Total Carb (g) = 47.7; Net Carb (g) = 47.7; Fat (g) = 8.6; Protein = 5.6

🍪 Sundae Strawberry ☞ serving size: 1 sundae = 153 g; Calories = 267.8; Total Carb (g) = 44.7; Net Carb (g) = 44.7; Fat (g) = 7.9; Protein = 6.3

🍪 Taco Bell Bean Burrito ☞ serving size: 1 each burrito = 185 g; Calories = 386.7; Total Carb (g) = 57.8; Net Carb (g) = 50; Fat (g) = 11.2; Protein = 13.6

🍪 Taco Bell Burrito Supreme With Beef ☞ serving size: 1 burrito = 241 g; Calories = 441; Total Carb (g) = 56.3; Net Carb (g) = 47.4; Fat (g) = 16.4; Protein = 16.9

🍪 Taco Bell Burrito Supreme With Chicken ☞ serving size: 1 item = 248 g; Calories = 443.9; Total Carb (g) = 50.9; Net Carb (g) = 44.9; Fat (g) = 15.9; Protein = 24.4

🍪 Taco Bell Burrito Supreme With Steak ☞ serving size: 1 item = 248 g; Calories = 453.8; Total Carb (g) = 50.4; Net Carb (g) = 44.4; Fat (g) = 18; Protein = 22.6

🍪 Taco Bell Nachos ☞ serving size: 1 serving = 80 g; Calories = 280; Total Carb (g) = 27.9; Net Carb (g) = 25.4; Fat (g) = 17.2; Protein = 3.5

🍪 Taco Bell Nachos Supreme ☞ serving size: 1 serving = 222 g; Calories = 495.1; Total Carb (g) = 47.5; Net Carb (g) = 39.3; Fat (g) = 27.7; Protein = 13.8

🍪 Taco Bell Original Taco With Beef Cheese And Lettuce ☞ serving size: 1 each taco = 69 g; Calories = 158; Total Carb (g) = 13.7; Net Carb (g) = 11; Fat (g) = 8.8; Protein = 6.1

🍪 Taco Bell Soft Taco With Beef Cheese And Lettuce ☞ serving size: 1 each taco = 102 g; Calories = 210.1; Total Carb (g) = 20.6; Net Carb (g) = 17.7; Fat (g) = 10; Protein = 9.4

🍪 Taco Bell Soft Taco With Chicken Cheese And Lettuce ☞

serving size: 1 each taco = 98 g; Calories = 185.2; Total Carb (g) = 19.3; Net Carb (g) = 18.1; Fat (g) = 6.2; Protein = 13

🍔 Taco Bell Soft Taco With Steak ☞ serving size: 1 item = 127 g; Calories = 285.8; Total Carb (g) = 21.9; Net Carb (g) = 19.8; Fat (g) = 15.4; Protein = 15

🍔 Taco Bell Taco Salad ☞ serving size: 1 item = 533 g; Calories = 906.1; Total Carb (g) = 80.5; Net Carb (g) = 64.5; Fat (g) = 48.9; Protein = 35.7

🍔 Taco With Beef Cheese And Lettuce Hard Shell ☞ serving size: 1 each taco = 69 g; Calories = 155.9; Total Carb (g) = 13.7; Net Carb (g) = 11; Fat (g) = 8.8; Protein = 6.1

🍔 Taco With Beef Cheese And Lettuce Soft ☞ serving size: 1 each taco = 102 g; Calories = 210.1; Total Carb (g) = 20.6; Net Carb (g) = 17.7; Fat (g) = 10; Protein = 9.4

🍔 Taco With Chicken Lettuce And Cheese Soft ☞ serving size: 1 each taco = 98 g; Calories = 185.2; Total Carb (g) = 19.3; Net Carb (g) = 18.1; Fat (g) = 6.2; Protein = 13

🍔 Taquito Or Flauta With Egg ☞ serving size: 1 small taquito = 36 g; Calories = 91.8; Total Carb (g) = 9.9; Net Carb (g) = 9.1; Fat (g) = 4.1; Protein = 3.6

🍔 Taquito Or Flauta With Egg And Breakfast Meat ☞ serving size: 1 small taquito = 36 g; Calories = 96.1; Total Carb (g) = 9.3; Net Carb (g) = 8.7; Fat (g) = 4.6; Protein = 4.1

🍔 Tomato Sandwich ☞ serving size: 1 sandwich = 134 g; Calories = 234.5; Total Carb (g) = 31.8; Net Carb (g) = 29.4; Fat (g) = 9.3; Protein = 5.9

🍔 Triple Cheeseburger 3 Medium Patties With Condiments On Bun From Fast Food / Restaurant ☞ serving size: 1 triple cheeseburger = 420 g; Calories = 1192.8; Total Carb (g) = 61.1; Net Carb (g) = 57.8; Fat (g) = 72.5; Protein = 73.7

🍔 Tuna Melt Sandwich ☞ serving size: 1 sandwich = 150 g; Calories = 348; Total Carb (g) = 25.6; Net Carb (g) = 24.1; Fat (g) = 20.3; Protein = 15.9

🍔 Tuna Salad Sandwich ☞ serving size: 1 sandwich = 157 g; Calories = 254.3; Total Carb (g) = 35.4; Net Carb (g) = 33.5; Fat (g) = 5.5; Protein = 16.1

🍔 Tuna Salad Sandwich With Lettuce ☞ serving size: 1 sandwich = 167 g; Calories = 255.5; Total Carb (g) = 35.8; Net Carb (g) = 33.8; Fat (g) = 5.6; Protein = 16.2

🍔 Turkey And Bacon Submarine Sandwich With Cheese Lettuce Tomato And Spread ☞ serving size: 1 submarine = 260 g; Calories = 577.2; Total Carb (g) = 45.4; Net Carb (g) = 42.8; Fat (g) = 29.8; Protein = 31.7

🍔 Turkey And Bacon Submarine Sandwich With Lettuce Tomato And Spread ☞ serving size: 1 submarine = 240 g; Calories = 494.4; Total Carb (g) = 46.7; Net Carb (g) = 44; Fat (g) = 22.7; Protein = 25

🍔 Turkey Ham And Roast Beef Club Sandwich With Lettuce Tomato And Spread ☞ serving size: 1 sandwich = 240 g; Calories = 398.4; Total Carb (g) = 36.4; Net Carb (g) = 34; Fat (g) = 19.3; Protein = 18.7

🍔 Turkey Or Chicken Burger Plain On Bun From Fast Food / Restaurant ☞ serving size: 1 sandwich = 145 g; Calories = 337.9; Total Carb (g) = 30.1; Net Carb (g) = 29.1; Fat (g) = 11.1; Protein = 28.9

🍔 Turkey Or Chicken Burger Plain On Wheat Bun ☞ serving size: 1 sandwich = 145 g; Calories = 329.2; Total Carb (g) = 27.2; Net Carb (g) = 24; Fat (g) = 11.1; Protein = 29.9

🍔 Turkey Or Chicken Burger Plain On White Bun ☞ serving size: 1 sandwich = 145 g; Calories = 337.9; Total Carb (g) = 30.1; Net Carb (g) = 29.1; Fat (g) = 11.1; Protein = 28.9

🍔 Turkey Or Chicken Burger With Condiments On Bun From Fast

Food / Restaurant ☞ serving size: 1 sandwich = 200 g; Calories = 380; Total Carb (g) = 33.5; Net Carb (g) = 31.9; Fat (g) = 14.4; Protein = 29

🍔 Turkey Or Chicken Burger With Condiments On Wheat Bun ☞ serving size: 1 sandwich = 200 g; Calories = 370; Total Carb (g) = 30.7; Net Carb (g) = 26.9; Fat (g) = 14.4; Protein = 30

🍔 Turkey Or Chicken Burger With Condiments On White Bun ☞ serving size: 1 sandwich = 200 g; Calories = 380; Total Carb (g) = 33.5; Net Carb (g) = 31.9; Fat (g) = 14.4; Protein = 29

🍔 Turkey Or Chicken Burger With Condiments On Whole Wheat Bun ☞ serving size: 1 sandwich = 200 g; Calories = 370; Total Carb (g) = 30.7; Net Carb (g) = 26.9; Fat (g) = 14.4; Protein = 30

🍔 Turkey Salad Or Turkey Spread Sandwich ☞ serving size: 1 sandwich = 141 g; Calories = 321.5; Total Carb (g) = 27.6; Net Carb (g) = 25.8; Fat (g) = 13.9; Protein = 19.9

🍔 Turkey Sandwich With Gravy ☞ serving size: 1 sandwich = 284 g; Calories = 383.4; Total Carb (g) = 33.1; Net Carb (g) = 31.2; Fat (g) = 8.6; Protein = 40.3

🍔 Turkey Sandwich With Spread ☞ serving size: 1 sandwich = 143 g; Calories = 318.9; Total Carb (g) = 26.7; Net Carb (g) = 25.3; Fat (g) = 9.9; Protein = 28.7

🍔 Vanilla Light Soft-Serve Ice Cream With Cone ☞ serving size: 1 item = 120 g; Calories = 195.6; Total Carb (g) = 31.6; Net Carb (g) = 31.5; Fat (g) = 5.8; Protein = 5.1

🍔 Vegetable Submarine Sandwich With Fat Free Spread ☞ serving size: 1 submarine = 240 g; Calories = 300; Total Carb (g) = 55.3; Net Carb (g) = 51.7; Fat (g) = 4.7; Protein = 9.3

🍔 Vegetable Submarine Sandwich With Spread ☞ serving size: 1 submarine = 167 g; Calories = 310.6; Total Carb (g) = 31.8; Net Carb (g) = 29.4; Fat (g) = 17.7; Protein = 6.3

🥞 Waffle Chocolate ☞ serving size: 1 miniature/bite size waffle = 10 g; Calories = 43.3; Total Carb (g) = 4.9; Net Carb (g) = 4.6; Fat (g) = 2.3; Protein = 0.9

🥞 Waffle Chocolate From Fast Food / Restaurant ☞ serving size: 1 miniature/bite size waffle = 10 g; Calories = 47.6; Total Carb (g) = 4.6; Net Carb (g) = 4.3; Fat (g) = 2.9; Protein = 0.9

🥞 Waffle Chocolate From Frozen ☞ serving size: 1 miniature/bite size waffle = 10 g; Calories = 32; Total Carb (g) = 4.9; Net Carb (g) = 4.6; Fat (g) = 1.1; Protein = 0.7

🥞 Waffle Cinnamon ☞ serving size: 1 miniature/bite size waffle = 10 g; Calories = 36.8; Total Carb (g) = 4.2; Net Carb (g) = 3.9; Fat (g) = 1.9; Protein = 0.9

🥞 Waffle Cornmeal ☞ serving size: 1 miniature/bite size waffle = 10 g; Calories = 26.4; Total Carb (g) = 3.3; Net Carb (g) = 3.2; Fat (g) = 1.1; Protein = 0.7

🥞 Waffle Fruit ☞ serving size: 1 miniature/bite size waffle = 10 g; Calories = 30.4; Total Carb (g) = 3.6; Net Carb (g) = 3.3; Fat (g) = 1.5; Protein = 0.7

🥞 Waffle Fruit From Fast Food / Restaurant ☞ serving size: 1 miniature/bite size waffle = 10 g; Calories = 35; Total Carb (g) = 3.5; Net Carb (g) = 3.2; Fat (g) = 2.1; Protein = 0.7

🥞 Waffle Fruit From Frozen ☞ serving size: 1 miniature/bite size waffle = 10 g; Calories = 29.6; Total Carb (g) = 4.7; Net Carb (g) = 4.4; Fat (g) = 0.9; Protein = 0.7

🥞 Waffle Plain ☞ serving size: 1 miniature/bite size waffle = 10 g; Calories = 36.8; Total Carb (g) = 4.2; Net Carb (g) = 3.9; Fat (g) = 1.9; Protein = 0.9

🥞 Waffle Plain From Fast Food / Restaurant ☞ serving size: 1 miniature/bite size waffle = 10 g; Calories = 42.2; Total Carb (g) = 3.9; Net Carb (g) = 3.7; Fat (g) = 2.6; Protein = 0.8

Waffle Plain Reduced Fat ☞ serving size: 1 miniature/bite size waffle = 10 g; Calories = 33.8; Total Carb (g) = 4.3; Net Carb (g) = 4; Fat (g) = 1.4; Protein = 0.9

Waffle Plain Reduced Fat From Frozen ☞ serving size: 1 miniature/bite size waffle = 10 g; Calories = 28.9; Total Carb (g) = 4.6; Net Carb (g) = 4.5; Fat (g) = 0.7; Protein = 0.9

Waffle Whole Grain ☞ serving size: 1 miniature/bite size waffle = 10 g; Calories = 36; Total Carb (g) = 3.9; Net Carb (g) = 3.5; Fat (g) = 1.9; Protein = 0.9

Waffle Whole Grain From Fast Food / Restaurant ☞ serving size: 1 miniature/bite size waffle = 10 g; Calories = 41.6; Total Carb (g) = 3.6; Net Carb (g) = 3.3; Fat (g) = 2.7; Protein = 0.9

Waffle Whole Grain From Frozen ☞ serving size: 1 miniature/bite size waffle = 10 g; Calories = 28.8; Total Carb (g) = 4.7; Net Carb (g) = 4.3; Fat (g) = 0.8; Protein = 0.7

Waffle Whole Grain Fruit From Frozen ☞ serving size: 1 miniature/bite size waffle = 10 g; Calories = 27.7; Total Carb (g) = 4.5; Net Carb (g) = 4.1; Fat (g) = 0.8; Protein = 0.7

Waffle Whole Grain Reduced Fat ☞ serving size: 1 miniature/bite size waffle = 10 g; Calories = 32.9; Total Carb (g) = 4; Net Carb (g) = 3.6; Fat (g) = 1.5; Protein = 1

Wendys Chicken Nuggets ☞ serving size: 5 pieces = 68 g; Calories = 221.7; Total Carb (g) = 9.7; Net Carb (g) = 9.7; Fat (g) = 15.3; Protein = 11.2

Wendys Classic Double With Cheese ☞ serving size: 1 item = 310 g; Calories = 747.1; Total Carb (g) = 36.3; Net Carb (g) = 32.9; Fat (g) = 44; Protein = 51.2

Wendys Classic Single Hamburger No Cheese ☞ serving size: 1 item = 218 g; Calories = 464.3; Total Carb (g) = 36.7; Net Carb (g) = 33.8; Fat (g) = 23.1; Protein = 27.5

🍔 Wendys Classic Single Hamburger With Cheese ☞ serving size: 1 item = 236 g; Calories = 521.6; Total Carb (g) = 33.5; Net Carb (g) = 30.2; Fat (g) = 27.4; Protein = 35.1

🍔 Wendys Crispy Chicken Sandwich ☞ serving size: 1 sandwich = 126 g; Calories = 350.3; Total Carb (g) = 33.2; Net Carb (g) = 33.2; Fat (g) = 17.6; Protein = 14.8

🍔 Wendys Daves Hot N Juicy 1/4 Lb Single ☞ serving size: 1 sandwich = 215 g; Calories = 576.2; Total Carb (g) = 38.1; Net Carb (g) = 35.8; Fat (g) = 34; Protein = 29.4

🍔 Wendys Double Stack With Cheese ☞ serving size: 1 sandwich = 146 g; Calories = 416.1; Total Carb (g) = 22.4; Net Carb (g) = 22.4; Fat (g) = 24.2; Protein = 27.1

🍔 Wendys French Fries ☞ serving size: 1 kid's meal serving = 71 g; Calories = 213.7; Total Carb (g) = 28.2; Net Carb (g) = 25.4; Fat (g) = 10; Protein = 2.7

🍔 Wendys Frosty Dairy Dessert ☞ serving size: 1 junior 6 oz. cup = 113 g; Calories = 149.2; Total Carb (g) = 26.7; Net Carb (g) = 23; Fat (g) = 2.9; Protein = 3.9

🍔 Wendys Homestyle Chicken Fillet Sandwich ☞ serving size: 1 item = 230 g; Calories = 492.2; Total Carb (g) = 49.6; Net Carb (g) = 46.6; Fat (g) = 18.6; Protein = 31.7

🍔 Wendys Jr. Hamburger With Cheese ☞ serving size: 1 item = 129 g; Calories = 330.2; Total Carb (g) = 32.2; Net Carb (g) = 30.4; Fat (g) = 14.8; Protein = 16.9

🍔 Wendys Jr. Hamburger Without Cheese ☞ serving size: 1 item = 117 g; Calories = 284.3; Total Carb (g) = 33.3; Net Carb (g) = 31.3; Fat (g) = 10.2; Protein = 14.8

🍔 Wendys Ultimate Chicken Grill Sandwich ☞ serving size: 1 item = 225 g; Calories = 402.8; Total Carb (g) = 42.5; Net Carb (g) = 40; Fat (g) = 11.3; Protein = 33.1

🦪 Wrap Sandwich Filled With Beef Patty Cheese And Spread And/or Sauce ☞ serving size: 1 snack wrap sandwich = 126 g; Calories = 340.2; Total Carb (g) = 23.8; Net Carb (g) = 22; Fat (g) = 19.6; Protein = 16.1

🦪 Wrap Sandwich Filled With Meat Poultry Or Fish And Vegetables ☞ serving size: 1 sandwich = 240 g; Calories = 448.8; Total Carb (g) = 32.1; Net Carb (g) = 29.2; Fat (g) = 22.3; Protein = 30.7

🦪 Wrap Sandwich Filled With Meat Poultry Or Fish Vegetables And Cheese ☞ serving size: 1 sandwich = 280 g; Calories = 574; Total Carb (g) = 39.1; Net Carb (g) = 36; Fat (g) = 31.3; Protein = 34.7

🦪 Wrap Sandwich Filled With Meat Poultry Or Fish Vegetables And Rice ☞ serving size: 1 sandwich = 433 g; Calories = 679.8; Total Carb (g) = 78.8; Net Carb (g) = 71.4; Fat (g) = 23.3; Protein = 39.4

🦪 Wrap Sandwich Filled With Meat Poultry Or Fish Vegetables Rice And Cheese ☞ serving size: 1 sandwich = 467 g; Calories = 761.2; Total Carb (g) = 85.2; Net Carb (g) = 76.8; Fat (g) = 29.1; Protein = 40.7

🦪 Wrap Sandwich Filled With Vegetables ☞ serving size: 1 sandwich = 273 g; Calories = 333.1; Total Carb (g) = 37.8; Net Carb (g) = 33.1; Fat (g) = 17; Protein = 8.7

🦪 Wrap Sandwich Filled With Vegetables And Rice ☞ serving size: 1 sandwich = 404 g; Calories = 549.4; Total Carb (g) = 80; Net Carb (g) = 71.5; Fat (g) = 20.1; Protein = 13.7

🦪 Yogurt Parfait Lowfat With Fruit And Granola ☞ serving size: 1 item = 149 g; Calories = 125.2; Total Carb (g) = 23.6; Net Carb (g) = 22; Fat (g) = 1.5; Protein = 5

17

FATS AND OILS

🥑 Almond Oil ☞ serving size: 1 tablespoon = 13.6 g; Calories = 120.2; Total Carb (g) = 0; Net Carb (g) = 0; Fat (g) = 13.6; Protein = 0

🥑 Animal Fat Or Drippings ☞ serving size: 1 cup = 205 g; Calories = 1724.1; Total Carb (g) = 0; Net Carb (g) = 0; Fat (g) = 189; Protein = 4.6

🥑 Apricot Kernel Oil ☞ serving size: 1 tablespoon = 13.6 g; Calories = 120.2; Total Carb (g) = 0; Net Carb (g) = 0; Fat (g) = 13.6; Protein = 0

🥑 Avocado Oil ☞ serving size: 1 tbsp = 14 g; Calories = 123.8; Total Carb (g) = 0; Net Carb (g) = 0; Fat (g) = 14; Protein = 0

🥑 Bacon Grease ☞ serving size: 1 tsp = 4.3 g; Calories = 38.6; Total Carb (g) = 0; Net Carb (g) = 0; Fat (g) = 4.3; Protein = 0

🥑 Beef Tallow ☞ serving size: 1 tbsp = 12.8 g; Calories = 115.5; Total Carb (g) = 0; Net Carb (g) = 0; Fat (g) = 12.8; Protein = 0

🥑 Butter Light Stick With Salt ☞ serving size: 1 tablespoon = 14 g; Calories = 69.9; Total Carb (g) = 0; Net Carb (g) = 0; Fat (g) = 7.7; Protein = 0.5

🍪 Butter Light Stick Without Salt ☞ serving size: 1 tablespoon = 14 g; Calories = 69.9; Total Carb (g) = 0; Net Carb (g) = 0; Fat (g) = 7.7; Protein = 0.5

🍪 Butter Replacement Without Fat Powder ☞ serving size: 1 cup = 80 g; Calories = 298.4; Total Carb (g) = 71.2; Net Carb (g) = 71.2; Fat (g) = 0.8; Protein = 1.6

🍪 Butter Whipped Tub Salted ☞ serving size: 1 cup = 151 g; Calories = 1084.2; Total Carb (g) = 4.3; Net Carb (g) = 4.3; Fat (g) = 118.2; Protein = 0.7

🍪 Butter-Margarine Blend Stick Salted ☞ serving size: 1 cup = 227 g; Calories = 1627.6; Total Carb (g) = 0.9; Net Carb (g) = 0.9; Fat (g) = 183.7; Protein = 1.1

🍪 Canola Oil ☞ serving size: 1 tbsp = 14 g; Calories = 123.8; Total Carb (g) = 0; Net Carb (g) = 0; Fat (g) = 14; Protein = 0

🍪 Cheese Cream Light Or Lite ☞ serving size: 1 cup = 240 g; Calories = 482.4; Total Carb (g) = 19.5; Net Carb (g) = 19.5; Fat (g) = 36.7; Protein = 18.8

🍪 Cheese Spread Cream Cheese Light Or Lite ☞ serving size: 1 cup = 240 g; Calories = 482.4; Total Carb (g) = 19.5; Net Carb (g) = 19.5; Fat (g) = 36.7; Protein = 18.8

🍪 Cocoa Butter ☞ serving size: 1 tablespoon = 13.6 g; Calories = 120.2; Total Carb (g) = 0; Net Carb (g) = 0; Fat (g) = 13.6; Protein = 0

🍪 Coconut Oil ☞ serving size: 1 tbsp = 13.6 g; Calories = 121.3; Total Carb (g) = 0; Net Carb (g) = 0; Fat (g) = 13.5; Protein = 0

🍪 Cod Liver Oil ☞ serving size: 1 tsp = 4.5 g; Calories = 40.6; Total Carb (g) = 0; Net Carb (g) = 0; Fat (g) = 4.5; Protein = 0

🍪 Coffee Creamer Liquid Fat Free Flavored ☞ serving size: 1 cup = 240 g; Calories = 360; Total Carb (g) = 76.4; Net Carb (g) = 76.4; Fat (g) = 6.3; Protein = 1.4

✅ Coleslaw Dressing ☞ serving size: 1 cup = 250 g; Calories = 975; Total Carb (g) = 59.5; Net Carb (g) = 59.3; Fat (g) = 83.5; Protein = 2.3

✅ Coleslaw Salad Dressing ☞ serving size: 1 tbsp = 16 g; Calories = 64.6; Total Carb (g) = 3.6; Net Carb (g) = 3.6; Fat (g) = 5.5; Protein = 0.1

✅ Corn Oil ☞ serving size: 1 tbsp = 13.6 g; Calories = 122.4; Total Carb (g) = 0; Net Carb (g) = 0; Fat (g) = 13.6; Protein = 0

✅ Cottonseed Oil ☞ serving size: 1 tablespoon = 13.6 g; Calories = 120.2; Total Carb (g) = 0; Net Carb (g) = 0; Fat (g) = 13.6; Protein = 0

✅ Cream Half And Half ☞ serving size: 1 cup = 240 g; Calories = 295.2; Total Carb (g) = 11.4; Net Carb (g) = 11.4; Fat (g) = 24.9; Protein = 7.5

✅ Cream Half And Half Flavored ☞ serving size: 1 cup = 240 g; Calories = 292.8; Total Carb (g) = 11.8; Net Carb (g) = 11.8; Fat (g) = 24.5; Protein = 7.4

✅ Cream Heavy ☞ serving size: 1 cup = 240 g; Calories = 816; Total Carb (g) = 6.6; Net Carb (g) = 6.6; Fat (g) = 86.6; Protein = 6.8

✅ Cream Light ☞ serving size: 1 cup = 240 g; Calories = 458.4; Total Carb (g) = 6.8; Net Carb (g) = 6.8; Fat (g) = 45.8; Protein = 7.1

✅ Cream Ns As To Light Heavy Or Half And Half ☞ serving size: 1 cup = 240 g; Calories = 295.2; Total Carb (g) = 11.4; Net Carb (g) = 11.4; Fat (g) = 24.9; Protein = 7.5

✅ Cream Whipped ☞ serving size: 1 cup = 120 g; Calories = 411.6; Total Carb (g) = 10.2; Net Carb (g) = 10.2; Fat (g) = 40.7; Protein = 3.2

✅ Creamy Dressing Made With Sour Cream And/or Buttermilk And Oil Reduced Calorie ☞ serving size: 1 tbsp = 15 g; Calories = 24; Total Carb (g) = 1.1; Net Carb (g) = 1.1; Fat (g) = 2.1; Protein = 0.2

✅ Creamy Dressing Made With Sour Cream And/or Buttermilk And Oil Reduced Calorie Cholesterol-Free ☞ serving size: 1 tbsp =

15 g; Calories = 21; Total Carb (g) = 2.4; Net Carb (g) = 2.4; Fat (g) = 1.2; Protein = 0.2

🍥 Creamy Dressing Made With Sour Cream And/or Buttermilk And Oil Reduced Calorie Fat-Free ☞ serving size: 1 tbsp = 17 g; Calories = 18.2; Total Carb (g) = 3.4; Net Carb (g) = 3.4; Fat (g) = 0.5; Protein = 0.2

🍥 Creamy Poppyseed Salad Dressing ☞ serving size: 2 tbsp = 33 g; Calories = 131.7; Total Carb (g) = 7.8; Net Carb (g) = 7.7; Fat (g) = 11; Protein = 0.3

🍥 Dressing Honey Mustard Fat-Free ☞ serving size: 2 tbsp (1 nlea serving) = 30 g; Calories = 50.7; Total Carb (g) = 11.5; Net Carb (g) = 11.2; Fat (g) = 0.4; Protein = 0.3

🍥 Fat Back Cooked ☞ serving size: 1 slice (2-1/4" x 1-3/4" x 1/4") = 26 g; Calories = 195; Total Carb (g) = 0; Net Carb (g) = 0; Fat (g) = 21.3; Protein = 0.7

🍥 Fat Goose ☞ serving size: 1 tbsp = 12.8 g; Calories = 115.2; Total Carb (g) = 0; Net Carb (g) = 0; Fat (g) = 12.8; Protein = 0

🍥 Fat Turkey ☞ serving size: 1 tbsp = 12.8 g; Calories = 115.2; Total Carb (g) = 0; Net Carb (g) = 0; Fat (g) = 12.8; Protein = 0

🍥 Fish Oil Menhaden Fully Hydrogenated ☞ serving size: 1 tbsp = 12.5 g; Calories = 112.8; Total Carb (g) = 0; Net Carb (g) = 0; Fat (g) = 12.5; Protein = 0

🍥 Flaxseed Oil ☞ serving size: 1 tbsp = 13.6 g; Calories = 120.2; Total Carb (g) = 0; Net Carb (g) = 0; Fat (g) = 13.6; Protein = 0

🍥 French Or Catalina Dressing ☞ serving size: 1 cup = 250 g; Calories = 1142.5; Total Carb (g) = 39; Net Carb (g) = 39; Fat (g) = 112; Protein = 1.9

🍥 Grapeseed Oil ☞ serving size: 1 tablespoon = 13.6 g; Calories = 120.2; Total Carb (g) = 0; Net Carb (g) = 0; Fat (g) = 13.6; Protein = 0

🍪 Hazelnut Oil ☞ serving size: 1 tablespoon = 13.6 g; Calories = 120.2; Total Carb (g) = 0; Net Carb (g) = 0; Fat (g) = 13.6; Protein = 0

🍪 Herring Oil ☞ serving size: 1 tbsp = 13.6 g; Calories = 122.7; Total Carb (g) = 0; Net Carb (g) = 0; Fat (g) = 13.6; Protein = 0

🍪 Honey Butter ☞ serving size: 1 cup = 288 g; Calories = 1353.6; Total Carb (g) = 142.2; Net Carb (g) = 141.9; Fat (g) = 93.7; Protein = 1.5

🍪 Honey Mustard Salad Dressing ☞ serving size: 2 tbsp = 30 g; Calories = 139.2; Total Carb (g) = 7; Net Carb (g) = 6.9; Fat (g) = 12.3; Protein = 0.3

🍪 Hydrogenated Soybean And Palm Oil ☞ serving size: 1 tbsp = 12.8 g; Calories = 113.2; Total Carb (g) = 0; Net Carb (g) = 0; Fat (g) = 12.8; Protein = 0

🍪 Italian Salad Dressing ☞ serving size: 1 tablespoon = 15 g; Calories = 15.3; Total Carb (g) = 1.5; Net Carb (g) = 1.5; Fat (g) = 1; Protein = 0.1

🍪 Korean Dressing Or Marinade ☞ serving size: 1 cup = 246 g; Calories = 831.5; Total Carb (g) = 31.9; Net Carb (g) = 30.6; Fat (g) = 75.6; Protein = 7.9

🍪 Lard ☞ serving size: 1 tbsp = 12.8 g; Calories = 115.5; Total Carb (g) = 0; Net Carb (g) = 0; Fat (g) = 12.8; Protein = 0

🍪 Lowfat French Salad Dressing ☞ serving size: 1 tablespoon = 16 g; Calories = 37.3; Total Carb (g) = 4.7; Net Carb (g) = 4.5; Fat (g) = 2.2; Protein = 0.1

🍪 Margarine ☞ serving size: 1 tsp = 4.7 g; Calories = 33.8; Total Carb (g) = 0; Net Carb (g) = 0; Fat (g) = 3.8; Protein = 0

🍪 Margarine (Unsalted) ☞ serving size: 1 tbsp = 14.2 g; Calories = 101.8; Total Carb (g) = 0.1; Net Carb (g) = 0.1; Fat (g) = 11.5; Protein = 0

🍪 Margarine 80% Fat Stick Includes Regular And Hydrogenated

Corn And Soybean Oils ☞ serving size: 1 tbsp = 14 g; Calories = 100.4; Total Carb (g) = 0.1; Net Carb (g) = 0.1; Fat (g) = 11.3; Protein = 0

🍴 Margarine 80% Fat Tub Canola Harvest Soft Spread (Canola Palm And Palm Kernel Oils) ☞ serving size: 1 tablespoon (1 nlea serving) = 14 g; Calories = 102.2; Total Carb (g) = 0.2; Net Carb (g) = 0.2; Fat (g) = 11.2; Protein = 0.1

🍴 Margarine Industrial Non-Dairy Cottonseed Soy Oil (Partially Hydrogenated) For Flaky Pastries ☞ serving size: 1 tbsp = 14 g; Calories = 100; Total Carb (g) = 0; Net Carb (g) = 0; Fat (g) = 11.2; Protein = 0.3

🍴 Margarine Industrial Soy And Partially Hydrogenated Soy Oil Use For Baking Sauces And Candy ☞ serving size: 1 tbsp = 14 g; Calories = 100; Total Carb (g) = 0.1; Net Carb (g) = 0.1; Fat (g) = 11.2; Protein = 0

🍴 Margarine Like Spread Whipped Tub Salted ☞ serving size: 1 tablespoon = 10 g; Calories = 53.3; Total Carb (g) = 0.1; Net Carb (g) = 0.1; Fat (g) = 6; Protein = 0

🍴 Margarine Margarine-Like Vegetable Oil Spread 67-70% Fat Tub ☞ serving size: 1 tbsp (1 nlea serving) = 14 g; Calories = 84.8; Total Carb (g) = 0.1; Net Carb (g) = 0.1; Fat (g) = 9.6; Protein = 0

🍴 Margarine Margarine-Type Vegetable Oil Spread 70% Fat Soybean And Partially Hydrogenated Soybean Stick ☞ serving size: 1 tbsp (1 nlea serving) = 14 g; Calories = 87.9; Total Carb (g) = 0.2; Net Carb (g) = 0.2; Fat (g) = 9.8; Protein = 0

🍴 Margarine Regular 80% Fat Composite Stick With Salt ☞ serving size: 1 tbsp = 14 g; Calories = 100.4; Total Carb (g) = 0.1; Net Carb (g) = 0.1; Fat (g) = 11.3; Protein = 0

🍴 Margarine Regular 80% Fat Composite Stick With Salt With Added Vitamin D ☞ serving size: 1 tablespoon = 14 g; Calories = 100.4; Total Carb (g) = 0.1; Net Carb (g) = 0.1; Fat (g) = 11.3; Protein = 0

🍳 Margarine Regular 80% Fat Composite Stick Without Salt With Added Vitamin D ☞ serving size: 1 tbsp = 14 g; Calories = 100.4; Total Carb (g) = 0.1; Net Carb (g) = 0.1; Fat (g) = 11.3; Protein = 0

🍳 Margarine Regular 80% Fat Composite Tub With Salt ☞ serving size: 1 tbsp = 14.2 g; Calories = 101.2; Total Carb (g) = 0.1; Net Carb (g) = 0.1; Fat (g) = 11.4; Protein = 0

🍳 Margarine Regular 80% Fat Composite Tub With Salt With Added Vitamin D ☞ serving size: 1 tbsp = 14 g; Calories = 99.8; Total Carb (g) = 0.1; Net Carb (g) = 0.1; Fat (g) = 11.2; Protein = 0

🍳 Margarine Regular 80% Fat Composite Tub Without Salt ☞ serving size: 1 tbsp = 14.2 g; Calories = 101.2; Total Carb (g) = 0.1; Net Carb (g) = 0.1; Fat (g) = 11.4; Protein = 0

🍳 Margarine Spread Approximately 48% Fat Tub ☞ serving size: 1 tbsp = 14 g; Calories = 56.1; Total Carb (g) = 0; Net Carb (g) = 0; Fat (g) = 6.2; Protein = 0

🍳 Margarine-Like Butter-Margarine Blend 80% Fat Stick Without Salt ☞ serving size: 1 tablespoon = 14 g; Calories = 100.5; Total Carb (g) = 0.1; Net Carb (g) = 0.1; Fat (g) = 11.3; Protein = 0.1

🍳 Margarine-Like Margarine-Butter Blend Soybean Oil And Butter ☞ serving size: 1 tbsp = 14.1 g; Calories = 102.5; Total Carb (g) = 0.1; Net Carb (g) = 0.1; Fat (g) = 11.3; Protein = 0

🍳 Margarine-Like Shortening Industrial Soy (Partially Hydrogenated) Cottonseed And Soy Principal Use Flaky Pastries ☞ serving size: 1 tbsp = 14 g; Calories = 87.9; Total Carb (g) = 0; Net Carb (g) = 0; Fat (g) = 9.9; Protein = 0

🍳 Margarine-Like Spread Benecol Light Spread ☞ serving size: 1 tablespoon (1 nlea serving) = 14 g; Calories = 50; Total Carb (g) = 0.8; Net Carb (g) = 0.8; Fat (g) = 5.4; Protein = 0

🍳 Margarine-Like Spread Liquid Salted ☞ serving size: 1 cup = 227 g; Calories = 1196.3; Total Carb (g) = 0; Net Carb (g) = 0; Fat (g) = 134.3; Protein = 1.4

🥄 Margarine-Like Spread Smart Balance Light Buttery Spread ☞ serving size: 1 tbsp = 14 g; Calories = 47.2; Total Carb (g) = 0.3; Net Carb (g) = 0.3; Fat (g) = 5.1; Protein = 0

🥄 Margarine-Like Spread Smart Balance Omega Plus Spread (With Plant Sterols & Fish Oil) ☞ serving size: 1 tablespoon = 14 g; Calories = 84.7; Total Carb (g) = 0; Net Carb (g) = 0; Fat (g) = 9.9; Protein = 0

🥄 Margarine-Like Spread Smart Balance Regular Buttery Spread With Flax Oil ☞ serving size: 1 tablespoon = 14 g; Calories = 81.6; Total Carb (g) = 0; Net Carb (g) = 0; Fat (g) = 9.1; Protein = 0

🥄 Margarine-Like Spread Smart Beat Smart Squeeze ☞ serving size: 1 tablespoon = 14 g; Calories = 6.6; Total Carb (g) = 1; Net Carb (g) = 1; Fat (g) = 0.3; Protein = 0

🥄 Margarine-Like Spread Smart Beat Super Light Without Saturated Fat ☞ serving size: 1 tablespoon = 14 g; Calories = 22.1; Total Carb (g) = 0; Net Carb (g) = 0; Fat (g) = 2.4; Protein = 0

🥄 Margarine-Like Spread With Yogurt 70% Fat Stick With Salt ☞ serving size: 1 tablespoon = 14 g; Calories = 88.2; Total Carb (g) = 0.1; Net Carb (g) = 0.1; Fat (g) = 9.8; Protein = 0

🥄 Margarine-Like Spread With Yogurt Approximately 40% Fat Tub With Salt ☞ serving size: 1 tablespoon = 14 g; Calories = 46.2; Total Carb (g) = 0.3; Net Carb (g) = 0.3; Fat (g) = 4.9; Protein = 0.3

🥄 Margarine-Like Vegetable Oil Spread 20% Fat With Salt ☞ serving size: 1 tbsp = 15 g; Calories = 26.3; Total Carb (g) = 0.1; Net Carb (g) = 0.1; Fat (g) = 2.9; Protein = 0

🥄 Margarine-Like Vegetable Oil Spread 20% Fat Without Salt ☞ serving size: 1 tbsp = 12.8 g; Calories = 22.4; Total Carb (g) = 0.1; Net Carb (g) = 0.1; Fat (g) = 2.5; Protein = 0

❋ Margarine-Like Vegetable Oil Spread 60% Fat Stick With Salt ☞ serving size: 1 tbsp = 14.3 g; Calories = 76.8; Total Carb (g) = 0.1; Net Carb (g) = 0.1; Fat (g) = 8.6; Protein = 0

❋ Margarine-Like Vegetable Oil Spread 60% Fat Stick With Salt With Added Vitamin D ☞ serving size: 1 tbsp = 14 g; Calories = 75.2; Total Carb (g) = 0.1; Net Carb (g) = 0.1; Fat (g) = 8.5; Protein = 0

❋ Margarine-Like Vegetable Oil Spread 60% Fat Stick/tub/bottle With Salt ☞ serving size: 1 tbsp = 14.3 g; Calories = 75.2; Total Carb (g) = 0; Net Carb (g) = 0; Fat (g) = 8.5; Protein = 0.1

❋ Margarine-Like Vegetable Oil Spread 60% Fat Stick/tub/bottle Without Salt ☞ serving size: 1 tbsp = 14 g; Calories = 74.6; Total Carb (g) = 0.1; Net Carb (g) = 0.1; Fat (g) = 8.4; Protein = 0

❋ Margarine-Like Vegetable Oil Spread 60% Fat Stick/tub/bottle Without Salt With Added Vitamin D ☞ serving size: 1 tbsp = 14 g; Calories = 75.9; Total Carb (g) = 0.1; Net Carb (g) = 0.1; Fat (g) = 8.4; Protein = 0

❋ Margarine-Like Vegetable Oil Spread 60% Fat Tub With Salt ☞ serving size: 1 tbsp = 14 g; Calories = 74.6; Total Carb (g) = 0.1; Net Carb (g) = 0.1; Fat (g) = 8.4; Protein = 0

❋ Margarine-Like Vegetable Oil Spread 60% Fat Tub With Salt With Added Vitamin D ☞ serving size: 1 tbsp = 14 g; Calories = 74.6; Total Carb (g) = 0.1; Net Carb (g) = 0.1; Fat (g) = 8.4; Protein = 0

❋ Margarine-Like Vegetable Oil Spread Approximately 37% Fat Unspecified Oils With Salt With Added Vitamin D ☞ serving size: 1 tbsp = 14.9 g; Calories = 50.5; Total Carb (g) = 0.1; Net Carb (g) = 0.1; Fat (g) = 5.6; Protein = 0.1

❋ Margarine-Like Vegetable Oil Spread Fat Free Liquid With Salt ☞ serving size: 1 tbsp = 15 g; Calories = 6.5; Total Carb (g) = 0.4; Net Carb (g) = 0.4; Fat (g) = 0.5; Protein = 0.2

❋ Margarine-Like Vegetable Oil Spread Fat-Free Tub ☞ serving

size: 1 tbsp = 14.6 g; Calories = 6.4; Total Carb (g) = 0.6; Net Carb (g) = 0.6; Fat (g) = 0.4; Protein = 0

🍃 Margarine-Like Vegetable Oil Spread Stick Or Tub Sweetened ☞ serving size: 1 tablespoon = 14 g; Calories = 74.8; Total Carb (g) = 2.3; Net Carb (g) = 2.3; Fat (g) = 7.3; Protein = 0

🍃 Margarine-Like Vegetable Oil Spread Unspecified Oils Approximately 37% Fat With Salt ☞ serving size: 1 tbsp = 14.9 g; Calories = 52; Total Carb (g) = 0.2; Net Carb (g) = 0.2; Fat (g) = 5.7; Protein = 0

🍃 Margarine-Like Vegetable Oil-Butter Spread Reduced Calorie Tub With Salt ☞ serving size: 1 tablespoon = 14 g; Calories = 63; Total Carb (g) = 0.1; Net Carb (g) = 0.1; Fat (g) = 7; Protein = 0.1

🍃 Margarine-Like Vegetable Oil-Butter Spread Tub With Salt ☞ serving size: 1 tablespoon = 14 g; Calories = 50.7; Total Carb (g) = 0.1; Net Carb (g) = 0.1; Fat (g) = 5.6; Protein = 0.1

🍃 Margarine-Like Vegetable-Oil Spread Stick/tub/bottle 60% Fat With Added Vitamin D ☞ serving size: 1 tbsp = 14 g; Calories = 74.9; Total Carb (g) = 0; Net Carb (g) = 0; Fat (g) = 8.3; Protein = 0.1

🍃 Mayonnaise Dressing No Cholesterol ☞ serving size: 1 tbsp = 15 g; Calories = 103.2; Total Carb (g) = 0.1; Net Carb (g) = 0.1; Fat (g) = 11.7; Protein = 0

🍃 Mayonnaise Low Sodium Low Calorie Or Diet ☞ serving size: 1 tbsp = 14 g; Calories = 32.3; Total Carb (g) = 2.2; Net Carb (g) = 2.2; Fat (g) = 2.7; Protein = 0

🍃 Mayonnaise Made With Tofu ☞ serving size: 1 tbsp = 15 g; Calories = 48.3; Total Carb (g) = 0.5; Net Carb (g) = 0.3; Fat (g) = 4.8; Protein = 0.9

🍃 Mayonnaise Reduced Fat With Olive Oil ☞ serving size: 1 tbsp = 15 g; Calories = 54.2; Total Carb (g) = 0; Net Carb (g) = 0; Fat (g) = 6; Protein = 0.1

🍃 Mayonnaise Reduced-Calorie Or Diet Cholesterol-Free ☞

serving size: 1 tbsp = 14.6 g; Calories = 48.6; Total Carb (g) = 1; Net Carb (g) = 1; Fat (g) = 4.9; Protein = 0.1

Mayonnaise Salad Dressing ☞ serving size: 1 tbsp = 14.7 g; Calories = 36.8; Total Carb (g) = 2.2; Net Carb (g) = 2.2; Fat (g) = 3.2; Protein = 0.1

Menhaden Oil ☞ serving size: 1 tbsp = 13.6 g; Calories = 122.7; Total Carb (g) = 0; Net Carb (g) = 0; Fat (g) = 13.6; Protein = 0

Mustard Oil ☞ serving size: 1 tbsp = 14 g; Calories = 123.8; Total Carb (g) = 0; Net Carb (g) = 0; Fat (g) = 14; Protein = 0

Oil Babassu ☞ serving size: 1 tbsp = 13.6 g; Calories = 120.2; Total Carb (g) = 0; Net Carb (g) = 0; Fat (g) = 13.6; Protein = 0

Oil Cooking And Salad Enova 80% Diglycerides ☞ serving size: 1 tbsp (1 nlea serving) = 14 g; Calories = 123.8; Total Carb (g) = 0; Net Carb (g) = 0; Fat (g) = 14; Protein = 0

Oil Corn And Canola ☞ serving size: 1 tbsp = 14 g; Calories = 123.8; Total Carb (g) = 0; Net Carb (g) = 0; Fat (g) = 14; Protein = 0

Oil Corn Peanut And Olive ☞ serving size: 1 tablespoon = 14 g; Calories = 123.8; Total Carb (g) = 0; Net Carb (g) = 0; Fat (g) = 14; Protein = 0

Oil Cupu Assu ☞ serving size: 1 tablespoon = 13.6 g; Calories = 120.2; Total Carb (g) = 0; Net Carb (g) = 0; Fat (g) = 13.6; Protein = 0

Oil Flaxseed Contains Added Sliced Flaxseed ☞ serving size: 1 tablespoon = 13.7 g; Calories = 120.3; Total Carb (g) = 0.1; Net Carb (g) = 0.1; Fat (g) = 13.6; Protein = 0.1

Oil Industrial Canola (Partially Hydrogenated) Oil For Deep Fat Frying ☞ serving size: 1 tablespoon = 13.6 g; Calories = 120.2; Total Carb (g) = 0; Net Carb (g) = 0; Fat (g) = 13.6; Protein = 0

Oil Industrial Canola For Salads Woks And Light Frying ☞

serving size: 1 tablespoon = 13.6 g; Calories = 120.2; Total Carb (g) = 0; Net Carb (g) = 0; Fat (g) = 13.6; Protein = 0

🥄 Oil Industrial Canola High Oleic ☞ serving size: 1 tablespoon = 14 g; Calories = 126; Total Carb (g) = 0; Net Carb (g) = 0; Fat (g) = 14; Protein = 0

🥄 Oil Industrial Canola With Antifoaming Agent Principal Uses Salads Woks And Light Frying ☞ serving size: 1 tablespoon = 13.6 g; Calories = 120.2; Total Carb (g) = 0; Net Carb (g) = 0; Fat (g) = 13.6; Protein = 0

🥄 Oil Industrial Coconut (Hydrogenated) Used For Whipped Toppings And Coffee Whiteners ☞ serving size: 1 tbsp = 13.6 g; Calories = 119.7; Total Carb (g) = 0; Net Carb (g) = 0; Fat (g) = 13.5; Protein = 0

🥄 Oil Industrial Coconut Confection Fat Typical Basis For Ice Cream Coatings ☞ serving size: 1 tbsp = 13.6 g; Calories = 120.2; Total Carb (g) = 0; Net Carb (g) = 0; Fat (g) = 13.6; Protein = 0

🥄 Oil Industrial Coconut Principal Uses Candy Coatings Oil Sprays Roasting Nuts ☞ serving size: 1 tbsp = 13.6 g; Calories = 120.2; Total Carb (g) = 0; Net Carb (g) = 0; Fat (g) = 13.6; Protein = 0

🥄 Oil Industrial Cottonseed Fully Hydrogenated ☞ serving size: 1 tablespoon = 13.6 g; Calories = 120.2; Total Carb (g) = 0; Net Carb (g) = 0; Fat (g) = 13.6; Protein = 0

🥄 Oil Industrial Mid-Oleic Sunflower ☞ serving size: 1 tablespoon = 13.6 g; Calories = 120.2; Total Carb (g) = 0; Net Carb (g) = 0; Fat (g) = 13.6; Protein = 0

🥄 Oil Industrial Palm And Palm Kernel Filling Fat (Non-Hydrogenated) ☞ serving size: 1 tbsp = 13.6 g; Calories = 119.7; Total Carb (g) = 0; Net Carb (g) = 0; Fat (g) = 13.5; Protein = 0

🥄 Oil Industrial Palm Kernel (Hydrogenated) Used For Whipped

Toppings Non-Dairy ☞ serving size: 1 tbsp = 13.6 g; Calories = 120.2; Total Carb (g) = 0; Net Carb (g) = 0; Fat (g) = 13.6; Protein = 0

Oil Industrial Palm Kernel (Hydrogenated) Confection Fat Intermediate Grade Product ☞ serving size: 1 tbsp = 13.6 g; Calories = 120.2; Total Carb (g) = 0; Net Carb (g) = 0; Fat (g) = 13.6; Protein = 0

Oil Industrial Palm Kernel (Hydrogenated) Confection Fat Uses Similar To 95 Degree Hard Butter ☞ serving size: 1 tbsp = 13.6 g; Calories = 120.2; Total Carb (g) = 0; Net Carb (g) = 0; Fat (g) = 13.6; Protein = 0

Oil Industrial Palm Kernel (Hydrogenated) Filling Fat ☞ serving size: 1 tbsp = 13.6 g; Calories = 120.2; Total Carb (g) = 0; Net Carb (g) = 0; Fat (g) = 13.6; Protein = 0

Oil Industrial Palm Kernel Confection Fat Uses Similar To High Quality Cocoa Butter ☞ serving size: 1 tbsp = 13.6 g; Calories = 120.2; Total Carb (g) = 0; Net Carb (g) = 0; Fat (g) = 13.6; Protein = 0

Oil Industrial Soy (Partially Hydrogenated) All Purpose ☞ serving size: 1 tbsp = 13.6 g; Calories = 120.2; Total Carb (g) = 0; Net Carb (g) = 0; Fat (g) = 13.6; Protein = 0

Oil Industrial Soy (Partially Hydrogenated) And Soy (Winterized) Pourable Clear Fry ☞ serving size: 1 tbsp = 13.6 g; Calories = 120.2; Total Carb (g) = 0; Net Carb (g) = 0; Fat (g) = 13.6; Protein = 0

Oil Industrial Soy (Partially Hydrogenated) Palm Principal Uses Icings And Fillings ☞ serving size: 1 tbsp = 13.6 g; Calories = 120.2; Total Carb (g) = 0; Net Carb (g) = 0; Fat (g) = 13.6; Protein = 0

Oil Industrial Soy (Partially Hydrogenated) And Cottonseed Principal Use As A Tortilla Shortening ☞ serving size: 1 tbsp = 13.6 g; Calories = 120.2; Total Carb (g) = 0; Net Carb (g) = 0; Fat (g) = 13.6; Protein = 0

Oil Industrial Soy (Partially Hydrogenated) Multiuse For Non-

Dairy Butter Flavor ☞ serving size: 1 tbsp = 13.6 g; Calories = 120.2; Total Carb (g) = 0; Net Carb (g) = 0; Fat (g) = 13.6; Protein = 0

☺ Oil Industrial Soy (Partially Hydrogenated) Principal Uses Popcorn And Flavoring Vegetables ☞ serving size: 1 tbsp = 13.6 g; Calories = 120.2; Total Carb (g) = 0; Net Carb (g) = 0; Fat (g) = 13.6; Protein = 0

☺ Oil Industrial Soy Fully Hydrogenated ☞ serving size: 1 tablespoon = 13.6 g; Calories = 120.2; Total Carb (g) = 0; Net Carb (g) = 0; Fat (g) = 13.6; Protein = 0

☺ Oil Industrial Soy Low Linolenic ☞ serving size: 1 tablespoon = 14 g; Calories = 126; Total Carb (g) = 0; Net Carb (g) = 0; Fat (g) = 14; Protein = 0

☺ Oil Industrial Soy Refined For Woks And Light Frying ☞ serving size: 1 tbsp = 13.6 g; Calories = 120.2; Total Carb (g) = 0; Net Carb (g) = 0; Fat (g) = 13.6; Protein = 0

☺ Oil Industrial Soy Ultra Low Linolenic ☞ serving size: 1 tablespoon = 13.6 g; Calories = 120.2; Total Carb (g) = 0; Net Carb (g) = 0; Fat (g) = 13.6; Protein = 0

☺ Oil Nutmeg Butter ☞ serving size: 1 tbsp = 13.6 g; Calories = 120.2; Total Carb (g) = 0; Net Carb (g) = 0; Fat (g) = 13.6; Protein = 0

☺ Oil Oat ☞ serving size: 1 tbsp = 13.6 g; Calories = 120.2; Total Carb (g) = 0; Net Carb (g) = 0; Fat (g) = 13.6; Protein = 0

☺ Oil Or Table Fat Nfs ☞ serving size: 1 cup = 224 g; Calories = 1711.4; Total Carb (g) = 0.4; Net Carb (g) = 0.4; Fat (g) = 193.3; Protein = 0.7

☺ Oil Pam Cooking Spray Original ☞ serving size: 1 spray , about 1/3 second (1 nlea serving) = 0.3 g; Calories = 2.4; Total Carb (g) = 0.1; Net Carb (g) = 0.1; Fat (g) = 0.2; Protein = 0

☺ Oil Safflower Salad Or Cooking High Oleic (Primary Safflower

Oil Of Commerce) ☞ serving size: 1 tablespoon = 13.6 g; Calories = 120.2; Total Carb (g) = 0; Net Carb (g) = 0; Fat (g) = 13.6; Protein = 0

🦪 Oil Safflower Salad Or Cooking Linoleic (Over 70%) ☞ serving size: 1 tbsp = 13.6 g; Calories = 120.2; Total Carb (g) = 0; Net Carb (g) = 0; Fat (g) = 13.6; Protein = 0

🦪 Oil Sheanut ☞ serving size: 1 tablespoon = 13.6 g; Calories = 120.2; Total Carb (g) = 0; Net Carb (g) = 0; Fat (g) = 13.6; Protein = 0

🦪 Oil Soybean Salad Or Cooking (Partially Hydrogenated) ☞ serving size: 1 tbsp = 13.6 g; Calories = 120.2; Total Carb (g) = 0; Net Carb (g) = 0; Fat (g) = 13.6; Protein = 0

🦪 Oil Soybean Salad Or Cooking (Partially Hydrogenated) And Cottonseed ☞ serving size: 1 tablespoon = 13.6 g; Calories = 120.2; Total Carb (g) = 0; Net Carb (g) = 0; Fat (g) = 13.6; Protein = 0

🦪 Oil Sunflower High Oleic (70% And Over) ☞ serving size: 1 tbsp = 14 g; Calories = 123.8; Total Carb (g) = 0; Net Carb (g) = 0; Fat (g) = 14; Protein = 0

🦪 Oil Sunflower Linoleic (Approx. 65%) ☞ serving size: 1 tbsp = 13.6 g; Calories = 120.2; Total Carb (g) = 0; Net Carb (g) = 0; Fat (g) = 13.6; Protein = 0

🦪 Oil Sunflower Linoleic (Less Than 60%) ☞ serving size: 1 tbsp = 13.6 g; Calories = 120.2; Total Carb (g) = 0; Net Carb (g) = 0; Fat (g) = 13.6; Protein = 0

🦪 Oil Sunflower Linoleic (Partially Hydrogenated) ☞ serving size: 1 tbsp = 13.6 g; Calories = 120.2; Total Carb (g) = 0; Net Carb (g) = 0; Fat (g) = 13.6; Protein = 0

🦪 Oil Ucuhuba Butter ☞ serving size: 1 tbsp = 13.6 g; Calories = 120.2; Total Carb (g) = 0; Net Carb (g) = 0; Fat (g) = 13.6; Protein = 0

🦪 Oil Vegetable Natreon Canola High Stability Non Trans High Oleic (70%) ☞ serving size: 1 tbsp = 14 g; Calories = 123.8; Total Carb (g) = 0; Net Carb (g) = 0; Fat (g) = 14; Protein = 0

Olive Oil ☞ serving size: 1 tablespoon = 13.5 g; Calories = 119.3; Total Carb (g) = 0; Net Carb (g) = 0; Fat (g) = 13.5; Protein = 0

Palm Kernel Oil ☞ serving size: 1 tablespoon = 13.6 g; Calories = 117.2; Total Carb (g) = 0; Net Carb (g) = 0; Fat (g) = 13.6; Protein = 0

Palm Oil ☞ serving size: 1 tbsp = 13.6 g; Calories = 120.2; Total Carb (g) = 0; Net Carb (g) = 0; Fat (g) = 13.6; Protein = 0

Peanut Oil ☞ serving size: 1 tbsp = 13.5 g; Calories = 119.3; Total Carb (g) = 0; Net Carb (g) = 0; Fat (g) = 13.5; Protein = 0

Poppyseed Oil ☞ serving size: 1 tablespoon = 13.6 g; Calories = 120.2; Total Carb (g) = 0; Net Carb (g) = 0; Fat (g) = 13.6; Protein = 0

Rendered Chicken Fat ☞ serving size: 1 tbsp = 12.8 g; Calories = 115.2; Total Carb (g) = 0; Net Carb (g) = 0; Fat (g) = 12.8; Protein = 0

Rice Bran Oil ☞ serving size: 1 tablespoon = 13.6 g; Calories = 120.2; Total Carb (g) = 0; Net Carb (g) = 0; Fat (g) = 13.6; Protein = 0

Russian Dressing ☞ serving size: 1 tbsp = 15 g; Calories = 53.3; Total Carb (g) = 4.8; Net Carb (g) = 4.7; Fat (g) = 3.9; Protein = 0.1

Salad Dressing Bacon And Tomato ☞ serving size: 1 tbsp = 15 g; Calories = 48.9; Total Carb (g) = 0.3; Net Carb (g) = 0.3; Fat (g) = 5.3; Protein = 0.3

Salad Dressing Blue Or Roquefort Cheese Dressing Commercial Regular ☞ serving size: 1 tbsp = 15 g; Calories = 72.6; Total Carb (g) = 0.7; Net Carb (g) = 0.7; Fat (g) = 7.7; Protein = 0.2

Salad Dressing Blue Or Roquefort Cheese Dressing Fat-Free ☞ serving size: 1 tbsp = 17 g; Calories = 19.6; Total Carb (g) = 4.4; Net Carb (g) = 4.1; Fat (g) = 0.2; Protein = 0.3

Salad Dressing Blue Or Roquefort Cheese Dressing Light ☞ serving size: 1 tbsp = 16 g; Calories = 13.8; Total Carb (g) = 2.1; Net Carb (g) = 2.1; Fat (g) = 0.4; Protein = 0.3

Salad Dressing Blue Or Roquefort Cheese Low Calorie ☞

serving size: 1 tbsp = 15 g; Calories = 14.9; Total Carb (g) = 0.4; Net Carb (g) = 0.4; Fat (g) = 1.1; Protein = 0.8

☞ Salad Dressing Buttermilk Lite ☞ serving size: 1 tablespoon = 15 g; Calories = 30.3; Total Carb (g) = 3.2; Net Carb (g) = 3; Fat (g) = 1.9; Protein = 0.2

☞ Salad Dressing Caesar Dressing Regular ☞ serving size: 1 tbsp = 14.7 g; Calories = 79.7; Total Carb (g) = 0.5; Net Carb (g) = 0.4; Fat (g) = 8.5; Protein = 0.3

☞ Salad Dressing Caesar Fat-Free ☞ serving size: 2 tbsp (1 nlea serving) = 34 g; Calories = 44.5; Total Carb (g) = 10.5; Net Carb (g) = 10.4; Fat (g) = 0.1; Protein = 0.5

☞ Salad Dressing Caesar Low Calorie ☞ serving size: 1 tbsp = 15 g; Calories = 16.5; Total Carb (g) = 2.8; Net Carb (g) = 2.8; Fat (g) = 0.7; Protein = 0.1

☞ Salad Dressing Coleslaw Dressing Reduced Fat ☞ serving size: 1 tbsp = 17 g; Calories = 55.9; Total Carb (g) = 6.8; Net Carb (g) = 6.7; Fat (g) = 3.4; Protein = 0

☞ Salad Dressing French Cottonseed Oil Home Recipe ☞ serving size: 1 tablespoon = 14 g; Calories = 88.3; Total Carb (g) = 0.5; Net Carb (g) = 0.5; Fat (g) = 9.8; Protein = 0

☞ Salad Dressing French Dressing Commercial Regular ☞ serving size: 1 tbsp = 16 g; Calories = 67; Total Carb (g) = 3; Net Carb (g) = 2.6; Fat (g) = 6.3; Protein = 0.1

☞ Salad Dressing French Dressing Commercial Regular Without Salt ☞ serving size: 1 tablespoon = 15 g; Calories = 68.9; Total Carb (g) = 2.3; Net Carb (g) = 2.3; Fat (g) = 6.7; Protein = 0.1

☞ Salad Dressing French Dressing Fat-Free ☞ serving size: 1 table-spoon = 16 g; Calories = 21.1; Total Carb (g) = 5.1; Net Carb (g) = 4.8; Fat (g) = 0; Protein = 0

☞ Salad Dressing French Dressing Reduced Calorie ☞ serving

size: 1 tbsp = 16 g; Calories = 36.3; Total Carb (g) = 4.3; Net Carb (g) = 4.3; Fat (g) = 2.1; Protein = 0.1

🍥 Salad Dressing French Dressing Reduced Fat ☞ serving size: 1 tablespoon = 16 g; Calories = 35.5; Total Carb (g) = 5; Net Carb (g) = 4.8; Fat (g) = 1.8; Protein = 0.1

🍥 Salad Dressing French Home Recipe ☞ serving size: 1 tablespoon = 14 g; Calories = 88.3; Total Carb (g) = 0.5; Net Carb (g) = 0.5; Fat (g) = 9.8; Protein = 0

🍥 Salad Dressing Green Goddess Regular ☞ serving size: 1 tbsp = 15 g; Calories = 64.1; Total Carb (g) = 1.1; Net Carb (g) = 1.1; Fat (g) = 6.5; Protein = 0.3

🍥 Salad Dressing Home Recipe Vinegar And Oil ☞ serving size: 1 tablespoon = 16 g; Calories = 71.8; Total Carb (g) = 0.4; Net Carb (g) = 0.4; Fat (g) = 8; Protein = 0

🍥 Salad Dressing Honey Mustard Dressing Reduced Calorie ☞ serving size: 2 tbsp (1 serving) = 30 g; Calories = 62.1; Total Carb (g) = 8.5; Net Carb (g) = 8.2; Fat (g) = 3; Protein = 0.3

🍥 Salad Dressing Italian Dressing Commercial Regular ☞ serving size: 1 tbsp = 14.7 g; Calories = 35.3; Total Carb (g) = 1.8; Net Carb (g) = 1.8; Fat (g) = 3.1; Protein = 0.1

🍥 Salad Dressing Italian Dressing Commercial Regular Without Salt ☞ serving size: 1 tablespoon = 14.7 g; Calories = 42.9; Total Carb (g) = 1.5; Net Carb (g) = 1.5; Fat (g) = 4.2; Protein = 0.1

🍥 Salad Dressing Italian Dressing Fat-Free ☞ serving size: 1 tbsp = 14 g; Calories = 6.6; Total Carb (g) = 1.2; Net Carb (g) = 1.1; Fat (g) = 0.1; Protein = 0.1

🍥 Salad Dressing Italian Dressing Reduced Calorie ☞ serving size: 1 tbsp = 14 g; Calories = 28; Total Carb (g) = 0.9; Net Carb (g) = 0.9; Fat (g) = 2.8; Protein = 0

🍥 Salad Dressing Italian Dressing Reduced Fat Without Salt ☞

serving size: 1 tablespoon = 15 g; Calories = 11.4; Total Carb (g) = 0.7; Net Carb (g) = 0.7; Fat (g) = 1; Protein = 0.1

✅ Salad Dressing Kraft Mayo Fat Free Mayonnaise Dressing ☞ serving size: 1 tbsp = 16 g; Calories = 10.2; Total Carb (g) = 2.5; Net Carb (g) = 2.2; Fat (g) = 0; Protein = 0

✅ Salad Dressing Kraft Mayo Light Mayonnaise ☞ serving size: 1 tbsp = 15 g; Calories = 50.1; Total Carb (g) = 1.3; Net Carb (g) = 1.3; Fat (g) = 4.9; Protein = 0.1

✅ Salad Dressing Kraft Miracle Whip Free Nonfat Dressing ☞ serving size: 1 tbsp = 16 g; Calories = 13.4; Total Carb (g) = 2.5; Net Carb (g) = 2.2; Fat (g) = 0.4; Protein = 0

✅ Salad Dressing Mayonnaise And Mayonnaise-Type Low Calorie ☞ serving size: 1 tbsp = 14.5 g; Calories = 38.1; Total Carb (g) = 3.5; Net Carb (g) = 3.5; Fat (g) = 2.8; Protein = 0.1

✅ Salad Dressing Mayonnaise Imitation Milk Cream ☞ serving size: 1 tablespoon = 15 g; Calories = 14.6; Total Carb (g) = 1.7; Net Carb (g) = 1.7; Fat (g) = 0.8; Protein = 0.3

✅ Salad Dressing Mayonnaise Imitation Soybean ☞ serving size: 1 tbsp = 15 g; Calories = 34.8; Total Carb (g) = 2.4; Net Carb (g) = 2.4; Fat (g) = 2.9; Protein = 0.1

✅ Salad Dressing Mayonnaise Imitation Soybean Without Cholesterol ☞ serving size: 1 tablespoon = 14.1 g; Calories = 68; Total Carb (g) = 2.2; Net Carb (g) = 2.2; Fat (g) = 6.7; Protein = 0

✅ Salad Dressing Mayonnaise Light ☞ serving size: 1 tablespoon = 15 g; Calories = 35.7; Total Carb (g) = 1.4; Net Carb (g) = 1.4; Fat (g) = 3.3; Protein = 0.1

✅ Salad Dressing Mayonnaise Light Smart Balance Omega Plus Light ☞ serving size: 1 tbsp (1 nlea serving) = 14 g; Calories = 46.6; Total Carb (g) = 1.3; Net Carb (g) = 1.3; Fat (g) = 4.8; Protein = 0.2

✅ Salad Dressing Mayonnaise Regular ☞ serving size: 1 tbsp = 13.8

g; Calories = 93.8; Total Carb (g) = 0.1; Net Carb (g) = 0.1; Fat (g) = 10.3; Protein = 0.1

🦪 Salad Dressing Mayonnaise Soybean And Safflower Oil With Salt ☞ serving size: 1 tablespoon = 13.8 g; Calories = 98.9; Total Carb (g) = 0.4; Net Carb (g) = 0.4; Fat (g) = 11; Protein = 0.2

🦪 Salad Dressing Mayonnaise Soybean Oil Without Salt ☞ serving size: 1 tablespoon = 13.8 g; Calories = 98.9; Total Carb (g) = 0.4; Net Carb (g) = 0.4; Fat (g) = 11; Protein = 0.2

🦪 Salad Dressing Mayonnaise-Like Fat-Free ☞ serving size: 1 tbsp = 16 g; Calories = 13.4; Total Carb (g) = 2.5; Net Carb (g) = 2.2; Fat (g) = 0.4; Protein = 0

🦪 Salad Dressing NFS For Sandwiches ☞ serving size: 1 cup = 237 g; Calories = 1407.8; Total Carb (g) = 8.1; Net Carb (g) = 8.1; Fat (g) = 152.2; Protein = 2.1

🦪 Salad Dressing Peppercorn Dressing Commercial Regular ☞ serving size: 1 tbsp = 13.4 g; Calories = 75.6; Total Carb (g) = 0.5; Net Carb (g) = 0.5; Fat (g) = 8.2; Protein = 0.2

🦪 Salad Dressing Ranch Dressing Fat-Free ☞ serving size: 1 tablespoon = 14 g; Calories = 16.7; Total Carb (g) = 3.7; Net Carb (g) = 3.7; Fat (g) = 0.3; Protein = 0

🦪 Salad Dressing Ranch Dressing Reduced Fat ☞ serving size: 1 tablespoon = 15 g; Calories = 29.4; Total Carb (g) = 3.2; Net Carb (g) = 3; Fat (g) = 1.9; Protein = 0.2

🦪 Salad Dressing Ranch Dressing Regular ☞ serving size: 1 tablespoon = 15 g; Calories = 64.5; Total Carb (g) = 0.9; Net Carb (g) = 0.9; Fat (g) = 6.7; Protein = 0.2

🦪 Salad Dressing Russian Dressing Low Calorie ☞ serving size: 1 tablespoon = 16 g; Calories = 22.6; Total Carb (g) = 4.4; Net Carb (g) = 4.4; Fat (g) = 0.6; Protein = 0.1

🦪 Salad Dressing Spray-Style Dressing Assorted Flavors ☞

serving size: 1 serving (approximately 10 sprays) = 8 g; Calories = 13.2; Total Carb (g) = 1.3; Net Carb (g) = 1.3; Fat (g) = 0.9; Protein = 0

Salad Dressing Sweet And Sour ☞ serving size: 1 tbsp = 16 g; Calories = 2.4; Total Carb (g) = 0.6; Net Carb (g) = 0.6; Fat (g) = 0; Protein = 0

Salad Dressing Thousand Island Dressing Fat-Free ☞ serving size: 1 tbsp = 16 g; Calories = 21.1; Total Carb (g) = 4.7; Net Carb (g) = 4.2; Fat (g) = 0.2; Protein = 0.1

Salad Dressing Thousand Island Dressing Reduced Fat ☞ serving size: 1 tablespoon = 15 g; Calories = 29.3; Total Carb (g) = 3.6; Net Carb (g) = 3.4; Fat (g) = 1.7; Protein = 0.1

Salmon Oil ☞ serving size: 1 tbsp = 13.6 g; Calories = 122.7; Total Carb (g) = 0; Net Carb (g) = 0; Fat (g) = 13.6; Protein = 0

Sandwich Spread With Chopped Pickle Regular Unspecified Oils ☞ serving size: 1 tablespoon = 15 g; Calories = 58.4; Total Carb (g) = 3.4; Net Carb (g) = 3.3; Fat (g) = 5.1; Protein = 0.1

Sardine Oil ☞ serving size: 1 tbsp = 13.6 g; Calories = 122.7; Total Carb (g) = 0; Net Carb (g) = 0; Fat (g) = 13.6; Protein = 0

Sesame Oil ☞ serving size: 1 tablespoon = 13.6 g; Calories = 120.2; Total Carb (g) = 0; Net Carb (g) = 0; Fat (g) = 13.6; Protein = 0

Sesame Seed Dressing ☞ serving size: 1 tablespoon = 15 g; Calories = 66.5; Total Carb (g) = 1.3; Net Carb (g) = 1.1; Fat (g) = 6.8; Protein = 0.5

Shortening ☞ serving size: 1 tbsp = 12.8 g; Calories = 115.2; Total Carb (g) = 0; Net Carb (g) = 0; Fat (g) = 12.8; Protein = 0

Shortening Bread Soybean (Hydrogenated) And Cottonseed ☞ serving size: 1 tablespoon = 12.8 g; Calories = 113.2; Total Carb (g) = 0; Net Carb (g) = 0; Fat (g) = 12.8; Protein = 0

Shortening Cake Mix Soybean (Hydrogenated) And Cottonseed

(Hydrogenated) ☞ serving size: 1 tbsp = 12.8 g; Calories = 113.2; Total Carb (g) = 0; Net Carb (g) = 0; Fat (g) = 12.8; Protein = 0

✐ Shortening Confectionery Coconut (Hydrogenated) And Or Palm Kernel (Hydrogenated) ☞ serving size: 1 tbsp = 12.8 g; Calories = 113.2; Total Carb (g) = 0; Net Carb (g) = 0; Fat (g) = 12.8; Protein = 0

✐ Shortening Confectionery Fractionated Palm ☞ serving size: 1 tbsp = 13.6 g; Calories = 120.2; Total Carb (g) = 0; Net Carb (g) = 0; Fat (g) = 13.6; Protein = 0

✐ Shortening Frying (Heavy Duty) Beef Tallow And Cottonseed ☞ serving size: 1 tbsp = 12.8 g; Calories = 115.2; Total Carb (g) = 0; Net Carb (g) = 0; Fat (g) = 12.8; Protein = 0

✐ Shortening Frying (Heavy Duty) Palm (Hydrogenated) ☞ serving size: 1 tbsp = 12.8 g; Calories = 113.2; Total Carb (g) = 0; Net Carb (g) = 0; Fat (g) = 12.8; Protein = 0

✐ Shortening Frying (Heavy Duty) Soybean (Hydrogenated) Linoleic (Less Than 1%) ☞ serving size: 1 tbsp = 12.8 g; Calories = 113.2; Total Carb (g) = 0; Net Carb (g) = 0; Fat (g) = 12.8; Protein = 0

✐ Shortening Household Lard And Vegetable Oil ☞ serving size: 1 tablespoon = 12.8 g; Calories = 115.2; Total Carb (g) = 0; Net Carb (g) = 0; Fat (g) = 12.8; Protein = 0

✐ Shortening Household Soybean (Hydrogenated) And Palm ☞ serving size: 1 tbsp = 12.8 g; Calories = 113.2; Total Carb (g) = 0; Net Carb (g) = 0; Fat (g) = 12.8; Protein = 0

✐ Shortening Household Soybean (Partially Hydrogenated)-Cottonseed (Partially Hydrogenated) ☞ serving size: 1 tbsp = 12.8 g; Calories = 113.2; Total Carb (g) = 0; Net Carb (g) = 0; Fat (g) = 12.8; Protein = 0

✐ Shortening Industrial Soy (Partially Hydrogenated) And Corn For Frying ☞ serving size: 1 tbsp = 12.8 g; Calories = 113.2; Total Carb (g) = 0; Net Carb (g) = 0; Fat (g) = 12.8; Protein = 0

🍳 Shortening Industrial Soy (Partially Hydrogenated) For Baking And Confections ☞ serving size: 1 tbsp = 12.8 g; Calories = 113.2; Total Carb (g) = 0; Net Carb (g) = 0; Fat (g) = 12.8; Protein = 0

🍳 Shortening Industrial Soy (Partially Hydrogenated) Pourable Liquid Fry Shortening ☞ serving size: 1 tbsp = 13.6 g; Calories = 120.2; Total Carb (g) = 0; Net Carb (g) = 0; Fat (g) = 13.6; Protein = 0

🍳 Shortening Industrial Soybean (Hydrogenated) And Cottonseed ☞ serving size: 1 tbsp = 12.8 g; Calories = 113.2; Total Carb (g) = 0; Net Carb (g) = 0; Fat (g) = 12.8; Protein = 0

🍳 Shortening Special Purpose For Baking Soybean (Hydrogenated) Palm And Cottonseed ☞ serving size: 1 tbsp = 12.8 g; Calories = 113.2; Total Carb (g) = 0; Net Carb (g) = 0; Fat (g) = 12.8; Protein = 0

🍳 Shortening Special Purpose For Cakes And Frostings Soybean (Hydrogenated) ☞ serving size: 1 tbsp = 12.8 g; Calories = 113.2; Total Carb (g) = 0; Net Carb (g) = 0; Fat (g) = 12.8; Protein = 0

🍳 Soybean Lecithin ☞ serving size: 1 tablespoon = 13.6 g; Calories = 103.8; Total Carb (g) = 0; Net Carb (g) = 0; Fat (g) = 13.6; Protein = 0

🍳 Soybean Oil ☞ serving size: 1 tbsp = 13.6 g; Calories = 120.2; Total Carb (g) = 0; Net Carb (g) = 0; Fat (g) = 13.6; Protein = 0

🍳 Table Fat Nfs ☞ serving size: 1 cup = 227 g; Calories = 1459.6; Total Carb (g) = 0.9; Net Carb (g) = 0.9; Fat (g) = 164.8; Protein = 1.3

🍳 Tartar Sauce Reduced Fat/calorie ☞ serving size: 1 cup = 224 g; Calories = 192.6; Total Carb (g) = 34.3; Net Carb (g) = 29.8; Fat (g) = 6.7; Protein = 0.9

🍳 Teaseed Oil ☞ serving size: 1 tablespoon = 13.6 g; Calories = 120.2; Total Carb (g) = 0; Net Carb (g) = 0; Fat (g) = 13.6; Protein = 0

🍳 Thousand Island ☞ serving size: 1 tbsp = 16 g; Calories = 60.6; Total Carb (g) = 2.3; Net Carb (g) = 2.2; Fat (g) = 5.6; Protein = 0.2

❦ Tomatoseed Oil ☞ serving size: 1 tablespoon = 13.6 g; Calories = 120.2; Total Carb (g) = 0; Net Carb (g) = 0; Fat (g) = 13.6; Protein = 0

❦ USDA Commodity Food Oil Vegetable Soybean Refined ☞ serving size: 1 tablespoon = 13.6 g; Calories = 120.2; Total Carb (g) = 0; Net Carb (g) = 0; Fat (g) = 13.6; Protein = 0

❦ Vegetable Oil Nfs ☞ serving size: 1 cup = 218 g; Calories = 1931.5; Total Carb (g) = 0; Net Carb (g) = 0; Fat (g) = 218; Protein = 0

❦ Vegetable Oil-Butter Spread Reduced Calorie ☞ serving size: 1 tbsp = 13 g; Calories = 60.5; Total Carb (g) = 0; Net Carb (g) = 0; Fat (g) = 6.9; Protein = 0

❦ Vegetable Oil-Butter Spread Stick Salted ☞ serving size: 1 cup = 227 g; Calories = 1209.9; Total Carb (g) = 0.2; Net Carb (g) = 0.2; Fat (g) = 136.2; Protein = 1.2

❦ Vegetable Shortening ☞ serving size: 1 tbsp = 12.8 g; Calories = 113.2; Total Carb (g) = 0; Net Carb (g) = 0; Fat (g) = 12.8; Protein = 0

❦ Walnut Oil ☞ serving size: 1 tbsp = 13.6 g; Calories = 120.2; Total Carb (g) = 0; Net Carb (g) = 0; Fat (g) = 13.6; Protein = 0

❦ Wheat Germ Oil ☞ serving size: 1 tsp = 4.5 g; Calories = 39.8; Total Carb (g) = 0; Net Carb (g) = 0; Fat (g) = 4.5; Protein = 0

❦ Yogurt Dressing ☞ serving size: 1 cup = 246 g; Calories = 541.2; Total Carb (g) = 28.9; Net Carb (g) = 28.7; Fat (g) = 44.9; Protein = 8.5

18

FISH AND SEAFOOD

🐟 Abalone (Cooked) ☞ serving size: 3 oz = 85 g; Calories = 160.7; Total Carb (g) = 9.4; Net Carb (g) = 9.4; Fat (g) = 5.8; Protein = 16.7

🐟 Abalone Cooked Ns As To Cooking Method ☞ serving size: 1 oz, boneless, cooked = 28 g; Calories = 44; Total Carb (g) = 2; Net Carb (g) = 2; Fat (g) = 1.3; Protein = 5.7

🐟 Abalone Floured Or Breaded Fried ☞ serving size: 1 oz, cooked = 28 g; Calories = 67.8; Total Carb (g) = 4.4; Net Carb (g) = 4.2; Fat (g) = 3.2; Protein = 5.1

🐟 Abalone Steamed Or Poached ☞ serving size: 1 oz, cooked = 28 g; Calories = 58.5; Total Carb (g) = 3.4; Net Carb (g) = 3.4; Fat (g) = 0.4; Protein = 9.5

🐟 Alaskan King Crab ☞ serving size: 1 leg = 134 g; Calories = 130; Total Carb (g) = 0; Net Carb (g) = 0; Fat (g) = 2.1; Protein = 25.9

🐟 Anchovies (Raw) ☞ serving size: 3 oz = 85 g; Calories = 111.4; Total Carb (g) = 0; Net Carb (g) = 0; Fat (g) = 4.1; Protein = 17.3

🐟 Atlantic Herring ☞ serving size: 1 fillet = 143 g; Calories = 290.3; Total Carb (g) = 0; Net Carb (g) = 0; Fat (g) = 16.6; Protein = 32.9

🐟 Atlantic Mackerel (Cooked) ☞ serving size: 1 fillet = 88 g; Calories = 230.6; Total Carb (g) = 0; Net Carb (g) = 0; Fat (g) = 15.7; Protein = 21

🐟 Atlantic Mackerel (Raw) ☞ serving size: 1 fillet = 112 g; Calories = 229.6; Total Carb (g) = 0; Net Carb (g) = 0; Fat (g) = 15.6; Protein = 20.8

🐟 Baked Conch ☞ serving size: 1 cup, sliced = 127 g; Calories = 165.1; Total Carb (g) = 2.2; Net Carb (g) = 2.2; Fat (g) = 1.5; Protein = 33.4

🐟 Barracuda Baked Or Broiled Fat Added In Cooking ☞ serving size: 1 small fillet = 113 g; Calories = 255.4; Total Carb (g) = 0.1; Net Carb (g) = 0.1; Fat (g) = 15.1; Protein = 27.8

🐟 Barracuda Baked Or Broiled Fat Not Added In Cooking ☞ serving size: 1 small fillet = 113 g; Calories = 224.9; Total Carb (g) = 0.1; Net Carb (g) = 0.1; Fat (g) = 11.2; Protein = 28.6

🐟 Barracuda Coated Baked Or Broiled Fat Added In Cooking ☞ serving size: 1 small fillet = 113 g; Calories = 298.3; Total Carb (g) = 14.2; Net Carb (g) = 13.5; Fat (g) = 15.5; Protein = 23.8

🐟 Barracuda Coated Baked Or Broiled Fat Not Added In Cooking ☞ serving size: 1 small fillet = 113 g; Calories = 253.1; Total Carb (g) = 14.8; Net Carb (g) = 14.1; Fat (g) = 9.6; Protein = 24.9

🐟 Barracuda Coated Fried ☞ serving size: 1 small fillet = 113 g; Calories = 315.3; Total Carb (g) = 11.1; Net Carb (g) = 10.5; Fat (g) = 19.3; Protein = 22.8

🐟 Barracuda Cooked Ns As To Cooking Method ☞ serving size: 1 small fillet = 113 g; Calories = 255.4; Total Carb (g) = 0.1; Net Carb (g) = 0.1; Fat (g) = 15.1; Protein = 27.8

🐟 Barracuda Steamed Or Poached ☞ serving size: 1 small fillet = 113 g; Calories = 224.9; Total Carb (g) = 0; Net Carb (g) = 0; Fat (g) = 11.2; Protein = 28.5

🐟 Bass Freshwater Mixed Species Cooked Dry Heat ☞ serving size: 1 fillet = 62 g; Calories = 90.5; Total Carb (g) = 0; Net Carb (g) = 0; Fat (g) = 2.9; Protein = 15

🐟 Biscayne Codfish Puerto Rican Style ☞ serving size: 1 cup = 175 g; Calories = 323.8; Total Carb (g) = 19.5; Net Carb (g) = 16.1; Fat (g) = 20.8; Protein = 16.1

🐟 Blue Crab ☞ serving size: 1 cup, flaked and pieces = 118 g; Calories = 97.9; Total Carb (g) = 0; Net Carb (g) = 0; Fat (g) = 0.9; Protein = 21.1

🐟 Blue Crab Cakes ☞ serving size: 1 cake = 60 g; Calories = 93; Total Carb (g) = 0.3; Net Carb (g) = 0.3; Fat (g) = 4.5; Protein = 12.1

🐟 Bluefin Tuna (Cooked) ☞ serving size: 3 oz = 85 g; Calories = 156.4; Total Carb (g) = 0; Net Carb (g) = 0; Fat (g) = 5.3; Protein = 25.4

🐟 Bluefin Tuna (Raw) ☞ serving size: 3 oz = 85 g; Calories = 122.4; Total Carb (g) = 0; Net Carb (g) = 0; Fat (g) = 4.2; Protein = 19.8

🐟 Bluefish Cooked Dry Heat ☞ serving size: 1 fillet = 117 g; Calories = 186; Total Carb (g) = 0; Net Carb (g) = 0; Fat (g) = 6.4; Protein = 30.1

🐟 Bluefish Raw ☞ serving size: 1 fillet = 150 g; Calories = 186; Total Carb (g) = 0; Net Carb (g) = 0; Fat (g) = 6.4; Protein = 30.1

🐟 Bouillabaisse ☞ serving size: 1 cup = 227 g; Calories = 222.5; Total Carb (g) = 4.9; Net Carb (g) = 4.2; Fat (g) = 8.4; Protein = 30.5

🐟 Burbot Cooked Dry Heat ☞ serving size: 1 fillet = 90 g; Calories = 103.5; Total Carb (g) = 0; Net Carb (g) = 0; Fat (g) = 0.9; Protein = 22.3

🐟 Burbot Raw ☞ serving size: 1 fillet = 116 g; Calories = 104.4; Total Carb (g) = 0; Net Carb (g) = 0; Fat (g) = 0.9; Protein = 22.4

🐟 Butterfish Cooked Dry Heat ☞ serving size: 1 fillet = 25 g; Calories = 46.8; Total Carb (g) = 0; Net Carb (g) = 0; Fat (g) = 2.6; Protein = 5.5

🐟 Butterfish Raw ☞ serving size: 1 fillet = 32 g; Calories = 46.7; Total Carb (g) = 0; Net Carb (g) = 0; Fat (g) = 2.6; Protein = 5.5

🐟 Cake Or Patty Ns As To Fish ☞ serving size: 1 cake or patty = 120 g; Calories = 244.8; Total Carb (g) = 15.2; Net Carb (g) = 14.1; Fat (g) = 12.8; Protein = 16.7

🐟 Canned Anchovies ☞ serving size: 1 oz, boneless = 28.4 g; Calories = 59.6; Total Carb (g) = 0; Net Carb (g) = 0; Fat (g) = 2.8; Protein = 8.2

🐟 Canned Atlantic Cod ☞ serving size: 3 oz = 85 g; Calories = 89.3; Total Carb (g) = 0; Net Carb (g) = 0; Fat (g) = 0.7; Protein = 19.4

🐟 Canned Blue Crab ☞ serving size: 1 cup = 135 g; Calories = 112.1; Total Carb (g) = 0; Net Carb (g) = 0; Fat (g) = 1; Protein = 24.1

🐟 Canned Clams ☞ serving size: 3 oz = 85 g; Calories = 120.7; Total Carb (g) = 5; Net Carb (g) = 5; Fat (g) = 1.4; Protein = 20.6

🐟 Canned Eastern Oysters ☞ serving size: 3 oz = 85 g; Calories = 57.8; Total Carb (g) = 3.3; Net Carb (g) = 3.3; Fat (g) = 2.1; Protein = 6

🐟 Canned Pink Salmon ☞ serving size: 3 oz = 85 g; Calories = 115.6; Total Carb (g) = 0; Net Carb (g) = 0; Fat (g) = 3.6; Protein = 20.9

🐟 Canned Pink Salmon (With Skin And Bones) ☞ serving size: 3 oz = 85 g; Calories = 117.3; Total Carb (g) = 0; Net Carb (g) = 0; Fat (g) = 4.3; Protein = 19.6

🐟 Canned Salmon ☞ serving size: 3 oz = 85 g; Calories = 142; Total Carb (g) = 0; Net Carb (g) = 0; Fat (g) = 6.3; Protein = 20.1

🐟 Canned Sardines ☞ serving size: 1 cup, drained = 149 g; Calories = 309.9; Total Carb (g) = 0; Net Carb (g) = 0; Fat (g) = 17.1; Protein = 36.7

🐟 Canned Shrimp ☞ serving size: 1 cup = 128 g; Calories = 128; Total Carb (g) = 0; Net Carb (g) = 0; Fat (g) = 1.7; Protein = 26.1

🦐 Canned Sockeye Salmon ☞ serving size: 3 oz = 85 g; Calories = 134.3; Total Carb (g) = 0; Net Carb (g) = 0; Fat (g) = 5; Protein = 22.4

🦐 Canned Sockeye Salmon (With Bones) ☞ serving size: 3 oz = 85 g; Calories = 130.1; Total Carb (g) = 0; Net Carb (g) = 0; Fat (g) = 6.2; Protein = 17.4

🦐 Canned Sockeye Salmon (With Skin And Bones) ☞ serving size: 3 oz = 85 g; Calories = 130.1; Total Carb (g) = 0; Net Carb (g) = 0; Fat (g) = 6.1; Protein = 17.5

🦐 Canned White Tuna (Oil Packed) ☞ serving size: 3 oz = 85 g; Calories = 158.1; Total Carb (g) = 0; Net Carb (g) = 0; Fat (g) = 6.9; Protein = 22.6

🦐 Canned White Tuna (Water Packed) ☞ serving size: 3 oz = 85 g; Calories = 108.8; Total Carb (g) = 0; Net Carb (g) = 0; Fat (g) = 2.5; Protein = 20.1

🦐 Carp Baked Or Broiled Fat Added In Cooking ☞ serving size: 1 small fillet = 170 g; Calories = 319.6; Total Carb (g) = 0.2; Net Carb (g) = 0.2; Fat (g) = 17.9; Protein = 37.1

🦐 Carp Baked Or Broiled Fat Not Added In Cooking ☞ serving size: 1 small fillet = 170 g; Calories = 272; Total Carb (g) = 0.2; Net Carb (g) = 0.2; Fat (g) = 12; Protein = 38.2

🦐 Carp Coated Baked Or Broiled Fat Added In Cooking ☞ serving size: 1 small fillet = 170 g; Calories = 399.5; Total Carb (g) = 21.3; Net Carb (g) = 20.3; Fat (g) = 19.7; Protein = 32.2

🦐 Carp Coated Baked Or Broiled Fat Not Added In Cooking ☞ serving size: 1 small fillet = 170 g; Calories = 329.8; Total Carb (g) = 22.3; Net Carb (g) = 21.3; Fat (g) = 10.6; Protein = 33.7

🦐 Carp Coated Fried ☞ serving size: 1 small fillet = 170 g; Calories = 430.1; Total Carb (g) = 16.8; Net Carb (g) = 15.7; Fat (g) = 25.7; Protein = 31

🐟 Carp Cooked Dry Heat ☞ serving size: 3 oz = 85 g; Calories = 137.7; Total Carb (g) = 0; Net Carb (g) = 0; Fat (g) = 6.1; Protein = 19.4

🐟 Carp Cooked Ns As To Cooking Method ☞ serving size: 1 small fillet = 170 g; Calories = 430.1; Total Carb (g) = 16.8; Net Carb (g) = 15.7; Fat (g) = 25.7; Protein = 31

🐟 Carp Raw ☞ serving size: 3 oz = 85 g; Calories = 108; Total Carb (g) = 0; Net Carb (g) = 0; Fat (g) = 4.8; Protein = 15.2

🐟 Carp Smoked ☞ serving size: 1 oz = 28 g; Calories = 55.4; Total Carb (g) = 0; Net Carb (g) = 0; Fat (g) = 2.5; Protein = 7.8

🐟 Carp Steamed Or Poached ☞ serving size: 1 small fillet = 170 g; Calories = 272; Total Carb (g) = 0; Net Carb (g) = 0; Fat (g) = 12; Protein = 38.1

🐟 Cassava Fritter Stuffed With Crab Meat Puerto Rican Style ☞ serving size: 1 empanada (5" x 2-1/2" x 1/2") = 126 g; Calories = 335.2; Total Carb (g) = 38.2; Net Carb (g) = 36.1; Fat (g) = 15.4; Protein = 11.2

🐟 Catfish Baked Or Broiled Made With Butter ☞ serving size: 1 small fillet = 113 g; Calories = 195.5; Total Carb (g) = 0.1; Net Carb (g) = 0.1; Fat (g) = 11.7; Protein = 21.1

🐟 Catfish Baked Or Broiled Made With Cooking Spray ☞ serving size: 1 small fillet = 113 g; Calories = 174; Total Carb (g) = 0.2; Net Carb (g) = 0.2; Fat (g) = 8.9; Protein = 21.6

🐟 Catfish Baked Or Broiled Made With Margarine ☞ serving size: 1 small fillet = 113 g; Calories = 187.6; Total Carb (g) = 0.2; Net Carb (g) = 0.2; Fat (g) = 10.8; Protein = 21

🐟 Catfish Baked Or Broiled Made With Oil ☞ serving size: 1 small fillet = 113 g; Calories = 201.1; Total Carb (g) = 0.1; Net Carb (g) = 0.1; Fat (g) = 12.4; Protein = 21.1

🐟 Catfish Baked Or Broiled Made Without Fat ☞ serving size: 1 small fillet = 113 g; Calories = 169.5; Total Carb (g) = 0.1; Net Carb (g) = 0.1; Fat (g) = 8.5; Protein = 21.7

🐟 Catfish Channel Cooked Breaded And Fried ☞ serving size: 1 fillet = 87 g; Calories = 199.2; Total Carb (g) = 7; Net Carb (g) = 6.4; Fat (g) = 11.6; Protein = 15.7

🐟 Catfish Channel Farmed Cooked Dry Heat ☞ serving size: 1 fillet = 143 g; Calories = 205.9; Total Carb (g) = 0; Net Carb (g) = 0; Fat (g) = 10.3; Protein = 26.4

🐟 Catfish Channel Farmed Raw ☞ serving size: 3 oz = 85 g; Calories = 101.2; Total Carb (g) = 0; Net Carb (g) = 0; Fat (g) = 5.1; Protein = 13

🐟 Catfish Channel Wild Raw ☞ serving size: 3 oz = 85 g; Calories = 80.8; Total Carb (g) = 0; Net Carb (g) = 0; Fat (g) = 2.4; Protein = 13.9

🐟 Catfish Coated Baked Or Broiled Made With Butter ☞ serving size: 1 small fillet = 113 g; Calories = 248.6; Total Carb (g) = 14.1; Net Carb (g) = 13.5; Fat (g) = 12.4; Protein = 18.7

🐟 Catfish Coated Baked Or Broiled Made With Cooking Spray ☞ serving size: 1 small fillet = 113 g; Calories = 213.6; Total Carb (g) = 14.9; Net Carb (g) = 14.2; Fat (g) = 7.7; Protein = 19.5

🐟 Catfish Coated Baked Or Broiled Made With Margarine ☞ serving size: 1 small fillet = 113 g; Calories = 236.2; Total Carb (g) = 14.2; Net Carb (g) = 13.5; Fat (g) = 11.1; Protein = 18.6

🐟 Catfish Coated Baked Or Broiled Made With Oil ☞ serving size: 1 small fillet = 113 g; Calories = 257.6; Total Carb (g) = 14.2; Net Carb (g) = 13.5; Fat (g) = 13.4; Protein = 18.7

🐟 Catfish Coated Baked Or Broiled Made Without Fat ☞ serving size: 1 small fillet = 113 g; Calories = 210.2; Total Carb (g) = 14.8; Net Carb (g) = 14.1; Fat (g) = 7.4; Protein = 19.5

🐟 Catfish Coated Fried Made With Butter ☞ serving size: 1 small fillet = 113 g; Calories = 261; Total Carb (g) = 11.1; Net Carb (g) = 10.5; Fat (g) = 15.5; Protein = 18.2

🐟 Catfish Coated Fried Made With Cooking Spray ☞ serving size:

1 small fillet = 113 g; Calories = 227.1; Total Carb (g) = 13.2; Net Carb (g) = 12.4; Fat (g) = 9.2; Protein = 21.2

🐟 Catfish Coated Fried Made With Margarine ☞ serving size: 1 small fillet = 113 g; Calories = 243; Total Carb (g) = 11.2; Net Carb (g) = 10.5; Fat (g) = 13.5; Protein = 18.1

🐟 Catfish Coated Fried Made With Oil ☞ serving size: 1 small fillet = 113 g; Calories = 278; Total Carb (g) = 11.1; Net Carb (g) = 10.5; Fat (g) = 17.4; Protein = 18.1

🐟 Catfish Coated Fried Made Without Fat ☞ serving size: 1 small fillet = 113 g; Calories = 224.9; Total Carb (g) = 13.1; Net Carb (g) = 12.3; Fat (g) = 8.9; Protein = 21.3

🐟 Catfish Cooked Ns As To Cooking Method ☞ serving size: 1 small fillet = 113 g; Calories = 278; Total Carb (g) = 11.1; Net Carb (g) = 10.5; Fat (g) = 17.4; Protein = 18.1

🐟 Catfish Steamed Or Poached ☞ serving size: 1 small fillet = 113 g; Calories = 169.5; Total Carb (g) = 0; Net Carb (g) = 0; Fat (g) = 8.4; Protein = 21.6

🐟 Caviar Black And Red Granular ☞ serving size: 1 tbsp = 16 g; Calories = 42.2; Total Carb (g) = 0.6; Net Carb (g) = 0.6; Fat (g) = 2.9; Protein = 3.9

🐟 Ceviche ☞ serving size: 1 cup = 250 g; Calories = 155; Total Carb (g) = 9; Net Carb (g) = 7.7; Fat (g) = 1.9; Protein = 25.9

🐟 Cisco Raw ☞ serving size: 1 fillet = 79 g; Calories = 77.4; Total Carb (g) = 0; Net Carb (g) = 0; Fat (g) = 1.5; Protein = 15

🐟 Cisco Smoked ☞ serving size: 1 oz = 28.4 g; Calories = 50.3; Total Carb (g) = 0; Net Carb (g) = 0; Fat (g) = 3.4; Protein = 4.7

🐟 Clam Cake Or Patty ☞ serving size: 1 cake or patty = 120 g; Calories = 295.2; Total Carb (g) = 8.1; Net Carb (g) = 7.9; Fat (g) = 18.4; Protein = 22.9

🦐 Clam Sauce White ☞ serving size: 1 cup = 240 g; Calories = 470.4; Total Carb (g) = 6.2; Net Carb (g) = 5.9; Fat (g) = 40.7; Protein = 20.6

🦐 Clams (Raw) ☞ serving size: 3 oz = 85 g; Calories = 73.1; Total Carb (g) = 3; Net Carb (g) = 3; Fat (g) = 0.8; Protein = 12.5

🦐 Clams Baked Or Broiled Fat Added In Cooking ☞ serving size: 1 oz, without shell, cooked = 28 g; Calories = 37.8; Total Carb (g) = 1.2; Net Carb (g) = 1.2; Fat (g) = 1.3; Protein = 4.9

🦐 Clams Baked Or Broiled Fat Not Added In Cooking ☞ serving size: 1 oz, without shell, cooked = 28 g; Calories = 29.7; Total Carb (g) = 1.3; Net Carb (g) = 1.3; Fat (g) = 0.3; Protein = 5.1

🦐 Clams Canned ☞ serving size: 1 oz = 28 g; Calories = 30.2; Total Carb (g) = 1.3; Net Carb (g) = 1.3; Fat (g) = 0.3; Protein = 5.1

🦐 Clams Casino ☞ serving size: 1 clam = 30 g; Calories = 35.4; Total Carb (g) = 3; Net Carb (g) = 2.6; Fat (g) = 1.4; Protein = 2.6

🦐 Clams Coated Baked Or Broiled Fat Added In Cooking ☞ serving size: 1 oz, without shell, cooked = 28 g; Calories = 53.8; Total Carb (g) = 4.3; Net Carb (g) = 4.2; Fat (g) = 2; Protein = 4.4

🦐 Clams Coated Baked Or Broiled Fat Not Added In Cooking ☞ serving size: 1 oz, without shell, cooked = 28 g; Calories = 42; Total Carb (g) = 4.5; Net Carb (g) = 4.4; Fat (g) = 0.5; Protein = 4.6

🦐 Clams Coated Fried ☞ serving size: 1 oz, without shell, cooked = 28 g; Calories = 63.3; Total Carb (g) = 3.7; Net Carb (g) = 3.6; Fat (g) = 3.2; Protein = 4.5

🦐 Clams Cooked Ns As To Cooking Method ☞ serving size: 1 oz, without shell, cooked = 28 g; Calories = 37.8; Total Carb (g) = 1.2; Net Carb (g) = 1.2; Fat (g) = 1.3; Protein = 4.9

🦐 Clams Smoked In Oil ☞ serving size: 1 oz = 28 g; Calories = 53.8; Total Carb (g) = 1.1; Net Carb (g) = 1.1; Fat (g) = 3.3; Protein = 4.7

🦐 Clams Steamed Or Boiled ☞ serving size: 1 oz, without shell, cooked = 28 g; Calories = 47.9; Total Carb (g) = 2; Net Carb (g) = 2; Fat (g) = 0.5; Protein = 8.2

🦐 Clams Stuffed ☞ serving size: 1 small (12 in 11 oz frozen package) = 26 g; Calories = 52; Total Carb (g) = 3.4; Net Carb (g) = 3.1; Fat (g) = 2.9; Protein = 3.1

🦐 Cod Atlantic Raw ☞ serving size: 3 oz = 85 g; Calories = 69.7; Total Carb (g) = 0; Net Carb (g) = 0; Fat (g) = 0.6; Protein = 15.1

🦐 Cod Cooked Ns As To Cooking Method ☞ serving size: 1 small fillet = 170 g; Calories = 198.9; Total Carb (g) = 0.2; Net Carb (g) = 0.2; Fat (g) = 7.1; Protein = 31.8

🦐 Cod Pacific Raw (May Have Been Previously Frozen) ☞ serving size: 1 fillet = 116 g; Calories = 80; Total Carb (g) = 0; Net Carb (g) = 0; Fat (g) = 0.5; Protein = 17.7

🦐 Cod Smoked ☞ serving size: 1 oz, boneless = 28 g; Calories = 30.2; Total Carb (g) = 0; Net Carb (g) = 0; Fat (g) = 0.2; Protein = 6.7

🦐 Cod Steamed Or Poached ☞ serving size: 1 small fillet = 170 g; Calories = 147.9; Total Carb (g) = 0; Net Carb (g) = 0; Fat (g) = 0.9; Protein = 32.6

🦐 Codfish Ball Or Cake ☞ serving size: 1 ball = 63 g; Calories = 112.1; Total Carb (g) = 8.2; Net Carb (g) = 7.6; Fat (g) = 4.7; Protein = 9

🦐 Cooked Alaska Pollock ☞ serving size: 1 fillet = 60 g; Calories = 66.6; Total Carb (g) = 0; Net Carb (g) = 0; Fat (g) = 0.7; Protein = 14.1

🦐 Cooked Atlantic Cod ☞ serving size: 3 oz = 85 g; Calories = 89.3; Total Carb (g) = 0; Net Carb (g) = 0; Fat (g) = 0.7; Protein = 19.4

🦐 Cooked Atlantic Perch ☞ serving size: 1 fillet = 50 g; Calories = 48; Total Carb (g) = 0; Net Carb (g) = 0; Fat (g) = 0.9; Protein = 9.3

🦐 Cooked Blue Mussels ☞ serving size: 3 oz = 85 g; Calories = 146.2; Total Carb (g) = 6.3; Net Carb (g) = 6.3; Fat (g) = 3.8; Protein = 20.2

🦐 Cooked Catfish ☞ serving size: 1 fillet = 143 g; Calories = 150.2; Total Carb (g) = 0; Net Carb (g) = 0; Fat (g) = 4.1; Protein = 26.4

🦐 Cooked Clams ☞ serving size: 3 oz = 85 g; Calories = 125.8; Total Carb (g) = 4.4; Net Carb (g) = 4.4; Fat (g) = 1.7; Protein = 21.7

🦐 Cooked Cod ☞ serving size: 3 oz = 85 g; Calories = 71.4; Total Carb (g) = 0; Net Carb (g) = 0; Fat (g) = 0.2; Protein = 17.4

🦐 Cooked Coho Salmon (Farmed) ☞ serving size: 1 fillet = 143 g; Calories = 254.5; Total Carb (g) = 0; Net Carb (g) = 0; Fat (g) = 11.8; Protein = 34.8

🦐 Cooked Coho Salmon (Wild Moist Heat) ☞ serving size: 3 oz = 85 g; Calories = 156.4; Total Carb (g) = 0; Net Carb (g) = 0; Fat (g) = 6.4; Protein = 23.3

🦐 Cooked Coho Salmon (Wild) ☞ serving size: 3 oz = 85 g; Calories = 118.2; Total Carb (g) = 0; Net Carb (g) = 0; Fat (g) = 3.7; Protein = 19.9

🦐 Cooked Crayfish ☞ serving size: 3 oz = 85 g; Calories = 74; Total Carb (g) = 0; Net Carb (g) = 0; Fat (g) = 1.1; Protein = 14.9

🦐 Cooked Cuttlefish ☞ serving size: 3 oz = 85 g; Calories = 134.3; Total Carb (g) = 1.4; Net Carb (g) = 1.4; Fat (g) = 1.2; Protein = 27.6

🦐 Cooked Dry Heat ☞ serving size: 1 fillet = 95 g; Calories = 106.4; Total Carb (g) = 0; Net Carb (g) = 0; Fat (g) = 0.8; Protein = 23.1

🦐 Cooked Dungeness Crab ☞ serving size: 3 oz = 85 g; Calories = 93.5; Total Carb (g) = 0.8; Net Carb (g) = 0.8; Fat (g) = 1.1; Protein = 19

🦐 Cooked Eastern Oysters (Farmed) ☞ serving size: 3 oz = 85 g; Calories = 67.2; Total Carb (g) = 6.2; Net Carb (g) = 6.2; Fat (g) = 1.8; Protein = 6

🦐 Cooked Eastern Oysters (Wild) ☞ serving size: 3 oz = 85 g; Calories = 67.2; Total Carb (g) = 3.6; Net Carb (g) = 3.6; Fat (g) = 2.3; Protein = 7.5

🐟 Cooked Eel ☞ serving size: 1 oz, boneless = 28.4 g; Calories = 67; Total Carb (g) = 0; Net Carb (g) = 0; Fat (g) = 4.3; Protein = 6.7

🐟 Cooked Grouper ☞ serving size: 3 oz = 85 g; Calories = 100.3; Total Carb (g) = 0; Net Carb (g) = 0; Fat (g) = 1.1; Protein = 21.1

🐟 Cooked Haddock ☞ serving size: 1 fillet = 150 g; Calories = 135; Total Carb (g) = 0; Net Carb (g) = 0; Fat (g) = 0.8; Protein = 30

🐟 Cooked Halibut ☞ serving size: 3 oz = 85 g; Calories = 94.4; Total Carb (g) = 0; Net Carb (g) = 0; Fat (g) = 1.4; Protein = 19.2

🐟 Cooked King Mackerel ☞ serving size: 3 oz = 85 g; Calories = 113.9; Total Carb (g) = 0; Net Carb (g) = 0; Fat (g) = 2.2; Protein = 22.1

🐟 Cooked Lingcod ☞ serving size: 3 oz = 85 g; Calories = 92.7; Total Carb (g) = 0; Net Carb (g) = 0; Fat (g) = 1.2; Protein = 19.2

🐟 Cooked Mahimahi ☞ serving size: 3 oz = 85 g; Calories = 92.7; Total Carb (g) = 0; Net Carb (g) = 0; Fat (g) = 0.8; Protein = 20.2

🐟 Cooked Northern Pike ☞ serving size: 3 oz = 85 g; Calories = 96.1; Total Carb (g) = 0; Net Carb (g) = 0; Fat (g) = 0.8; Protein = 21

🐟 Cooked Orange Roughy ☞ serving size: 3 oz = 85 g; Calories = 89.3; Total Carb (g) = 0; Net Carb (g) = 0; Fat (g) = 0.8; Protein = 19.2

🐟 Cooked Pacific Cod ☞ serving size: 1 fillet = 90 g; Calories = 76.5; Total Carb (g) = 0; Net Carb (g) = 0; Fat (g) = 0.5; Protein = 16.9

🐟 Cooked Pacific Herring ☞ serving size: 1 fillet = 144 g; Calories = 360; Total Carb (g) = 0; Net Carb (g) = 0; Fat (g) = 25.6; Protein = 30.3

🐟 Cooked Pacific Oysters ☞ serving size: 1 medium = 25 g; Calories = 40.8; Total Carb (g) = 2.5; Net Carb (g) = 2.5; Fat (g) = 1.2; Protein = 4.7

🐟 Cooked Pollock ☞ serving size: 3 oz = 85 g; Calories = 100.3; Total Carb (g) = 0; Net Carb (g) = 0; Fat (g) = 1.1; Protein = 21.2

🐟 Cooked Pompano ☞ serving size: 1 fillet = 88 g; Calories = 185.7; Total Carb (g) = 0; Net Carb (g) = 0; Fat (g) = 10.7; Protein = 20.9

🐟 Cooked Rainbow Trout ☞ serving size: 1 fillet = 71 g; Calories = 119.3; Total Carb (g) = 0; Net Carb (g) = 0; Fat (g) = 5.2; Protein = 16.9

🐟 Cooked Sablefish ☞ serving size: 3 oz = 85 g; Calories = 212.5; Total Carb (g) = 0; Net Carb (g) = 0; Fat (g) = 16.7; Protein = 14.6

🐟 Cooked Sea Bass ☞ serving size: 1 fillet = 101 g; Calories = 125.2; Total Carb (g) = 0; Net Carb (g) = 0; Fat (g) = 2.6; Protein = 23.9

🐟 Cooked Shrimp ☞ serving size: 3 oz = 85 g; Calories = 101.2; Total Carb (g) = 1.3; Net Carb (g) = 1.3; Fat (g) = 1.5; Protein = 19.4

🐟 Cooked Skipjack ☞ serving size: 3 oz = 85 g; Calories = 112.2; Total Carb (g) = 0; Net Carb (g) = 0; Fat (g) = 1.1; Protein = 24

🐟 Cooked Smelt ☞ serving size: 3 oz = 85 g; Calories = 105.4; Total Carb (g) = 0; Net Carb (g) = 0; Fat (g) = 2.6; Protein = 19.2

🐟 Cooked Snapper ☞ serving size: 3 oz = 85 g; Calories = 108.8; Total Carb (g) = 0; Net Carb (g) = 0; Fat (g) = 1.5; Protein = 22.4

🐟 Cooked Sockeye Salmon ☞ serving size: 3 oz = 85 g; Calories = 132.6; Total Carb (g) = 0; Net Carb (g) = 0; Fat (g) = 4.7; Protein = 22.5

🐟 Cooked Spiny Lobster ☞ serving size: 3 oz = 85 g; Calories = 121.6; Total Carb (g) = 2.7; Net Carb (g) = 2.7; Fat (g) = 1.7; Protein = 22.5

🐟 Cooked Striped Bass ☞ serving size: 1 fillet = 124 g; Calories = 153.8; Total Carb (g) = 0; Net Carb (g) = 0; Fat (g) = 3.7; Protein = 28.2

🐟 Cooked Sturgeon ☞ serving size: 3 oz = 85 g; Calories = 114.8; Total Carb (g) = 0; Net Carb (g) = 0; Fat (g) = 4.4; Protein = 17.6

🐟 Cooked Swordfish ☞ serving size: 3 oz = 85 g; Calories = 146.2; Total Carb (g) = 0; Net Carb (g) = 0; Fat (g) = 6.7; Protein = 19.9

🐟 Cooked Tilapia ☞ serving size: 1 fillet = 87 g; Calories = 111.4; Total Carb (g) = 0; Net Carb (g) = 0; Fat (g) = 2.3; Protein = 22.8

🐟 Cooked Tilefish ☞ serving size: 1/2 fillet = 150 g; Calories = 220.5; Total Carb (g) = 0; Net Carb (g) = 0; Fat (g) = 7; Protein = 36.7

🐟 Cooked Trout ☞ serving size: 1 fillet = 143 g; Calories = 214.5; Total Carb (g) = 0; Net Carb (g) = 0; Fat (g) = 8.3; Protein = 32.8

🐟 Cooked Turbot ☞ serving size: 3 oz = 85 g; Calories = 103.7; Total Carb (g) = 0; Net Carb (g) = 0; Fat (g) = 3.2; Protein = 17.5

🐟 Cooked Walleye Pike ☞ serving size: 1 fillet = 124 g; Calories = 147.6; Total Carb (g) = 0; Net Carb (g) = 0; Fat (g) = 1.9; Protein = 30.4

🐟 Cooked Whitefish ☞ serving size: 3 oz = 85 g; Calories = 146.2; Total Carb (g) = 0; Net Carb (g) = 0; Fat (g) = 6.4; Protein = 20.8

🐟 Cooked Whiting ☞ serving size: 1 fillet = 72 g; Calories = 83.5; Total Carb (g) = 0; Net Carb (g) = 0; Fat (g) = 1.2; Protein = 16.9

🐟 Cooked Wild Eastern Oysters ☞ serving size: 3 oz = 85 g; Calories = 86.7; Total Carb (g) = 4.6; Net Carb (g) = 4.6; Fat (g) = 2.9; Protein = 9.7

🐟 Cooked Yellowfin Tuna ☞ serving size: 3 oz = 85 g; Calories = 110.5; Total Carb (g) = 0; Net Carb (g) = 0; Fat (g) = 0.5; Protein = 24.8

🐟 Cooked Yellowtail ☞ serving size: 1/2 fillet = 146 g; Calories = 273; Total Carb (g) = 0; Net Carb (g) = 0; Fat (g) = 9.8; Protein = 43.3

🐟 Crab Cooked Ns As To Cooking Method ☞ serving size: 1 oz, without shell, cooked = 28 g; Calories = 23; Total Carb (g) = 0; Net Carb (g) = 0; Fat (g) = 0.2; Protein = 5

🐟 Crab Deviled ☞ serving size: 1 cup = 175 g; Calories = 327.3; Total Carb (g) = 23.2; Net Carb (g) = 22.2; Fat (g) = 16.8; Protein = 20.9

🐟 Crab Hard Shell Steamed ☞ serving size: 1 cup, cooked, flaked and pieces = 118 g; Calories = 96.8; Total Carb (g) = 0; Net Carb (g) = 0; Fat (g) = 0.9; Protein = 21

🦐 Crab Imperial ☞ serving size: 1 cup = 259 g; Calories = 354.8; Total Carb (g) = 8.3; Net Carb (g) = 7.8; Fat (g) = 19; Protein = 36.1

🦐 Crayfish ☞ serving size: 3 oz = 85 g; Calories = 69.7; Total Carb (g) = 0; Net Carb (g) = 0; Fat (g) = 1; Protein = 14.3

🦐 Croaker Atlantic Raw ☞ serving size: 1 fillet = 79 g; Calories = 82.2; Total Carb (g) = 0; Net Carb (g) = 0; Fat (g) = 2.5; Protein = 14.1

🦐 Croaker Cooked Ns As To Cooking Method ☞ serving size: 1 small fillet = 113 g; Calories = 180.8; Total Carb (g) = 0.1; Net Carb (g) = 0.1; Fat (g) = 8.5; Protein = 24.6

🦐 Croaker Steamed Or Poached ☞ serving size: 1 small fillet = 113 g; Calories = 148; Total Carb (g) = 0; Net Carb (g) = 0; Fat (g) = 4.5; Protein = 25.3

🦐 Crustaceans Crab Alaska King Raw ☞ serving size: 3 oz = 85 g; Calories = 71.4; Total Carb (g) = 0; Net Carb (g) = 0; Fat (g) = 0.5; Protein = 15.6

🦐 Crustaceans Crab Blue Raw ☞ serving size: 3 oz = 85 g; Calories = 74; Total Carb (g) = 0; Net Carb (g) = 0; Fat (g) = 0.9; Protein = 15.4

🦐 Crustaceans Crayfish Mixed Species Farmed Raw ☞ serving size: 3 oz = 85 g; Calories = 61.2; Total Carb (g) = 0; Net Carb (g) = 0; Fat (g) = 0.8; Protein = 12.6

🦐 Crustaceans Crayfish Mixed Species Wild Raw ☞ serving size: 3 oz = 85 g; Calories = 65.5; Total Carb (g) = 0; Net Carb (g) = 0; Fat (g) = 0.8; Protein = 13.6

🦐 Crustaceans Lobster Northern Raw ☞ serving size: 1 lobster = 150 g; Calories = 115.5; Total Carb (g) = 0; Net Carb (g) = 0; Fat (g) = 1.1; Protein = 24.8

🦐 Crustaceans Shrimp Cooked (Not Previously Frozen) ☞ serving size: 3 oz = 85 g; Calories = 84.2; Total Carb (g) = 0.2; Net Carb (g) = 0.2; Fat (g) = 0.2; Protein = 20.4

🦐 Crustaceans Shrimp Mixed Species Cooked Breaded And Fried ☞ serving size: 3 oz = 85 g; Calories = 205.7; Total Carb (g) = 9.8; Net Carb (g) = 9.4; Fat (g) = 10.4; Protein = 18.2

🦐 Crustaceans Shrimp Mixed Species Imitation Made From Surimi ☞ serving size: 3 oz = 85 g; Calories = 85.9; Total Carb (g) = 7.8; Net Carb (g) = 7.8; Fat (g) = 1.3; Protein = 10.5

🦐 Crustaceans Shrimp Mixed Species Raw (May Have Been Previously Frozen) ☞ serving size: 1 medium = 6 g; Calories = 4.3; Total Carb (g) = 0.1; Net Carb (g) = 0.1; Fat (g) = 0.1; Protein = 0.8

🦐 Crustaceans Shrimp Raw (Not Previously Frozen) ☞ serving size: 3 oz = 85 g; Calories = 72.3; Total Carb (g) = 0; Net Carb (g) = 0; Fat (g) = 0.4; Protein = 17.1

🦐 Crustaceans Spiny Lobster Mixed Species Raw ☞ serving size: 3 oz = 85 g; Calories = 95.2; Total Carb (g) = 2.1; Net Carb (g) = 2.1; Fat (g) = 1.3; Protein = 17.5

🦐 Curry ☞ serving size: 1 cup = 236 g; Calories = 165.2; Total Carb (g) = 16.1; Net Carb (g) = 12.1; Fat (g) = 6.9; Protein = 10.6

🦐 Cusk Raw ☞ serving size: 1 fillet = 122 g; Calories = 106.1; Total Carb (g) = 0; Net Carb (g) = 0; Fat (g) = 0.8; Protein = 23.2

🦐 Drum Freshwater Raw ☞ serving size: 3 oz = 85 g; Calories = 101.2; Total Carb (g) = 0; Net Carb (g) = 0; Fat (g) = 4.2; Protein = 14.9

🦐 Dungeness Crab (Raw) ☞ serving size: 3 oz = 85 g; Calories = 73.1; Total Carb (g) = 0.6; Net Carb (g) = 0.6; Fat (g) = 0.8; Protein = 14.8

🦐 Eel Cooked Ns As To Cooking Method ☞ serving size: 1 oz, boneless, cooked = 28 g; Calories = 83.4; Total Carb (g) = 2.6; Net Carb (g) = 2.5; Fat (g) = 5.6; Protein = 5.2

🦐 Eel Mixed Species Raw ☞ serving size: 3 oz = 85 g; Calories = 156.4; Total Carb (g) = 0; Net Carb (g) = 0; Fat (g) = 9.9; Protein = 15.7

🐟 Eel Smoked ☞ serving size: 1 oz, boneless = 28 g; Calories = 80.4; Total Carb (g) = 0; Net Carb (g) = 0; Fat (g) = 5.1; Protein = 8

🐟 Eel Steamed Or Poached ☞ serving size: 1 oz, boneless, raw (yield after cooking) = 23 g; Calories = 53.1; Total Carb (g) = 0; Net Carb (g) = 0; Fat (g) = 3.4; Protein = 5.3

🐟 Farmed Atlantic Salmon ☞ serving size: 3 oz = 85 g; Calories = 175.1; Total Carb (g) = 0; Net Carb (g) = 0; Fat (g) = 10.5; Protein = 18.8

🐟 Farmed Atlantic Salmon (Raw) ☞ serving size: 3 oz = 85 g; Calories = 176.8; Total Carb (g) = 0; Net Carb (g) = 0; Fat (g) = 11.4; Protein = 17.4

🐟 Flat Fish (Flounder Or Sole) ☞ serving size: 1 fillet = 127 g; Calories = 109.2; Total Carb (g) = 0; Net Carb (g) = 0; Fat (g) = 3; Protein = 19.4

🐟 Flatfish (Flounder And Sole Species) Raw ☞ serving size: 1 oz, boneless = 28.4 g; Calories = 19.9; Total Carb (g) = 0; Net Carb (g) = 0; Fat (g) = 0.6; Protein = 3.5

🐟 Flounder Cooked Ns As To Cooking Method ☞ serving size: 1 small fillet = 113 g; Calories = 230.5; Total Carb (g) = 11.1; Net Carb (g) = 10.5; Fat (g) = 13.5; Protein = 15.4

🐟 Flounder Smoked ☞ serving size: 1 oz, boneless = 28 g; Calories = 47.3; Total Carb (g) = 0; Net Carb (g) = 0; Fat (g) = 1.3; Protein = 8.4

🐟 Flounder Steamed Or Poached ☞ serving size: 1 small fillet = 113 g; Calories = 99.4; Total Carb (g) = 0; Net Carb (g) = 0; Fat (g) = 2.8; Protein = 17.6

🐟 Fresh Water Bass (Raw) ☞ serving size: 1 fillet = 79 g; Calories = 90.1; Total Carb (g) = 0; Net Carb (g) = 0; Fat (g) = 2.9; Protein = 14.9

🐟 Frog Legs Ns As To Cooking Method ☞ serving size: 1 oz, boneless, cooked = 28 g; Calories = 59.9; Total Carb (g) = 2.9; Net Carb (g) = 2.7; Fat (g) = 3.1; Protein = 4.9

🦑 Frog Legs Raw ☞ serving size: 1 leg = 45 g; Calories = 32.9; Total Carb (g) = 0; Net Carb (g) = 0; Fat (g) = 0.1; Protein = 7.4

🦑 Frog Legs Steamed ☞ serving size: 1 oz, boneless, cooked = 28 g; Calories = 25.8; Total Carb (g) = 0; Net Carb (g) = 0; Fat (g) = 0.1; Protein = 5.8

🦑 Gefilte Fish ☞ serving size: 1 cup = 227 g; Calories = 256.5; Total Carb (g) = 2.3; Net Carb (g) = 2.1; Fat (g) = 8.6; Protein = 39.8

🦑 Gefiltefish Commercial Sweet Recipe ☞ serving size: 1 piece = 42 g; Calories = 35.3; Total Carb (g) = 3.1; Net Carb (g) = 3.1; Fat (g) = 0.7; Protein = 3.8

🦑 Grouper Mixed Species Raw ☞ serving size: 3 oz = 85 g; Calories = 78.2; Total Carb (g) = 0; Net Carb (g) = 0; Fat (g) = 0.9; Protein = 16.5

🦑 Gumbo No Rice ☞ serving size: 1 cup = 244 g; Calories = 200.1; Total Carb (g) = 9.5; Net Carb (g) = 7.1; Fat (g) = 8.9; Protein = 20.9

🦑 Gumbo With Rice ☞ serving size: 1 cup = 244 g; Calories = 214.7; Total Carb (g) = 15.7; Net Carb (g) = 13.5; Fat (g) = 8.3; Protein = 20

🦑 Haddock Cake Or Patty ☞ serving size: 1 cake or patty = 120 g; Calories = 244.8; Total Carb (g) = 15.2; Net Carb (g) = 14.1; Fat (g) = 12.8; Protein = 16.7

🦑 Haddock Cooked Ns As To Cooking Method ☞ serving size: 1 small fillet = 170 g; Calories = 209.1; Total Carb (g) = 0.2; Net Carb (g) = 0.2; Fat (g) = 7.2; Protein = 34

🦑 Haddock Raw ☞ serving size: 3 oz = 85 g; Calories = 62.9; Total Carb (g) = 0; Net Carb (g) = 0; Fat (g) = 0.4; Protein = 13.9

🦑 Haddock Steamed Or Poached ☞ serving size: 1 small fillet = 170 g; Calories = 158.1; Total Carb (g) = 0; Net Carb (g) = 0; Fat (g) = 1; Protein = 34.9

🦑 Halibut Atlantic And Pacific Raw ☞ serving size: 3 oz = 85 g;

Calories = 77.4; Total Carb (g) = 0; Net Carb (g) = 0; Fat (g) = 1.1; Protein = 15.8

🐟 Halibut Cooked Ns As To Cooking Method ☞ serving size: 1 small fillet = 170 g; Calories = 244.8; Total Carb (g) = 0.2; Net Carb (g) = 0.2; Fat (g) = 9; Protein = 38.6

🐟 Halibut Greenland Cooked Dry Heat ☞ serving size: 3 oz = 85 g; Calories = 203.2; Total Carb (g) = 0; Net Carb (g) = 0; Fat (g) = 15.1; Protein = 15.7

🐟 Halibut Greenland Raw ☞ serving size: 3 oz = 85 g; Calories = 158.1; Total Carb (g) = 0; Net Carb (g) = 0; Fat (g) = 11.8; Protein = 12.2

🐟 Halibut Smoked ☞ serving size: 1 oz, boneless = 28 g; Calories = 61.3; Total Carb (g) = 0; Net Carb (g) = 0; Fat (g) = 0.9; Protein = 12.5

🐟 Halibut Steamed Or Poached ☞ serving size: 1 small fillet = 170 g; Calories = 193.8; Total Carb (g) = 0; Net Carb (g) = 0; Fat (g) = 2.8; Protein = 39.7

🐟 Herring Atlantic Raw ☞ serving size: 1 oz, boneless = 28.4 g; Calories = 44.9; Total Carb (g) = 0; Net Carb (g) = 0; Fat (g) = 2.6; Protein = 5.1

🐟 Herring Cooked Ns As To Cooking Method ☞ serving size: 1 oz, boneless, raw (yield after cooking) = 23 g; Calories = 52; Total Carb (g) = 0; Net Carb (g) = 0; Fat (g) = 3.4; Protein = 5.1

🐟 Herring Dried Salted ☞ serving size: 1 oz, boneless = 28 g; Calories = 137.2; Total Carb (g) = 0; Net Carb (g) = 0; Fat (g) = 7.9; Protein = 15.6

🐟 Herring Pacific Raw ☞ serving size: 3 oz = 85 g; Calories = 165.8; Total Carb (g) = 0; Net Carb (g) = 0; Fat (g) = 11.8; Protein = 13.9

🐟 Imitation Crab Meat ☞ serving size: 3 oz = 85 g; Calories = 80.8; Total Carb (g) = 12.8; Net Carb (g) = 12.3; Fat (g) = 0.4; Protein = 6.5

🐟 Lau Lau ☞ serving size: 1 lau lau = 214 g; Calories = 299.6; Total Carb (g) = 0; Net Carb (g) = 0; Fat (g) = 17.8; Protein = 32.6

🐟 Ling Cooked Dry Heat ☞ serving size: 3 oz = 85 g; Calories = 94.4; Total Carb (g) = 0; Net Carb (g) = 0; Fat (g) = 0.7; Protein = 20.7

🐟 Ling Raw ☞ serving size: 3 oz = 85 g; Calories = 74; Total Carb (g) = 0; Net Carb (g) = 0; Fat (g) = 0.5; Protein = 16.1

🐟 Lingcod Raw ☞ serving size: 3 oz = 85 g; Calories = 72.3; Total Carb (g) = 0; Net Carb (g) = 0; Fat (g) = 0.9; Protein = 15

🐟 Lobster Cooked Ns As To Cooking Method ☞ serving size: 1 small lobster (1 lb live weight) (yield after cooking, shell removed) = 118 g; Calories = 103.8; Total Carb (g) = 0; Net Carb (g) = 0; Fat (g) = 1; Protein = 22.3

🐟 Lobster Gumbo ☞ serving size: 1 cup = 244 g; Calories = 144; Total Carb (g) = 11.3; Net Carb (g) = 9.1; Fat (g) = 4.3; Protein = 15.1

🐟 Lobster Newburg ☞ serving size: 1 cup = 244 g; Calories = 588; Total Carb (g) = 8.8; Net Carb (g) = 8.5; Fat (g) = 49.1; Protein = 28.3

🐟 Lomi Salmon ☞ serving size: 1 cup = 234 g; Calories = 140.4; Total Carb (g) = 7.8; Net Carb (g) = 5.4; Fat (g) = 4.4; Protein = 17.7

🐟 Mackerel Cake Or Patty ☞ serving size: 1 cake or patty = 120 g; Calories = 309.6; Total Carb (g) = 15.8; Net Carb (g) = 14.6; Fat (g) = 18.1; Protein = 19.8

🐟 Mackerel Cooked Ns As To Cooking Method ☞ serving size: 1 small fillet = 170 g; Calories = 448.8; Total Carb (g) = 0.2; Net Carb (g) = 0.2; Fat (g) = 31; Protein = 39.7

🐟 Mackerel Jack Canned Drained Solids ☞ serving size: 1 oz, boneless = 28.4 g; Calories = 44.3; Total Carb (g) = 0; Net Carb (g) = 0; Fat (g) = 1.8; Protein = 6.6

🐟 Mackerel King Raw ☞ serving size: 3 oz = 85 g; Calories = 89.3; Total Carb (g) = 0; Net Carb (g) = 0; Fat (g) = 1.7; Protein = 17.2

🐟 Mackerel Pickled ☞ serving size: 1 oz, boneless = 28 g; Calories = 60.8; Total Carb (g) = 1.1; Net Carb (g) = 1; Fat (g) = 4.8; Protein = 3.1

🐟 Mackerel Raw ☞ serving size: 1 oz, boneless, raw = 28 g; Calories = 52.9; Total Carb (g) = 0; Net Carb (g) = 0; Fat (g) = 3.3; Protein = 5.3

🐟 Mackerel Salted ☞ serving size: 1 piece (5-1/2 inch x 1-1/2 inch x 1/2 inch) = 80 g; Calories = 244; Total Carb (g) = 0; Net Carb (g) = 0; Fat (g) = 20.1; Protein = 14.8

🐟 Mackerel Smoked ☞ serving size: 1 oz, boneless = 28 g; Calories = 56; Total Carb (g) = 0; Net Carb (g) = 0; Fat (g) = 2.8; Protein = 7.2

🐟 Mackerel Spanish Cooked Dry Heat ☞ serving size: 1 fillet = 146 g; Calories = 230.7; Total Carb (g) = 0; Net Carb (g) = 0; Fat (g) = 9.2; Protein = 34.4

🐟 Mackerel Spanish Raw ☞ serving size: 3 oz = 85 g; Calories = 118.2; Total Carb (g) = 0; Net Carb (g) = 0; Fat (g) = 5.4; Protein = 16.4

🐟 Mahimahi Raw ☞ serving size: 3 oz = 85 g; Calories = 72.3; Total Carb (g) = 0; Net Carb (g) = 0; Fat (g) = 0.6; Protein = 15.7

🐟 Milkfish Cooked Dry Heat ☞ serving size: 3 oz = 85 g; Calories = 161.5; Total Carb (g) = 0; Net Carb (g) = 0; Fat (g) = 7.3; Protein = 22.4

🐟 Milkfish Raw ☞ serving size: 3 oz = 85 g; Calories = 125.8; Total Carb (g) = 0; Net Carb (g) = 0; Fat (g) = 5.7; Protein = 17.5

🐟 Mollusks Abalone Mixed Species Raw ☞ serving size: 3 oz = 85 g; Calories = 89.3; Total Carb (g) = 5.1; Net Carb (g) = 5.1; Fat (g) = 0.7; Protein = 14.5

🐟 Mollusks Clam Mixed Species Canned Liquid ☞ serving size: 3 oz = 85 g; Calories = 1.7; Total Carb (g) = 0.1; Net Carb (g) = 0.1; Fat (g) = 0; Protein = 0.3

🐟 Mollusks Clam Mixed Species Cooked Breaded And Fried ☞ serving size: 3 oz = 85 g; Calories = 171.7; Total Carb (g) = 8.8; Net Carb (g) = 8.8; Fat (g) = 9.5; Protein = 12.1

🦑 Mollusks Cuttlefish Mixed Species Raw ☞ serving size: 3 oz = 85 g; Calories = 67.2; Total Carb (g) = 0.7; Net Carb (g) = 0.7; Fat (g) = 0.6; Protein = 13.8

🦑 Mollusks Mussel Blue Raw ☞ serving size: 1 cup = 150 g; Calories = 129; Total Carb (g) = 5.5; Net Carb (g) = 5.5; Fat (g) = 3.4; Protein = 17.9

🦑 Mollusks Octopus Common Raw ☞ serving size: 3 oz = 85 g; Calories = 69.7; Total Carb (g) = 1.9; Net Carb (g) = 1.9; Fat (g) = 0.9; Protein = 12.7

🦑 Mollusks Oyster Eastern Cooked Breaded And Fried ☞ serving size: 3 oz = 85 g; Calories = 169.2; Total Carb (g) = 9.9; Net Carb (g) = 9.9; Fat (g) = 10.7; Protein = 7.5

🦑 Mollusks Oyster Eastern Wild Raw ☞ serving size: 6 medium = 84 g; Calories = 42.8; Total Carb (g) = 2.3; Net Carb (g) = 2.3; Fat (g) = 1.4; Protein = 4.8

🦑 Mollusks Scallop Mixed Species Cooked Breaded And Fried ☞ serving size: 2 large = 31 g; Calories = 67; Total Carb (g) = 3.1; Net Carb (g) = 3.1; Fat (g) = 3.4; Protein = 5.6

🦑 Mollusks Scallop Mixed Species Imitation Made From Surimi ☞ serving size: 3 oz = 85 g; Calories = 84.2; Total Carb (g) = 9; Net Carb (g) = 9; Fat (g) = 0.4; Protein = 10.9

🦑 Mollusks Snail Raw ☞ serving size: 3 oz = 85 g; Calories = 76.5; Total Carb (g) = 1.7; Net Carb (g) = 1.7; Fat (g) = 1.2; Protein = 13.7

🦑 Mollusks Whelk Unspecified Raw ☞ serving size: 3 oz = 85 g; Calories = 116.5; Total Carb (g) = 6.6; Net Carb (g) = 6.6; Fat (g) = 0.3; Protein = 20.3

🦑 Monkfish Cooked Dry Heat ☞ serving size: 3 oz = 85 g; Calories = 82.5; Total Carb (g) = 0; Net Carb (g) = 0; Fat (g) = 1.7; Protein = 15.8

🦑 Monkfish Raw ☞ serving size: 3 oz = 85 g; Calories = 64.6; Total Carb (g) = 0; Net Carb (g) = 0; Fat (g) = 1.3; Protein = 12.3

🦐 Moochim ☞ serving size: 1 tablespoon = 5 g; Calories = 17; Total Carb (g) = 0.5; Net Carb (g) = 0.5; Fat (g) = 0.8; Protein = 1.9

🦐 Mullet Cooked Ns As To Cooking Method ☞ serving size: 1 small fillet = 113 g; Calories = 275.7; Total Carb (g) = 11.1; Net Carb (g) = 10.5; Fat (g) = 15.3; Protein = 22.1

🦐 Mullet Steamed Or Poached ☞ serving size: 1 small fillet = 113 g; Calories = 166.1; Total Carb (g) = 0; Net Carb (g) = 0; Fat (g) = 5.4; Protein = 27.5

🦐 Mullet Striped Cooked Dry Heat ☞ serving size: 1 fillet = 93 g; Calories = 139.5; Total Carb (g) = 0; Net Carb (g) = 0; Fat (g) = 4.5; Protein = 23.1

🦐 Mullet Striped Raw ☞ serving size: 1 oz = 28.4 g; Calories = 33.2; Total Carb (g) = 0; Net Carb (g) = 0; Fat (g) = 1.1; Protein = 5.5

🦐 Mussels Cooked Ns As To Cooking Method ☞ serving size: 1 oz, cooked = 28 g; Calories = 47.9; Total Carb (g) = 2.1; Net Carb (g) = 2.1; Fat (g) = 1.3; Protein = 6.6

🦐 Mussels Steamed Or Poached ☞ serving size: 1 oz, cooked = 28 g; Calories = 47.9; Total Carb (g) = 2.1; Net Carb (g) = 2.1; Fat (g) = 1.3; Protein = 6.6

🦐 Ocean Perch Atlantic Raw ☞ serving size: 1 oz, boneless = 28.4 g; Calories = 22.4; Total Carb (g) = 0; Net Carb (g) = 0; Fat (g) = 0.4; Protein = 4.4

🦐 Ocean Perch Cooked Ns As To Cooking Method ☞ serving size: 1 small fillet = 113 g; Calories = 145.8; Total Carb (g) = 0.1; Net Carb (g) = 0.1; Fat (g) = 6.3; Protein = 21.2

🦐 Ocean Perch Steamed Or Poached ☞ serving size: 1 small fillet = 113 g; Calories = 111.9; Total Carb (g) = 0; Net Carb (g) = 0; Fat (g) = 2.2; Protein = 21.8

🦐 Octopus Cooked Ns As To Cooking Method ☞ serving size: 1 oz, boneless, cooked = 28 g; Calories = 62.2; Total Carb (g) = 3.4; Net Carb (g) = 3.2; Fat (g) = 3.3; Protein = 4.6

🦑 Octopus Dried ☞ serving size: 1 oz = 28 g; Calories = 87.1; Total Carb (g) = 2.3; Net Carb (g) = 2.3; Fat (g) = 1.1; Protein = 15.8

🦑 Octopus Smoked ☞ serving size: 1 oz, boneless, cooked = 28 g; Calories = 45.9; Total Carb (g) = 1.2; Net Carb (g) = 1.2; Fat (g) = 0.6; Protein = 8.4

🦑 Octopus Steamed ☞ serving size: 1 oz, boneless, cooked = 28 g; Calories = 45.6; Total Carb (g) = 1.2; Net Carb (g) = 1.2; Fat (g) = 0.6; Protein = 8.3

🦑 Oyster Fritter ☞ serving size: 1 fritter = 40 g; Calories = 78.4; Total Carb (g) = 2.1; Net Carb (g) = 2; Fat (g) = 6.5; Protein = 2.8

🦑 Oyster Pie ☞ serving size: 1 pie = 656 g; Calories = 1607.2; Total Carb (g) = 130; Net Carb (g) = 124.8; Fat (g) = 104.9; Protein = 35.2

🦑 Oysters Cooked Ns As To Cooking Method ☞ serving size: 1 oz, without shell, cooked = 28 g; Calories = 54.6; Total Carb (g) = 3.5; Net Carb (g) = 3.4; Fat (g) = 3.4; Protein = 2.3

🦑 Oysters Rockefeller ☞ serving size: 1 oyster, no shell = 24 g; Calories = 30.5; Total Carb (g) = 2.2; Net Carb (g) = 1.8; Fat (g) = 1.7; Protein = 1.8

🦑 Oysters Smoked ☞ serving size: 1 oz = 28 g; Calories = 23; Total Carb (g) = 1.2; Net Carb (g) = 1.2; Fat (g) = 0.8; Protein = 2.6

🦑 Oysters Steamed ☞ serving size: 1 oz, without shell, cooked = 28 g; Calories = 28.6; Total Carb (g) = 1.5; Net Carb (g) = 1.5; Fat (g) = 1; Protein = 3.2

🦑 Perch Cooked Ns As To Cooking Method ☞ serving size: 1 small fillet = 113 g; Calories = 250.9; Total Carb (g) = 11.1; Net Carb (g) = 10.5; Fat (g) = 12.6; Protein = 22.1

🦑 Perch Mixed Species Cooked Dry Heat ☞ serving size: 1 fillet =

46 g; Calories = 53.8; Total Carb (g) = 0; Net Carb (g) = 0; Fat (g) = 0.5; Protein = 11.4

🐟 Perch Mixed Species Raw ☞ serving size: 1 fillet = 60 g; Calories = 54.6; Total Carb (g) = 0; Net Carb (g) = 0; Fat (g) = 0.6; Protein = 11.6

🐟 Perch Steamed Or Poached ☞ serving size: 1 small fillet = 113 g; Calories = 128.8; Total Carb (g) = 0; Net Carb (g) = 0; Fat (g) = 1.3; Protein = 27.6

🐟 Pike Cooked Ns As To Cooking Method ☞ serving size: 1 small fillet = 170 g; Calories = 401.2; Total Carb (g) = 23.6; Net Carb (g) = 22.1; Fat (g) = 18.9; Protein = 32.6

🐟 Pike Northern Raw ☞ serving size: 3 oz = 85 g; Calories = 74.8; Total Carb (g) = 0; Net Carb (g) = 0; Fat (g) = 0.6; Protein = 16.4

🐟 Pike Steamed Or Poached ☞ serving size: 1 small fillet = 170 g; Calories = 188.7; Total Carb (g) = 0; Net Carb (g) = 0; Fat (g) = 1.5; Protein = 41.2

🐟 Pike Walleye Raw ☞ serving size: 3 oz = 85 g; Calories = 79.1; Total Carb (g) = 0; Net Carb (g) = 0; Fat (g) = 1; Protein = 16.3

🐟 Pink Salmon (Raw) ☞ serving size: 3 oz = 85 g; Calories = 108; Total Carb (g) = 0; Net Carb (g) = 0; Fat (g) = 3.7; Protein = 17.4

🐟 Pollock Alaska Cooked (Not Previously Frozen) ☞ serving size: 3 oz = 85 g; Calories = 73.6; Total Carb (g) = 0; Net Carb (g) = 0; Fat (g) = 0.9; Protein = 16.5

🐟 Pollock Alaska Raw (May Have Been Previously Frozen) ☞ serving size: 1 fillet = 77 g; Calories = 43.1; Total Carb (g) = 0; Net Carb (g) = 0; Fat (g) = 0.3; Protein = 9.4

🐟 Pollock Alaska Raw (Not Previously Frozen) ☞ serving size: 3 oz = 85 g; Calories = 64.6; Total Carb (g) = 0; Net Carb (g) = 0; Fat (g) = 0.7; Protein = 14.6

🐟 Pollock Atlantic Raw ☞ serving size: 3 oz = 85 g; Calories = 78.2; Total Carb (g) = 0; Net Carb (g) = 0; Fat (g) = 0.8; Protein = 16.5

🐟 Pompano Cooked Ns As To Cooking Method ☞ serving size: 1 small fillet = 113 g; Calories = 263.3; Total Carb (g) = 0.1; Net Carb (g) = 0.1; Fat (g) = 17.2; Protein = 25.6

🐟 Pompano Florida Raw ☞ serving size: 1 oz, boneless = 28.4 g; Calories = 46.6; Total Carb (g) = 0; Net Carb (g) = 0; Fat (g) = 2.7; Protein = 5.3

🐟 Pompano Smoked ☞ serving size: 1 oz, boneless = 28 g; Calories = 53.8; Total Carb (g) = 0; Net Carb (g) = 0; Fat (g) = 3.1; Protein = 6

🐟 Porgy Cooked Ns As To Cooking Method ☞ serving size: 1 small fillet = 113 g; Calories = 181.9; Total Carb (g) = 0.1; Net Carb (g) = 0.1; Fat (g) = 7.9; Protein = 26.1

🐟 Porgy Steamed Or Poached ☞ serving size: 1 small fillet = 113 g; Calories = 149.2; Total Carb (g) = 0; Net Carb (g) = 0; Fat (g) = 3.9; Protein = 26.8

🐟 Pout Ocean Cooked Dry Heat ☞ serving size: 1/2 fillet = 137 g; Calories = 139.7; Total Carb (g) = 0; Net Carb (g) = 0; Fat (g) = 1.6; Protein = 29.2

🐟 Pout Ocean Raw ☞ serving size: 3 oz = 85 g; Calories = 67.2; Total Carb (g) = 0; Net Carb (g) = 0; Fat (g) = 0.8; Protein = 14.1

🐟 Queen Crab (Cooked) ☞ serving size: 3 oz = 85 g; Calories = 97.8; Total Carb (g) = 0; Net Carb (g) = 0; Fat (g) = 1.3; Protein = 20.2

🐟 Queen Crab (Raw) ☞ serving size: 3 oz = 85 g; Calories = 76.5; Total Carb (g) = 0; Net Carb (g) = 0; Fat (g) = 1; Protein = 15.7

🐟 Rainbow Trout (Raw) ☞ serving size: 1 fillet = 79 g; Calories = 111.4; Total Carb (g) = 0; Net Carb (g) = 0; Fat (g) = 4.9; Protein = 15.8

🐟 Ray Cooked Ns As To Cooking Method ☞ serving size: 1 oz,

boneless, raw (yield after cooking) = 23 g; Calories = 44.2; Total Carb (g) = 0; Net Carb (g) = 0; Fat (g) = 2.1; Protein = 5.9

🦐 Ray Steamed Or Poached ☞ serving size: 1 oz, boneless, raw (yield after cooking) = 23 g; Calories = 37.5; Total Carb (g) = 0; Net Carb (g) = 0; Fat (g) = 1.3; Protein = 6.1

🦐 Rockfish Pacific Mixed Species Cooked Dry Heat ☞ serving size: 1 fillet = 149 g; Calories = 162.4; Total Carb (g) = 0; Net Carb (g) = 0; Fat (g) = 2.4; Protein = 33.1

🦐 Rockfish Pacific Mixed Species Raw ☞ serving size: 3 oz = 85 g; Calories = 76.5; Total Carb (g) = 0; Net Carb (g) = 0; Fat (g) = 1.1; Protein = 15.6

🦐 Roe ☞ serving size: 1 tbsp = 14 g; Calories = 20; Total Carb (g) = 0.2; Net Carb (g) = 0.2; Fat (g) = 0.9; Protein = 3.1

🦐 Roe (Cooked) ☞ serving size: 1 oz = 28.4 g; Calories = 57.9; Total Carb (g) = 0.6; Net Carb (g) = 0.6; Fat (g) = 2.3; Protein = 8.1

🦐 Roe Shad Cooked ☞ serving size: 1 oz = 28 g; Calories = 58.2; Total Carb (g) = 0.5; Net Carb (g) = 0.5; Fat (g) = 3.2; Protein = 7.7

🦐 Roughy Orange Raw ☞ serving size: 3 oz = 85 g; Calories = 64.6; Total Carb (g) = 0; Net Carb (g) = 0; Fat (g) = 0.6; Protein = 14

🦐 Sablefish Raw ☞ serving size: 3 oz = 85 g; Calories = 165.8; Total Carb (g) = 0; Net Carb (g) = 0; Fat (g) = 13; Protein = 11.4

🦐 Sablefish Smoked ☞ serving size: 1 oz = 28.4 g; Calories = 73; Total Carb (g) = 0; Net Carb (g) = 0; Fat (g) = 5.7; Protein = 5

🦐 Salmon Cake Or Patty ☞ serving size: 1 ball = 63 g; Calories = 155; Total Carb (g) = 1.6; Net Carb (g) = 1.5; Fat (g) = 11.4; Protein = 10.8

🦐 Salmon Canned ☞ serving size: 1 oz = 28 g; Calories = 38.4; Total Carb (g) = 0; Net Carb (g) = 0; Fat (g) = 1.5; Protein = 5.8

🦐 Salmon Chinook Cooked Dry Heat ☞ serving size: 3 oz = 85 g;

Calories = 196.4; Total Carb (g) = 0; Net Carb (g) = 0; Fat (g) = 11.4; Protein = 21.9

🐟 Salmon Chinook Raw ☞ serving size: 3 oz = 85 g; Calories = 152.2; Total Carb (g) = 0; Net Carb (g) = 0; Fat (g) = 8.9; Protein = 16.9

🐟 Salmon Chinook Smoked (Lox) Regular ☞ serving size: 1 oz = 28.4 g; Calories = 33.2; Total Carb (g) = 0; Net Carb (g) = 0; Fat (g) = 1.2; Protein = 5.2

🐟 Salmon Chum Raw ☞ serving size: 3 oz = 85 g; Calories = 102; Total Carb (g) = 0; Net Carb (g) = 0; Fat (g) = 3.2; Protein = 17.1

🐟 Salmon Coho Wild Raw ☞ serving size: 3 oz = 85 g; Calories = 124.1; Total Carb (g) = 0; Net Carb (g) = 0; Fat (g) = 5; Protein = 18.4

🐟 Salmon Cooked Ns As To Cooking Method ☞ serving size: 1 small fillet = 170 g; Calories = 319.6; Total Carb (g) = 0.2; Net Carb (g) = 0.2; Fat (g) = 15.4; Protein = 42.6

🐟 Salmon Dried ☞ serving size: 1 oz, boneless = 28 g; Calories = 111.2; Total Carb (g) = 0; Net Carb (g) = 0; Fat (g) = 3.9; Protein = 17.9

🐟 Salmon Loaf ☞ serving size: 1 slice = 105 g; Calories = 201.6; Total Carb (g) = 9.6; Net Carb (g) = 9.1; Fat (g) = 10.4; Protein = 16.5

🐟 Salmon Pink Canned Total Can Contents ☞ serving size: 3 oz = 85 g; Calories = 109.7; Total Carb (g) = 0; Net Carb (g) = 0; Fat (g) = 4.2; Protein = 16.7

🐟 Salmon Pink Canned Without Salt Solids With Bone And Liquid ☞ serving size: 3 oz = 85 g; Calories = 118.2; Total Carb (g) = 0; Net Carb (g) = 0; Fat (g) = 5.1; Protein = 16.8

🐟 Salmon Pink Cooked Dry Heat ☞ serving size: 3 oz = 85 g; Calories = 130.1; Total Carb (g) = 0; Net Carb (g) = 0; Fat (g) = 4.5; Protein = 20.9

🐟 Salmon Salad ☞ serving size: 1 cup = 208 g; Calories = 441; Total Carb (g) = 5.5; Net Carb (g) = 4.7; Fat (g) = 36.1; Protein = 22.6

🦐 Salmon Sockeye Raw ☞ serving size: 1 oz, boneless = 28.4 g; Calories = 37.2; Total Carb (g) = 0; Net Carb (g) = 0; Fat (g) = 1.3; Protein = 6.3

🦐 Salmon Steamed Or Poached ☞ serving size: 1 small fillet = 170 g; Calories = 272; Total Carb (g) = 0; Net Carb (g) = 0; Fat (g) = 9.4; Protein = 43.8

🦐 Sardine Pacific Canned In Tomato Sauce Drained Solids With Bone ☞ serving size: 1 cup = 89 g; Calories = 164.7; Total Carb (g) = 0.5; Net Carb (g) = 0.4; Fat (g) = 9.3; Protein = 18.6

🦐 Sardines Dried ☞ serving size: 1 oz = 28 g; Calories = 113.7; Total Carb (g) = 0; Net Carb (g) = 0; Fat (g) = 6.5; Protein = 12.9

🦐 Scallops ☞ serving size: 3 oz = 85 g; Calories = 94.4; Total Carb (g) = 4.6; Net Carb (g) = 4.6; Fat (g) = 0.7; Protein = 17.5

🦐 Scallops Cooked Ns As To Cooking Method ☞ serving size: 1 oz, cooked = 28 g; Calories = 31.9; Total Carb (g) = 1.1; Net Carb (g) = 1.1; Fat (g) = 1.2; Protein = 4

🦐 Scup Raw ☞ serving size: 3 oz = 85 g; Calories = 89.3; Total Carb (g) = 0; Net Carb (g) = 0; Fat (g) = 2.3; Protein = 16.1

🦐 Sea Bass Cooked Ns As To Cooking Method ☞ serving size: 1 small fillet = 113 g; Calories = 171.8; Total Carb (g) = 0.1; Net Carb (g) = 0.1; Fat (g) = 6.9; Protein = 25.5

🦐 Sea Bass Mixed Species Raw ☞ serving size: 1 fillet = 129 g; Calories = 125.1; Total Carb (g) = 0; Net Carb (g) = 0; Fat (g) = 2.6; Protein = 23.8

🦐 Sea Bass Pickled ☞ serving size: 1 oz, boneless = 28 g; Calories = 43.4; Total Carb (g) = 1.1; Net Carb (g) = 1; Fat (g) = 2.9; Protein = 3.1

🦐 Seafood Newburg ☞ serving size: 1 cup = 244 g; Calories = 597.8; Total Carb (g) = 9.3; Net Carb (g) = 9.1; Fat (g) = 49.4; Protein = 29.3

🦐 Seatrout Mixed Species Cooked Dry Heat ☞ serving size: 3 oz =

85 g; Calories = 113.1; Total Carb (g) = 0; Net Carb (g) = 0; Fat (g) = 3.9; Protein = 18.2

🐟 Seatrout Mixed Species Raw ☞ serving size: 3 oz = 85 g; Calories = 88.4; Total Carb (g) = 0; Net Carb (g) = 0; Fat (g) = 3.1; Protein = 14.2

🐟 Shad American Cooked Dry Heat ☞ serving size: 1 fillet = 144 g; Calories = 362.9; Total Carb (g) = 0; Net Carb (g) = 0; Fat (g) = 25.4; Protein = 31.3

🐟 Shad American Raw ☞ serving size: 3 oz = 85 g; Calories = 167.5; Total Carb (g) = 0; Net Carb (g) = 0; Fat (g) = 11.7; Protein = 14.4

🐟 Shark Cooked Ns As To Cooking Method ☞ serving size: 1 small fillet = 170 g; Calories = 326.4; Total Carb (g) = 0.2; Net Carb (g) = 0.2; Fat (g) = 15.6; Protein = 43.6

🐟 Shark Mixed Species Raw ☞ serving size: 3 oz = 85 g; Calories = 110.5; Total Carb (g) = 0; Net Carb (g) = 0; Fat (g) = 3.8; Protein = 17.8

🐟 Shark Steamed Or Poached ☞ serving size: 1 small fillet = 170 g; Calories = 277.1; Total Carb (g) = 0; Net Carb (g) = 0; Fat (g) = 9.6; Protein = 44.9

🐟 Sheepshead Cooked Dry Heat ☞ serving size: 3 oz = 85 g; Calories = 107.1; Total Carb (g) = 0; Net Carb (g) = 0; Fat (g) = 1.4; Protein = 22.1

🐟 Sheepshead Raw ☞ serving size: 3 oz = 85 g; Calories = 91.8; Total Carb (g) = 0; Net Carb (g) = 0; Fat (g) = 2.1; Protein = 17.2

🐟 Shrimp Cake Or Patty ☞ serving size: 1 cake or patty = 120 g; Calories = 276; Total Carb (g) = 4.4; Net Carb (g) = 4.2; Fat (g) = 18.5; Protein = 21.7

🐟 Shrimp Cocktail ☞ serving size: 1 cup = 230 g; Calories = 278.3; Total Carb (g) = 24.8; Net Carb (g) = 23.4; Fat (g) = 3.4; Protein = 35.4

🐟 Shrimp Cooked Ns As To Cooking Method ☞ serving size: 1 tiny shrimp ("popcorn") = 1 g; Calories = 2.1; Total Carb (g) = 0.1; Net Carb (g) = 0.1; Fat (g) = 0.1; Protein = 0.2

🦐 Shrimp Creole No Rice ☞ serving size: 1 cup = 246 g; Calories = 305; Total Carb (g) = 11; Net Carb (g) = 8.6; Fat (g) = 12.8; Protein = 35.2

🦐 Shrimp Creole With Rice ☞ serving size: 1 cup = 243 g; Calories = 301.3; Total Carb (g) = 28.9; Net Carb (g) = 27; Fat (g) = 8.9; Protein = 24.6

🦐 Shrimp Curry ☞ serving size: 1 cup = 236 g; Calories = 177; Total Carb (g) = 16.9; Net Carb (g) = 12.8; Fat (g) = 7.4; Protein = 11.8

🦐 Shrimp Dried ☞ serving size: 1 oz = 28 g; Calories = 70.8; Total Carb (g) = 0; Net Carb (g) = 0; Fat (g) = 1; Protein = 14.5

🦐 Skipjack Tuna (Raw) ☞ serving size: 3 oz = 85 g; Calories = 87.6; Total Carb (g) = 0; Net Carb (g) = 0; Fat (g) = 0.9; Protein = 18.7

🦐 Smelt Rainbow Raw ☞ serving size: 3 oz = 85 g; Calories = 82.5; Total Carb (g) = 0; Net Carb (g) = 0; Fat (g) = 2.1; Protein = 15

🦐 Smoked Haddock ☞ serving size: 1 oz, boneless = 28.4 g; Calories = 32.9; Total Carb (g) = 0; Net Carb (g) = 0; Fat (g) = 0.3; Protein = 7.2

🦐 Smoked Salmon ☞ serving size: 1 oz, boneless = 28.4 g; Calories = 33.2; Total Carb (g) = 0; Net Carb (g) = 0; Fat (g) = 1.2; Protein = 5.2

🦐 Smoked Sturgeon ☞ serving size: 1 oz = 28.4 g; Calories = 49.1; Total Carb (g) = 0; Net Carb (g) = 0; Fat (g) = 1.3; Protein = 8.9

🦐 Smoked Whitefish ☞ serving size: 1 cup, cooked = 136 g; Calories = 146.9; Total Carb (g) = 0; Net Carb (g) = 0; Fat (g) = 1.3; Protein = 31.8

🦐 Snails Cooked Ns As To Cooking Method ☞ serving size: 1 oz, without shell, cooked = 28 g; Calories = 38.9; Total Carb (g) = 0.7; Net Carb (g) = 0.7; Fat (g) = 1.5; Protein = 5.4

🦐 Snapper Mixed Species Raw ☞ serving size: 3 oz = 85 g; Calories = 85; Total Carb (g) = 0; Net Carb (g) = 0; Fat (g) = 1.1; Protein = 17.4

🐟 Spot Cooked Dry Heat ☞ serving size: 1 fillet = 50 g; Calories = 79; Total Carb (g) = 0; Net Carb (g) = 0; Fat (g) = 3.1; Protein = 11.9

🐟 Spot Raw ☞ serving size: 1 fillet = 64 g; Calories = 78.7; Total Carb (g) = 0; Net Carb (g) = 0; Fat (g) = 3.1; Protein = 11.9

🐟 Squid (Raw) ☞ serving size: 1 oz, boneless = 28.4 g; Calories = 26.1; Total Carb (g) = 0.9; Net Carb (g) = 0.9; Fat (g) = 0.4; Protein = 4.4

🐟 Squid Dried ☞ serving size: 1 oz, boneless = 28 g; Calories = 97.4; Total Carb (g) = 3.3; Net Carb (g) = 3.3; Fat (g) = 1.5; Protein = 16.5

🐟 Squid Pickled ☞ serving size: 1 oz, boneless = 28 g; Calories = 26; Total Carb (g) = 0.8; Net Carb (g) = 0.8; Fat (g) = 0.4; Protein = 4.2

🐟 Squid Steamed Or Boiled ☞ serving size: 1 oz, boneless, cooked = 28 g; Calories = 51.2; Total Carb (g) = 1.7; Net Carb (g) = 1.7; Fat (g) = 0.8; Protein = 8.7

🐟 Stewed Codfish No Potatoes Puerto Rican Style ☞ serving size: 1 cup = 227 g; Calories = 238.4; Total Carb (g) = 10.1; Net Carb (g) = 7.6; Fat (g) = 9.7; Protein = 27.5

🐟 Stewed Codfish Puerto Rican Style ☞ serving size: 1 cup = 200 g; Calories = 226; Total Carb (g) = 17.3; Net Carb (g) = 14.7; Fat (g) = 7.8; Protein = 21.9

🐟 Stewed Salmon Puerto Rican Style ☞ serving size: 1 cup = 212 g; Calories = 307.4; Total Carb (g) = 18; Net Carb (g) = 15.2; Fat (g) = 14.7; Protein = 25.5

🐟 Sticks Frozen Prepared ☞ serving size: 1 piece (4 inch x 2 inch x 1/2 inch) = 57 g; Calories = 157.9; Total Carb (g) = 12.4; Net Carb (g) = 11.5; Fat (g) = 9.3; Protein = 6.3

🐟 Striped Bass (Raw) ☞ serving size: 3 oz = 85 g; Calories = 82.5; Total Carb (g) = 0; Net Carb (g) = 0; Fat (g) = 2; Protein = 15.1

🐟 Sturgeon Cooked Ns As To Cooking Method ☞ serving size: 1

oz, boneless, raw (yield after cooking) = 23 g; Calories = 37; Total Carb (g) = 0; Net Carb (g) = 0; Fat (g) = 2; Protein = 4.5

🐟 Sturgeon Mixed Species Raw ☞ serving size: 3 oz = 85 g; Calories = 89.3; Total Carb (g) = 0; Net Carb (g) = 0; Fat (g) = 3.4; Protein = 13.7

🐟 Sturgeon Steamed ☞ serving size: 1 oz, boneless, raw (yield after cooking) = 23 g; Calories = 30.4; Total Carb (g) = 0; Net Carb (g) = 0; Fat (g) = 1.2; Protein = 4.7

🐟 Sucker White Cooked Dry Heat ☞ serving size: 1 fillet = 124 g; Calories = 147.6; Total Carb (g) = 0; Net Carb (g) = 0; Fat (g) = 3.7; Protein = 26.7

🐟 Sucker White Raw ☞ serving size: 3 oz = 85 g; Calories = 78.2; Total Carb (g) = 0; Net Carb (g) = 0; Fat (g) = 2; Protein = 14.3

🐟 Sunfish Pumpkin Seed Cooked Dry Heat ☞ serving size: 1 fillet = 37 g; Calories = 42.2; Total Carb (g) = 0; Net Carb (g) = 0; Fat (g) = 0.3; Protein = 9.2

🐟 Sunfish Pumpkin Seed Raw ☞ serving size: 1 fillet = 48 g; Calories = 42.7; Total Carb (g) = 0; Net Carb (g) = 0; Fat (g) = 0.3; Protein = 9.3

🐟 Surimi ☞ serving size: 1 oz = 28.4 g; Calories = 28.1; Total Carb (g) = 2; Net Carb (g) = 2; Fat (g) = 0.3; Protein = 4.3

🐟 Swordfish Cooked Ns As To Cooking Method ☞ serving size: 1 small fillet = 170 g; Calories = 355.3; Total Carb (g) = 0.2; Net Carb (g) = 0.2; Fat (g) = 20.1; Protein = 40.9

🐟 Swordfish Raw ☞ serving size: 3 oz = 85 g; Calories = 122.4; Total Carb (g) = 0; Net Carb (g) = 0; Fat (g) = 5.7; Protein = 16.7

🐟 Swordfish Steamed Or Poached ☞ serving size: 1 small fillet = 170 g; Calories = 307.7; Total Carb (g) = 0; Net Carb (g) = 0; Fat (g) = 14.2; Protein = 42

🦐 Tilapia Cooked Ns As To Cooking Method ☞ serving size: 1 small fillet = 113 g; Calories = 169.5; Total Carb (g) = 0.1; Net Carb (g) = 0.1; Fat (g) = 6.5; Protein = 27.8

🦐 Tilapia Steamed Or Poached ☞ serving size: 1 small fillet = 113 g; Calories = 136.7; Total Carb (g) = 0; Net Carb (g) = 0; Fat (g) = 2.4; Protein = 28.5

🦐 Tilefish Raw ☞ serving size: 3 oz = 85 g; Calories = 81.6; Total Carb (g) = 0; Net Carb (g) = 0; Fat (g) = 2; Protein = 14.9

🦐 Timbale Or Mousse ☞ serving size: 1 cup = 175 g; Calories = 259; Total Carb (g) = 3.1; Net Carb (g) = 3.1; Fat (g) = 19.2; Protein = 17.9

🦐 Trout Brook Raw New York State ☞ serving size: 1 filet = 149 g; Calories = 163.9; Total Carb (g) = 0; Net Carb (g) = 0; Fat (g) = 4.1; Protein = 31.6

🦐 Trout Cooked Ns As To Cooking Method ☞ serving size: 1 small fillet = 113 g; Calories = 231.7; Total Carb (g) = 0.1; Net Carb (g) = 0.1; Fat (g) = 12.7; Protein = 27.6

🦐 Trout Mixed Species Cooked Dry Heat ☞ serving size: 1 fillet = 62 g; Calories = 117.8; Total Carb (g) = 0; Net Carb (g) = 0; Fat (g) = 5.3; Protein = 16.5

🦐 Trout Mixed Species Raw ☞ serving size: 1 fillet = 79 g; Calories = 116.9; Total Carb (g) = 0; Net Carb (g) = 0; Fat (g) = 5.2; Protein = 16.4

🦐 Trout Rainbow Wild Raw ☞ serving size: 3 oz = 85 g; Calories = 101.2; Total Carb (g) = 0; Net Carb (g) = 0; Fat (g) = 2.9; Protein = 17.4

🦐 Trout Smoked ☞ serving size: 1 oz, boneless = 28 g; Calories = 70.3; Total Carb (g) = 0; Net Carb (g) = 0; Fat (g) = 3.1; Protein = 9.9

🦐 Trout Steamed Or Poached ☞ serving size: 1 small fillet = 113 g; Calories = 200; Total Carb (g) = 0; Net Carb (g) = 0; Fat (g) = 8.8; Protein = 28.3

🦐 Tuna Cake Or Patty ☞ serving size: 1 cake or patty = 120 g; Calo-

ries = 247.2; Total Carb (g) = 3.1; Net Carb (g) = 2.8; Fat (g) = 17.9; Protein = 18.8

🐟 Tuna Fresh Cooked Ns As To Cooking Method ☞ serving size: 1 small fillet = 170 g; Calories = 282.2; Total Carb (g) = 0.2; Net Carb (g) = 0.2; Fat (g) = 7.3; Protein = 50.8

🐟 Tuna Fresh Dried ☞ serving size: 1 cup, nfs = 42 g; Calories = 143.2; Total Carb (g) = 0; Net Carb (g) = 0; Fat (g) = 0.6; Protein = 32

🐟 Tuna Fresh Smoked ☞ serving size: 1 oz, boneless = 28 g; Calories = 56; Total Carb (g) = 0; Net Carb (g) = 0; Fat (g) = 2.8; Protein = 7.2

🐟 Tuna Fresh Steamed Or Poached ☞ serving size: 1 small fillet = 170 g; Calories = 232.9; Total Carb (g) = 0; Net Carb (g) = 0; Fat (g) = 1.1; Protein = 52.2

🐟 Tuna Light Canned In Oil Drained Solids ☞ serving size: 1 cup, solid or chunks = 146 g; Calories = 289.1; Total Carb (g) = 0; Net Carb (g) = 0; Fat (g) = 12; Protein = 42.5

🐟 Tuna Light Canned In Oil Without Salt Drained Solids ☞ serving size: 3 oz = 85 g; Calories = 168.3; Total Carb (g) = 0; Net Carb (g) = 0; Fat (g) = 7; Protein = 24.8

🐟 Tuna Light Canned In Water Drained Solids ☞ serving size: 1 oz = 28.4 g; Calories = 24.4; Total Carb (g) = 0; Net Carb (g) = 0; Fat (g) = 0.3; Protein = 5.5

🐟 Tuna Light Canned In Water Without Salt Drained Solids ☞ serving size: 3 oz = 85 g; Calories = 98.6; Total Carb (g) = 0; Net Carb (g) = 0; Fat (g) = 0.7; Protein = 21.7

🐟 Tuna Loaf ☞ serving size: 1 slice = 105 g; Calories = 243.6; Total Carb (g) = 9.8; Net Carb (g) = 9.3; Fat (g) = 12.4; Protein = 22

🐟 Tuna Pot Pie ☞ serving size: 1 pie = 769 g; Calories = 1691.8; Total Carb (g) = 125.5; Net Carb (g) = 115.5; Fat (g) = 101.3; Protein = 68.9

🐟 Tuna White Canned In Oil Without Salt Drained Solids ☞ serving size: 3 oz = 85 g; Calories = 158.1; Total Carb (g) = 0; Net Carb (g) = 0; Fat (g) = 6.9; Protein = 22.6

🐟 Tuna White Canned In Water Without Salt Drained Solids ☞ serving size: 3 oz = 85 g; Calories = 108.8; Total Carb (g) = 0; Net Carb (g) = 0; Fat (g) = 2.5; Protein = 20.1

🐟 Turbot European Raw ☞ serving size: 3 oz = 85 g; Calories = 80.8; Total Carb (g) = 0; Net Carb (g) = 0; Fat (g) = 2.5; Protein = 13.6

🐟 Turtle Cooked Ns As To Cooking Method ☞ serving size: 1 oz, boneless, cooked = 28 g; Calories = 38.6; Total Carb (g) = 0; Net Carb (g) = 0; Fat (g) = 1.2; Protein = 6.6

🐟 Turtle Green Raw ☞ serving size: 3 oz = 85 g; Calories = 75.7; Total Carb (g) = 0; Net Carb (g) = 0; Fat (g) = 0.4; Protein = 16.8

🐟 USDA Commodity Salmon Nuggets Breaded Frozen Heated ☞ serving size: 1 oz = 28.4 g; Calories = 60.2; Total Carb (g) = 4; Net Carb (g) = 4; Fat (g) = 3.3; Protein = 3.6

🐟 USDA Commodity Salmon Nuggets Cooked As Purchased Unheated ☞ serving size: 1 oz = 28.4 g; Calories = 53.7; Total Carb (g) = 3.4; Net Carb (g) = 3.4; Fat (g) = 3; Protein = 3.4

🐟 Whelk (Cooked) ☞ serving size: 3 oz = 85 g; Calories = 233.8; Total Carb (g) = 13.2; Net Carb (g) = 13.2; Fat (g) = 0.7; Protein = 40.5

🐟 Whitefish (Raw) ☞ serving size: 3 oz = 85 g; Calories = 113.9; Total Carb (g) = 0; Net Carb (g) = 0; Fat (g) = 5; Protein = 16.2

🐟 Whiting Cooked Ns As To Cooking Method ☞ serving size: 1 small fillet = 113 g; Calories = 249.7; Total Carb (g) = 11.1; Net Carb (g) = 10.5; Fat (g) = 12.9; Protein = 21

🐟 Whiting Steamed Or Poached ☞ serving size: 1 oz, boneless, raw (yield after cooking) = 23 g; Calories = 26; Total Carb (g) = 0; Net Carb (g) = 0; Fat (g) = 0.4; Protein = 5.3

🐟 Wild Atlantic Salmon (Cooked) ☞ serving size: 3 oz = 85 g; Calories = 154.7; Total Carb (g) = 0; Net Carb (g) = 0; Fat (g) = 6.9; Protein = 21.6

🐟 Wild Atlantic Salmon (Raw) ☞ serving size: 3 oz = 85 g; Calories = 120.7; Total Carb (g) = 0; Net Carb (g) = 0; Fat (g) = 5.4; Protein = 16.9

🐟 Wolffish Atlantic Cooked Dry Heat ☞ serving size: 1/2 fillet = 119 g; Calories = 146.4; Total Carb (g) = 0; Net Carb (g) = 0; Fat (g) = 3.6; Protein = 26.7

🐟 Wolffish Atlantic Raw ☞ serving size: 3 oz = 85 g; Calories = 81.6; Total Carb (g) = 0; Net Carb (g) = 0; Fat (g) = 2; Protein = 14.9

🐟 Yellowfin Tuna (Raw) ☞ serving size: 1 oz, boneless = 28.4 g; Calories = 31; Total Carb (g) = 0; Net Carb (g) = 0; Fat (g) = 0.1; Protein = 6.9

🐟 Yellowtail (Raw) ☞ serving size: 3 oz = 85 g; Calories = 124.1; Total Carb (g) = 0; Net Carb (g) = 0; Fat (g) = 4.5; Protein = 19.7

19

FRUITS & FRUITS PRODUCTS

🍈 Abiyuch ☞ serving size: 1/2 cup = 114 g; Calories = 78.7; Total Carb (g) = 20.1; Net Carb (g) = 14; Fat (g) = 0.1; Protein = 1.7

🍈 Acerola Cherries (West Indian Cherry) ☞ serving size: 1 cup = 98 g; Calories = 31.4; Total Carb (g) = 7.5; Net Carb (g) = 6.5; Fat (g) = 0.3; Protein = 0.4

🍈 Acerola Juice Raw ☞ serving size: 1 cup = 242 g; Calories = 55.7; Total Carb (g) = 11.6; Net Carb (g) = 10.9; Fat (g) = 0.7; Protein = 1

🍈 Ambrosia ☞ serving size: 1 cup = 193 g; Calories = 135.1; Total Carb (g) = 31.2; Net Carb (g) = 26.8; Fat (g) = 1.9; Protein = 1.7

🍈 Apple Baked Ns As To Added Sweetener ☞ serving size: 1 apple with liquid = 171 g; Calories = 162.5; Total Carb (g) = 42.4; Net Carb (g) = 38.5; Fat (g) = 0.3; Protein = 0.4

🍈 Apple Baked Unsweetened ☞ serving size: 1 apple with liquid = 161 g; Calories = 90.2; Total Carb (g) = 23.9; Net Carb (g) = 19.7; Fat (g) = 0.3; Protein = 0.5

🍈 Apple Baked With Sugar ☞ serving size: 1 apple with liquid = 171

g; Calories = 162.5; Total Carb (g) = 42.4; Net Carb (g) = 38.5; Fat (g) = 0.3; Protein = 0.4

Apple Candied ☞ serving size: 1 small apple = 198 g; Calories = 255.4; Total Carb (g) = 56.6; Net Carb (g) = 53; Fat (g) = 4; Protein = 2.5

Apple Chips ☞ serving size: 1 cup = 28 g; Calories = 128.8; Total Carb (g) = 20.6; Net Carb (g) = 17.9; Fat (g) = 6.1; Protein = 0.3

Apple Dried Cooked Ns As To Sweetened Or Unsweetened; Sweetened Ns As To Type Of Sweetener ☞ serving size: 1 cup = 255 g; Calories = 234.6; Total Carb (g) = 62.2; Net Carb (g) = 57.6; Fat (g) = 0.2; Protein = 0.5

Apple Dried Cooked With Sugar ☞ serving size: 1 cup = 280 g; Calories = 257.6; Total Carb (g) = 68.3; Net Carb (g) = 63.3; Fat (g) = 0.2; Protein = 0.6

Apple Fried ☞ serving size: 1 cup = 179 g; Calories = 247; Total Carb (g) = 43.1; Net Carb (g) = 39.1; Fat (g) = 9.6; Protein = 0.5

Apple Juice ☞ serving size: 1 cup = 248 g; Calories = 114.1; Total Carb (g) = 28; Net Carb (g) = 27.5; Fat (g) = 0.3; Protein = 0.3

Apple Pickled ☞ serving size: 1 apple = 29 g; Calories = 36.5; Total Carb (g) = 9.3; Net Carb (g) = 8.9; Fat (g) = 0; Protein = 0.1

Apple Rings Fried ☞ serving size: 1 ring = 19 g; Calories = 22.6; Total Carb (g) = 3.7; Net Carb (g) = 3.2; Fat (g) = 1; Protein = 0.1

Apples ☞ serving size: 1 cup, quartered or chopped = 125 g; Calories = 65; Total Carb (g) = 17.3; Net Carb (g) = 14.3; Fat (g) = 0.2; Protein = 0.3

Apples (Without Skin) ☞ serving size: 1 cup slices = 110 g; Calories = 52.8; Total Carb (g) = 14; Net Carb (g) = 12.6; Fat (g) = 0.1; Protein = 0.3

Apples Canned Sweetened Sliced Drained Heated ☞ serving

size: 1 cup slices = 204 g; Calories = 136.7; Total Carb (g) = 34.4; Net Carb (g) = 30.3; Fat (g) = 0.9; Protein = 0.4

Apples Dehydrated (Low Moisture) Sulfured Stewed ☞ serving size: 1 cup = 193 g; Calories = 142.8; Total Carb (g) = 38.4; Net Carb (g) = 33.4; Fat (g) = 0.2; Protein = 0.5

Apples Dehydrated (Low Moisture) Sulfured Uncooked ☞ serving size: 1 cup = 60 g; Calories = 207.6; Total Carb (g) = 56.1; Net Carb (g) = 48.7; Fat (g) = 0.4; Protein = 0.8

Apples Dried Sulfured Stewed With Added Sugar ☞ serving size: 1 cup = 280 g; Calories = 232.4; Total Carb (g) = 58; Net Carb (g) = 52.7; Fat (g) = 0.2; Protein = 0.6

Apples Dried Sulfured Stewed Without Added Sugar ☞ serving size: 1 cup = 255 g; Calories = 145.4; Total Carb (g) = 39.1; Net Carb (g) = 34; Fat (g) = 0.2; Protein = 0.6

Apples Frozen Unsweetened Heated ☞ serving size: 1 cup slices = 206 g; Calories = 96.8; Total Carb (g) = 24.7; Net Carb (g) = 22; Fat (g) = 0.7; Protein = 0.6

Apples Frozen Unsweetened Unheated ☞ serving size: 1 cup slices = 173 g; Calories = 83; Total Carb (g) = 21.3; Net Carb (g) = 19.1; Fat (g) = 0.6; Protein = 0.5

Apples Raw Without Skin Cooked Boiled ☞ serving size: 1 cup slices = 171 g; Calories = 90.6; Total Carb (g) = 23.3; Net Carb (g) = 19.2; Fat (g) = 0.6; Protein = 0.4

Apples Raw Without Skin Cooked Microwave ☞ serving size: 1 cup slices = 170 g; Calories = 95.2; Total Carb (g) = 24.5; Net Carb (g) = 19.7; Fat (g) = 0.7; Protein = 0.5

Applesauce Canned Sweetened With Salt ☞ serving size: 1 cup = 255 g; Calories = 193.8; Total Carb (g) = 50.8; Net Carb (g) = 47.7; Fat (g) = 0.5; Protein = 0.5

Applesauce Canned Sweetened Without Salt (Includes USDA

Commodity) ☞ serving size: 1 cup = 246 g; Calories = 167.3; Total Carb (g) = 43; Net Carb (g) = 40.1; Fat (g) = 0.4; Protein = 0.4

◔ Applesauce Canned Unsweetened With Added Ascorbic Acid ☞ serving size: 1 cup = 244 g; Calories = 102.5; Total Carb (g) = 27.5; Net Carb (g) = 24.8; Fat (g) = 0.2; Protein = 0.4

◔ Applesauce Canned Unsweetened Without Added Ascorbic Acid (Includes USDA Commodity) ☞ serving size: 1 cup = 244 g; Calories = 102.5; Total Carb (g) = 27.5; Net Carb (g) = 24.8; Fat (g) = 0.2; Protein = 0.4

◔ Apricot Dried Cooked Ns As To Sweetened Or Unsweetened; Sweetened Ns As To Type Of Sweetener ☞ serving size: 1 cup = 250 g; Calories = 292.5; Total Carb (g) = 76.2; Net Carb (g) = 70.5; Fat (g) = 0.4; Protein = 2.7

◔ Apricot Dried Cooked With Sugar ☞ serving size: 1 cup, nfs = 270 g; Calories = 315.9; Total Carb (g) = 82.3; Net Carb (g) = 76.1; Fat (g) = 0.4; Protein = 2.9

◔ Apricot Nectar Canned Without Added Ascorbic Acid ☞ serving size: 1 cup = 251 g; Calories = 140.6; Total Carb (g) = 34.2; Net Carb (g) = 34; Fat (g) = 1.1; Protein = 0.4

◔ Apricots ☞ serving size: 1 cup, halves = 155 g; Calories = 74.4; Total Carb (g) = 17.2; Net Carb (g) = 14.1; Fat (g) = 0.6; Protein = 2.2

◔ Apricots Canned Extra Heavy Syrup Pack Without Skin Solids And Liquids ☞ serving size: 1 cup, whole, without pits = 246 g; Calories = 236.2; Total Carb (g) = 61.1; Net Carb (g) = 57.2; Fat (g) = 0.1; Protein = 1.4

◔ Apricots Canned Extra Light Syrup Pack With Skin Solids And Liquids ☞ serving size: 1 cup, halves = 247 g; Calories = 121; Total Carb (g) = 30.9; Net Carb (g) = 26.9; Fat (g) = 0.3; Protein = 1.5

◔ Apricots Canned Heavy Syrup Drained ☞ serving size: 1 cup, halves = 219 g; Calories = 181.8; Total Carb (g) = 46.7; Net Carb (g) = 40.8; Fat (g) = 0.2; Protein = 1.4

Apricots Canned Heavy Syrup Pack With Skin Solids And Liquids ☞ serving size: 1 cup, halves = 258 g; Calories = 214.1; Total Carb (g) = 55.4; Net Carb (g) = 51.3; Fat (g) = 0.2; Protein = 1.4

Apricots Canned Heavy Syrup Pack Without Skin Solids And Liquids ☞ serving size: 1 cup, whole, without pits = 258 g; Calories = 214.1; Total Carb (g) = 55.3; Net Carb (g) = 51.2; Fat (g) = 0.2; Protein = 1.3

Apricots Canned Juice Pack With Skin Solids And Liquids ☞ serving size: 1 cup, halves = 244 g; Calories = 117.1; Total Carb (g) = 30.1; Net Carb (g) = 26.2; Fat (g) = 0.1; Protein = 1.5

Apricots Canned Light Syrup Pack With Skin Solids And Liquids ☞ serving size: 1 cup, halves = 253 g; Calories = 159.4; Total Carb (g) = 41.7; Net Carb (g) = 37.7; Fat (g) = 0.1; Protein = 1.3

Apricots Canned Water Pack With Skin Solids And Liquids ☞ serving size: 1 cup, halves = 243 g; Calories = 65.6; Total Carb (g) = 15.5; Net Carb (g) = 11.6; Fat (g) = 0.4; Protein = 1.7

Apricots Canned Water Pack Without Skin Solids And Liquids ☞ serving size: 1 cup, whole, without pits = 227 g; Calories = 49.9; Total Carb (g) = 12.4; Net Carb (g) = 9.9; Fat (g) = 0.1; Protein = 1.6

Apricots Dehydrated (Low-Moisture) Sulfured Stewed ☞ serving size: 1 cup = 249 g; Calories = 313.7; Total Carb (g) = 81.2; Net Carb (g) = 81.2; Fat (g) = 0.6; Protein = 4.8

Apricots Dried Sulfured Stewed With Added Sugar ☞ serving size: 1 cup, halves = 270 g; Calories = 305.1; Total Carb (g) = 79; Net Carb (g) = 67.9; Fat (g) = 0.4; Protein = 3.2

Apricots Dried Sulfured Stewed Without Added Sugar ☞ serving size: 1 cup, halves = 250 g; Calories = 212.5; Total Carb (g) = 55.4; Net Carb (g) = 48.9; Fat (g) = 0.5; Protein = 3

◯ Apricots Frozen Sweetened ☞ serving size: 1 cup = 242 g; Calories = 237.2; Total Carb (g) = 60.7; Net Carb (g) = 55.4; Fat (g) = 0.2; Protein = 1.7

◯ Asian Pears ☞ serving size: 1 fruit 2-1/4 inch high x 2-1/2 inch dia = 122 g; Calories = 51.2; Total Carb (g) = 13; Net Carb (g) = 8.6; Fat (g) = 0.3; Protein = 0.6

◯ Avocados ☞ serving size: 1 cup, cubes = 150 g; Calories = 240; Total Carb (g) = 12.8; Net Carb (g) = 2.8; Fat (g) = 22; Protein = 3

◯ Banana Baked ☞ serving size: 1 banana (7-1/4" long) = 128 g; Calories = 162.6; Total Carb (g) = 41.7; Net Carb (g) = 38; Fat (g) = 0.5; Protein = 1.6

◯ Banana Batter-Dipped Fried ☞ serving size: 1 small = 108 g; Calories = 332.6; Total Carb (g) = 42.5; Net Carb (g) = 40.1; Fat (g) = 16.4; Protein = 5.2

◯ Banana Red Fried ☞ serving size: 1 fruit (7-1/4" long) = 94 g; Calories = 138.2; Total Carb (g) = 22.6; Net Carb (g) = 20; Fat (g) = 6; Protein = 1.1

◯ Banana Ripe Fried ☞ serving size: 1 small = 73 g; Calories = 107.3; Total Carb (g) = 17.5; Net Carb (g) = 15.5; Fat (g) = 4.7; Protein = 0.8

◯ Banana Whip ☞ serving size: 1 cup = 130 g; Calories = 176.8; Total Carb (g) = 39.3; Net Carb (g) = 37.1; Fat (g) = 0.4; Protein = 6.4

◯ Bananas ☞ serving size: 1 cup, mashed = 225 g; Calories = 200.3; Total Carb (g) = 51.4; Net Carb (g) = 45.5; Fat (g) = 0.7; Protein = 2.5

◯ Bartlett Pears ☞ serving size: 1 cup, sliced = 140 g; Calories = 88.2; Total Carb (g) = 21; Net Carb (g) = 16.7; Fat (g) = 0.2; Protein = 0.6

◯ Beans String Green Pickled ☞ serving size: 1 cup = 135 g; Calories = 37.8; Total Carb (g) = 8.2; Net Carb (g) = 5.1; Fat (g) = 0.3; Protein = 2.1

Blackberries ☞ serving size: 1 cup = 144 g; Calories = 61.9; Total Carb (g) = 13.8; Net Carb (g) = 6.2; Fat (g) = 0.7; Protein = 2

Blackberries Canned Heavy Syrup Solids And Liquids ☞ serving size: 1 cup = 256 g; Calories = 235.5; Total Carb (g) = 59.1; Net Carb (g) = 50.4; Fat (g) = 0.4; Protein = 3.4

Blackberries Frozen Sweetened Ns As To Type Of Sweetener ☞ serving size: 1 cup = 145 g; Calories = 143.6; Total Carb (g) = 35.8; Net Carb (g) = 29.3; Fat (g) = 0.6; Protein = 1.5

Blackberries Frozen Unsweetened ☞ serving size: 1 cup, unthawed = 151 g; Calories = 96.6; Total Carb (g) = 23.7; Net Carb (g) = 16.1; Fat (g) = 0.7; Protein = 1.8

Blackberry Juice Canned ☞ serving size: 1 cup = 250 g; Calories = 95; Total Carb (g) = 19.5; Net Carb (g) = 19.3; Fat (g) = 1.5; Protein = 0.8

Blueberries ☞ serving size: 1 cup = 148 g; Calories = 84.4; Total Carb (g) = 21.5; Net Carb (g) = 17.9; Fat (g) = 0.5; Protein = 1.1

Blueberries (Frozen) ☞ serving size: 1 cup, unthawed = 155 g; Calories = 79.1; Total Carb (g) = 18.9; Net Carb (g) = 14.7; Fat (g) = 1; Protein = 0.7

Blueberries Canned Heavy Syrup Solids And Liquids ☞ serving size: 1 cup = 256 g; Calories = 225.3; Total Carb (g) = 56.5; Net Carb (g) = 52.4; Fat (g) = 0.8; Protein = 1.7

Blueberries Canned Light Syrup Drained ☞ serving size: 1 cup = 244 g; Calories = 214.7; Total Carb (g) = 55.3; Net Carb (g) = 49; Fat (g) = 1; Protein = 2.5

Blueberries Cooked Or Canned Unsweetened Water Pack ☞ serving size: 1 cup = 244 g; Calories = 92.7; Total Carb (g) = 23.7; Net Carb (g) = 19.8; Fat (g) = 0.5; Protein = 1.2

Blueberries Frozen Sweetened ☞ serving size: 1 cup, thawed =

230 g; Calories = 195.5; Total Carb (g) = 50.5; Net Carb (g) = 45.4; Fat (g) = 0.3; Protein = 0.9

🫐 Blueberries Wild Canned Heavy Syrup Drained ☞ serving size: 1 cup = 319 g; Calories = 341.3; Total Carb (g) = 90.3; Net Carb (g) = 74.7; Fat (g) = 1.1; Protein = 1.8

🫐 Bosc Pear ☞ serving size: 1 cup, sliced = 140 g; Calories = 93.8; Total Carb (g) = 22.5; Net Carb (g) = 18.2; Fat (g) = 0.1; Protein = 0.5

🫐 Boysenberries (Frozen) ☞ serving size: 1 cup, unthawed = 132 g; Calories = 66; Total Carb (g) = 16.1; Net Carb (g) = 9.1; Fat (g) = 0.3; Protein = 1.5

🫐 Boysenberries Canned Heavy Syrup ☞ serving size: 1 cup = 256 g; Calories = 225.3; Total Carb (g) = 57.1; Net Carb (g) = 50.5; Fat (g) = 0.3; Protein = 2.5

🫐 Breadfruit ☞ serving size: 1 cup = 220 g; Calories = 226.6; Total Carb (g) = 59.7; Net Carb (g) = 48.9; Fat (g) = 0.5; Protein = 2.4

🫐 Cabbage Red Pickled ☞ serving size: 1 cup = 150 g; Calories = 66; Total Carb (g) = 12.9; Net Carb (g) = 11.1; Fat (g) = 0.2; Protein = 1.2

🫐 California Avocados ☞ serving size: 1 cup, pureed = 230 g; Calories = 384.1; Total Carb (g) = 19.9; Net Carb (g) = 4.2; Fat (g) = 35.4; Protein = 4.5

🫐 California Grapefruit ☞ serving size: 1 cup sections, with juice = 230 g; Calories = 85.1; Total Carb (g) = 22.3; Net Carb (g) = 22.3; Fat (g) = 0.2; Protein = 1.2

🫐 California Valencia Oranges ☞ serving size: 1 cup sections, without membranes = 180 g; Calories = 88.2; Total Carb (g) = 21.4; Net Carb (g) = 16.9; Fat (g) = 0.5; Protein = 1.9

🫐 Canned Orange Juice ☞ serving size: 1 cup = 249 g; Calories = 117; Total Carb (g) = 27.4; Net Carb (g) = 26.7; Fat (g) = 0.4; Protein = 1.7

🍈 Cantaloupe Melons ☞ serving size: 1 cup, balls = 177 g; Calories = 60.2; Total Carb (g) = 14.4; Net Carb (g) = 12.9; Fat (g) = 0.3; Protein = 1.5

🍈 Carissa ☞ serving size: 1 cup slices = 150 g; Calories = 93; Total Carb (g) = 20.5; Net Carb (g) = 20.5; Fat (g) = 2; Protein = 0.8

🍈 Casaba Melon ☞ serving size: 1 cup, cubes = 170 g; Calories = 47.6; Total Carb (g) = 11.2; Net Carb (g) = 9.7; Fat (g) = 0.2; Protein = 1.9

🍈 Cauliflower Pickled ☞ serving size: 1 cup = 125 g; Calories = 53.8; Total Carb (g) = 12; Net Carb (g) = 9.8; Fat (g) = 0.4; Protein = 1.9

🍈 Celery Pickled ☞ serving size: 1 cup = 150 g; Calories = 24; Total Carb (g) = 4; Net Carb (g) = 1.9; Fat (g) = 0.2; Protein = 0.9

🍈 Cherimoya ☞ serving size: 1 cup, pieces = 160 g; Calories = 120; Total Carb (g) = 28.3; Net Carb (g) = 23.5; Fat (g) = 1.1; Protein = 2.5

🍈 Cherries (Sweet) ☞ serving size: 1 cup, with pits, yields = 138 g; Calories = 86.9; Total Carb (g) = 22.1; Net Carb (g) = 19.2; Fat (g) = 0.3; Protein = 1.5

🍈 Cherries Sweet Canned Water Pack Solids And Liquids ☞ serving size: 1 cup, pitted = 248 g; Calories = 114.1; Total Carb (g) = 29.2; Net Carb (g) = 25.4; Fat (g) = 0.3; Protein = 1.9

🍈 Cherries Tart Dried Sweetened ☞ serving size: 1/4 cup = 40 g; Calories = 133.2; Total Carb (g) = 32.2; Net Carb (g) = 31.2; Fat (g) = 0.3; Protein = 0.5

🍈 Chinese Preserved Sweet Vegetable ☞ serving size: 1 slice = 12 g; Calories = 44.5; Total Carb (g) = 11.5; Net Carb (g) = 11.4; Fat (g) = 0; Protein = 0.1

🍈 Clementines ☞ serving size: 1 fruit = 74 g; Calories = 34.8; Total Carb (g) = 8.9; Net Carb (g) = 7.6; Fat (g) = 0.1; Protein = 0.6

🍈 Corn Relish ☞ serving size: 1 cup = 245 g; Calories = 205.8; Total Carb (g) = 46.6; Net Carb (g) = 42.7; Fat (g) = 1.4; Protein = 4.2

◐ Crabapples ☞ serving size: 1 cup slices = 110 g; Calories = 83.6; Total Carb (g) = 22; Net Carb (g) = 22; Fat (g) = 0.3; Protein = 0.4

◐ Cranberries ☞ serving size: 1 cup, chopped = 110 g; Calories = 50.6; Total Carb (g) = 13.2; Net Carb (g) = 9.2; Fat (g) = 0.1; Protein = 0.5

◐ Cranberry Juice Blend 100% Juice Bottled With Added Vitamin C And Calcium ☞ serving size: 6 (3/4) fl oz = 200 g; Calories = 90; Total Carb (g) = 21.8; Net Carb (g) = 21.6; Fat (g) = 0.2; Protein = 0.5

◐ Cranberry Juice Unsweetened ☞ serving size: 1 cup = 253 g; Calories = 116.4; Total Carb (g) = 30.9; Net Carb (g) = 30.6; Fat (g) = 0.3; Protein = 1

◐ Dates (Deglet Noor) ☞ serving size: 1 cup, chopped = 147 g; Calories = 414.5; Total Carb (g) = 110.3; Net Carb (g) = 98.5; Fat (g) = 0.6; Protein = 3.6

◐ Dried Apples ☞ serving size: 1 cup = 86 g; Calories = 209; Total Carb (g) = 56.7; Net Carb (g) = 49.2; Fat (g) = 0.3; Protein = 0.8

◐ Dried Apricots ☞ serving size: 1 cup, halves = 130 g; Calories = 313.3; Total Carb (g) = 81.4; Net Carb (g) = 71.9; Fat (g) = 0.7; Protein = 4.4

◐ Dried Bananas ☞ serving size: 1 cup = 100 g; Calories = 346; Total Carb (g) = 88.3; Net Carb (g) = 78.4; Fat (g) = 1.8; Protein = 3.9

◐ Dried Blueberries (Sweetened) ☞ serving size: 1/4 cup = 40 g; Calories = 126.8; Total Carb (g) = 32; Net Carb (g) = 29; Fat (g) = 1; Protein = 1

◐ Dried Cranberries (Sweetened) ☞ serving size: 1/4 cup = 40 g; Calories = 123.2; Total Carb (g) = 33.1; Net Carb (g) = 31; Fat (g) = 0.4; Protein = 0.1

◐ Dried Figs ☞ serving size: 1 cup = 149 g; Calories = 371; Total Carb (g) = 95.2; Net Carb (g) = 80.6; Fat (g) = 1.4; Protein = 4.9

Dried Litchis ☞ serving size: 1 fruit = 2.5 g; Calories = 6.9; Total Carb (g) = 1.8; Net Carb (g) = 1.7; Fat (g) = 0; Protein = 0.1

Dried Longans ☞ serving size: 1 fruit = 1.7 g; Calories = 4.9; Total Carb (g) = 1.3; Net Carb (g) = 1.3; Fat (g) = 0; Protein = 0.1

Dried Peaches ☞ serving size: 1 cup, halves = 160 g; Calories = 382.4; Total Carb (g) = 98.1; Net Carb (g) = 85; Fat (g) = 1.2; Protein = 5.8

Dried Peaches (Low-Moisture) ☞ serving size: 1 cup = 116 g; Calories = 377; Total Carb (g) = 96.5; Net Carb (g) = 96.5; Fat (g) = 1.2; Protein = 5.7

Dried Pears ☞ serving size: 1 cup, halves = 180 g; Calories = 471.6; Total Carb (g) = 125.5; Net Carb (g) = 112; Fat (g) = 1.1; Protein = 3.4

Durian ☞ serving size: 1 cup, chopped or diced = 243 g; Calories = 357.2; Total Carb (g) = 65.8; Net Carb (g) = 56.6; Fat (g) = 13; Protein = 3.6

Elderberries ☞ serving size: 1 cup = 145 g; Calories = 105.9; Total Carb (g) = 26.7; Net Carb (g) = 16.5; Fat (g) = 0.7; Protein = 1

European Black Currants ☞ serving size: 1 cup = 112 g; Calories = 70.6; Total Carb (g) = 17.2; Net Carb (g) = 17.2; Fat (g) = 0.5; Protein = 1.6

Feijoa ☞ serving size: 1 cup, pureed = 243 g; Calories = 148.2; Total Carb (g) = 37; Net Carb (g) = 21.4; Fat (g) = 1; Protein = 1.7

Fig Dried Cooked Ns As To Sweetened Or Unsweetened; Sweetened Ns As To Type Of Sweetener ☞ serving size: 1 cup = 259 g; Calories = 354.8; Total Carb (g) = 91.5; Net Carb (g) = 81.7; Fat (g) = 0.9; Protein = 3.3

Fig Dried Cooked With Sugar ☞ serving size: 1 cup = 270 g; Calories = 369.9; Total Carb (g) = 95.4; Net Carb (g) = 85.1; Fat (g) = 1; Protein = 3.4

◎ Figs ☞ serving size: 1 large (2-1/2 inch dia) = 64 g; Calories = 47.4; Total Carb (g) = 12.3; Net Carb (g) = 10.4; Fat (g) = 0.2; Protein = 0.5

◎ Figs Canned Extra Heavy Syrup Pack Solids And Liquids ☞ serving size: 1 cup = 261 g; Calories = 279.3; Total Carb (g) = 72.7; Net Carb (g) = 72.7; Fat (g) = 0.3; Protein = 1

◎ Figs Canned Heavy Syrup Pack Solids And Liquids ☞ serving size: 1 cup = 259 g; Calories = 227.9; Total Carb (g) = 59.3; Net Carb (g) = 53.6; Fat (g) = 0.3; Protein = 1

◎ Figs Canned Light Syrup Pack Solids And Liquids ☞ serving size: 1 cup = 252 g; Calories = 173.9; Total Carb (g) = 45.2; Net Carb (g) = 40.7; Fat (g) = 0.3; Protein = 1

◎ Figs Canned Water Pack Solids And Liquids ☞ serving size: 1 cup = 248 g; Calories = 131.4; Total Carb (g) = 34.7; Net Carb (g) = 29.2; Fat (g) = 0.3; Protein = 1

◎ Figs Dried Stewed ☞ serving size: 1 cup = 259 g; Calories = 277.1; Total Carb (g) = 71.4; Net Carb (g) = 60.5; Fat (g) = 1; Protein = 3.7

◎ Florida Avocados ☞ serving size: 1 cup, pureed = 230 g; Calories = 276; Total Carb (g) = 18; Net Carb (g) = 5.1; Fat (g) = 23.1; Protein = 5.1

◎ Florida Grapefruit ☞ serving size: 1 cup sections, with juice = 230 g; Calories = 69; Total Carb (g) = 17.3; Net Carb (g) = 14.7; Fat (g) = 0.2; Protein = 1.3

◎ Florida Oranges ☞ serving size: 1 cup sections, without membranes = 185 g; Calories = 85.1; Total Carb (g) = 21.4; Net Carb (g) = 16.9; Fat (g) = 0.4; Protein = 1.3

◎ Fortified Fruit Juice Smoothie ☞ serving size: 8 fl oz = 240 g; Calories = 170.4; Total Carb (g) = 40; Net Carb (g) = 33.1; Fat (g) = 0; Protein = 1

◎ Fried Dwarf Banana Puerto Rican Style ☞ serving size: 1 banana (4" x 1-1/2" x 1-1/2") = 36 g; Calories = 55.8; Total Carb (g) = 7.6; Net Carb (g) = 6.7; Fat (g) = 3.1; Protein = 0.4

Fried Dwarf Banana With Cheese Puerto Rican Style ☞ serving size: 1 banana (4" x 1-1/2" x 1-1/2") = 40 g; Calories = 84; Total Carb (g) = 9.6; Net Carb (g) = 8.5; Fat (g) = 5; Protein = 1.4

Fried Yellow Plantains ☞ serving size: 1 cup = 169 g; Calories = 398.8; Total Carb (g) = 68.9; Net Carb (g) = 63.5; Fat (g) = 12.7; Protein = 2.4

Frozen Raspberries ☞ serving size: 1 cup, unthawed = 140 g; Calories = 78.4; Total Carb (g) = 17.6; Net Carb (g) = 11.6; Fat (g) = 1.1; Protein = 1.6

Frozen Strawberries ☞ serving size: 1 cup, thawed = 221 g; Calories = 77.4; Total Carb (g) = 20.2; Net Carb (g) = 15.5; Fat (g) = 0.2; Protein = 1

Fruit Cocktail (Peach And Pineapple And Pear And Grape And Cherry) Canned Extra Heavy Syrup Solids And Liquids ☞ serving size: 1/2 cup = 130 g; Calories = 114.4; Total Carb (g) = 29.8; Net Carb (g) = 28.3; Fat (g) = 0.1; Protein = 0.5

Fruit Cocktail (Peach And Pineapple And Pear And Grape And Cherry) Canned Extra Light Syrup Solids And Liquids ☞ serving size: 1/2 cup = 123 g; Calories = 55.4; Total Carb (g) = 14.3; Net Carb (g) = 13; Fat (g) = 0.1; Protein = 0.5

Fruit Cocktail (Peach And Pineapple And Pear And Grape And Cherry) Canned Heavy Syrup Solids And Liquids ☞ serving size: 1 cup = 248 g; Calories = 181; Total Carb (g) = 46.9; Net Carb (g) = 44.4; Fat (g) = 0.2; Protein = 1

Fruit Cocktail (Peach And Pineapple And Pear And Grape And Cherry) Canned Juice Pack Solids And Liquids ☞ serving size: 1 cup = 237 g; Calories = 109; Total Carb (g) = 28.1; Net Carb (g) = 25.7; Fat (g) = 0; Protein = 1.1

Fruit Cocktail (Peach And Pineapple And Pear And Grape And Cherry) Canned Light Syrup Solids And Liquids ☞ serving size: 1

cup = 242 g; Calories = 137.9; Total Carb (g) = 36.1; Net Carb (g) = 33.7; Fat (g) = 0.2; Protein = 1

Fruit Cocktail (Peach And Pineapple And Pear And Grape And Cherry) Canned Water Pack Solids And Liquids ☞ serving size: 1 cup = 237 g; Calories = 75.8; Total Carb (g) = 20.2; Net Carb (g) = 17.8; Fat (g) = 0.1; Protein = 1

Fruit Cocktail Canned Heavy Syrup Drained ☞ serving size: 1 cup = 214 g; Calories = 149.8; Total Carb (g) = 40.2; Net Carb (g) = 36.6; Fat (g) = 0.2; Protein = 1

Fruit Cocktail Or Mix Frozen ☞ serving size: 1 cup = 215 g; Calories = 105.4; Total Carb (g) = 25.8; Net Carb (g) = 20.4; Fat (g) = 0.7; Protein = 2.1

Fruit Dessert With Cream And/or Pudding And Nuts ☞ serving size: 1 cup = 178 g; Calories = 361.3; Total Carb (g) = 51.6; Net Carb (g) = 50.1; Fat (g) = 17.8; Protein = 2.7

Fruit Juice Smoothie Bolthouse Farms Berry Boost ☞ serving size: 1 cup = 252 g; Calories = 115.9; Total Carb (g) = 27.5; Net Carb (g) = 27.5; Fat (g) = 0.1; Protein = 1.6

Fruit Juice Smoothie Bolthouse Farms Green Goodness ☞ serving size: 1 cup = 230 g; Calories = 128.8; Total Carb (g) = 30; Net Carb (g) = 28.6; Fat (g) = 0.8; Protein = 1.5

Fruit Juice Smoothie Bolthouse Farms Strawberry Banana ☞ serving size: 1 cup = 233 g; Calories = 121.2; Total Carb (g) = 28.8; Net Carb (g) = 27.4; Fat (g) = 0.7; Protein = 1

Fruit Juice Smoothie Naked Juice Green Machine ☞ serving size: 1 cup = 275 g; Calories = 145.8; Total Carb (g) = 34.5; Net Carb (g) = 32.5; Fat (g) = 0.7; Protein = 1.7

Fruit Juice Smoothie Naked Juice Mighty Mango ☞ serving size: 8 fl oz = 240 g; Calories = 151.2; Total Carb (g) = 36; Net Carb (g) = 36; Fat (g) = 0; Protein = 1

Fruit Juice Smoothie Naked Juice Strawberry Banana ☞ serving size: 1 cup = 228 g; Calories = 114; Total Carb (g) = 26.6; Net Carb (g) = 25.2; Fat (g) = 0.6; Protein = 1.1

Fruit Juice Smoothie Odwalla Original Superfood ☞ serving size: 1 cup = 227 g; Calories = 113.5; Total Carb (g) = 26.1; Net Carb (g) = 24.8; Fat (g) = 0.8; Protein = 1.4

Fruit Juice Smoothie Odwalla Strawberry Banana ☞ serving size: 1 cup = 233 g; Calories = 111.8; Total Carb (g) = 25.8; Net Carb (g) = 24.4; Fat (g) = 0.8; Protein = 1.2

Fruit Ns As To Type ☞ serving size: 1 fruit = 138 g; Calories = 95.2; Total Carb (g) = 24.5; Net Carb (g) = 21.3; Fat (g) = 0.3; Protein = 1.1

Fruit Salad (Peach And Pear And Apricot And Pineapple And Cherry) Canned Extra Heavy Syrup Solids And Liquids ☞ serving size: 1 cup = 259 g; Calories = 227.9; Total Carb (g) = 59; Net Carb (g) = 56.4; Fat (g) = 0.2; Protein = 0.9

Fruit Salad (Peach And Pear And Apricot And Pineapple And Cherry) Canned Juice Pack Solids And Liquids ☞ serving size: 1 cup = 249 g; Calories = 124.5; Total Carb (g) = 32.5; Net Carb (g) = 30; Fat (g) = 0.1; Protein = 1.3

Fruit Salad (Peach And Pear And Apricot And Pineapple And Cherry) Canned Light Syrup Solids And Liquids ☞ serving size: 1 cup = 252 g; Calories = 146.2; Total Carb (g) = 38.2; Net Carb (g) = 35.6; Fat (g) = 0.2; Protein = 0.9

Fruit Salad (Peach And Pear And Apricot And Pineapple And Cherry) Canned Water Pack Solids And Liquids ☞ serving size: 1 cup = 245 g; Calories = 73.5; Total Carb (g) = 19.3; Net Carb (g) = 16.8; Fat (g) = 0.2; Protein = 0.9

Fruit Salad (Pineapple And Papaya And Banana And Guava) Tropical Canned Heavy Syrup Solids And Liquids ☞ serving size: 1

cup = 257 g; Calories = 221; Total Carb (g) = 57.5; Net Carb (g) = 54.1; Fat (g) = 0.3; Protein = 1.1

🜊 Fruit Salad Excluding Citrus Fruits With Marshmallows ☞ serving size: 1 cup = 171 g; Calories = 408.7; Total Carb (g) = 29.5; Net Carb (g) = 26.4; Fat (g) = 32.7; Protein = 3.2

🜊 Fruit Salad Excluding Citrus Fruits With Nondairy Whipped Topping ☞ serving size: 1 cup = 175 g; Calories = 243.3; Total Carb (g) = 29.6; Net Carb (g) = 25.8; Fat (g) = 14.5; Protein = 3.6

🜊 Fruit Salad Excluding Citrus Fruits With Pudding ☞ serving size: 1 cup = 182 g; Calories = 227.5; Total Carb (g) = 32.4; Net Carb (g) = 29.2; Fat (g) = 11.2; Protein = 3.6

🜊 Fruit Salad Excluding Citrus Fruits With Salad Dressing Or Mayonnaise ☞ serving size: 1 cup = 188 g; Calories = 441.8; Total Carb (g) = 25; Net Carb (g) = 21.4; Fat (g) = 38.2; Protein = 3.6

🜊 Fruit Salad Excluding Citrus Fruits With Whipped Cream ☞ serving size: 1 cup = 182 g; Calories = 273; Total Carb (g) = 26.9; Net Carb (g) = 23.1; Fat (g) = 18.7; Protein = 4

🜊 Fruit Salad Fresh Or Raw Excluding Citrus Fruits No Dressing ☞ serving size: 1 cup = 175 g; Calories = 92.8; Total Carb (g) = 23.7; Net Carb (g) = 20.7; Fat (g) = 0.5; Protein = 1.2

🜊 Fruit Salad Fresh Or Raw Including Citrus Fruits No Dressing ☞ serving size: 1 cup = 175 g; Calories = 91; Total Carb (g) = 23; Net Carb (g) = 19.7; Fat (g) = 0.4; Protein = 1.3

🜊 Fruit Salad Including Citrus Fruit With Whipped Cream ☞ serving size: 1 cup = 182 g; Calories = 267.5; Total Carb (g) = 26.2; Net Carb (g) = 22; Fat (g) = 18.3; Protein = 4.2

🜊 Fruit Salad Including Citrus Fruits With Marshmallows ☞ serving size: 1 cup = 171 g; Calories = 401.9; Total Carb (g) = 28.9; Net Carb (g) = 25.4; Fat (g) = 32.1; Protein = 3.3

🜊 Fruit Salad Including Citrus Fruits With Nondairy Whipped

Topping ☞ serving size: 1 cup = 175 g; Calories = 238; Total Carb (g) = 28.8; Net Carb (g) = 24.6; Fat (g) = 14.1; Protein = 3.7

Fruit Salad Including Citrus Fruits With Pudding ☞ serving size: 1 cup = 182 g; Calories = 223.9; Total Carb (g) = 31.7; Net Carb (g) = 27.9; Fat (g) = 10.9; Protein = 3.7

Fruit Salad Including Citrus Fruits With Salad Dressing Or Mayonnaise ☞ serving size: 1 cup = 188 g; Calories = 432.4; Total Carb (g) = 24.3; Net Carb (g) = 20.4; Fat (g) = 37.5; Protein = 3.7

Fruit Salad Puerto Rican Style ☞ serving size: 1 cup = 247 g; Calories = 143.3; Total Carb (g) = 36.4; Net Carb (g) = 32.7; Fat (g) = 0.5; Protein = 1.7

Fuji Apples ☞ serving size: 1 cup, sliced = 109 g; Calories = 68.7; Total Carb (g) = 16.6; Net Carb (g) = 14.3; Fat (g) = 0.2; Protein = 0.2

Fuyu Persimmon ☞ serving size: 1 fruit (2-1/2 inch dia) = 168 g; Calories = 117.6; Total Carb (g) = 31.2; Net Carb (g) = 25.2; Fat (g) = 0.3; Protein = 1

Gala Apples ☞ serving size: 1 cup, sliced = 109 g; Calories = 62.1; Total Carb (g) = 14.9; Net Carb (g) = 12.4; Fat (g) = 0.1; Protein = 0.3

Goji Berries Dried ☞ serving size: 5 tbsp = 28 g; Calories = 97.7; Total Carb (g) = 21.6; Net Carb (g) = 17.9; Fat (g) = 0.1; Protein = 4

Golden Delicious Apples ☞ serving size: 1 cup, sliced = 109 g; Calories = 62.1; Total Carb (g) = 14.8; Net Carb (g) = 12.2; Fat (g) = 0.2; Protein = 0.3

Golden Seedless Raisins ☞ serving size: 1 cup, packed = 165 g; Calories = 496.7; Total Carb (g) = 132; Net Carb (g) = 126.6; Fat (g) = 0.3; Protein = 5.4

Gooseberries ☞ serving size: 1 cup = 150 g; Calories = 66; Total Carb (g) = 15.3; Net Carb (g) = 8.8; Fat (g) = 0.9; Protein = 1.3

Gooseberries Canned Light Syrup Pack Solids And Liquids ☞

serving size: 1 cup = 252 g; Calories = 184; Total Carb (g) = 47.3; Net Carb (g) = 41.2; Fat (g) = 0.5; Protein = 1.6

Granny Smith Apples ☞ serving size: 1 cup, sliced = 109 g; Calories = 63.2; Total Carb (g) = 14.8; Net Carb (g) = 11.8; Fat (g) = 0.2; Protein = 0.5

Grape Juice ☞ serving size: 1 cup = 253 g; Calories = 151.8; Total Carb (g) = 37.4; Net Carb (g) = 36.9; Fat (g) = 0.3; Protein = 0.9

Grape Juice (With Added Vitamin C) ☞ serving size: 1 cup = 253 g; Calories = 151.8; Total Carb (g) = 37.4; Net Carb (g) = 36.9; Fat (g) = 0.3; Protein = 0.9

Grape Juice Canned Or Bottled Unsweetened With Added Ascorbic Acid And Calcium ☞ serving size: 1 cup = 253 g; Calories = 156.9; Total Carb (g) = 37.4; Net Carb (g) = 36.9; Fat (g) = 0.3; Protein = 0.9

Grapefruit ☞ serving size: 1 cup sections, with juice = 230 g; Calories = 73.6; Total Carb (g) = 18.6; Net Carb (g) = 16.1; Fat (g) = 0.2; Protein = 1.5

Grapefruit And Orange Sections Cooked Canned Or Frozen In Light Syrup ☞ serving size: 1 cup = 254 g; Calories = 152.4; Total Carb (g) = 39; Net Carb (g) = 36.5; Fat (g) = 0.2; Protein = 1.5

Grapefruit And Orange Sections Cooked Canned Or Frozen Ns As To Added Sweetener ☞ serving size: 1 cup = 254 g; Calories = 152.4; Total Carb (g) = 39; Net Carb (g) = 36.5; Fat (g) = 0.2; Protein = 1.5

Grapefruit And Orange Sections Cooked Canned Or Frozen Unsweetened Water Pack ☞ serving size: 1 cup = 244 g; Calories = 65.9; Total Carb (g) = 16.3; Net Carb (g) = 13.4; Fat (g) = 0.2; Protein = 1.3

Grapefruit And Orange Sections Raw ☞ serving size: 1 section =

16 g; Calories = 6.4; Total Carb (g) = 1.6; Net Carb (g) = 1.3; Fat (g) = 0; Protein = 0.1

🌐 Grapefruit Juice ☞ serving size: 8 fl oz = 240 g; Calories = 93.6; Total Carb (g) = 18.6; Net Carb (g) = 17.9; Fat (g) = 1.6; Protein = 1.2

🌐 Grapefruit Juice 100% With Calcium Added ☞ serving size: 1 fl oz (no ice) = 31 g; Calories = 11.8; Total Carb (g) = 2.7; Net Carb (g) = 2.7; Fat (g) = 0; Protein = 0.2

🌐 Grapefruit Juice White Bottled Unsweetened Ocean Spray ☞ serving size: 1 cup = 247 g; Calories = 91.4; Total Carb (g) = 18.6; Net Carb (g) = 17.1; Fat (g) = 1.6; Protein = 1.3

🌐 Grapefruit Juice White Canned Or Bottled Unsweetened ☞ serving size: 1 cup = 247 g; Calories = 91.4; Total Carb (g) = 18.6; Net Carb (g) = 17.1; Fat (g) = 1.6; Protein = 1.4

🌐 Grapefruit Juice White Canned Sweetened ☞ serving size: 1 cup = 250 g; Calories = 115; Total Carb (g) = 27.8; Net Carb (g) = 27.6; Fat (g) = 0.2; Protein = 1.5

🌐 Grapefruit Juice White Frozen Concentrate Unsweetened Diluted With 3 Volume Water ☞ serving size: 1 cup = 247 g; Calories = 101.3; Total Carb (g) = 24; Net Carb (g) = 23.8; Fat (g) = 0.3; Protein = 1.4

🌐 Grapefruit Juice White Frozen Concentrate Unsweetened Undiluted ☞ serving size: 1 can (6 fl oz) = 207 g; Calories = 302.2; Total Carb (g) = 71.5; Net Carb (g) = 70.7; Fat (g) = 1; Protein = 4.1

🌐 Grapefruit Sections Canned Juice Pack Solids And Liquids ☞ serving size: 1 cup = 249 g; Calories = 92.1; Total Carb (g) = 22.9; Net Carb (g) = 21.9; Fat (g) = 0.2; Protein = 1.7

🌐 Grapefruit Sections Canned Light Syrup Pack Solids And Liquids ☞ serving size: 1 cup = 254 g; Calories = 152.4; Total Carb (g) = 39.2; Net Carb (g) = 38.2; Fat (g) = 0.3; Protein = 1.4

🌐 Grapefruit Sections Canned Water Pack Solids And Liquids ☞

serving size: 1 cup = 244 g; Calories = 87.8; Total Carb (g) = 22.3; Net Carb (g) = 21.4; Fat (g) = 0.2; Protein = 1.4

Grapes ☞ serving size: 1 cup = 92 g; Calories = 61.6; Total Carb (g) = 15.8; Net Carb (g) = 15; Fat (g) = 0.3; Protein = 0.6

Grapes Canned Thompson Seedless Heavy Syrup Pack Solids And Liquids ☞ serving size: 1 cup = 256 g; Calories = 194.6; Total Carb (g) = 50.3; Net Carb (g) = 48.8; Fat (g) = 0.3; Protein = 1.2

Grapes Canned Thompson Seedless Water Pack Solids And Liquids ☞ serving size: 1 cup = 245 g; Calories = 98; Total Carb (g) = 25.2; Net Carb (g) = 23.8; Fat (g) = 0.3; Protein = 1.2

Green Anjou Pear ☞ serving size: 1 cup, sliced = 140 g; Calories = 92.4; Total Carb (g) = 22.1; Net Carb (g) = 17.8; Fat (g) = 0.1; Protein = 0.6

Green Olives ☞ serving size: 1 olive = 2.7 g; Calories = 3.9; Total Carb (g) = 0.1; Net Carb (g) = 0; Fat (g) = 0.4; Protein = 0

Groundcherries ☞ serving size: 1 cup = 140 g; Calories = 74.2; Total Carb (g) = 15.7; Net Carb (g) = 15.7; Fat (g) = 1; Protein = 2.7

Guanabana Nectar Canned ☞ serving size: 1 cup = 251 g; Calories = 148.1; Total Carb (g) = 37.5; Net Carb (g) = 37.2; Fat (g) = 0.4; Protein = 0.3

Guava Nectar Canned With Added Ascorbic Acid ☞ serving size: 1 cup = 251 g; Calories = 158.1; Total Carb (g) = 40.8; Net Carb (g) = 38.3; Fat (g) = 0.2; Protein = 0.2

Guava Nectar With Sucralose Canned ☞ serving size: fl oz = 335 g; Calories = 160.8; Total Carb (g) = 44.6; Net Carb (g) = 40.5; Fat (g) = 0.2; Protein = 1

Guava Sauce Cooked ☞ serving size: 1 cup = 238 g; Calories = 85.7; Total Carb (g) = 22.6; Net Carb (g) = 14; Fat (g) = 0.3; Protein = 0.8

◔ Guava Shell Canned In Heavy Syrup ☞ serving size: 1 cup = 310 g; Calories = 337.9; Total Carb (g) = 80.1; Net Carb (g) = 68.3; Fat (g) = 2.1; Protein = 5.6

◔ Guavas ☞ serving size: 1 cup = 165 g; Calories = 112.2; Total Carb (g) = 23.6; Net Carb (g) = 14.7; Fat (g) = 1.6; Protein = 4.2

◔ Honeydew Melon ☞ serving size: 1 cup, diced (approx 20 pieces per cup) = 170 g; Calories = 61.2; Total Carb (g) = 15.5; Net Carb (g) = 14.1; Fat (g) = 0.2; Protein = 0.9

◔ Horned Melon (Kiwano) ☞ serving size: 1 cup = 233 g; Calories = 102.5; Total Carb (g) = 17.6; Net Carb (g) = 17.6; Fat (g) = 2.9; Protein = 4.2

◔ Jackfruit ☞ serving size: 1 cup, sliced = 165 g; Calories = 156.8; Total Carb (g) = 38.4; Net Carb (g) = 35.9; Fat (g) = 1.1; Protein = 2.8

◔ Jackfruit Canned Syrup Pack ☞ serving size: 1 cup, drained = 178 g; Calories = 163.8; Total Carb (g) = 42.6; Net Carb (g) = 41; Fat (g) = 0.3; Protein = 0.6

◔ Java Plum ☞ serving size: 1 cup = 135 g; Calories = 81; Total Carb (g) = 21; Net Carb (g) = 21; Fat (g) = 0.3; Protein = 1

◔ Juice Apple And Grape Blend With Added Ascorbic Acid ☞ serving size: 8 fl oz = 250 g; Calories = 125; Total Carb (g) = 31.2; Net Carb (g) = 30.7; Fat (g) = 0.3; Protein = 0.4

◔ Juice Apple Grape And Pear Blend With Added Ascorbic Acid And Calcium ☞ serving size: 8 fl oz = 250 g; Calories = 130; Total Carb (g) = 32.4; Net Carb (g) = 31.9; Fat (g) = 0.3; Protein = 0.4

◔ Jumbo Olives ☞ serving size: 1 super colossal = 15 g; Calories = 12.2; Total Carb (g) = 0.8; Net Carb (g) = 0.5; Fat (g) = 1; Protein = 0.2

◔ Kiwifruit ☞ serving size: 1 cup, sliced = 180 g; Calories = 109.8; Total Carb (g) = 26.4; Net Carb (g) = 21; Fat (g) = 0.9; Protein = 2.1

◔ Kiwifruit Zespri Sungold Raw ☞ serving size: 1 fruit = 81 g; Calories = 51; Total Carb (g) = 12.8; Net Carb (g) = 11.7; Fat (g) = 0.2; Protein = 0.8

🦪 Kumquat Cooked Or Canned In Syrup ☞ serving size: 1 kumquat = 14 g; Calories = 13.7; Total Carb (g) = 3.3; Net Carb (g) = 2.7; Fat (g) = 0.1; Protein = 0.2

🦪 Kumquats ☞ serving size: 1 fruit without refuse = 19 g; Calories = 13.5; Total Carb (g) = 3; Net Carb (g) = 1.8; Fat (g) = 0.2; Protein = 0.4

🦪 Lemon Juice From Concentrate Bottled Concord ☞ serving size: 1 tbsp = 15 g; Calories = 3.6; Total Carb (g) = 0.8; Net Carb (g) = 0.8; Fat (g) = 0; Protein = 0.1

🦪 Lemon Juice From Concentrate Bottled Real Lemon ☞ serving size: 1 tbsp = 15 g; Calories = 2.6; Total Carb (g) = 0.9; Net Carb (g) = 0.7; Fat (g) = 0; Protein = 0.1

🦪 Lemon Juice From Concentrate Canned Or Bottled ☞ serving size: 1 tbsp = 15 g; Calories = 2.6; Total Carb (g) = 0.8; Net Carb (g) = 0.7; Fat (g) = 0; Protein = 0.1

🦪 Lemon Juice Raw ☞ serving size: 1 cup = 244 g; Calories = 53.7; Total Carb (g) = 16.8; Net Carb (g) = 16.1; Fat (g) = 0.6; Protein = 0.9

🦪 Lemon Peel Raw ☞ serving size: 1 tbsp = 6 g; Calories = 2.8; Total Carb (g) = 1; Net Carb (g) = 0.3; Fat (g) = 0; Protein = 0.1

🦪 Lemons ☞ serving size: 1 cup, sections = 212 g; Calories = 61.5; Total Carb (g) = 19.8; Net Carb (g) = 13.8; Fat (g) = 0.6; Protein = 2.3

🦪 Lime Juice ☞ serving size: 1 cup = 242 g; Calories = 60.5; Total Carb (g) = 20.4; Net Carb (g) = 19.4; Fat (g) = 0.2; Protein = 1

🦪 Lime Juice Canned Or Bottled Unsweetened ☞ serving size: 1 cup = 246 g; Calories = 51.7; Total Carb (g) = 16.5; Net Carb (g) = 15.5; Fat (g) = 0.6; Protein = 0.6

🦪 Limes ☞ serving size: 1 fruit (2 inch dia) = 67 g; Calories = 20.1; Total Carb (g) = 7.1; Net Carb (g) = 5.2; Fat (g) = 0.1; Protein = 0.5

🍈 Litchis ☞ serving size: 1 cup = 190 g; Calories = 125.4; Total Carb (g) = 31.4; Net Carb (g) = 28.9; Fat (g) = 0.8; Protein = 1.6

🍈 Loganberries (Frozen) ☞ serving size: 1 cup, unthawed = 147 g; Calories = 80.9; Total Carb (g) = 19.1; Net Carb (g) = 11.4; Fat (g) = 0.5; Protein = 2.2

🍈 Longans ☞ serving size: 1 fruit without refuse = 3.2 g; Calories = 1.9; Total Carb (g) = 0.5; Net Carb (g) = 0.5; Fat (g) = 0; Protein = 0

🍈 Loquats ☞ serving size: 1 cup, cubed = 149 g; Calories = 70; Total Carb (g) = 18.1; Net Carb (g) = 15.6; Fat (g) = 0.3; Protein = 0.6

🍈 Low-Moisture Dried Apricots ☞ serving size: 1 cup = 119 g; Calories = 380.8; Total Carb (g) = 98.6; Net Carb (g) = 98.6; Fat (g) = 0.7; Protein = 5.8

🍈 Lychee Cooked Or Canned In Sugar Or Syrup ☞ serving size: 1 lychee with liquid = 21 g; Calories = 20; Total Carb (g) = 5.1; Net Carb (g) = 4.9; Fat (g) = 0.1; Protein = 0.1

🍈 Mamey Sapote ☞ serving size: 1 cup 1 inch pieces = 175 g; Calories = 217; Total Carb (g) = 56.2; Net Carb (g) = 46.7; Fat (g) = 0.8; Protein = 2.5

🍈 Mammy Apple ☞ serving size: 1 fruit without refuse = 846 g; Calories = 431.5; Total Carb (g) = 105.8; Net Carb (g) = 80.4; Fat (g) = 4.2; Protein = 4.2

🍈 Mango Cooked ☞ serving size: 1 oz = 28 g; Calories = 16.8; Total Carb (g) = 4.2; Net Carb (g) = 3.8; Fat (g) = 0.1; Protein = 0.2

🍈 Mango Nectar Canned ☞ serving size: 1 cup = 251 g; Calories = 128; Total Carb (g) = 32.9; Net Carb (g) = 32.2; Fat (g) = 0.2; Protein = 0.3

🍈 Mango Pickled ☞ serving size: 1 slice = 28 g; Calories = 37; Total Carb (g) = 9.2; Net Carb (g) = 8.9; Fat (g) = 0.1; Protein = 0.2

🍶 Mangos ☞ serving size: 1 cup pieces = 165 g; Calories = 99; Total Carb (g) = 24.7; Net Carb (g) = 22.1; Fat (g) = 0.6; Protein = 1.4

🍶 Mangosteen Canned Syrup Pack ☞ serving size: 1 cup, drained = 196 g; Calories = 143.1; Total Carb (g) = 35.1; Net Carb (g) = 31.6; Fat (g) = 1.1; Protein = 0.8

🍶 Maraschino Cherries (Canned) ☞ serving size: 1 cherry (nlea serving) = 5 g; Calories = 8.3; Total Carb (g) = 2.1; Net Carb (g) = 1.9; Fat (g) = 0; Protein = 0

🍶 Medjool Dates ☞ serving size: 1 date, pitted = 24 g; Calories = 66.5; Total Carb (g) = 18; Net Carb (g) = 16.4; Fat (g) = 0; Protein = 0.4

🍶 Melon Balls ☞ serving size: 1 cup, unthawed = 173 g; Calories = 57.1; Total Carb (g) = 13.7; Net Carb (g) = 12.5; Fat (g) = 0.4; Protein = 1.5

🍶 Mulberries ☞ serving size: 1 cup = 140 g; Calories = 60.2; Total Carb (g) = 13.7; Net Carb (g) = 11.3; Fat (g) = 0.6; Protein = 2

🍶 Muscadine Grapes ☞ serving size: 1 grape = 6 g; Calories = 3.4; Total Carb (g) = 0.8; Net Carb (g) = 0.6; Fat (g) = 0; Protein = 0.1

🍶 Mushrooms Pickled ☞ serving size: 1 cup = 156 g; Calories = 32.8; Total Carb (g) = 4.5; Net Carb (g) = 3.1; Fat (g) = 0.5; Protein = 4.1

🍶 Nance Canned Syrup Drained ☞ serving size: 3 fruit without pits = 11.1 g; Calories = 10.5; Total Carb (g) = 2.5; Net Carb (g) = 1.8; Fat (g) = 0.1; Protein = 0.1

🍶 Nance Frozen Unsweetened ☞ serving size: 1 cup without pits, thawed = 112 g; Calories = 81.8; Total Carb (g) = 19; Net Carb (g) = 10.6; Fat (g) = 1.3; Protein = 0.7

🍶 Naranjilla (Lulo) Pulp Frozen Unsweetened ☞ serving size: 1 cup thawed = 120 g; Calories = 30; Total Carb (g) = 7.1; Net Carb (g) = 5.8; Fat (g) = 0.3; Protein = 0.5

🍶 Navel Oranges ☞ serving size: 1 cup sections, without

membranes = 165 g; Calories = 80.9; Total Carb (g) = 20.7; Net Carb (g) = 17.1; Fat (g) = 0.3; Protein = 1.5

Nectarine Cooked ☞ serving size: 1 cup = 262 g; Calories = 222.7; Total Carb (g) = 55.5; Net Carb (g) = 51.3; Fat (g) = 0.8; Protein = 2.6

Nectarines ☞ serving size: 1 cup slices = 143 g; Calories = 62.9; Total Carb (g) = 15.1; Net Carb (g) = 12.7; Fat (g) = 0.5; Protein = 1.5

Oheloberries ☞ serving size: 1 cup = 140 g; Calories = 39.2; Total Carb (g) = 9.6; Net Carb (g) = 9.6; Fat (g) = 0.3; Protein = 0.5

Okra Pickled ☞ serving size: 1 pod = 11 g; Calories = 3.3; Total Carb (g) = 0.7; Net Carb (g) = 0.4; Fat (g) = 0; Protein = 0.2

Olives ☞ serving size: 1 tbsp = 8.4 g; Calories = 9.7; Total Carb (g) = 0.5; Net Carb (g) = 0.4; Fat (g) = 0.9; Protein = 0.1

Olives Black ☞ serving size: 1 slice = 1 g; Calories = 1.1; Total Carb (g) = 0.1; Net Carb (g) = 0; Fat (g) = 0.1; Protein = 0

Olives Green Stuffed ☞ serving size: 1 cup = 147 g; Calories = 188.2; Total Carb (g) = 5.9; Net Carb (g) = 1.4; Fat (g) = 19.4; Protein = 1.5

Olives Nfs ☞ serving size: 1 slice = 1 g; Calories = 1.2; Total Carb (g) = 0.1; Net Carb (g) = 0; Fat (g) = 0.1; Protein = 0

Orange Juice ☞ serving size: 1 cup = 248 g; Calories = 111.6; Total Carb (g) = 25.8; Net Carb (g) = 25.3; Fat (g) = 0.5; Protein = 1.7

Orange Juice 100% Nfs ☞ serving size: 1 fl oz (no ice) = 31 g; Calories = 14.9; Total Carb (g) = 3.6; Net Carb (g) = 3.5; Fat (g) = 0; Protein = 0.2

Orange Juice Chilled Includes From Concentrate With Added Calcium And Vitamins A D E ☞ serving size: 1 cup = 249 g; Calories = 122; Total Carb (g) = 28.7; Net Carb (g) = 28; Fat (g) = 0.3; Protein = 1.7

Orange Juice From Concentrate ☞ serving size: 1 cup = 249 g;

Calories = 122; Total Carb (g) = 28.7; Net Carb (g) = 28; Fat (g) = 0.3; Protein = 1.7

🜪 Orange Juice Frozen Concentrate Unsweetened Diluted With 3 Volume Water ☞ serving size: 1 cup = 249 g; Calories = 92.1; Total Carb (g) = 21.9; Net Carb (g) = 21.4; Fat (g) = 0.2; Protein = 1.5

🜪 Orange Juice Frozen Concentrate Unsweetened Diluted With 3 Volume Water With Added Calcium ☞ serving size: 1 cup = 249 g; Calories = 92.1; Total Carb (g) = 21.1; Net Carb (g) = 20.6; Fat (g) = 0.2; Protein = 1.5

🜪 Orange Juice Frozen Concentrate Unsweetened Undiluted ☞ serving size: 1 cup = 262 g; Calories = 387.8; Total Carb (g) = 92.2; Net Carb (g) = 89.6; Fat (g) = 0.7; Protein = 6.3

🜪 Orange Juice Frozen Concentrate Unsweetened Undiluted With Added Calcium ☞ serving size: 1 cup = 262 g; Calories = 385.1; Total Carb (g) = 88.7; Net Carb (g) = 86.1; Fat (g) = 0.7; Protein = 6.3

🜪 Orange Juice With Added Calcium ☞ serving size: 1 cup = 249 g; Calories = 117; Total Carb (g) = 28.1; Net Carb (g) = 27.3; Fat (g) = 0.3; Protein = 1.7

🜪 Orange Juice With Added Calcium And Vitamin D ☞ serving size: 1 cup = 249 g; Calories = 117; Total Carb (g) = 28.1; Net Carb (g) = 27.3; Fat (g) = 0.3; Protein = 1.7

🜪 Orange Peel Raw ☞ serving size: 1 tbsp = 6 g; Calories = 5.8; Total Carb (g) = 1.5; Net Carb (g) = 0.9; Fat (g) = 0; Protein = 0.1

🜪 Orange Pineapple Juice Blend ☞ serving size: 8 fl oz = 246 g; Calories = 125.5; Total Carb (g) = 30; Net Carb (g) = 29.5; Fat (g) = 0.2; Protein = 1

🜪 Orange Sections Canned Juice Pack ☞ serving size: 1 cup = 204 g; Calories = 95.9; Total Carb (g) = 23.5; Net Carb (g) = 20; Fat (g) = 0.3; Protein = 1.7

🜪 Orange-Grapefruit Juice Canned Or Bottled Unsweetened ☞

serving size: 1 cup = 247 g; Calories = 106.2; Total Carb (g) = 25.4; Net Carb (g) = 25.1; Fat (g) = 0.3; Protein = 1.5

Oranges ☞ serving size: 1 cup, sections = 180 g; Calories = 84.6; Total Carb (g) = 21.2; Net Carb (g) = 16.8; Fat (g) = 0.2; Protein = 1.7

Oranges Raw With Peel ☞ serving size: 1 cup = 170 g; Calories = 107.1; Total Carb (g) = 26.4; Net Carb (g) = 18.7; Fat (g) = 0.5; Protein = 2.2

Papaya ☞ serving size: 1 cup 1 inch pieces = 145 g; Calories = 62.4; Total Carb (g) = 15.7; Net Carb (g) = 13.2; Fat (g) = 0.4; Protein = 0.7

Papaya Canned Heavy Syrup Drained ☞ serving size: 1 piece = 39 g; Calories = 80.3; Total Carb (g) = 21.8; Net Carb (g) = 21.2; Fat (g) = 0.2; Protein = 0.1

Papaya Cooked Or Canned In Sugar Or Syrup ☞ serving size: 1 cup = 244 g; Calories = 192.8; Total Carb (g) = 49.4; Net Carb (g) = 46.7; Fat (g) = 0.4; Protein = 0.8

Papaya Dried ☞ serving size: 1 strip = 23 g; Calories = 68.1; Total Carb (g) = 17.4; Net Carb (g) = 16.1; Fat (g) = 0.2; Protein = 0.4

Papaya Green Cooked ☞ serving size: 1 cup = 244 g; Calories = 104.9; Total Carb (g) = 26.4; Net Carb (g) = 22.3; Fat (g) = 0.6; Protein = 1.2

Papaya Nectar Canned ☞ serving size: 1 cup = 250 g; Calories = 142.5; Total Carb (g) = 36.3; Net Carb (g) = 34.8; Fat (g) = 0.4; Protein = 0.4

Passion Fruit (Granadilla) ☞ serving size: 1 cup = 236 g; Calories = 228.9; Total Carb (g) = 55.2; Net Carb (g) = 30.6; Fat (g) = 1.7; Protein = 5.2

Peach Dried Cooked Ns As To Sweetened Or Unsweetened; Sweetened Ns As To Type Of Sweetener ☞ serving size: 1 cup = 258 g; Calories = 283.8; Total Carb (g) = 73; Net Carb (g) = 66.8; Fat (g) = 0.6; Protein = 2.7

Peach Dried Cooked With Sugar ☞ serving size: 1 cup = 270 g; Calories = 297; Total Carb (g) = 76.4; Net Carb (g) = 69.9; Fat (g) = 0.6; Protein = 2.8

Peach Nectar Canned With Added Ascorbic Acid ☞ serving size: 1 cup = 249 g; Calories = 124.5; Total Carb (g) = 29.7; Net Carb (g) = 29.5; Fat (g) = 1.3; Protein = 0.5

Peach Nectar Canned Without Added Ascorbic Acid ☞ serving size: 1 cup = 249 g; Calories = 122; Total Carb (g) = 28.9; Net Carb (g) = 28.7; Fat (g) = 1.4; Protein = 0.3

Peach Pickled ☞ serving size: 1 fruit = 88 g; Calories = 103.8; Total Carb (g) = 25.7; Net Carb (g) = 24.8; Fat (g) = 0.2; Protein = 0.6

Peaches Canned Extra Heavy Syrup Pack Solids And Liquids ☞ serving size: 1 cup, halves or slices = 262 g; Calories = 251.5; Total Carb (g) = 68.3; Net Carb (g) = 65.7; Fat (g) = 0.1; Protein = 1.2

Peaches Canned Extra Light Syrup Solids And Liquids ☞ serving size: 1 cup, halves or slices = 247 g; Calories = 103.7; Total Carb (g) = 27.4; Net Carb (g) = 25; Fat (g) = 0.3; Protein = 1

Peaches Canned Heavy Syrup Drained ☞ serving size: 1 cup = 222 g; Calories = 159.8; Total Carb (g) = 40.9; Net Carb (g) = 38.3; Fat (g) = 0.4; Protein = 1.2

Peaches Canned Heavy Syrup Pack Solids And Liquids ☞ serving size: 1 cup = 262 g; Calories = 193.9; Total Carb (g) = 52.2; Net Carb (g) = 48.8; Fat (g) = 0.3; Protein = 1.2

Peaches Canned Juice Pack Solids And Liquids ☞ serving size: 1 cup = 250 g; Calories = 110; Total Carb (g) = 28.9; Net Carb (g) = 25.7; Fat (g) = 0.1; Protein = 1.6

Peaches Canned Light Syrup Pack Solids And Liquids ☞ serving size: 1 cup, halves or slices = 251 g; Calories = 135.5; Total Carb (g) = 36.5; Net Carb (g) = 33.3; Fat (g) = 0.1; Protein = 1.1

Peaches Canned Water Pack Solids And Liquids ☞ serving size:

1 cup, halves or slices = 244 g; Calories = 58.6; Total Carb (g) = 14.9; Net Carb (g) = 11.7; Fat (g) = 0.2; Protein = 1.1

Peaches Dehydrated (Low-Moisture) Sulfured Stewed ☞ serving size: 1 cup = 242 g; Calories = 321.9; Total Carb (g) = 82.6; Net Carb (g) = 82.6; Fat (g) = 1; Protein = 4.9

Peaches Dried Sulfured Stewed With Added Sugar ☞ serving size: 1 cup = 270 g; Calories = 278.1; Total Carb (g) = 71.8; Net Carb (g) = 65.3; Fat (g) = 0.6; Protein = 2.9

Peaches Dried Sulfured Stewed Without Added Sugar ☞ serving size: 1 cup = 258 g; Calories = 198.7; Total Carb (g) = 50.8; Net Carb (g) = 43.8; Fat (g) = 0.7; Protein = 3

Peaches Frozen Sliced Sweetened ☞ serving size: 1 cup, thawed = 250 g; Calories = 235; Total Carb (g) = 60; Net Carb (g) = 55.5; Fat (g) = 0.3; Protein = 1.6

Peaches Spiced Canned Heavy Syrup Pack Solids And Liquids ☞ serving size: 1 cup, whole = 242 g; Calories = 181.5; Total Carb (g) = 48.6; Net Carb (g) = 45.5; Fat (g) = 0.2; Protein = 1

Pear Dried Cooked Ns As To Sweetened Or Unsweetened; Sweetened Ns As To Type Of Sweetener ☞ serving size: 1 cup = 255 g; Calories = 395.3; Total Carb (g) = 104.3; Net Carb (g) = 89.8; Fat (g) = 0.7; Protein = 2.1

Pear Dried Cooked With Sugar ☞ serving size: 1 cup = 280 g; Calories = 434; Total Carb (g) = 114.5; Net Carb (g) = 98.6; Fat (g) = 0.8; Protein = 2.3

Pear Nectar Canned With Added Ascorbic Acid ☞ serving size: 1 cup = 250 g; Calories = 150; Total Carb (g) = 39.4; Net Carb (g) = 37.9; Fat (g) = 0; Protein = 0.3

Pear Nectar Canned Without Added Ascorbic Acid ☞ serving size: 1 cup = 250 g; Calories = 150; Total Carb (g) = 39.4; Net Carb (g) = 37.9; Fat (g) = 0; Protein = 0.3

🍐 Pears ☞ serving size: 1 cup, slices = 140 g; Calories = 79.8; Total Carb (g) = 21.3; Net Carb (g) = 17; Fat (g) = 0.2; Protein = 0.5

🍐 Pears Canned Extra Light Syrup Pack Solids And Liquids ☞ serving size: 1 cup, halves = 247 g; Calories = 116.1; Total Carb (g) = 30.1; Net Carb (g) = 26.2; Fat (g) = 0.3; Protein = 0.7

🍐 Pears Canned Heavy Syrup Drained ☞ serving size: 1 cup = 201 g; Calories = 148.7; Total Carb (g) = 38.4; Net Carb (g) = 32.9; Fat (g) = 0.4; Protein = 0.5

🍐 Pears Canned Heavy Syrup Pack Solids And Liquids ☞ serving size: 1 cup = 266 g; Calories = 196.8; Total Carb (g) = 51; Net Carb (g) = 46.7; Fat (g) = 0.4; Protein = 0.5

🍐 Pears Canned In Syrup ☞ serving size: 1 cup, halves = 266 g; Calories = 258; Total Carb (g) = 67.2; Net Carb (g) = 62.9; Fat (g) = 0.4; Protein = 0.5

🍐 Pears Canned Juice Pack Solids And Liquids ☞ serving size: 1 cup, halves = 248 g; Calories = 124; Total Carb (g) = 32.1; Net Carb (g) = 28.1; Fat (g) = 0.2; Protein = 0.8

🍐 Pears Canned Light Syrup Pack Solids And Liquids ☞ serving size: 1 cup, halves = 251 g; Calories = 143.1; Total Carb (g) = 38.1; Net Carb (g) = 34.1; Fat (g) = 0.1; Protein = 0.5

🍐 Pears Canned Water Pack Solids And Liquids ☞ serving size: 1 cup, halves = 244 g; Calories = 70.8; Total Carb (g) = 19.1; Net Carb (g) = 15.2; Fat (g) = 0.1; Protein = 0.5

🍐 Pears Dried Sulfured Stewed With Added Sugar ☞ serving size: 1 cup, halves = 280 g; Calories = 392; Total Carb (g) = 104; Net Carb (g) = 87.8; Fat (g) = 0.8; Protein = 2.4

🍐 Pears Dried Sulfured Stewed Without Added Sugar ☞ serving size: 1 cup, halves = 255 g; Calories = 323.9; Total Carb (g) = 86.2; Net Carb (g) = 69.9; Fat (g) = 0.8; Protein = 2.3

🌑 Peppers Pickled ☞ serving size: 1 cup = 135 g; Calories = 54; Total Carb (g) = 12.2; Net Carb (g) = 10; Fat (g) = 0.3; Protein = 1.1

🌑 Persimmons Japanese Dried ☞ serving size: 1 fruit without refuse = 34 g; Calories = 93.2; Total Carb (g) = 25; Net Carb (g) = 20; Fat (g) = 0.2; Protein = 0.5

🌑 Persimmons Native Raw ☞ serving size: 1 fruit without refuse = 25 g; Calories = 31.8; Total Carb (g) = 8.4; Net Carb (g) = 8.4; Fat (g) = 0.1; Protein = 0.2

🌑 Pickled Green Bananas Puerto Rican Style ☞ serving size: 1 cup = 150 g; Calories = 480; Total Carb (g) = 22.6; Net Carb (g) = 19.9; Fat (g) = 44.3; Protein = 1.4

🌑 Pineapple ☞ serving size: 1 cup, chunks = 165 g; Calories = 82.5; Total Carb (g) = 21.7; Net Carb (g) = 19.3; Fat (g) = 0.2; Protein = 0.9

🌑 Pineapple (Traditional) ☞ serving size: 1 cup, chunks = 165 g; Calories = 74.3; Total Carb (g) = 19.5; Net Carb (g) = 19.5; Fat (g) = 0.2; Protein = 0.9

🌑 Pineapple Canned Extra Heavy Syrup Pack Solids And Liquids ☞ serving size: 1 cup, crushed, sliced, or chunks = 260 g; Calories = 215.8; Total Carb (g) = 55.9; Net Carb (g) = 53.8; Fat (g) = 0.3; Protein = 0.9

🌑 Pineapple Canned Heavy Syrup Pack Solids And Liquids ☞ serving size: 1 cup, crushed, sliced, or chunks = 254 g; Calories = 198.1; Total Carb (g) = 51.3; Net Carb (g) = 49.3; Fat (g) = 0.3; Protein = 0.9

🌑 Pineapple Canned Juice Pack Drained ☞ serving size: 1 cup, chunks = 181 g; Calories = 108.6; Total Carb (g) = 28.2; Net Carb (g) = 25.8; Fat (g) = 0.2; Protein = 0.9

🌑 Pineapple Canned Juice Pack Solids And Liquids ☞ serving size: 1 cup, crushed, sliced, or chunks = 249 g; Calories = 149.4; Total Carb (g) = 39.1; Net Carb (g) = 37.1; Fat (g) = 0.2; Protein = 1.1

Pineapple Canned Light Syrup Pack Solids And Liquids ☞ serving size: 1 cup, crushed, sliced, or chunks = 252 g; Calories = 131; Total Carb (g) = 33.9; Net Carb (g) = 31.9; Fat (g) = 0.3; Protein = 0.9

Pineapple Canned Water Pack Solids And Liquids ☞ serving size: 1 cup, crushed, sliced, or chunks = 246 g; Calories = 78.7; Total Carb (g) = 20.4; Net Carb (g) = 18.5; Fat (g) = 0.2; Protein = 1.1

Pineapple Dried ☞ serving size: 1 piece = 28 g; Calories = 75.3; Total Carb (g) = 19.6; Net Carb (g) = 18.5; Fat (g) = 0.1; Protein = 0.4

Pineapple Frozen Chunks Sweetened ☞ serving size: 1 cup, chunks = 245 g; Calories = 210.7; Total Carb (g) = 54.4; Net Carb (g) = 51.7; Fat (g) = 0.3; Protein = 1

Pineapple Juice Canned Not From Concentrate Unsweetened With Added Vitamins A C And E ☞ serving size: 1 cup = 250 g; Calories = 125; Total Carb (g) = 30.5; Net Carb (g) = 30; Fat (g) = 0.4; Protein = 0.9

Pineapple Juice Canned Or Bottled Unsweetened With Added Ascorbic Acid ☞ serving size: 1 cup = 250 g; Calories = 132.5; Total Carb (g) = 32.2; Net Carb (g) = 31.7; Fat (g) = 0.3; Protein = 0.9

Pineapple Juice Canned Or Bottled Unsweetened Without Added Ascorbic Acid ☞ serving size: 1 cup = 250 g; Calories = 132.5; Total Carb (g) = 32.2; Net Carb (g) = 31.7; Fat (g) = 0.3; Protein = 0.9

Pineapple Juice Frozen Concentrate Unsweetened Diluted With 3 Volume Water ☞ serving size: 1 cup = 250 g; Calories = 127.5; Total Carb (g) = 31.7; Net Carb (g) = 31.2; Fat (g) = 0.1; Protein = 1

Pineapple Juice Frozen Concentrate Unsweetened Undiluted ☞ serving size: 1 can (6 fl oz) = 216 g; Calories = 386.6; Total Carb (g) = 95.7; Net Carb (g) = 94.2; Fat (g) = 0.2; Protein = 2.8

Pineapple Raw Extra Sweet Variety ☞ serving size: 1 cup, chunks = 165 g; Calories = 84.2; Total Carb (g) = 22.3; Net Carb (g) = 20; Fat (g) = 0.2; Protein = 0.9

Pineapple Salad With Dressing ☞ serving size: 1 serving (lettuce, 1 cup diced pineapple, dressing) = 184 g; Calories = 176.6; Total Carb (g) = 21.9; Net Carb (g) = 19.5; Fat (g) = 10.5; Protein = 1.1

Pink Grapefruit ☞ serving size: 1 cup sections, with juice = 230 g; Calories = 96.6; Total Carb (g) = 24.5; Net Carb (g) = 20.8; Fat (g) = 0.3; Protein = 1.8

Pink Grapefruit Juice ☞ serving size: 1 cup = 247 g; Calories = 96.3; Total Carb (g) = 22.7; Net Carb (g) = 22.7; Fat (g) = 0.3; Protein = 1.2

Pitanga ☞ serving size: 1 cup = 173 g; Calories = 57.1; Total Carb (g) = 13; Net Carb (g) = 13; Fat (g) = 0.7; Protein = 1.4

Plantains ☞ serving size: 1 cup, sliced = 148 g; Calories = 180.6; Total Carb (g) = 47.2; Net Carb (g) = 44.7; Fat (g) = 0.5; Protein = 1.9

Plantains Cooked ☞ serving size: 1 cup, mashed = 200 g; Calories = 310; Total Carb (g) = 82.7; Net Carb (g) = 78.3; Fat (g) = 0.3; Protein = 3

Plantains Green Fried ☞ serving size: 1 cup = 118 g; Calories = 364.6; Total Carb (g) = 58; Net Carb (g) = 53.9; Fat (g) = 13.9; Protein = 1.8

Plum Pickled ☞ serving size: 1 plum = 28 g; Calories = 34.4; Total Carb (g) = 8.6; Net Carb (g) = 8.3; Fat (g) = 0.1; Protein = 0.1

Plums ☞ serving size: 1 cup, sliced = 165 g; Calories = 75.9; Total Carb (g) = 18.8; Net Carb (g) = 16.5; Fat (g) = 0.5; Protein = 1.2

Plums Canned Heavy Syrup Drained ☞ serving size: 1 cup, with pits, yields = 183 g; Calories = 162.9; Total Carb (g) = 42.3; Net Carb (g) = 39.6; Fat (g) = 0.3; Protein = 0.8

Plums Canned Purple Extra Heavy Syrup Pack Solids And Liquids ☞ serving size: 1 cup, pitted = 261 g; Calories = 263.6; Total Carb (g) = 68.7; Net Carb (g) = 66.1; Fat (g) = 0.3; Protein = 0.9

🫐 Plums Canned Purple Heavy Syrup Pack Solids And Liquids ☞ serving size: 1 cup, pitted = 258 g; Calories = 229.6; Total Carb (g) = 60; Net Carb (g) = 57.6; Fat (g) = 0.3; Protein = 0.9

🫐 Plums Canned Purple Juice Pack Solids And Liquids ☞ serving size: 1 cup, pitted = 252 g; Calories = 146.2; Total Carb (g) = 38.2; Net Carb (g) = 35.9; Fat (g) = 0.1; Protein = 1.3

🫐 Plums Canned Purple Light Syrup Pack Solids And Liquids ☞ serving size: 1 cup, pitted = 252 g; Calories = 158.8; Total Carb (g) = 41; Net Carb (g) = 38.8; Fat (g) = 0.3; Protein = 0.9

🫐 Plums Canned Purple Water Pack Solids And Liquids ☞ serving size: 1 cup, pitted = 249 g; Calories = 102.1; Total Carb (g) = 27.5; Net Carb (g) = 25.2; Fat (g) = 0; Protein = 1

🫐 Plums Dried (Prunes) Stewed With Added Sugar ☞ serving size: 1 cup, pitted = 248 g; Calories = 307.5; Total Carb (g) = 81.5; Net Carb (g) = 72.1; Fat (g) = 0.6; Protein = 2.7

🫐 Plums Dried (Prunes) Stewed Without Added Sugar ☞ serving size: 1 cup, pitted = 248 g; Calories = 265.4; Total Carb (g) = 69.6; Net Carb (g) = 62; Fat (g) = 0.4; Protein = 2.4

🫐 Pomegranate Juice Bottled ☞ serving size: 1 cup = 249 g; Calories = 134.5; Total Carb (g) = 32.7; Net Carb (g) = 32.4; Fat (g) = 0.7; Protein = 0.4

🫐 Pomegranates ☞ serving size: 1/2 cup arils (seed/juice sacs) = 87 g; Calories = 72.2; Total Carb (g) = 16.3; Net Carb (g) = 12.8; Fat (g) = 1; Protein = 1.5

🫐 Prickly Pears ☞ serving size: 1 cup = 149 g; Calories = 61.1; Total Carb (g) = 14.3; Net Carb (g) = 8.9; Fat (g) = 0.8; Protein = 1.1

🫐 Prune Dried Cooked Ns As To Sweetened Or Unsweetened; Sweetened Ns As To Type Of Sweetener ☞ serving size: 1 prune = 10 g; Calories = 13.7; Total Carb (g) = 3.6; Net Carb (g) = 3.3; Fat (g) = 0; Protein = 0.1

🫐 Prune Dried Cooked With Sugar ☞ serving size: 1 prune = 10 g; Calories = 13.7; Total Carb (g) = 3.6; Net Carb (g) = 3.3; Fat (g) = 0; Protein = 0.1

🫐 Prune Puree ☞ serving size: 2 tbsp = 36 g; Calories = 92.5; Total Carb (g) = 23.4; Net Carb (g) = 22.3; Fat (g) = 0.1; Protein = 0.8

🫐 Prune Whip ☞ serving size: 1 cup = 130 g; Calories = 191.1; Total Carb (g) = 43.9; Net Carb (g) = 41.2; Fat (g) = 0.3; Protein = 6.1

🫐 Prunes (Dried Plums) ☞ serving size: 1 cup, pitted = 174 g; Calories = 417.6; Total Carb (g) = 111.2; Net Carb (g) = 98.8; Fat (g) = 0.7; Protein = 3.8

🫐 Prunes (Low-Moisture) ☞ serving size: 1 cup = 132 g; Calories = 447.5; Total Carb (g) = 117.6; Net Carb (g) = 117.6; Fat (g) = 1; Protein = 4.9

🫐 Prunes Canned Heavy Syrup Pack Solids And Liquids ☞ serving size: 1 cup = 234 g; Calories = 245.7; Total Carb (g) = 65.1; Net Carb (g) = 56.2; Fat (g) = 0.5; Protein = 2

🫐 Prunes Dehydrated (Low-Moisture) Stewed ☞ serving size: 1 cup = 280 g; Calories = 316.4; Total Carb (g) = 83.2; Net Carb (g) = 83.2; Fat (g) = 0.7; Protein = 3.4

🫐 Pummelo ☞ serving size: 1 cup, sections = 190 g; Calories = 72.2; Total Carb (g) = 18.3; Net Carb (g) = 16.4; Fat (g) = 0.1; Protein = 1.4

🫐 Purple Passion Fruit Juice ☞ serving size: 1 cup = 247 g; Calories = 126; Total Carb (g) = 33.6; Net Carb (g) = 33.1; Fat (g) = 0.1; Protein = 1

🫐 Quinces ☞ serving size: 1 fruit without refuse = 92 g; Calories = 52.4; Total Carb (g) = 14.1; Net Carb (g) = 12.3; Fat (g) = 0.1; Protein = 0.4

🫐 Raisins ☞ serving size: 1 cup, packed = 165 g; Calories = 493.4; Total Carb (g) = 130.9; Net Carb (g) = 123.5; Fat (g) = 0.4; Protein = 5.5

🫐 Raisins Cooked ☞ serving size: 1 cup = 295 g; Calories = 646.1; Total Carb (g) = 169.3; Net Carb (g) = 164.3; Fat (g) = 0.6; Protein = 4.2

🫐 Raisins Seeded ☞ serving size: 1 cup, packed = 165 g; Calories = 488.4; Total Carb (g) = 129.5; Net Carb (g) = 118.3; Fat (g) = 0.9; Protein = 4.2

🫐 Rambutan Canned Syrup Pack ☞ serving size: 1 cup, drained = 150 g; Calories = 123; Total Carb (g) = 31.3; Net Carb (g) = 30; Fat (g) = 0.3; Protein = 1

🫐 Raspberries ☞ serving size: 1 cup = 123 g; Calories = 64; Total Carb (g) = 14.7; Net Carb (g) = 6.7; Fat (g) = 0.8; Protein = 1.5

🫐 Raspberries Canned Red Heavy Syrup Pack Solids And Liquids ☞ serving size: 1 cup = 256 g; Calories = 233; Total Carb (g) = 59.8; Net Carb (g) = 51.4; Fat (g) = 0.3; Protein = 2.1

🫐 Raspberries Cooked Or Canned Unsweetened Water Pack ☞ serving size: 1 cup = 243 g; Calories = 85.1; Total Carb (g) = 19.4; Net Carb (g) = 8.8; Fat (g) = 1.1; Protein = 1.9

🫐 Raspberries Frozen Red Sweetened ☞ serving size: 1 cup, thawed = 250 g; Calories = 257.5; Total Carb (g) = 65.4; Net Carb (g) = 54.4; Fat (g) = 0.4; Protein = 1.8

🫐 Raspberries Frozen Unsweetened ☞ serving size: 1 cup = 250 g; Calories = 130; Total Carb (g) = 29.9; Net Carb (g) = 13.6; Fat (g) = 1.6; Protein = 3

🫐 Red And White Currants ☞ serving size: 1 cup = 112 g; Calories = 62.7; Total Carb (g) = 15.5; Net Carb (g) = 10.6; Fat (g) = 0.2; Protein = 1.6

🫐 Red Anjou Pears ☞ serving size: 1 small = 126 g; Calories = 78.1; Total Carb (g) = 18.8; Net Carb (g) = 15; Fat (g) = 0.2; Protein = 0.4

🫐 Red Delicious Apples ☞ serving size: 1 cup, sliced = 109 g; Calories = 64.3; Total Carb (g) = 15.3; Net Carb (g) = 12.8; Fat (g) = 0.2; Protein = 0.3

Red Or Green Grapes (European) ☞ serving size: 1 cup = 151 g; Calories = 104.2; Total Carb (g) = 27.3; Net Carb (g) = 26; Fat (g) = 0.2; Protein = 1.1

Rhubarb ☞ serving size: 1 cup, diced = 122 g; Calories = 25.6; Total Carb (g) = 5.5; Net Carb (g) = 3.3; Fat (g) = 0.2; Protein = 1.1

Rhubarb Cooked Or Canned Drained Solids ☞ serving size: 1 cup = 240 g; Calories = 278.4; Total Carb (g) = 74.9; Net Carb (g) = 70.1; Fat (g) = 0.1; Protein = 0.9

Rhubarb Cooked Or Canned In Light Syrup ☞ serving size: 1 cup = 240 g; Calories = 144; Total Carb (g) = 36.7; Net Carb (g) = 32.8; Fat (g) = 0.2; Protein = 1.2

Rhubarb Cooked Or Canned Unsweetened ☞ serving size: 1 cup = 240 g; Calories = 50.4; Total Carb (g) = 10.9; Net Carb (g) = 6.6; Fat (g) = 0.5; Protein = 2.2

Rhubarb Frozen Cooked With Sugar ☞ serving size: 1 cup = 240 g; Calories = 278.4; Total Carb (g) = 74.9; Net Carb (g) = 70.1; Fat (g) = 0.1; Protein = 0.9

Rhubarb Frozen Uncooked ☞ serving size: 1 cup, diced = 137 g; Calories = 28.8; Total Carb (g) = 7; Net Carb (g) = 4.5; Fat (g) = 0.2; Protein = 0.8

Roselle ☞ serving size: 1 cup, without refuse = 57 g; Calories = 27.9; Total Carb (g) = 6.5; Net Carb (g) = 6.5; Fat (g) = 0.4; Protein = 0.6

Rowal ☞ serving size: 1/2 cup = 114 g; Calories = 126.5; Total Carb (g) = 27.3; Net Carb (g) = 20.2; Fat (g) = 2.3; Protein = 2.6

Ruby Red Grapefruit Juice Blend (Grapefruit Grape Apple) Ocean Spray Bottled With Added Vitamin C ☞ serving size: 8 fl oz = 248 g; Calories = 109.1; Total Carb (g) = 26.1; Net Carb (g) = 25.6; Fat (g) = 0.3; Protein = 1.2

Sapodilla ☞ serving size: 1 cup, pulp = 241 g; Calories = 200; Total Carb (g) = 48.1; Net Carb (g) = 35.3; Fat (g) = 2.7; Protein = 1.1

Sauerkraut Cooked Fat Added In Cooking ☞ serving size: 1 cup = 147 g; Calories = 45.6; Total Carb (g) = 6.2; Net Carb (g) = 2.1; Fat (g) = 2.3; Protein = 1.3

Sauerkraut Cooked Ns As To Fat Added In Cooking ☞ serving size: 1 cup = 142 g; Calories = 55.4; Total Carb (g) = 5.9; Net Carb (g) = 1.9; Fat (g) = 3.5; Protein = 1.3

Seaweed Pickled ☞ serving size: 1 cup = 150 g; Calories = 234; Total Carb (g) = 56.4; Net Carb (g) = 55.9; Fat (g) = 0.3; Protein = 2

Shredded Coconut Meat (Sweetened) ☞ serving size: 1 cup = 256 g; Calories = 181.8; Total Carb (g) = 44.7; Net Carb (g) = 42.1; Fat (g) = 0.1; Protein = 1.6

Sour Red Cherries ☞ serving size: 1 cup, without pits = 155 g; Calories = 77.5; Total Carb (g) = 18.9; Net Carb (g) = 16.4; Fat (g) = 0.5; Protein = 1.6

Sour Red Cherries (Frozen) ☞ serving size: 1 cup, unthawed = 155 g; Calories = 71.3; Total Carb (g) = 17.1; Net Carb (g) = 14.6; Fat (g) = 0.7; Protein = 1.4

Soursop ☞ serving size: 1 cup, pulp = 225 g; Calories = 148.5; Total Carb (g) = 37.9; Net Carb (g) = 30.5; Fat (g) = 0.7; Protein = 2.3

Starfruit (Carambola) ☞ serving size: 1 cup, cubes = 132 g; Calories = 40.9; Total Carb (g) = 8.9; Net Carb (g) = 5.2; Fat (g) = 0.4; Protein = 1.4

Starfruit Cooked With Sugar ☞ serving size: 1 cup = 205 g; Calories = 141.5; Total Carb (g) = 34.3; Net Carb (g) = 29.2; Fat (g) = 0.6; Protein = 1.9

Strawberries ☞ serving size: 1 cup, halves = 152 g; Calories = 48.6; Total Carb (g) = 11.7; Net Carb (g) = 8.6; Fat (g) = 0.5; Protein = 1

Strawberries Canned Heavy Syrup Pack Solids And Liquids ☞ serving size: 1 cup = 254 g; Calories = 233.7; Total Carb (g) = 59.8; Net Carb (g) = 55.5; Fat (g) = 0.7; Protein = 1.4

🍓 Strawberries Cooked Or Canned Unsweetened Water Pack ☞ serving size: 1 cup = 242 g; Calories = 50.8; Total Carb (g) = 12.5; Net Carb (g) = 9.3; Fat (g) = 0.5; Protein = 1.1

🍓 Strawberries Frozen Sweetened Sliced ☞ serving size: 1 cup, thawed = 255 g; Calories = 244.8; Total Carb (g) = 66.1; Net Carb (g) = 61.3; Fat (g) = 0.3; Protein = 1.4

🍓 Strawberries Raw With Sugar ☞ serving size: 1 cup, nfs = 160 g; Calories = 80; Total Carb (g) = 19.7; Net Carb (g) = 16.6; Fat (g) = 0.5; Protein = 1

🍓 Strawberry Guavas ☞ serving size: 1 cup = 244 g; Calories = 168.4; Total Carb (g) = 42.4; Net Carb (g) = 29.2; Fat (g) = 1.5; Protein = 1.4

🍏 Sugar Apples ☞ serving size: 1 cup, pulp = 250 g; Calories = 235; Total Carb (g) = 59.1; Net Carb (g) = 48.1; Fat (g) = 0.7; Protein = 5.2

🍈 Tamarind Nectar Canned ☞ serving size: 1 cup = 251 g; Calories = 143.1; Total Carb (g) = 37; Net Carb (g) = 35.7; Fat (g) = 0.3; Protein = 0.2

🍈 Tamarinds ☞ serving size: 1 cup, pulp = 120 g; Calories = 286.8; Total Carb (g) = 75; Net Carb (g) = 68.9; Fat (g) = 0.7; Protein = 3.4

🍊 Tangerine Juice ☞ serving size: 1 cup = 247 g; Calories = 106.2; Total Carb (g) = 25; Net Carb (g) = 24.5; Fat (g) = 0.5; Protein = 1.2

🍊 Tangerines ☞ serving size: 1 cup, sections = 195 g; Calories = 103.4; Total Carb (g) = 26; Net Carb (g) = 22.5; Fat (g) = 0.6; Protein = 1.6

🍊 Tangerines (Mandarin Oranges) Canned Juice Pack ☞ serving size: 1 cup = 249 g; Calories = 92.1; Total Carb (g) = 23.8; Net Carb (g) = 22.1; Fat (g) = 0.1; Protein = 1.5

🍊 Tangerines (Mandarin Oranges) Canned Juice Pack Drained ☞ serving size: 1 cup = 189 g; Calories = 71.8; Total Carb (g) = 17.8; Net Carb (g) = 15.5; Fat (g) = 0.1; Protein = 1.4

🫐 Tangerines (Mandarin Oranges) Canned Light Syrup Pack ☞ serving size: 1 cup = 252 g; Calories = 153.7; Total Carb (g) = 40.8; Net Carb (g) = 39; Fat (g) = 0.3; Protein = 1.1

🫐 Tomato Green Pickled ☞ serving size: 1 tomato (2-3/8" dia) = 74 g; Calories = 26.6; Total Carb (g) = 6.1; Net Carb (g) = 5.3; Fat (g) = 0.2; Protein = 0.8

🫐 Tsukemono Japanese Pickles ☞ serving size: 1 cup = 135 g; Calories = 39.2; Total Carb (g) = 7.3; Net Carb (g) = 3.8; Fat (g) = 0.3; Protein = 1.8

🫐 Turnip Pickled ☞ serving size: 1 cup = 155 g; Calories = 66.7; Total Carb (g) = 15.4; Net Carb (g) = 12.9; Fat (g) = 0.2; Protein = 1.3

🫐 Vegetable Relish ☞ serving size: 1 cup = 140 g; Calories = 50.4; Total Carb (g) = 12.1; Net Carb (g) = 11.1; Fat (g) = 0.2; Protein = 1

🫐 Vegetables Pickled ☞ serving size: 1 cup = 163 g; Calories = 44; Total Carb (g) = 9.1; Net Carb (g) = 6.1; Fat (g) = 0.3; Protein = 1.7

🫐 Vegetables Pickled Hawaiian Style ☞ serving size: 1 cup = 150 g; Calories = 52.5; Total Carb (g) = 10.3; Net Carb (g) = 6.4; Fat (g) = 0.6; Protein = 1.6

🫐 Watermelon ☞ serving size: 1 cup, balls = 154 g; Calories = 46.2; Total Carb (g) = 11.6; Net Carb (g) = 11; Fat (g) = 0.2; Protein = 0.9

🫐 White California Grapefruit ☞ serving size: 1 cup sections, with juice = 230 g; Calories = 85.1; Total Carb (g) = 20.9; Net Carb (g) = 20.9; Fat (g) = 0.2; Protein = 2

🫐 White Florida Grapefruit ☞ serving size: 1 cup sections, with juice = 230 g; Calories = 73.6; Total Carb (g) = 18.8; Net Carb (g) = 18.8; Fat (g) = 0.2; Protein = 1.5

🫐 White Grapefruit ☞ serving size: 1 cup sections, with juice = 230 g; Calories = 75.9; Total Carb (g) = 19.3; Net Carb (g) = 16.8; Fat (g) = 0.2; Protein = 1.6

🔵 White Grapefruit Juice ☞ serving size: 1 cup = 247 g; Calories = 96.3; Total Carb (g) = 22.7; Net Carb (g) = 22.5; Fat (g) = 0.3; Protein = 1.2

🔵 Wild Blueberries (Frozen) ☞ serving size: 1 cup, frozen = 140 g; Calories = 79.8; Total Carb (g) = 19.4; Net Carb (g) = 13.2; Fat (g) = 0.2; Protein = 0

🔵 Yellow Passion Fruit Juice ☞ serving size: 1 cup = 247 g; Calories = 148.2; Total Carb (g) = 35.7; Net Carb (g) = 35.2; Fat (g) = 0.4; Protein = 1.7

🔵 Yellow Peaches ☞ serving size: 1 cup slices = 154 g; Calories = 60.1; Total Carb (g) = 14.7; Net Carb (g) = 12.4; Fat (g) = 0.4; Protein = 1.4

🔵 Zante Currants ☞ serving size: 1 cup = 144 g; Calories = 417.6; Total Carb (g) = 110.9; Net Carb (g) = 104.5; Fat (g) = 0.3; Protein = 4.9

🔵 Zucchini Pickled ☞ serving size: 1 cup = 170 g; Calories = 64.6; Total Carb (g) = 14; Net Carb (g) = 12.2; Fat (g) = 0.5; Protein = 1.8

20

GRAINS AND PASTA

🕷 Amaranth Grain Uncooked ☞ serving size: 1 cup = 193 g; Calories = 716; Total Carb (g) = 125.9; Net Carb (g) = 113; Fat (g) = 13.6; Protein = 26.2

🕷 Arrowroot Flour ☞ serving size: 1 cup = 128 g; Calories = 457; Total Carb (g) = 112.8; Net Carb (g) = 108.5; Fat (g) = 0.1; Protein = 0.4

🕷 Barley Ns As To Fat Added In Cooking ☞ serving size: 1 cup, cooked = 170 g; Calories = 207.4; Total Carb (g) = 47.8; Net Carb (g) = 41.3; Fat (g) = 0.8; Protein = 3.8

🕷 Barley Pearled Raw ☞ serving size: 1 cup = 200 g; Calories = 704; Total Carb (g) = 155.4; Net Carb (g) = 124.2; Fat (g) = 2.3; Protein = 19.8

🕷 Brown Rice ☞ serving size: 1 cup = 202 g; Calories = 248.5; Total Carb (g) = 51.7; Net Carb (g) = 48.4; Fat (g) = 2; Protein = 5.5

🕷 Buckwheat (Uncooked) ☞ serving size: 1 cup = 170 g; Calories = 583.1; Total Carb (g) = 121.6; Net Carb (g) = 104.6; Fat (g) = 5.8; Protein = 22.5

🕷 Buckwheat Flour Whole-Groat ☞ serving size: 1 cup = 120 g;

Calories = 402; Total Carb (g) = 84.7; Net Carb (g) = 72.7; Fat (g) = 3.7; Protein = 15.1

⚜ Buckwheat Groats Ns As To Fat Added In Cooking ☞ serving size: 1 cup, cooked = 170 g; Calories = 156.4; Total Carb (g) = 33.8; Net Carb (g) = 29.2; Fat (g) = 1.1; Protein = 5.7

⚜ Buckwheat Groats Roasted Dry ☞ serving size: 1 cup = 164 g; Calories = 567.4; Total Carb (g) = 122.9; Net Carb (g) = 106; Fat (g) = 4.4; Protein = 19.2

⚜ Bulgur Dry ☞ serving size: 1 cup = 140 g; Calories = 478.8; Total Carb (g) = 106.2; Net Carb (g) = 88.7; Fat (g) = 1.9; Protein = 17.2

⚜ Bulgur Ns As To Fat Added In Cooking ☞ serving size: 1 cup, cooked = 140 g; Calories = 116.2; Total Carb (g) = 25.9; Net Carb (g) = 19.6; Fat (g) = 0.3; Protein = 4.3

⚜ Canned Hominy ☞ serving size: 1 cup = 165 g; Calories = 118.8; Total Carb (g) = 23.5; Net Carb (g) = 19.4; Fat (g) = 1.5; Protein = 2.4

⚜ Congee ☞ serving size: 1 cup = 249 g; Calories = 82.2; Total Carb (g) = 17.8; Net Carb (g) = 17.6; Fat (g) = 0.2; Protein = 1.7

⚜ Cooked Amaranth ☞ serving size: 1 cup = 246 g; Calories = 250.9; Total Carb (g) = 46; Net Carb (g) = 40.8; Fat (g) = 3.9; Protein = 9.4

⚜ Cooked Brown Rice ☞ serving size: 1 cup = 195 g; Calories = 218.4; Total Carb (g) = 45.8; Net Carb (g) = 42.3; Fat (g) = 1.6; Protein = 4.5

⚜ Cooked Bulgur ☞ serving size: 1 cup = 182 g; Calories = 151.1; Total Carb (g) = 33.8; Net Carb (g) = 25.6; Fat (g) = 0.4; Protein = 5.6

⚜ Cooked Couscous ☞ serving size: 1 cup, cooked = 157 g; Calories = 175.8; Total Carb (g) = 36.5; Net Carb (g) = 34.3; Fat (g) = 0.3; Protein = 6

⚜ Cooked Japanese Somen ☞ serving size: 1 cup = 176 g; Calories =

230.6; Total Carb (g) = 48.5; Net Carb (g) = 48.5; Fat (g) = 0.3; Protein = 7

🌑 Cooked Millet ☞ serving size: 1 cup = 174 g; Calories = 207.1; Total Carb (g) = 41.2; Net Carb (g) = 38.9; Fat (g) = 1.7; Protein = 6.1

🌑 Cooked Oat Bran ☞ serving size: 1 cup = 219 g; Calories = 87.6; Total Carb (g) = 25.1; Net Carb (g) = 19.4; Fat (g) = 1.9; Protein = 7

🌑 Cooked Oatmeal ☞ serving size: 1 cup = 234 g; Calories = 166.1; Total Carb (g) = 28.1; Net Carb (g) = 24.1; Fat (g) = 3.6; Protein = 5.9

🌑 Cooked Pasta (Unenriched) ☞ serving size: 1 cup spaghetti not packed = 124 g; Calories = 195.9; Total Carb (g) = 38.3; Net Carb (g) = 36; Fat (g) = 1.2; Protein = 7.2

🌑 Cooked Pearled Barley ☞ serving size: 1 cup = 157 g; Calories = 193.1; Total Carb (g) = 44.3; Net Carb (g) = 38.3; Fat (g) = 0.7; Protein = 3.6

🌑 Cooked Spelt ☞ serving size: 1 cup = 194 g; Calories = 246.4; Total Carb (g) = 51.3; Net Carb (g) = 43.7; Fat (g) = 1.7; Protein = 10.7

🌑 Cooked Teff ☞ serving size: 1 cup = 252 g; Calories = 254.5; Total Carb (g) = 50.1; Net Carb (g) = 43; Fat (g) = 1.6; Protein = 9.8

🌑 Cooked Wild Rice ☞ serving size: 1 cup = 164 g; Calories = 165.6; Total Carb (g) = 35; Net Carb (g) = 32.1; Fat (g) = 0.6; Protein = 6.5

🌑 Corn Bran Crude ☞ serving size: 1 cup = 76 g; Calories = 170.2; Total Carb (g) = 65.1; Net Carb (g) = 5.1; Fat (g) = 0.7; Protein = 6.4

🌑 Corn Flour Masa Enriched White ☞ serving size: 1 cup = 114 g; Calories = 413.8; Total Carb (g) = 87.3; Net Carb (g) = 80; Fat (g) = 4.2; Protein = 9.6

🌑 Corn Grain White ☞ serving size: 1 cup = 166 g; Calories = 605.9; Total Carb (g) = 123.3; Net Carb (g) = 123.3; Fat (g) = 7.9; Protein = 15.6

🌑 Corn Grain Yellow ☞ serving size: 1 cup = 166 g; Calories = 605.9; Total Carb (g) = 123.3; Net Carb (g) = 111.2; Fat (g) = 7.9; Protein = 15.6

🦂 Cornmeal Degermed Enriched White ☞ serving size: 1 cup = 157 g; Calories = 580.9; Total Carb (g) = 124.7; Net Carb (g) = 118.6; Fat (g) = 2.8; Protein = 11.2

🦂 Cornmeal Degermed Enriched Yellow ☞ serving size: 1 cup = 157 g; Calories = 580.9; Total Carb (g) = 124.7; Net Carb (g) = 118.6; Fat (g) = 2.8; Protein = 11.2

🦂 Cornstarch ☞ serving size: 1 cup = 128 g; Calories = 487.7; Total Carb (g) = 116.8; Net Carb (g) = 115.7; Fat (g) = 0.1; Protein = 0.3

🦂 Couscous Dry ☞ serving size: 1 cup = 173 g; Calories = 650.5; Total Carb (g) = 134; Net Carb (g) = 125.3; Fat (g) = 1.1; Protein = 22.1

🦂 Couscous Plain Cooked ☞ serving size: 1 cup, cooked = 160 g; Calories = 177.6; Total Carb (g) = 37; Net Carb (g) = 34.7; Fat (g) = 0.3; Protein = 6

🦂 Hominy Canned Yellow ☞ serving size: 1 cup = 160 g; Calories = 115.2; Total Carb (g) = 22.8; Net Carb (g) = 18.8; Fat (g) = 1.4; Protein = 2.4

🦂 Japanese Soba Noodles (Buckwheat) ☞ serving size: 1 cup = 114 g; Calories = 112.9; Total Carb (g) = 24.4; Net Carb (g) = 24.4; Fat (g) = 0.1; Protein = 5.8

🦂 Kamut Cooked ☞ serving size: 1 cup = 172 g; Calories = 227; Total Carb (g) = 47.5; Net Carb (g) = 40.1; Fat (g) = 1.4; Protein = 9.8

🦂 Long Rice Noodles Made From Mung Beans Cooked ☞ serving size: 1 cup, cooked = 190 g; Calories = 159.6; Total Carb (g) = 39.3; Net Carb (g) = 39.1; Fat (g) = 0; Protein = 0.1

🦂 Macaroni Vegetable Enriched Cooked ☞ serving size: 1 cup spiral shaped = 134 g; Calories = 171.5; Total Carb (g) = 35.7; Net Carb (g) = 29.9; Fat (g) = 0.2; Protein = 6.1

🦂 Macaroni Vegetable Enriched Dry ☞ serving size: 1 cup spiral shaped = 84 g; Calories = 308.3; Total Carb (g) = 62.9; Net Carb (g) = 59.3; Fat (g) = 0.9; Protein = 11

🦠 Millet Flour ☞ serving size: 1 cup = 119 g; Calories = 454.6; Total Carb (g) = 89.4; Net Carb (g) = 85.2; Fat (g) = 5.1; Protein = 12.8

🦠 Millet Ns As To Fat Added In Cooking ☞ serving size: 1 cup, cooked = 170 g; Calories = 200.6; Total Carb (g) = 40.1; Net Carb (g) = 37.9; Fat (g) = 1.7; Protein = 6

🦠 Millet Raw ☞ serving size: 1 cup = 200 g; Calories = 756; Total Carb (g) = 145.7; Net Carb (g) = 128.7; Fat (g) = 8.4; Protein = 22

🦠 Noodles Chinese Chow Mein ☞ serving size: 1/2 cup dry = 28 g; Calories = 131.9; Total Carb (g) = 17.8; Net Carb (g) = 15.9; Fat (g) = 6; Protein = 3.1

🦠 Noodles Cooked ☞ serving size: 1 cup, cooked = 160 g; Calories = 219.2; Total Carb (g) = 40; Net Carb (g) = 38.1; Fat (g) = 3.3; Protein = 7.2

🦠 Noodles Egg Cooked Enriched With Added Salt ☞ serving size: 1 cup = 160 g; Calories = 220.8; Total Carb (g) = 40.3; Net Carb (g) = 38.3; Fat (g) = 3.3; Protein = 7.3

🦠 Noodles Egg Cooked Unenriched With Added Salt ☞ serving size: 1 cup = 160 g; Calories = 220.8; Total Carb (g) = 40.3; Net Carb (g) = 38.3; Fat (g) = 3.3; Protein = 7.3

🦠 Noodles Flat Crunchy Chinese Restaurant ☞ serving size: 1 cup = 45 g; Calories = 234.5; Total Carb (g) = 23.4; Net Carb (g) = 22.5; Fat (g) = 14.3; Protein = 4.7

🦠 Noodles Japanese Soba Dry ☞ serving size: 2 oz = 57 g; Calories = 191.5; Total Carb (g) = 42.5; Net Carb (g) = 42.5; Fat (g) = 0.4; Protein = 8.2

🦠 Noodles Japanese Somen Dry ☞ serving size: 2 oz = 57 g; Calories = 202.9; Total Carb (g) = 42.2; Net Carb (g) = 39.8; Fat (g) = 0.5; Protein = 6.5

🦠 Noodles Whole Grain Cooked ☞ serving size: 1 cup, cooked =

160 g; Calories = 236.8; Total Carb (g) = 47.9; Net Carb (g) = 41.6; Fat (g) = 2.7; Protein = 9.5

🌟 Oat Bran ☞ serving size: 1 cup = 94 g; Calories = 231.2; Total Carb (g) = 62.3; Net Carb (g) = 47.8; Fat (g) = 6.6; Protein = 16.3

🌟 Oat Flour Partially Debranned ☞ serving size: 1 cup = 104 g; Calories = 420.2; Total Carb (g) = 68.3; Net Carb (g) = 61.6; Fat (g) = 9.5; Protein = 15.3

🌟 Pasta Cooked ☞ serving size: 1 cup, cooked = 140 g; Calories = 219.8; Total Carb (g) = 43; Net Carb (g) = 40.4; Fat (g) = 1.3; Protein = 8.1

🌟 Pasta Dry Enriched ☞ serving size: 1 cup spaghetti = 91 g; Calories = 337.6; Total Carb (g) = 68; Net Carb (g) = 65; Fat (g) = 1.4; Protein = 11.9

🌟 Pasta Dry Unenriched ☞ serving size: 1 cup spaghetti = 91 g; Calories = 337.6; Total Carb (g) = 68; Net Carb (g) = 65; Fat (g) = 1.4; Protein = 11.9

🌟 Pasta Fresh-Refrigerated Plain As Purchased ☞ serving size: 4 (1/2) oz = 128 g; Calories = 368.6; Total Carb (g) = 70.1; Net Carb (g) = 70.1; Fat (g) = 2.9; Protein = 14.5

🌟 Pasta Fresh-Refrigerated Plain Cooked ☞ serving size: 2 oz = 128 g; Calories = 167.7; Total Carb (g) = 31.9; Net Carb (g) = 31.9; Fat (g) = 1.3; Protein = 6.6

🌟 Pasta Fresh-Refrigerated Spinach As Purchased ☞ serving size: 4 (1/2) oz = 128 g; Calories = 369.9; Total Carb (g) = 71.3; Net Carb (g) = 71.3; Fat (g) = 2.7; Protein = 14.4

🌟 Pasta Fresh-Refrigerated Spinach Cooked ☞ serving size: 2 oz = 57 g; Calories = 74.1; Total Carb (g) = 14.3; Net Carb (g) = 14.3; Fat (g) = 0.5; Protein = 2.9

🌟 Pasta Gluten-Free Brown Rice Flour Cooked Tinkyada ☞

serving size: 1 cup spaghetti not packed = 169 g; Calories = 233.2; Total Carb (g) = 54.4; Net Carb (g) = 51.6; Fat (g) = 2.8; Protein = 5.9

🐾 Pasta Gluten-Free Corn And Rice Flour Cooked ☞ serving size: 1 cup spaghetti = 141 g; Calories = 252.4; Total Carb (g) = 53.7; Net Carb (g) = 51.7; Fat (g) = 1.4; Protein = 4.5

🐾 Pasta Gluten-Free Corn Dry ☞ serving size: 1 cup = 105 g; Calories = 374.9; Total Carb (g) = 83.2; Net Carb (g) = 71.7; Fat (g) = 2.2; Protein = 7.8

🐾 Pasta Gluten-Free Corn Flour And Quinoa Flour Cooked Ancient Harvest ☞ serving size: 1 cup spaghetti packed = 166 g; Calories = 252.3; Total Carb (g) = 51.6; Net Carb (g) = 46.2; Fat (g) = 3.4; Protein = 5.4

🐾 Pasta Gluten-Free Rice Flour And Rice Bran Extract Cooked De Boles ☞ serving size: 1 cup spaghetti = 121 g; Calories = 242; Total Carb (g) = 49.3; Net Carb (g) = 47; Fat (g) = 2.1; Protein = 5.1

🐾 Pasta Homemade Made With Egg Cooked ☞ serving size: 2 oz = 57 g; Calories = 74.1; Total Carb (g) = 13.4; Net Carb (g) = 13.4; Fat (g) = 1; Protein = 3

🐾 Pasta Homemade Made Without Egg Cooked ☞ serving size: 2 oz = 57 g; Calories = 70.7; Total Carb (g) = 14.3; Net Carb (g) = 14.3; Fat (g) = 0.6; Protein = 2.5

🐾 Pasta Vegetable Cooked ☞ serving size: 1 cup, cooked = 140 g; Calories = 179.2; Total Carb (g) = 37.2; Net Carb (g) = 31.2; Fat (g) = 0.2; Protein = 6.3

🐾 Pasta Whole Grain 51% Whole Wheat Remaining Enriched Semolina Cooked ☞ serving size: 1 cup spaghetti not packed = 116 g; Calories = 181; Total Carb (g) = 35.8; Net Carb (g) = 30.6; Fat (g) = 1.7; Protein = 6.6

🐾 Pasta Whole Grain 51% Whole Wheat Remaining Enriched Semolina Dry ☞ serving size: 1 cup spaghetti = 91 g; Calories =

328.5; Total Carb (g) = 66.7; Net Carb (g) = 56.4; Fat (g) = 2.3; Protein = 12

🌑 Pasta Whole Grain 51% Whole Wheat Remaining Unenriched Semolina Cooked ☞ serving size: 1 cup spaghetti not packed = 116 g; Calories = 184.4; Total Carb (g) = 36.6; Net Carb (g) = 31.2; Fat (g) = 1.7; Protein = 6.8

🌑 Pasta Whole Grain 51% Whole Wheat Remaining Unenriched Semolina Dry ☞ serving size: 1 cup spaghetti = 91 g; Calories = 329.4; Total Carb (g) = 66.5; Net Carb (g) = 57.3; Fat (g) = 2.4; Protein = 12.3

🌑 Pasta Whole Grain Cooked ☞ serving size: 1 cup, cooked = 140 g; Calories = 207.2; Total Carb (g) = 41.9; Net Carb (g) = 36.4; Fat (g) = 2.4; Protein = 8.3

🌑 Pasta Whole-Wheat Dry ☞ serving size: 1 cup spaghetti = 91 g; Calories = 320.3; Total Carb (g) = 66.8; Net Carb (g) = 58.4; Fat (g) = 2.7; Protein = 12.6

🌑 Quinoa Cooked ☞ serving size: 1 cup = 185 g; Calories = 222; Total Carb (g) = 39.4; Net Carb (g) = 34.2; Fat (g) = 3.6; Protein = 8.1

🌑 Quinoa Fat Added In Cooking ☞ serving size: 1 cup, cooked = 170 g; Calories = 238; Total Carb (g) = 34.4; Net Carb (g) = 29.8; Fat (g) = 8.1; Protein = 7.1

🌑 Quinoa Fat Not Added In Cooking ☞ serving size: 1 cup, cooked = 170 g; Calories = 204; Total Carb (g) = 36.1; Net Carb (g) = 31.3; Fat (g) = 3.3; Protein = 7.5

🌑 Quinoa Ns As To Fat Added In Cooking ☞ serving size: 1 cup, cooked = 170 g; Calories = 238; Total Carb (g) = 34.4; Net Carb (g) = 29.8; Fat (g) = 8.1; Protein = 7.1

🌑 Quinoa Uncooked ☞ serving size: 1 cup = 170 g; Calories = 625.6; Total Carb (g) = 109.1; Net Carb (g) = 97.2; Fat (g) = 10.3; Protein = 24

🌑 Rice Bran ☞ serving size: 1 cup = 118 g; Calories = 372.9; Total Carb (g) = 58.6; Net Carb (g) = 33.9; Fat (g) = 24.6; Protein = 15.8

🌑 Rice Brown Cooked Ns As To Fat Added In Cooking ☞ serving size: 1 cup, cooked = 196 g; Calories = 239.1; Total Carb (g) = 49.9; Net Carb (g) = 46.8; Fat (g) = 1.9; Protein = 5.4

🌑 Rice Brown Long-Grain Raw ☞ serving size: 1 cup = 185 g; Calories = 679; Total Carb (g) = 141.1; Net Carb (g) = 134.4; Fat (g) = 5.9; Protein = 14

🌑 Rice Brown Medium-Grain Raw ☞ serving size: 1 cup = 190 g; Calories = 687.8; Total Carb (g) = 144.7; Net Carb (g) = 138.3; Fat (g) = 5.1; Protein = 14.3

🌑 Rice Brown Parboiled Cooked Uncle Bens ☞ serving size: 1 cup = 155 g; Calories = 227.9; Total Carb (g) = 48.6; Net Carb (g) = 45.9; Fat (g) = 1.3; Protein = 4.8

🌑 Rice Brown Parboiled Dry Uncle Bens ☞ serving size: 1/4 cup = 48 g; Calories = 177.6; Total Carb (g) = 37.8; Net Carb (g) = 36.1; Fat (g) = 1.3; Protein = 3.7

🌑 Rice Cooked Nfs ☞ serving size: 1 cup, cooked = 158 g; Calories = 203.8; Total Carb (g) = 44.2; Net Carb (g) = 43.6; Fat (g) = 0.4; Protein = 4.2

🌑 Rice Cooked With Milk ☞ serving size: 1 cup, cooked = 200 g; Calories = 286; Total Carb (g) = 50.1; Net Carb (g) = 49.5; Fat (g) = 4.4; Protein = 10.1

🌑 Rice Flour Brown ☞ serving size: 1 cup = 158 g; Calories = 573.5; Total Carb (g) = 120.8; Net Carb (g) = 113.6; Fat (g) = 4.4; Protein = 11.4

🌑 Rice Flour White Unenriched ☞ serving size: 1 cup = 158 g; Calories = 578.3; Total Carb (g) = 126.6; Net Carb (g) = 122.8; Fat (g) = 2.2; Protein = 9.4

🌑 Rice Noodles (Cooked) ☞ serving size: 1 cup = 176 g; Calories =

190.1; Total Carb (g) = 42.3; Net Carb (g) = 40.5; Fat (g) = 0.4; Protein = 3.2

☀ Rice Noodles Dry ☞ serving size: 2 oz = 57 g; Calories = 207.5; Total Carb (g) = 45.7; Net Carb (g) = 44.8; Fat (g) = 0.3; Protein = 3.4

☀ Rice Sweet Cooked With Honey ☞ serving size: 1 cup, cooked = 175 g; Calories = 245; Total Carb (g) = 54.8; Net Carb (g) = 54.1; Fat (g) = 0.5; Protein = 4.4

☀ Rice White Cooked Ns As To Fat Added In Cooking ☞ serving size: 1 cup, cooked = 163 g; Calories = 210.3; Total Carb (g) = 45.6; Net Carb (g) = 45; Fat (g) = 0.5; Protein = 4.4

☀ Rice White Long-Grain Regular Raw Enriched ☞ serving size: 1 cup = 185 g; Calories = 675.3; Total Carb (g) = 147.9; Net Carb (g) = 145.5; Fat (g) = 1.2; Protein = 13.2

☀ Rice White Long-Grain Regular Raw Unenriched ☞ serving size: 1 cup = 185 g; Calories = 675.3; Total Carb (g) = 147.9; Net Carb (g) = 145.5; Fat (g) = 1.2; Protein = 13.2

☀ Rice White Medium-Grain Raw Enriched ☞ serving size: 1 cup = 195 g; Calories = 702; Total Carb (g) = 154.7; Net Carb (g) = 152; Fat (g) = 1.1; Protein = 12.9

☀ Rice White Medium-Grain Raw Unenriched ☞ serving size: 1 cup = 195 g; Calories = 702; Total Carb (g) = 154.7; Net Carb (g) = 154.7; Fat (g) = 1.1; Protein = 12.9

☀ Rice White Short-Grain Raw Unenriched ☞ serving size: 1 cup = 200 g; Calories = 716; Total Carb (g) = 158.3; Net Carb (g) = 158.3; Fat (g) = 1; Protein = 13

☀ Rice Wild 100% Cooked Ns As To Fat Added In Cooking ☞ serving size: 1 cup, cooked = 164 g; Calories = 198.4; Total Carb (g) = 33.9; Net Carb (g) = 31.1; Fat (g) = 4.9; Protein = 6.3

☀ Roasted Buckwheat Groats ☞ serving size: 1 cup = 168 g; Calories = 154.6; Total Carb (g) = 33.5; Net Carb (g) = 29; Fat (g) = 1; Protein = 5.7

🌑 Rye Flour Dark ☞ serving size: 1 cup = 128 g; Calories = 416; Total Carb (g) = 87.9; Net Carb (g) = 57.4; Fat (g) = 2.8; Protein = 20.4

🌑 Rye Flour Light ☞ serving size: 1 cup = 102 g; Calories = 364.1; Total Carb (g) = 78.2; Net Carb (g) = 70.1; Fat (g) = 1.4; Protein = 10

🌑 Rye Flour Medium ☞ serving size: 1 cup = 102 g; Calories = 356; Total Carb (g) = 76.9; Net Carb (g) = 64.9; Fat (g) = 1.6; Protein = 11.1

🌑 Rye Grain ☞ serving size: 1 cup = 169 g; Calories = 571.2; Total Carb (g) = 128.2; Net Carb (g) = 102.7; Fat (g) = 2.8; Protein = 17.5

🌑 Semolina Enriched ☞ serving size: 1 cup = 167 g; Calories = 601.2; Total Carb (g) = 121.6; Net Carb (g) = 115.1; Fat (g) = 1.8; Protein = 21.2

🌑 Semolina Unenriched ☞ serving size: 1 cup = 167 g; Calories = 601.2; Total Carb (g) = 121.6; Net Carb (g) = 115.1; Fat (g) = 1.8; Protein = 21.2

🌑 Sorghum Flour Refined Unenriched ☞ serving size: 1 cup = 161 g; Calories = 574.8; Total Carb (g) = 123.7; Net Carb (g) = 120.7; Fat (g) = 2; Protein = 15.3

🌑 Sorghum Grain ☞ serving size: 1 cup = 192 g; Calories = 631.7; Total Carb (g) = 138.4; Net Carb (g) = 125.6; Fat (g) = 6.6; Protein = 20.4

🌑 Spaghetti Protein-Fortified Cooked Enriched (N X 6.25) ☞ serving size: 1 cup = 140 g; Calories = 229.6; Total Carb (g) = 43.2; Net Carb (g) = 40.4; Fat (g) = 0.3; Protein = 12.4

🌑 Spaghetti Protein-Fortified Dry Enriched (N X 6.25) ☞ serving size: 2 oz = 57 g; Calories = 213.2; Total Carb (g) = 37.4; Net Carb (g) = 36.1; Fat (g) = 1.3; Protein = 12.4

🌑 Spaghetti Spinach Cooked ☞ serving size: 1 cup = 140 g; Calories = 182; Total Carb (g) = 36.6; Net Carb (g) = 36.6; Fat (g) = 0.9; Protein = 6.4

🌑 Spaghetti Spinach Dry ☞ serving size: 2 oz = 57 g; Calories = 212; Total Carb (g) = 42.6; Net Carb (g) = 36.6; Fat (g) = 0.9; Protein = 7.6

🌑 Spelt Uncooked ☞ serving size: 1 cup = 174 g; Calories = 588.1; Total Carb (g) = 122.1; Net Carb (g) = 103.5; Fat (g) = 4.2; Protein = 25.4

🌑 Spinach Egg Noodles (Cooked) ☞ serving size: 1 cup = 160 g; Calories = 211.2; Total Carb (g) = 38.8; Net Carb (g) = 35.1; Fat (g) = 2.5; Protein = 8.1

🌑 Tapioca Pearl Dry ☞ serving size: 1 cup = 152 g; Calories = 544.2; Total Carb (g) = 134.8; Net Carb (g) = 133.4; Fat (g) = 0; Protein = 0.3

🌑 Teff Uncooked ☞ serving size: 1 cup = 193 g; Calories = 708.3; Total Carb (g) = 141.1; Net Carb (g) = 125.7; Fat (g) = 4.6; Protein = 25.7

🌑 Triticale ☞ serving size: 1 cup = 192 g; Calories = 645.1; Total Carb (g) = 138.5; Net Carb (g) = 138.5; Fat (g) = 4; Protein = 25.1

🌑 Triticale Flour Whole-Grain ☞ serving size: 1 cup = 130 g; Calories = 439.4; Total Carb (g) = 95.1; Net Carb (g) = 76.1; Fat (g) = 2.4; Protein = 17.1

🌑 Uncooked Oats ☞ serving size: 1 cup = 156 g; Calories = 606.8; Total Carb (g) = 103.4; Net Carb (g) = 86.9; Fat (g) = 10.8; Protein = 26.4

🌑 Uncooked Whole-Grain Cornmeal ☞ serving size: 1 cup = 122 g; Calories = 441.6; Total Carb (g) = 93.8; Net Carb (g) = 84.9; Fat (g) = 4.4; Protein = 9.9

🌑 Uncooked Yellow Cornmeal ☞ serving size: 1 cup = 122 g; Calories = 441.6; Total Carb (g) = 93.8; Net Carb (g) = 84.9; Fat (g) = 4.4; Protein = 9.9

🌑 Vermicelli Made From Soybeans ☞ serving size: 1 cup = 140 g; Calories = 176.4; Total Carb (g) = 44; Net Carb (g) = 41.9; Fat (g) = 0.1; Protein = 0.1

🐾 Wheat Bran Crude ☞ serving size: 1 cup = 58 g; Calories = 125.3; Total Carb (g) = 37.4; Net Carb (g) = 12.6; Fat (g) = 2.5; Protein = 9

🐾 Wheat Durum ☞ serving size: 1 cup = 192 g; Calories = 650.9; Total Carb (g) = 136.6; Net Carb (g) = 136.6; Fat (g) = 4.7; Protein = 26.3

🐾 Wheat Flour White All-Purpose Enriched Bleached ☞ serving size: 1 cup = 125 g; Calories = 455; Total Carb (g) = 95.4; Net Carb (g) = 92; Fat (g) = 1.2; Protein = 12.9

🐾 Wheat Flour White All-Purpose Enriched Calcium-Fortified ☞ serving size: 1 cup = 125 g; Calories = 455; Total Carb (g) = 95.4; Net Carb (g) = 92; Fat (g) = 1.2; Protein = 12.9

🐾 Wheat Flour White All-Purpose Enriched Unbleached ☞ serving size: 1 cup = 125 g; Calories = 455; Total Carb (g) = 95.4; Net Carb (g) = 92; Fat (g) = 1.2; Protein = 12.9

🐾 Wheat Flour White All-Purpose Self-Rising Enriched ☞ serving size: 1 cup = 125 g; Calories = 442.5; Total Carb (g) = 92.8; Net Carb (g) = 89.4; Fat (g) = 1.2; Protein = 12.4

🐾 Wheat Flour White All-Purpose Unenriched ☞ serving size: 1 cup = 125 g; Calories = 455; Total Carb (g) = 95.4; Net Carb (g) = 92; Fat (g) = 1.2; Protein = 12.9

🐾 Wheat Flour White Bread Enriched ☞ serving size: 1 cup = 137 g; Calories = 494.6; Total Carb (g) = 99.4; Net Carb (g) = 96.1; Fat (g) = 2.3; Protein = 16.4

🐾 Wheat Flour White Cake Enriched ☞ serving size: 1 cup unsifted, dipped = 137 g; Calories = 495.9; Total Carb (g) = 106.9; Net Carb (g) = 104.6; Fat (g) = 1.2; Protein = 11.2

🐾 Wheat Flour White Tortilla Mix Enriched ☞ serving size: 1 cup = 111 g; Calories = 449.6; Total Carb (g) = 74.5; Net Carb (g) = 74.5; Fat (g) = 11.8; Protein = 10.7

🐾 Wheat Flour Whole-Grain ☞ serving size: 1 cup = 120 g; Calories

= 408; Total Carb (g) = 86.4; Net Carb (g) = 73.5; Fat (g) = 3; Protein = 15.9

✹ Wheat Flours Bread Unenriched ☞ serving size: 1 cup unsifted, dipped = 137 g; Calories = 494.6; Total Carb (g) = 99.4; Net Carb (g) = 96.1; Fat (g) = 2.3; Protein = 16.4

✹ Wheat Germ Crude ☞ serving size: 1 cup = 115 g; Calories = 414; Total Carb (g) = 59.6; Net Carb (g) = 44.4; Fat (g) = 11.2; Protein = 26.6

✹ Wheat Hard Red Spring ☞ serving size: 1 cup = 192 g; Calories = 631.7; Total Carb (g) = 130.6; Net Carb (g) = 107.2; Fat (g) = 3.7; Protein = 29.6

✹ Wheat Hard Red Winter ☞ serving size: 1 cup = 192 g; Calories = 627.8; Total Carb (g) = 136.7; Net Carb (g) = 113.2; Fat (g) = 3; Protein = 24.2

✹ Wheat Hard White ☞ serving size: 1 cup = 192 g; Calories = 656.6; Total Carb (g) = 145.7; Net Carb (g) = 122.3; Fat (g) = 3.3; Protein = 21.7

✹ Wheat Kamut Khorasan Uncooked ☞ serving size: 1 cup = 186 g; Calories = 626.8; Total Carb (g) = 131.3; Net Carb (g) = 110.6; Fat (g) = 4; Protein = 27

✹ Wheat Soft Red Winter ☞ serving size: 1 cup = 168 g; Calories = 556.1; Total Carb (g) = 124.7; Net Carb (g) = 103.7; Fat (g) = 2.6; Protein = 17.4

✹ Wheat Soft White ☞ serving size: 1 cup = 168 g; Calories = 571.2; Total Carb (g) = 126.6; Net Carb (g) = 105.3; Fat (g) = 3.3; Protein = 18

✹ Wheat Sprouted ☞ serving size: 1 cup = 108 g; Calories = 213.8; Total Carb (g) = 45.9; Net Carb (g) = 44.7; Fat (g) = 1.4; Protein = 8.1

✹ White Rice ☞ serving size: 1 cup = 158 g; Calories = 205.4; Total Carb (g) = 44.5; Net Carb (g) = 43.9; Fat (g) = 0.4; Protein = 4.3

✹ Whole Grain Sorghum Flour ☞ serving size: 1 cup = 121 g; Calo-

ries = 434.4; Total Carb (g) = 92.7; Net Carb (g) = 84.8; Fat (g) = 4; Protein = 10.2

❁ Whole Wheat Pasta ☞ serving size: 1 cup spaghetti not packed = 117 g; Calories = 174.3; Total Carb (g) = 35.2; Net Carb (g) = 30.6; Fat (g) = 2; Protein = 7

❁ Wild Rice Raw ☞ serving size: 1 cup = 160 g; Calories = 571.2; Total Carb (g) = 119.8; Net Carb (g) = 109.9; Fat (g) = 1.7; Protein = 23.6

❁ Yellow Cornmeal (Grits) ☞ serving size: 1 cup = 233 g; Calories = 151.5; Total Carb (g) = 32.3; Net Carb (g) = 30.7; Fat (g) = 0.9; Protein = 2.9

❁ Yellow Rice Cooked Ns As To Fat Added In Cooking ☞ serving size: 1 cup, cooked = 158 g; Calories = 139; Total Carb (g) = 30.2; Net Carb (g) = 29.4; Fat (g) = 0.7; Protein = 2.8

21

MEATS AND POULTRY

Bacon (Pan-Fried) ☞ serving size: 1 slice = 11.5 g; Calories = 53.8; Total Carb (g) = 0.2; Net Carb (g) = 0.2; Fat (g) = 4; Protein = 3.9

Bacon (Raw) ☞ serving size: 1 slice raw = 28 g; Calories = 110; Total Carb (g) = 0; Net Carb (g) = 0; Fat (g) = 10.4; Protein = 3.8

Bacon And Beef Sticks ☞ serving size: 1 oz = 28 g; Calories = 144.8; Total Carb (g) = 0.2; Net Carb (g) = 0.2; Fat (g) = 12.4; Protein = 8.2

Bacon Pre-Sliced Reduced/low Sodium Unprepared ☞ serving size: 1 slice = 26 g; Calories = 105.8; Total Carb (g) = 0.2; Net Carb (g) = 0.2; Fat (g) = 10.2; Protein = 3.3

Bacon Turkey Low Sodium ☞ serving size: 1 serving = 15 g; Calories = 38; Total Carb (g) = 0.7; Net Carb (g) = 0.7; Fat (g) = 3; Protein = 2

Barbecue Loaf Pork Beef ☞ serving size: 1 oz = 28.4 g; Calories = 49.1; Total Carb (g) = 1.8; Net Carb (g) = 1.8; Fat (g) = 2.5; Protein = 4.5

Bear Cooked ☞ serving size: 1 oz, boneless, cooked = 28 g; Calories = 72.2; Total Carb (g) = 0; Net Carb (g) = 0; Fat (g) = 3.7; Protein = 9

🦫 Beaver Cooked ☞ serving size: 1 oz, boneless, cooked = 28 g; Calories = 59.1; Total Carb (g) = 0; Net Carb (g) = 0; Fat (g) = 1.9; Protein = 9.7

🦫 Beef Australian Imported Grass-Fed Seam Fat Raw ☞ serving size: 1 oz = 28.4 g; Calories = 159.6; Total Carb (g) = 0.3; Net Carb (g) = 0.3; Fat (g) = 16.4; Protein = 2.7

🦫 Beef Australian Imported Wagyu Loin Tenderloin Steak/roast Boneless Separable Lean Only Aust. Marble Score 9 Raw ☞ serving size: 4 oz = 114 g; Calories = 270.2; Total Carb (g) = 0.7; Net Carb (g) = 0.7; Fat (g) = 20.2; Protein = 21.5

🦫 Beef Australian Imported Wagyu Loin Top Loin Steak/roast Boneless Separable Lean And Fat Aust. Marble Score 4/5 Raw ☞ serving size: 4 oz = 114 g; Calories = 329.5; Total Carb (g) = 0.1; Net Carb (g) = 0.1; Fat (g) = 27.6; Protein = 20.1

🦫 Beef Baloney (Bologna) ☞ serving size: 1 slice = 30 g; Calories = 89.7; Total Carb (g) = 1.3; Net Carb (g) = 1.3; Fat (g) = 7.8; Protein = 3.3

🦫 Beef Bologna Reduced Sodium ☞ serving size: 1 cup pieces = 138 g; Calories = 427.8; Total Carb (g) = 2.8; Net Carb (g) = 2.8; Fat (g) = 39.2; Protein = 16.2

🦫 Beef Bottom Sirloin Tri-Tip Roast Separable Lean Only Trimmed To 0 Inch Fat Select Raw ☞ serving size: 3 oz = 85 g; Calories = 109.7; Total Carb (g) = 0; Net Carb (g) = 0; Fat (g) = 3.6; Protein = 18.1

🦫 Beef Brisket Cooked Lean And Fat Eaten ☞ serving size: 1 thin slice (approx 4-1/2" x 2-1/2" x 1/8") = 21 g; Calories = 60.7; Total Carb (g) = 0; Net Carb (g) = 0; Fat (g) = 4.1; Protein = 5.6

🦫 Beef Brisket Flat Half Separable Lean Only Trimmed To 1/8

Inch Fat Select Raw ☞ serving size: 1 oz = 28.4 g; Calories = 35.2; Total Carb (g) = 0; Net Carb (g) = 0; Fat (g) = 1; Protein = 6.1

🍖 Beef Brisket Point Half Separable Lean And Fat Trimmed To 0 Inch Fat All Grades Cooked Braised ☞ serving size: 3 oz = 85 g; Calories = 304.3; Total Carb (g) = 0; Net Carb (g) = 0; Fat (g) = 24.2; Protein = 20

🍖 Beef Brisket Whole Separable Lean Only Trimmed To 0 Inch Fat All Grades Cooked Braised ☞ serving size: 3 oz = 85 g; Calories = 185.3; Total Carb (g) = 0; Net Carb (g) = 0; Fat (g) = 8.6; Protein = 25.3

🍖 Beef Burgundy ☞ serving size: 1 cup = 244 g; Calories = 356.2; Total Carb (g) = 9.9; Net Carb (g) = 8.2; Fat (g) = 14.5; Protein = 45.1

🍖 Beef Carcass Separable Lean And Fat Choice Raw ☞ serving size: 1 oz = 28.4 g; Calories = 82.6; Total Carb (g) = 0; Net Carb (g) = 0; Fat (g) = 6.8; Protein = 4.9

🍖 Beef Carcass Separable Lean And Fat Select Raw ☞ serving size: 1 oz = 28.4 g; Calories = 79; Total Carb (g) = 0; Net Carb (g) = 0; Fat (g) = 6.4; Protein = 5

🍖 Beef Chuck Arm Pot Roast Separable Lean And Fat Trimmed To 0 Inch Fat All Grades Cooked Braised ☞ serving size: 3 oz = 85 g; Calories = 252.5; Total Carb (g) = 0; Net Carb (g) = 0; Fat (g) = 16.3; Protein = 24.6

🍖 Beef Chuck For Stew Separable Lean And Fat Select Raw ☞ serving size: 3 oz = 85 g; Calories = 105.4; Total Carb (g) = 0.2; Net Carb (g) = 0.2; Fat (g) = 3.4; Protein = 18.6

🍖 Beef Chuck Mock Tender Steak Boneless Separable Lean And Fat Trimmed To 0 Inch Fat All Grades Cooked Braised ☞ serving size: 1 steak = 141 g; Calories = 310.2; Total Carb (g) = 0; Net Carb (g) = 0; Fat (g) = 14.4; Protein = 45.2

🐾 Beef Chuck Pot Roast ☞ serving size: 3 oz = 85 g; Calories = 180.2; Total Carb (g) = 0; Net Carb (g) = 0; Fat (g) = 6.5; Protein = 28.4

🐾 Beef Chuck Short Ribs Boneless Separable Lean And Fat Trimmed To 0 Inch Fat All Grades Cooked Braised ☞ serving size: 3 oz = 85 g; Calories = 259.3; Total Carb (g) = 0; Net Carb (g) = 0; Fat (g) = 19.2; Protein = 21.7

🐾 Beef Chuck Top Blade Separable Lean And Fat Trimmed To 0 Inch Fat All Grades Cooked Broiled ☞ serving size: 3 oz = 85 g; Calories = 183.6; Total Carb (g) = 0; Net Carb (g) = 0; Fat (g) = 10; Protein = 21.9

🐾 Beef Chuck Under Blade Center Steak Boneless Denver Cut Separable Lean Only Trimmed To 0 Inch Fat Select Raw ☞ serving size: 3 oz = 85 g; Calories = 133.5; Total Carb (g) = 0.2; Net Carb (g) = 0.2; Fat (g) = 7.3; Protein = 16.8

🐾 Beef Composite Of Trimmed Retail Cuts Separable Lean And Fat Trimmed To 0 Inch Fat All Grades Cooked ☞ serving size: 3 oz = 85 g; Calories = 195.5; Total Carb (g) = 0; Net Carb (g) = 0; Fat (g) = 10.6; Protein = 24.1

🐾 Beef Composite Separable Lean Only Trimmed To 1/8 Inch Fat Choice Cooked ☞ serving size: 3 oz = 85 g; Calories = 172.6; Total Carb (g) = 0; Net Carb (g) = 0; Fat (g) = 7.8; Protein = 24.4

🐾 Beef Cow Head Cooked ☞ serving size: 1 oz, boneless, cooked = 28 g; Calories = 72; Total Carb (g) = 0; Net Carb (g) = 0; Fat (g) = 4.6; Protein = 7.3

🐾 Beef Cured Breakfast Strips Cooked ☞ serving size: 3 slices = 34 g; Calories = 152.7; Total Carb (g) = 0.5; Net Carb (g) = 0.5; Fat (g) = 11.7; Protein = 10.6

🐾 Beef Cured Breakfast Strips Raw Or Unheated ☞ serving size: 3 slices = 68 g; Calories = 276.1; Total Carb (g) = 0.5; Net Carb (g) = 0.5; Fat (g) = 26.4; Protein = 8.5

🐾 Beef Cured Corned Beef Brisket Cooked ☞ serving size: 3 oz = 85 g; Calories = 213.4; Total Carb (g) = 0.4; Net Carb (g) = 0.4; Fat (g) = 16.1; Protein = 15.4

🐾 Beef Cured Corned Beef Brisket Raw ☞ serving size: 1 oz = 28.4 g; Calories = 56.2; Total Carb (g) = 0; Net Carb (g) = 0; Fat (g) = 4.2; Protein = 4.2

🐾 Beef Cured Corned Beef Canned ☞ serving size: 1 oz = 28.4 g; Calories = 71; Total Carb (g) = 0; Net Carb (g) = 0; Fat (g) = 4.2; Protein = 7.7

🐾 Beef Cured Dried ☞ serving size: 10 slices = 28 g; Calories = 42.8; Total Carb (g) = 0.8; Net Carb (g) = 0.8; Fat (g) = 0.5; Protein = 8.7

🐾 Beef Cured Luncheon Meat Jellied ☞ serving size: 1 slice (1 oz) (4 inch x 4 inch x 3/32 inch thick) = 28 g; Calories = 31.1; Total Carb (g) = 0; Net Carb (g) = 0; Fat (g) = 0.9; Protein = 5.3

🐾 Beef Cured Pastrami ☞ serving size: 1 package, 2.5 oz = 71 g; Calories = 104.4; Total Carb (g) = 0.3; Net Carb (g) = 0.3; Fat (g) = 4.1; Protein = 15.5

🐾 Beef Cured Sausage Cooked Smoked ☞ serving size: 1 sausage = 43 g; Calories = 134.2; Total Carb (g) = 1; Net Carb (g) = 1; Fat (g) = 11.6; Protein = 6.1

🐾 Beef Flank Steak Separable Lean And Fat Trimmed To 0 Inch Fat All Grades Cooked Broiled ☞ serving size: 3 oz = 85 g; Calories = 163.2; Total Carb (g) = 0; Net Carb (g) = 0; Fat (g) = 7; Protein = 23.5

🐾 Beef Goulash ☞ serving size: 1 cup = 249 g; Calories = 254; Total Carb (g) = 7; Net Carb (g) = 6; Fat (g) = 9.4; Protein = 34.1

🐾 Beef Grass-Fed Ground Raw ☞ serving size: 1 serving = 85 g; Calories = 168.3; Total Carb (g) = 0; Net Carb (g) = 0; Fat (g) = 10.8; Protein = 16.5

🐾 Beef Ground 70% Lean Meat / 30% Fat Loaf Cooked Baked ☞

serving size: 3 oz = 85 g; Calories = 204.9; Total Carb (g) = 0; Net Carb (g) = 0; Fat (g) = 13.1; Protein = 20.3

👉 Beef Ground 75% Lean Meat / 25% Fat Raw ☞ serving size: 4 oz = 113 g; Calories = 331.1; Total Carb (g) = 0; Net Carb (g) = 0; Fat (g) = 28.3; Protein = 17.8

👉 Beef Ground 80% Lean Meat / 20% Fat Raw ☞ serving size: 4 oz = 113 g; Calories = 287; Total Carb (g) = 0; Net Carb (g) = 0; Fat (g) = 22.6; Protein = 19.4

👉 Beef Ground 85% Lean Meat / 15% Fat Crumbles Cooked Pan-Browned ☞ serving size: 3 oz = 85 g; Calories = 217.6; Total Carb (g) = 0; Net Carb (g) = 0; Fat (g) = 13; Protein = 23.6

👉 Beef Ground 90% Lean Meat / 10% Fat Raw ☞ serving size: 4 oz = 113 g; Calories = 198.9; Total Carb (g) = 0; Net Carb (g) = 0; Fat (g) = 11.3; Protein = 22.6

👉 Beef Ground 93% Lean Meat / 7% Fat Crumbles Cooked Pan-Browned ☞ serving size: 3 oz = 85 g; Calories = 177.7; Total Carb (g) = 0; Net Carb (g) = 0; Fat (g) = 8.1; Protein = 24.6

👉 Beef Ground 95% Lean Meat / 5% Fat Raw ☞ serving size: 4 oz = 113 g; Calories = 154.8; Total Carb (g) = 0; Net Carb (g) = 0; Fat (g) = 5.7; Protein = 24.2

👉 Beef Ground 97% Lean Meat / 3% Fat Crumbles Cooked Pan-Browned ☞ serving size: 3 oz = 85 g; Calories = 148.8; Total Carb (g) = 0; Net Carb (g) = 0; Fat (g) = 4.6; Protein = 25

👉 Beef Ground Patties Frozen Cooked Broiled ☞ serving size: 3 oz = 85 g; Calories = 250.8; Total Carb (g) = 0; Net Carb (g) = 0; Fat (g) = 18.6; Protein = 19.6

👉 Beef Ground Unspecified Fat Content Cooked ☞ serving size: 3 oz = 85 g; Calories = 204; Total Carb (g) = 0.5; Net Carb (g) = 0.5; Fat (g) = 12.4; Protein = 21.3

👉 Beef Liver Braised ☞ serving size: 1 oz, raw (yield after cooking)

= 19 g; Calories = 35.9; Total Carb (g) = 1; Net Carb (g) = 1; Fat (g) = 1; Protein = 5.5

🐾 Beef Liver Fried ☞ serving size: 1 oz, raw (yield after cooking) = 21 g; Calories = 36.5; Total Carb (g) = 1.1; Net Carb (g) = 1.1; Fat (g) = 1; Protein = 5.5

🐾 Beef Loin Bottom Sirloin Butt Tri-Tip Roast Separable Lean Only Trimmed To 0 Inch Fat All Grades Cooked Roasted ☞ serving size: 1 serving = 85 g; Calories = 154.7; Total Carb (g) = 0; Net Carb (g) = 0; Fat (g) = 7.1; Protein = 22.7

🐾 Beef Loin Bottom Sirloin Butt Tri-Tip Steak Separable Lean And Fat Trimmed To 0 Inch Fat All Grades Cooked Broiled ☞ serving size: 3 oz = 85 g; Calories = 225.3; Total Carb (g) = 0; Net Carb (g) = 0; Fat (g) = 12.9; Protein = 25.5

🐾 Beef Loin Tenderloin Roast Boneless Separable Lean And Fat Trimmed To 0 Inch Fat All Grades Cooked Roasted ☞ serving size: 3 oz = 85 g; Calories = 155.6; Total Carb (g) = 0; Net Carb (g) = 0; Fat (g) = 6.9; Protein = 23.2

🐾 Beef Loin Top Loin Separable Lean And Fat Trimmed To 1/8 Inch Fat All Grades Cooked Grilled ☞ serving size: 3 oz = 85 g; Calories = 224.4; Total Carb (g) = 0; Net Carb (g) = 0; Fat (g) = 14.3; Protein = 22.5

🐾 Beef New Zealand Imported Ribs Prepared Raw ☞ serving size: 4 oz = 113 g; Calories = 165; Total Carb (g) = 0; Net Carb (g) = 0; Fat (g) = 7.7; Protein = 24.1

🐾 Beef Ns As To Cut Cooked Lean And Fat Eaten ☞ serving size: 1 oz, boneless, cooked = 28 g; Calories = 65.8; Total Carb (g) = 0; Net Carb (g) = 0; Fat (g) = 3.8; Protein = 7.6

🐾 Beef Ns As To Cut Cooked Lean Only Eaten ☞ serving size: 1 oz, boneless, cooked, lean only = 28 g; Calories = 51.5; Total Carb (g) = 0; Net Carb (g) = 0; Fat (g) = 1.9; Protein = 8.2

🐄 Beef Ns As To Cut Cooked Ns As To Fat Eaten ☞ serving size: 1 oz, boneless, cooked = 28 g; Calories = 51.5; Total Carb (g) = 0; Net Carb (g) = 0; Fat (g) = 1.9; Protein = 8.2

🐄 Beef Ns As To Cut Fried Ns To Fat Eaten ☞ serving size: 1 oz, boneless, cooked = 28 g; Calories = 51.5; Total Carb (g) = 0; Net Carb (g) = 0; Fat (g) = 1.9; Protein = 8.2

🐄 Beef Oxtails Cooked ☞ serving size: 1 oz, with bone, cooked (yield after bone removed) = 16 g; Calories = 40.2; Total Carb (g) = 0; Net Carb (g) = 0; Fat (g) = 2.1; Protein = 4.9

🐄 Beef Round Top Round Roast Boneless Separable Lean Only Trimmed To 0 Inch Fat Select Raw ☞ serving size: 3 oz = 85 g; Calories = 98.6; Total Carb (g) = 0; Net Carb (g) = 0; Fat (g) = 2.1; Protein = 20.1

🐄 Beef Round Top Round Separable Lean And Fat Trimmed To 0 Inch Fat All Grades Cooked Braised ☞ serving size: 3 oz = 85 g; Calories = 177.7; Total Carb (g) = 0; Net Carb (g) = 0; Fat (g) = 5.4; Protein = 30.3

🐄 Beef Sausage ☞ serving size: 1 patty = 35 g; Calories = 141.8; Total Carb (g) = 0; Net Carb (g) = 0; Fat (g) = 13.2; Protein = 5.4

🐄 Beef Sausage Fresh Cooked ☞ serving size: 1 serving = 43 g; Calories = 142.8; Total Carb (g) = 0.2; Net Carb (g) = 0.2; Fat (g) = 12; Protein = 7.8

🐄 Beef Sloppy Joe No Bun ☞ serving size: 1 cup = 251 g; Calories = 346.4; Total Carb (g) = 22; Net Carb (g) = 19.7; Fat (g) = 17; Protein = 27.1

🐄 Beef Steak Ns As To Cooking Method Ns As To Fat Eaten ☞ serving size: 1 oz, with bone, cooked (yield after bone removed) = 23 g; Calories = 42.3; Total Carb (g) = 0; Net Carb (g) = 0; Fat (g) = 1.6; Protein = 6.7

🐄 Berliner Sausage ☞ serving size: 1 slice = 23 g; Calories = 52.9;

Total Carb (g) = 0.6; Net Carb (g) = 0.6; Fat (g) = 4; Protein = 3.5

🐾 Bison Cooked ☞ serving size: 1 cup, cooked = 134 g; Calories = 190.3; Total Carb (g) = 0; Net Carb (g) = 0; Fat (g) = 3.2; Protein = 38

🐾 Bison Ground Grass-Fed Raw ☞ serving size: 1 patty (cooked from 4 oz raw) = 85 g; Calories = 124.1; Total Carb (g) = 0; Net Carb (g) = 0; Fat (g) = 6.1; Protein = 17.2

🐾 Blood Sausage ☞ serving size: 4 slices = 100 g; Calories = 379; Total Carb (g) = 1.3; Net Carb (g) = 1.3; Fat (g) = 34.5; Protein = 14.6

🐾 Bockwurst Pork Veal Raw ☞ serving size: 1 sausage = 91 g; Calories = 273.9; Total Carb (g) = 2.7; Net Carb (g) = 1.8; Fat (g) = 23.5; Protein = 12.8

🐾 Bologna Beef And Pork Low Fat ☞ serving size: 1 cup pieces = 138 g; Calories = 317.4; Total Carb (g) = 3.6; Net Carb (g) = 3.6; Fat (g) = 26.6; Protein = 15.9

🐾 Bratwurst Beef And Pork Smoked ☞ serving size: 1 serving 2.33 oz = 66 g; Calories = 196; Total Carb (g) = 1.3; Net Carb (g) = 1.3; Fat (g) = 17.4; Protein = 8.1

🐾 Brunswick Stew ☞ serving size: 1 cup = 243 g; Calories = 291.6; Total Carb (g) = 18.2; Net Carb (g) = 15.3; Fat (g) = 12.3; Protein = 27.6

🐾 Buffalo Sirloin Steak ☞ serving size: 1 serving (3 oz) = 85 g; Calories = 145.4; Total Carb (g) = 0; Net Carb (g) = 0; Fat (g) = 4.8; Protein = 23.8

🐾 Canada Goose Breast Meat Skinless Raw ☞ serving size: 3 oz = 85 g; Calories = 113.1; Total Carb (g) = 0; Net Carb (g) = 0; Fat (g) = 3.4; Protein = 20.7

🐾 Canadian Bacon (Pan-Fried) ☞ serving size: 1 slice = 13.8 g; Calories = 20.1; Total Carb (g) = 0.3; Net Carb (g) = 0.3; Fat (g) = 0.4; Protein = 3.9

🐾 Canadian Bacon (Raw) ☞ serving size: 3 oz = 85 g; Calories =

93.5; Total Carb (g) = 1.1; Net Carb (g) = 1.1; Fat (g) = 2.2; Protein = 17.3

🍖 Canned Ham ☞ serving size: 1 oz = 28.4 g; Calories = 67.9; Total Carb (g) = 0.1; Net Carb (g) = 0.1; Fat (g) = 5.4; Protein = 4.6

🍖 Caribou Cooked ☞ serving size: 1 oz, boneless, cooked = 28 g; Calories = 46.5; Total Carb (g) = 0; Net Carb (g) = 0; Fat (g) = 1.2; Protein = 8.3

🍖 Cassava Pasteles Puerto Rican Style ☞ serving size: 1 pastel (6" x 2" x 1/2") = 145 g; Calories = 368.3; Total Carb (g) = 27.6; Net Carb (g) = 25.7; Fat (g) = 24.6; Protein = 9.7

🍖 Cheesefurter Cheese Smokie Pork Beef ☞ serving size: 2 (1/3) links = 100 g; Calories = 328; Total Carb (g) = 1.5; Net Carb (g) = 1.5; Fat (g) = 29; Protein = 14.1

🍖 Chicken "wings" Boneless With Hot Sauce From Fast Food / Restaurant ☞ serving size: 1 boneless wing = 35 g; Calories = 98.4; Total Carb (g) = 7; Net Carb (g) = 6.7; Fat (g) = 5.9; Protein = 4.3

🍖 Chicken "wings" Boneless With Hot Sauce From Other Sources ☞ serving size: 1 boneless wing = 35 g; Calories = 80.9; Total Carb (g) = 7; Net Carb (g) = 6.5; Fat (g) = 4.1; Protein = 4

🍖 Chicken "wings" Plain From Fast Food / Restaurant ☞ serving size: 1 drummette = 22 g; Calories = 70.8; Total Carb (g) = 3.3; Net Carb (g) = 3.2; Fat (g) = 4.7; Protein = 3.9

🍖 Chicken Broiler Rotisserie BBQ Back Meat And Skin ☞ serving size: 3 oz = 85 g; Calories = 213.4; Total Carb (g) = 0.3; Net Carb (g) = 0.3; Fat (g) = 16; Protein = 17.3

🍖 Chicken Broiler Rotisserie BBQ Back Meat Only ☞ serving size: 3 oz = 85 g; Calories = 180.2; Total Carb (g) = 0.3; Net Carb (g) = 0.3; Fat (g) = 11.8; Protein = 18.6

🍖 Chicken Broiler Rotisserie BBQ Breast Meat And Skin ☞ serving size: 3 oz = 85 g; Calories = 148.8; Total Carb (g) = 0.1; Net Carb (g) = 0.1; Fat (g) = 6.5; Protein = 22.4

🍖 Chicken Broiler Rotisserie BBQ Breast Meat Only ☞ serving size: 3 oz = 85 g; Calories = 122.4; Total Carb (g) = 0; Net Carb (g) = 0; Fat (g) = 3; Protein = 23.8

🍖 Chicken Broiler Rotisserie BBQ Drumstick Meat And Skin ☞ serving size: 1 drumstick = 71 g; Calories = 146.3; Total Carb (g) = 0.1; Net Carb (g) = 0.1; Fat (g) = 8.1; Protein = 18.2

🍖 Chicken Broiler Rotisserie BBQ Drumstick Meat Only ☞ serving size: 1 drumstick = 71 g; Calories = 122.1; Total Carb (g) = 0; Net Carb (g) = 0; Fat (g) = 4.8; Protein = 19.7

🍖 Chicken Broiler Rotisserie BBQ Skin ☞ serving size: 1 serving = 85 g; Calories = 321.3; Total Carb (g) = 0.6; Net Carb (g) = 0.6; Fat (g) = 29.9; Protein = 12.9

🍖 Chicken Broiler Rotisserie BBQ Thigh Meat And Skin ☞ serving size: 1 thigh = 95 g; Calories = 214.7; Total Carb (g) = 0.1; Net Carb (g) = 0.1; Fat (g) = 14.3; Protein = 21.4

🍖 Chicken Broiler Rotisserie BBQ Thigh Meat Only ☞ serving size: 1 thigh = 95 g; Calories = 183.4; Total Carb (g) = 0; Net Carb (g) = 0; Fat (g) = 10.2; Protein = 22.9

🍖 Chicken Fillet Grilled ☞ serving size: 1 fillet = 100 g; Calories = 145; Total Carb (g) = 2.4; Net Carb (g) = 2.3; Fat (g) = 5.2; Protein = 22.2

🍖 Chicken Ground Raw ☞ serving size: 4 oz crumbled = 112 g; Calories = 160.2; Total Carb (g) = 0; Net Carb (g) = 0; Fat (g) = 9.1; Protein = 19.5

🍖 Chicken Heart All Classes Cooked Simmered ☞ serving size: 1 cup, chopped or diced = 145 g; Calories = 268.3; Total Carb (g) = 0.2; Net Carb (g) = 0.2; Fat (g) = 11.5; Protein = 38.3

🍖 Chicken Heart All Classes Raw ☞ serving size: 1 heart = 6.1 g; Calories = 9.3; Total Carb (g) = 0; Net Carb (g) = 0; Fat (g) = 0.6; Protein = 1

🍖 Chicken Hotdog ☞ serving size: 3 oz = 85 g; Calories = 189.6; Total Carb (g) = 2.3; Net Carb (g) = 2.3; Fat (g) = 13.8; Protein = 13.2

🍖 Chicken Leg Drumstick And Thigh Stewed Skin Not Eaten ☞ serving size: 1 cup, cooked, diced = 135 g; Calories = 221.4; Total Carb (g) = 0; Net Carb (g) = 0; Fat (g) = 10.1; Protein = 32.6

🍖 Chicken Liver All Classes Cooked Pan-Fried ☞ serving size: 1 liver = 44 g; Calories = 75.7; Total Carb (g) = 0.5; Net Carb (g) = 0.5; Fat (g) = 2.8; Protein = 11.3

🍖 Chorizo ☞ serving size: 1 oz = 28.4 g; Calories = 84.1; Total Carb (g) = 1.1; Net Carb (g) = 1.1; Fat (g) = 7.1; Protein = 3.9

🍖 Cornish Game Hen Cooked Skin Eaten ☞ serving size: 1 hen (1-1/4 lb, raw) (yield after cooking, bone removed) = 305 g; Calories = 783.9; Total Carb (g) = 0; Net Carb (g) = 0; Fat (g) = 55.1; Protein = 67.3

🍖 Cornish Game Hen Cooked Skin Not Eaten ☞ serving size: 1 hen (1-1/4 lb, raw) (yield after cooking, bone and skin removed) = 250 g; Calories = 332.5; Total Carb (g) = 0; Net Carb (g) = 0; Fat (g) = 9.6; Protein = 57.8

🍖 Deer Chop Cooked ☞ serving size: 1 oz, with bone, cooked (yield after bone removed) = 23 g; Calories = 44.4; Total Carb (g) = 0; Net Carb (g) = 0; Fat (g) = 1.9; Protein = 6.5

🍖 Dove Cooked (Includes Squab) ☞ serving size: 1 cup, chopped or diced = 140 g; Calories = 298.2; Total Carb (g) = 0; Net Carb (g) = 0; Fat (g) = 18.2; Protein = 33.5

🍖 Dove Cooked Ns As To Cooking Method ☞ serving size: 1 dove (yield after cooking, bone removed) = 110 g; Calories = 233.2; Total Carb (g) = 0; Net Carb (g) = 0; Fat (g) = 14.3; Protein = 26.2

🍖 Dove Fried ☞ serving size: 1 dove (yield after cooking, bone removed) = 110 g; Calories = 245.3; Total Carb (g) = 1.6; Net Carb (g) = 1.6; Fat (g) = 15.2; Protein = 25.4

🍖 Dry Pork And Beef Salami ☞ serving size: 1 slice = 9.8 g; Calories = 37; Total Carb (g) = 0.1; Net Carb (g) = 0.1; Fat (g) = 3.1; Protein = 2.1

🐾 Dry Pork Salami ☞ serving size: 1 package (4 oz) = 113 g; Calories = 459.9; Total Carb (g) = 1.8; Net Carb (g) = 1.8; Fat (g) = 38.1; Protein = 25.5

🐾 Duck Coated Fried ☞ serving size: 1 leg (drumstick and thigh) (yield after cooking, bone removed) = 115 g; Calories = 258.8; Total Carb (g) = 9.1; Net Carb (g) = 8.9; Fat (g) = 12.6; Protein = 25.7

🐾 Duck Cooked Skin Eaten ☞ serving size: 1/2 duck (yield after cooking, bone removed) = 380 g; Calories = 1276.8; Total Carb (g) = 0; Net Carb (g) = 0; Fat (g) = 107.3; Protein = 71.9

🐾 Duck Cooked Skin Not Eaten ☞ serving size: 1/2 duck (yield after cooking, bone and skin removed) = 220 g; Calories = 440; Total Carb (g) = 0; Net Carb (g) = 0; Fat (g) = 24.5; Protein = 51.4

🐾 Duck Domesticated Liver Raw ☞ serving size: 1 liver = 44 g; Calories = 59.8; Total Carb (g) = 1.6; Net Carb (g) = 1.6; Fat (g) = 2; Protein = 8.3

🐾 Duck Domesticated Meat And Skin Cooked Roasted ☞ serving size: 1 cup, chopped or diced = 140 g; Calories = 471.8; Total Carb (g) = 0; Net Carb (g) = 0; Fat (g) = 39.7; Protein = 26.6

🐾 Duck Domesticated Meat And Skin Raw ☞ serving size: 3 oz = 85 g; Calories = 343.4; Total Carb (g) = 0; Net Carb (g) = 0; Fat (g) = 33.4; Protein = 9.8

🐾 Duck Domesticated Meat Only Raw ☞ serving size: 1 unit (yield from 1 lb ready-to-cook duck) = 137 g; Calories = 185; Total Carb (g) = 1.3; Net Carb (g) = 1.3; Fat (g) = 8.2; Protein = 25

🐾 Duck Pressed Chinese ☞ serving size: 1 oz, cooked = 28 g; Calories = 42.8; Total Carb (g) = 1.9; Net Carb (g) = 1.8; Fat (g) = 3.3; Protein = 1.5

🐾 Emu Fan Fillet Raw ☞ serving size: 1 serving (3 oz) = 85 g; Calories = 87.6; Total Carb (g) = 0; Net Carb (g) = 0; Fat (g) = 0.7; Protein = 19.1

🐾 Emu Inside Drum Raw ☞ serving size: 3 oz = 85 g; Calories = 91.8; Total Carb (g) = 0; Net Carb (g) = 0; Fat (g) = 1.3; Protein = 18.9

🐾 Emu Inside Drums Cooked Broiled ☞ serving size: 1 serving (3 oz) = 85 g; Calories = 132.6; Total Carb (g) = 0; Net Carb (g) = 0; Fat (g) = 1.7; Protein = 27.5

🐾 Emu Outside Drum Raw ☞ serving size: 3 oz = 85 g; Calories = 87.6; Total Carb (g) = 0; Net Carb (g) = 0; Fat (g) = 0.4; Protein = 19.6

🐾 Emu Oyster Raw ☞ serving size: 3 oz = 85 g; Calories = 119.9; Total Carb (g) = 0; Net Carb (g) = 0; Fat (g) = 4.1; Protein = 19.4

🐾 Emu Steak ☞ serving size: 1 serving (3 oz) = 85 g; Calories = 130.9; Total Carb (g) = 0; Net Carb (g) = 0; Fat (g) = 2; Protein = 26.6

🐾 Fat Free Ground Turkey ☞ serving size: 3 oz = 85 g; Calories = 128.4; Total Carb (g) = 0; Net Carb (g) = 0; Fat (g) = 2.3; Protein = 26.9

🐾 Frankfurter Beef Heated ☞ serving size: 1 frankfurter = 48 g; Calories = 154.6; Total Carb (g) = 1.3; Net Carb (g) = 1.3; Fat (g) = 14.1; Protein = 5.6

🐾 Game Meat Beaver Raw ☞ serving size: 1 oz = 28.4 g; Calories = 41.5; Total Carb (g) = 0; Net Carb (g) = 0; Fat (g) = 1.4; Protein = 6.8

🐾 Game Meat Beefalo Composite Of Cuts Cooked Roasted ☞ serving size: 3 oz = 85 g; Calories = 159.8; Total Carb (g) = 0; Net Carb (g) = 0; Fat (g) = 5.4; Protein = 26.1

🐾 Game Meat Beefalo Composite Of Cuts Raw ☞ serving size: 1 oz = 28.4 g; Calories = 40.6; Total Carb (g) = 0; Net Carb (g) = 0; Fat (g) = 1.4; Protein = 6.6

🐾 Game Meat Bison Chuck Shoulder Clod Separable Lean Only Cooked Braised ☞ serving size: 1 serving (3 oz) = 85 g; Calories = 164.1; Total Carb (g) = 0; Net Carb (g) = 0; Fat (g) = 4.6; Protein = 28.7

🥩 Game Meat Bison Chuck Shoulder Clod Separable Lean Only Raw ☞ serving size: 1 serving (3 oz) = 85 g; Calories = 101.2; Total Carb (g) = 0; Net Carb (g) = 0; Fat (g) = 2.7; Protein = 18

🥩 Ground Beef Patty Cooked ☞ serving size: 1 miniature patty = 20 g; Calories = 54.4; Total Carb (g) = 0; Net Carb (g) = 0; Fat (g) = 3.6; Protein = 5.1

🥩 Ground Beef Raw ☞ serving size: 1 oz = 28 g; Calories = 69.2; Total Carb (g) = 0; Net Carb (g) = 0; Fat (g) = 5.3; Protein = 4.9

🥩 Ham Smoked Or Cured Canned Ns As To Fat Eaten ☞ serving size: 1 thin slice (approx 4-1/2" x 2-1/2" x 1/8") = 21 g; Calories = 27.7; Total Carb (g) = 0.2; Net Carb (g) = 0.2; Fat (g) = 1.3; Protein = 3.7

🥩 Ham Stroganoff ☞ serving size: 1 cup = 244 g; Calories = 317.2; Total Carb (g) = 12.1; Net Carb (g) = 10.4; Fat (g) = 22.1; Protein = 18.4

🥩 Lamb Ribs ☞ serving size: 3 oz = 85 g; Calories = 305.2; Total Carb (g) = 0; Net Carb (g) = 0; Fat (g) = 25.4; Protein = 18

🥩 Lamb Roast Cooked Ns As To Fat Eaten ☞ serving size: 1 thin slice (approx 3" dia x 1/8") = 14 g; Calories = 37.1; Total Carb (g) = 0; Net Carb (g) = 0; Fat (g) = 2.5; Protein = 3.3

🥩 Lamb Shank ☞ serving size: 3 oz = 85 g; Calories = 153; Total Carb (g) = 0; Net Carb (g) = 0; Fat (g) = 5.7; Protein = 23.9

🥩 Lamb Sirloin ☞ serving size: 3 oz = 85 g; Calories = 173.4; Total Carb (g) = 0; Net Carb (g) = 0; Fat (g) = 7.8; Protein = 24.1

🥩 Lamb Variety Meats And By-Products Brain Cooked Braised ☞ serving size: 3 oz = 85 g; Calories = 123.3; Total Carb (g) = 0; Net Carb (g) = 0; Fat (g) = 8.6; Protein = 10.7

🥩 Lamb Variety Meats And By-Products Brain Cooked Pan-Fried ☞ serving size: 3 oz = 85 g; Calories = 232.1; Total Carb (g) = 0; Net Carb (g) = 0; Fat (g) = 18.9; Protein = 14.4

🥩 Lamb Variety Meats And By-Products Brain Raw ☞ serving size:

1 oz = 28.4 g; Calories = 34.6; Total Carb (g) = 0; Net Carb (g) = 0; Fat (g) = 2.4; Protein = 3

🍖 Lamb Variety Meats And By-Products Heart Cooked Braised ☞ serving size: 3 oz = 85 g; Calories = 157.3; Total Carb (g) = 1.6; Net Carb (g) = 1.6; Fat (g) = 6.7; Protein = 21.2

🍖 Lamb Variety Meats And By-Products Heart Raw ☞ serving size: 1 oz = 28.4 g; Calories = 34.6; Total Carb (g) = 0.1; Net Carb (g) = 0.1; Fat (g) = 1.6; Protein = 4.7

🍖 Lamb Variety Meats And By-Products Kidneys Cooked Braised ☞ serving size: 3 oz = 85 g; Calories = 116.5; Total Carb (g) = 0.8; Net Carb (g) = 0.8; Fat (g) = 3.1; Protein = 20.1

🍖 Lamb Variety Meats And By-Products Kidneys Raw ☞ serving size: 1 oz = 28.4 g; Calories = 27.5; Total Carb (g) = 0.2; Net Carb (g) = 0.2; Fat (g) = 0.8; Protein = 4.5

🍖 Lamb Variety Meats And By-Products Liver Cooked Braised ☞ serving size: 3 oz = 85 g; Calories = 187; Total Carb (g) = 2.2; Net Carb (g) = 2.2; Fat (g) = 7.5; Protein = 26

🍖 Lamb Variety Meats And By-Products Liver Raw ☞ serving size: 1 oz = 28.4 g; Calories = 39.5; Total Carb (g) = 0.5; Net Carb (g) = 0.5; Fat (g) = 1.4; Protein = 5.8

🍖 Lamb Variety Meats And By-Products Lungs Cooked Braised ☞ serving size: 3 oz = 85 g; Calories = 96.1; Total Carb (g) = 0; Net Carb (g) = 0; Fat (g) = 2.6; Protein = 16.9

🍖 Lamb Variety Meats And By-Products Lungs Raw ☞ serving size: 1 oz = 28.4 g; Calories = 27; Total Carb (g) = 0; Net Carb (g) = 0; Fat (g) = 0.7; Protein = 4.7

🍖 Lamb Variety Meats And By-Products Mechanically Separated Raw ☞ serving size: 1 oz = 28.4 g; Calories = 78.4; Total Carb (g) = 0; Net Carb (g) = 0; Fat (g) = 6.7; Protein = 4.3

🍖 Lamb Variety Meats And By-Products Pancreas Cooked Braised

☞ serving size: 3 oz = 85 g; Calories = 198.9; Total Carb (g) = 0; Net Carb (g) = 0; Fat (g) = 12.9; Protein = 19.4

🍖 Lamb Variety Meats And By-Products Pancreas Raw ☞ serving size: 1 oz = 28.4 g; Calories = 43.2; Total Carb (g) = 0; Net Carb (g) = 0; Fat (g) = 2.8; Protein = 4.2

🍖 Lamb Variety Meats And By-Products Spleen Cooked Braised ☞ serving size: 3 oz = 85 g; Calories = 132.6; Total Carb (g) = 0; Net Carb (g) = 0; Fat (g) = 4.1; Protein = 22.5

🍖 Lamb Variety Meats And By-Products Spleen Raw ☞ serving size: 1 oz = 28.4 g; Calories = 28.7; Total Carb (g) = 0; Net Carb (g) = 0; Fat (g) = 0.9; Protein = 4.9

🍖 Lamb Variety Meats And By-Products Tongue Cooked Braised ☞ serving size: 3 oz = 85 g; Calories = 233.8; Total Carb (g) = 0; Net Carb (g) = 0; Fat (g) = 17.2; Protein = 18.3

🍖 Lamb Variety Meats And By-Products Tongue Raw ☞ serving size: 1 oz = 28.4 g; Calories = 63; Total Carb (g) = 0; Net Carb (g) = 0; Fat (g) = 4.9; Protein = 4.5

🍖 Lean Chicken Breast (Cooked) ☞ serving size: 3 oz = 85 g; Calories = 133.5; Total Carb (g) = 0; Net Carb (g) = 0; Fat (g) = 2.8; Protein = 27.3

🍖 Lean Cured Ham ☞ serving size: 1 cup = 140 g; Calories = 203; Total Carb (g) = 2.1; Net Carb (g) = 2.1; Fat (g) = 7.7; Protein = 29.3

🍖 Lean Grass Fed Beef Strip Steak ☞ serving size: 3 oz = 85 g; Calories = 99.5; Total Carb (g) = 0; Net Carb (g) = 0; Fat (g) = 2.3; Protein = 19.6

🍖 Lowfat Pastrami ☞ serving size: 1 serving 6 slices = 57 g; Calories = 54.2; Total Carb (g) = 0.9; Net Carb (g) = 0.9; Fat (g) = 0.7; Protein = 11.2

🍖 Luncheon Meat Pork And Chicken Minced Canned Includes Spam Lite ☞ serving size: 2 oz (1 serving) = 56 g; Calories =

109.8; Total Carb (g) = 0.8; Net Carb (g) = 0.8; Fat (g) = 7.8; Protein = 8.5

🦐 Luncheon Meat Pork Canned ☞ serving size: 1 oz = 28.4 g; Calories = 94.9; Total Carb (g) = 0.6; Net Carb (g) = 0.6; Fat (g) = 8.6; Protein = 3.6

🦐 Meat Loaf Made With Beef ☞ serving size: 1 small or thin slice = 86 g; Calories = 171.1; Total Carb (g) = 6.2; Net Carb (g) = 5.8; Fat (g) = 9.2; Protein = 15

🦐 Meat Loaf Made With Beef And Pork ☞ serving size: 1 small or thin slice = 86 g; Calories = 168.6; Total Carb (g) = 6.2; Net Carb (g) = 5.8; Fat (g) = 9; Protein = 14.8

🦐 Meat Loaf Ns As To Type Of Meat ☞ serving size: 1 small or thin slice = 86 g; Calories = 173.7; Total Carb (g) = 6.2; Net Carb (g) = 5.8; Fat (g) = 9.4; Protein = 15

🦐 Meat Loaf Puerto Rican Style ☞ serving size: 1 serving (3" x 1" x 2") = 95 g; Calories = 306.9; Total Carb (g) = 10.1; Net Carb (g) = 9.5; Fat (g) = 20.7; Protein = 18.8

🦐 Mortadella Beef Pork ☞ serving size: 1 oz = 28.4 g; Calories = 88.3; Total Carb (g) = 0.9; Net Carb (g) = 0.9; Fat (g) = 7.2; Protein = 4.7

🦐 Ostrich Cooked ☞ serving size: 1 oz, cooked = 28 g; Calories = 48.7; Total Carb (g) = 0; Net Carb (g) = 0; Fat (g) = 2; Protein = 7.3

🦐 Ostrich Fan Raw ☞ serving size: 1 serving (cooked from 4oz raw) = 85 g; Calories = 99.5; Total Carb (g) = 0; Net Carb (g) = 0; Fat (g) = 2.3; Protein = 18.5

🦐 Ostrich Ground Cooked Pan-Broiled ☞ serving size: 1 patty = 93 g; Calories = 162.8; Total Carb (g) = 0; Net Carb (g) = 0; Fat (g) = 6.6; Protein = 24.3

🦐 Ostrich Ground Raw ☞ serving size: 1 patty = 109 g; Calories = 179.9; Total Carb (g) = 0; Net Carb (g) = 0; Fat (g) = 9.5; Protein = 22

🍖 Ostrich Top Loin Raw ☞ serving size: 1 serving (cooked from 4 oz raw) = 85 g; Calories = 101.2; Total Carb (g) = 0; Net Carb (g) = 0; Fat (g) = 2.5; Protein = 18.4

🍖 Pastrami Turkey ☞ serving size: 2 slices = 57 g; Calories = 79.2; Total Carb (g) = 1.9; Net Carb (g) = 1.9; Fat (g) = 3.5; Protein = 9.3

🍖 Pate Chicken Liver Canned ☞ serving size: 1 tbsp = 13 g; Calories = 26.1; Total Carb (g) = 0.9; Net Carb (g) = 0.9; Fat (g) = 1.7; Protein = 1.8

🍖 Pate De Foie Gras Canned (Goose Liver Pate) Smoked ☞ serving size: 1 tbsp = 13 g; Calories = 60.1; Total Carb (g) = 0.6; Net Carb (g) = 0.6; Fat (g) = 5.7; Protein = 1.5

🍖 Pate Goose Liver Smoked Canned ☞ serving size: 1 tbsp = 13 g; Calories = 60.1; Total Carb (g) = 0.6; Net Carb (g) = 0.6; Fat (g) = 5.7; Protein = 1.5

🍖 Pate Liver Not Specified Canned ☞ serving size: 1 tbsp = 13 g; Calories = 41.5; Total Carb (g) = 0.2; Net Carb (g) = 0.2; Fat (g) = 3.6; Protein = 1.9

🍖 Pate Truffle Flavor ☞ serving size: 1 serving 2 oz = 56 g; Calories = 183.1; Total Carb (g) = 3.5; Net Carb (g) = 3.5; Fat (g) = 16; Protein = 6.3

🍖 Pepper Steak ☞ serving size: 1 cup = 217 g; Calories = 310.3; Total Carb (g) = 9.5; Net Carb (g) = 7.9; Fat (g) = 19.5; Protein = 25.7

🍖 Peppered Loaf Pork Beef ☞ serving size: 3 (1/2) slices = 100 g; Calories = 149; Total Carb (g) = 4.5; Net Carb (g) = 4.5; Fat (g) = 6.4; Protein = 17.3

🍖 Pepperoni ☞ serving size: 3 oz = 85 g; Calories = 428.4; Total Carb (g) = 1; Net Carb (g) = 1; Fat (g) = 39.3; Protein = 16.4

🍖 Pheasant Breast Meat Only Raw ☞ serving size: 3 oz = 85 g; Calories = 113.1; Total Carb (g) = 0; Net Carb (g) = 0; Fat (g) = 2.8; Protein = 20.7

🍃 Pheasant Cooked ☞ serving size: 1/2 pheasant breast (yield after cooking, bone removed) = 130 g; Calories = 309.4; Total Carb (g) = 0; Net Carb (g) = 0; Fat (g) = 15.7; Protein = 41.9

🍃 Pheasant Cooked Total Edible ☞ serving size: 1 cup, chopped or diced = 140 g; Calories = 334.6; Total Carb (g) = 0; Net Carb (g) = 0; Fat (g) = 16.9; Protein = 45.4

🍃 Pheasant Leg Meat Only Raw ☞ serving size: 1 unit (yield from 1 lb ready-to-eat pheasant) = 99 g; Calories = 132.7; Total Carb (g) = 0; Net Carb (g) = 0; Fat (g) = 4.3; Protein = 22

🍃 Pheasant Raw Meat And Skin ☞ serving size: 3 oz = 85 g; Calories = 153.9; Total Carb (g) = 0; Net Carb (g) = 0; Fat (g) = 7.9; Protein = 19.3

🍃 Pork Fresh Ground Raw ☞ serving size: 1 oz = 28.4 g; Calories = 74.7; Total Carb (g) = 0; Net Carb (g) = 0; Fat (g) = 6; Protein = 4.8

🍃 Salami ☞ serving size: 1 oz = 28 g; Calories = 119; Total Carb (g) = 0.3; Net Carb (g) = 0.3; Fat (g) = 10.4; Protein = 6.1

🍃 Salami Cooked Beef ☞ serving size: 1 slice = 26 g; Calories = 67.9; Total Carb (g) = 0.5; Net Carb (g) = 0.5; Fat (g) = 5.8; Protein = 3.3

🍃 Salami Cooked Beef And Pork ☞ serving size: 1 slice round = 12.3 g; Calories = 41.3; Total Carb (g) = 0.3; Net Carb (g) = 0.3; Fat (g) = 3.2; Protein = 2.7

🍃 Salami Italian Pork And Beef Dry Sliced 50% Less Sodium ☞ serving size: 1 serving 5 slices = 28 g; Calories = 98; Total Carb (g) = 1.8; Net Carb (g) = 1.8; Fat (g) = 7.4; Protein = 6.1

🍃 Salami Pork Beef Less Sodium ☞ serving size: 3 (1/2) oz = 100 g; Calories = 396; Total Carb (g) = 15.4; Net Carb (g) = 15.2; Fat (g) = 30.5; Protein = 15

🍃 Salisbury Steak Baked With Tomato Sauce Vegetable Diet Frozen Meal ☞ serving size: 1 meal (9.5 oz) = 269 g; Calories = 285.1; Total Carb (g) = 13.1; Net Carb (g) = 10.9; Fat (g) = 15.2; Protein = 23.8

🍖 Salisbury Steak Dinner NFS Frozen Meal ☞ serving size: 1 meal (11 oz) = 312 g; Calories = 458.6; Total Carb (g) = 35.1; Net Carb (g) = 31; Fat (g) = 26.3; Protein = 21.6

🍖 Skirt Steak ☞ serving size: 3 oz = 85 g; Calories = 227.8; Total Carb (g) = 0; Net Carb (g) = 0; Fat (g) = 14.5; Protein = 24.4

🍖 Squab (Pigeon) Light Meat Without Skin Raw ☞ serving size: 1 breast, bone removed = 101 g; Calories = 135.3; Total Carb (g) = 0; Net Carb (g) = 0; Fat (g) = 4.6; Protein = 22

🍖 Squab (Pigeon) Meat And Skin Raw ☞ serving size: 3 oz = 85 g; Calories = 249.9; Total Carb (g) = 0; Net Carb (g) = 0; Fat (g) = 20.2; Protein = 15.7

🍖 Squab (Pigeon) Meat Only Raw ☞ serving size: 1 unit (yield from 1 lb ready-to-cook squab) = 251 g; Calories = 356.4; Total Carb (g) = 0; Net Carb (g) = 0; Fat (g) = 18.8; Protein = 43.9

🍖 Squirrel Cooked ☞ serving size: 1 oz, with bone, cooked (yield after bone removed) = 23 g; Calories = 39.6; Total Carb (g) = 0; Net Carb (g) = 0; Fat (g) = 1.1; Protein = 7.1

🍖 Tripe Cooked ☞ serving size: 1 oz, raw (yield after cooking) = 16 g; Calories = 14.2; Total Carb (g) = 0; Net Carb (g) = 0; Fat (g) = 0.6; Protein = 2

🍖 Turkey All Classes Back Meat And Skin Cooked Roasted ☞ serving size: 1 cup, chopped or diced = 140 g; Calories = 341.6; Total Carb (g) = 0.2; Net Carb (g) = 0.2; Fat (g) = 20.1; Protein = 37.2

🍖 Turkey All Classes Breast Meat And Skin Cooked Roasted ☞ serving size: 1 unit (yield from 1 lb ready-to-cook turkey) = 112 g; Calories = 211.7; Total Carb (g) = 0; Net Carb (g) = 0; Fat (g) = 8.3; Protein = 32.2

🍖 Turkey All Classes Breast Meat And Skin Raw ☞ serving size: 1 unit (yield from 1 lb ready-to-cook turkey) = 146 g; Calories = 229.2; Total Carb (g) = 0; Net Carb (g) = 0; Fat (g) = 10.3; Protein = 32

🦃 Turkey All Classes Leg Meat And Skin Cooked Roasted ☞ serving size: 1 unit (yield from 1 lb ready-to-cook turkey) = 71 g; Calories = 147.7; Total Carb (g) = 0; Net Carb (g) = 0; Fat (g) = 7; Protein = 19.8

🦃 Turkey All Classes Leg Meat And Skin Raw ☞ serving size: 1 unit (yield from 1 lb ready-to-cook turkey) = 105 g; Calories = 151.2; Total Carb (g) = 0; Net Carb (g) = 0; Fat (g) = 7.1; Protein = 20.5

🦃 Turkey All Classes Wing Meat And Skin Cooked Roasted ☞ serving size: 1 unit (yield from 1 lb ready-to-cook turkey) = 24 g; Calories = 55; Total Carb (g) = 0; Net Carb (g) = 0; Fat (g) = 3; Protein = 6.6

🦃 Turkey All Classes Wing Meat And Skin Raw ☞ serving size: 1 unit (yield from 1 lb ready-to-cook turkey) = 33 g; Calories = 65; Total Carb (g) = 0; Net Carb (g) = 0; Fat (g) = 4.1; Protein = 6.7

🦃 Turkey And Gravy Frozen ☞ serving size: 3 oz = 85 g; Calories = 57; Total Carb (g) = 3.9; Net Carb (g) = 3.9; Fat (g) = 2.2; Protein = 5

🦃 Turkey And Pork Sausage Fresh Bulk Patty Or Link Cooked ☞ serving size: 1 cup, cooked = 130 g; Calories = 399.1; Total Carb (g) = 0.9; Net Carb (g) = 0.9; Fat (g) = 29.9; Protein = 29.5

🦃 Turkey Back ☞ serving size: 1 back (yield after cooking, bone removed) = 525 g; Calories = 1065.8; Total Carb (g) = 0; Net Carb (g) = 0; Fat (g) = 59.1; Protein = 134.3

🦃 Turkey Breast From Whole Bird Meat Only Raw ☞ serving size: 4 oz = 114 g; Calories = 130; Total Carb (g) = 0.2; Net Carb (g) = 0.2; Fat (g) = 1.7; Protein = 27

🦃 Turkey Breast Smoked Lemon Pepper Flavor 97% Fat-Free ☞ serving size: 1 slice = 28 g; Calories = 26.6; Total Carb (g) = 0.4; Net Carb (g) = 0.4; Fat (g) = 0.2; Protein = 5.9

🦃 Turkey Canned Meat Only With Broth ☞ serving size: 1 cup,

drained = 135 g; Calories = 228.2; Total Carb (g) = 2; Net Carb (g) = 2; Fat (g) = 9.3; Protein = 32

🖎 Turkey Dark Meat From Whole Meat And Skin Cooked Roasted ☞ serving size: 1 serving = 85 g; Calories = 175.1; Total Carb (g) = 0.1; Net Carb (g) = 0.1; Fat (g) = 8.5; Protein = 23.2

🖎 Turkey Dark Meat From Whole Meat And Skin With Added Solution Cooked Roasted ☞ serving size: 3 oz = 85 g; Calories = 169.2; Total Carb (g) = 0; Net Carb (g) = 0; Fat (g) = 9.2; Protein = 21.7

🖎 Turkey Dark Meat From Whole Meat And Skin With Added Solution Raw ☞ serving size: 4 oz = 114 g; Calories = 192.7; Total Carb (g) = 0.2; Net Carb (g) = 0.2; Fat (g) = 12.4; Protein = 20.3

🖎 Veal Breast Plate Half Boneless Separable Lean And Fat Cooked Braised ☞ serving size: 3 oz = 85 g; Calories = 239.7; Total Carb (g) = 0; Net Carb (g) = 0; Fat (g) = 16.1; Protein = 22

🖎 Veal Chop Ns As To Cooking Method Lean And Fat Eaten ☞ serving size: 1 small chop (4.75 oz, with bone, raw) (yield after cooking, bone removed) = 78 g; Calories = 167.7; Total Carb (g) = 0; Net Carb (g) = 0; Fat (g) = 9.5; Protein = 19.2

🖎 Veal Chop Ns As To Cooking Method Lean Only Eaten ☞ serving size: 1 small chop (4.75 oz, with bone, raw) (yield after cooking, bone and fat removed) = 62 g; Calories = 107.9; Total Carb (g) = 0; Net Carb (g) = 0; Fat (g) = 4.3; Protein = 16.2

🖎 Veal Cordon Bleu ☞ serving size: 1 roll (with ham and sauce) = 229 g; Calories = 593.1; Total Carb (g) = 22; Net Carb (g) = 20.4; Fat (g) = 33.9; Protein = 47.4

🖎 Veal Ground Or Patty Cooked ☞ serving size: 1 small patty (3.2 oz, raw, 5 patties per lb) (yield after cooking) = 54 g; Calories = 92.3; Total Carb (g) = 0; Net Carb (g) = 0; Fat (g) = 4.1; Protein = 13.1

🖎 Veal Ground Raw ☞ serving size: 3 oz = 85 g; Calories = 167.5; Total Carb (g) = 0; Net Carb (g) = 0; Fat (g) = 11.1; Protein = 15.8

🍖 Veal Ns As To Cut Cooked Lean And Fat Eaten ☞ serving size: 1 oz, with bone, cooked (yield after bone removed) = 23 g; Calories = 52.7; Total Carb (g) = 0; Net Carb (g) = 0; Fat (g) = 2.6; Protein = 6.9

🍖 Veal Ns As To Cut Cooked Lean Only Eaten ☞ serving size: 1 oz, with bone, cooked, lean only (yield after bone removed) = 22 g; Calories = 42.7; Total Carb (g) = 0; Net Carb (g) = 0; Fat (g) = 1.4; Protein = 7

🍖 Veal Ns As To Cut Cooked Ns As To Fat Eaten ☞ serving size: 1 oz, with bone, cooked (yield after bone removed) = 23 g; Calories = 52.7; Total Carb (g) = 0; Net Carb (g) = 0; Fat (g) = 2.6; Protein = 6.9

🍖 Venison/deer Cured ☞ serving size: 1 oz, boneless, cooked = 28 g; Calories = 52.4; Total Carb (g) = 0; Net Carb (g) = 0; Fat (g) = 1.1; Protein = 9.8

🍖 Venison/deer Jerky ☞ serving size: 1 strip or stick (4" long) = 14 g; Calories = 55.4; Total Carb (g) = 2.1; Net Carb (g) = 2.1; Fat (g) = 3.1; Protein = 4.5

🍖 Venison/deer Nfs ☞ serving size: 1 oz, boneless, cooked = 28 g; Calories = 53.2; Total Carb (g) = 0; Net Carb (g) = 0; Fat (g) = 1.1; Protein = 10.1

🍖 Venison/deer Steak Cooked Ns As To Cooking Method ☞ serving size: 1 oz, boneless, cooked = 28 g; Calories = 42; Total Carb (g) = 0; Net Carb (g) = 0; Fat (g) = 0.7; Protein = 8.3

🍖 Venison/deer Stewed ☞ serving size: 1 oz, boneless, cooked = 28 g; Calories = 53.2; Total Carb (g) = 0; Net Carb (g) = 0; Fat (g) = 1.1; Protein = 10.1

🍖 Vienna Sausages Stewed With Potatoes Puerto Rican Style ☞ serving size: 1 cup = 175 g; Calories = 376.3; Total Carb (g) = 22.9; Net Carb (g) = 20; Fat (g) = 28.2; Protein = 8.9

22

NUTS AND SEEDS

⬤ Acorns (Dried) ☞ serving size: 1 oz = 28.4 g; Calories = 144.6; Total Carb (g) = 15.2; Net Carb (g) = 15.2; Fat (g) = 8.9; Protein = 2.3

⬤ Almond Butter ☞ serving size: 1 tbsp = 16 g; Calories = 98.2; Total Carb (g) = 3; Net Carb (g) = 1.4; Fat (g) = 8.9; Protein = 3.4

⬤ Almond Paste ☞ serving size: 1 oz = 28.4 g; Calories = 130.1; Total Carb (g) = 13.6; Net Carb (g) = 12.2; Fat (g) = 7.9; Protein = 2.6

⬤ Almonds ☞ serving size: 1 cup, whole = 143 g; Calories = 828; Total Carb (g) = 30.8; Net Carb (g) = 12.9; Fat (g) = 71.4; Protein = 30.2

⬤ Almonds Flavored ☞ serving size: 1 nut = 1 g; Calories = 6; Total Carb (g) = 0.2; Net Carb (g) = 0.1; Fat (g) = 0.5; Protein = 0.2

⬤ Almonds Honey Roasted ☞ serving size: 1 nut = 1 g; Calories = 5.8; Total Carb (g) = 0.4; Net Carb (g) = 0.3; Fat (g) = 0.5; Protein = 0.1

⬤ Almonds Salted ☞ serving size: 1 nut = 1 g; Calories = 6; Total Carb (g) = 0.2; Net Carb (g) = 0.1; Fat (g) = 0.5; Protein = 0.2

⬤ Almonds Unsalted ☞ serving size: 1 nut = 1 g; Calories = 6.1; Total Carb (g) = 0.2; Net Carb (g) = 0.1; Fat (g) = 0.5; Protein = 0.2

● Black Walnuts (Dried) ☞ serving size: 1 cup, chopped = 125 g; Calories = 773.8; Total Carb (g) = 12; Net Carb (g) = 3.5; Fat (g) = 74.2; Protein = 30.1

● Boiled Chestnuts ☞ serving size: 1 oz = 28.4 g; Calories = 37.2; Total Carb (g) = 7.9; Net Carb (g) = 7.9; Fat (g) = 0.4; Protein = 0.6

● Boiled Chinese Chestnuts ☞ serving size: 1 oz = 28.4 g; Calories = 43.5; Total Carb (g) = 9.6; Net Carb (g) = 9.6; Fat (g) = 0.2; Protein = 0.8

● Boiled Japanese Chestnuts ☞ serving size: 1 oz = 28.4 g; Calories = 15.9; Total Carb (g) = 3.6; Net Carb (g) = 3.6; Fat (g) = 0.1; Protein = 0.2

● Brazilnuts ☞ serving size: 1 cup, whole = 133 g; Calories = 876.5; Total Carb (g) = 15.6; Net Carb (g) = 5.6; Fat (g) = 89.2; Protein = 19.1

● Breadfruit Nuts (Seeds) ☞ serving size: 1 oz = 28.4 g; Calories = 47.7; Total Carb (g) = 9.1; Net Carb (g) = 7.7; Fat (g) = 0.7; Protein = 1.5

● Butternuts (Dried) ☞ serving size: 1 cup = 120 g; Calories = 734.4; Total Carb (g) = 14.5; Net Carb (g) = 8.8; Fat (g) = 68.4; Protein = 29.9

● Cashew Butter ☞ serving size: 1 tbsp = 16 g; Calories = 93.9; Total Carb (g) = 4.4; Net Carb (g) = 4.1; Fat (g) = 7.9; Protein = 2.8

● Cashews (Raw) ☞ serving size: 1 oz = 28.4 g; Calories = 157.1; Total Carb (g) = 8.6; Net Carb (g) = 7.6; Fat (g) = 12.5; Protein = 5.2

● Cashews Lightly Salted ☞ serving size: 1 nut = 2 g; Calories = 11.6; Total Carb (g) = 0.6; Net Carb (g) = 0.6; Fat (g) = 1; Protein = 0.3

● Cashews Unsalted ☞ serving size: 1 nut = 2 g; Calories = 11.7; Total Carb (g) = 0.6; Net Carb (g) = 0.6; Fat (g) = 1; Protein = 0.3

● Chestnuts ☞ serving size: 1 oz = 28.4 g; Calories = 55.7; Total Carb (g) = 12.5; Net Carb (g) = 12.5; Fat (g) = 0.4; Protein = 0.5

● Chia Seeds ☞ serving size: 1 oz = 28.4 g; Calories = 138; Total Carb (g) = 12; Net Carb (g) = 2.2; Fat (g) = 8.7; Protein = 4.7

● Chinese Chestnuts ☞ serving size: 1 oz = 28.4 g; Calories = 63.6; Total Carb (g) = 13.9; Net Carb (g) = 13.9; Fat (g) = 0.3; Protein = 1.2

● Coconut Milk ☞ serving size: 1 cup = 226 g; Calories = 445.2; Total Carb (g) = 6.4; Net Carb (g) = 6.4; Fat (g) = 48.2; Protein = 4.6

● Coconut Water ☞ serving size: 1 cup = 240 g; Calories = 45.6; Total Carb (g) = 8.9; Net Carb (g) = 6.3; Fat (g) = 0.5; Protein = 1.7

● Dried Beechnuts ☞ serving size: 1 oz = 28.4 g; Calories = 163.6; Total Carb (g) = 9.5; Net Carb (g) = 9.5; Fat (g) = 14.2; Protein = 1.8

● Dried Chinese Chestnuts ☞ serving size: 1 oz = 28.4 g; Calories = 103.1; Total Carb (g) = 22.7; Net Carb (g) = 22.7; Fat (g) = 0.5; Protein = 1.9

● Dried Coconut ☞ serving size: 1 oz = 28.4 g; Calories = 168.1; Total Carb (g) = 12.6; Net Carb (g) = 12.6; Fat (g) = 13.4; Protein = 1.5

● Dried Coconut (Unsweetened) ☞ serving size: 1 oz = 28.4 g; Calories = 187.4; Total Carb (g) = 6.7; Net Carb (g) = 2.1; Fat (g) = 18.3; Protein = 2

● Dried Ginkgo Nuts ☞ serving size: 1 oz = 28.4 g; Calories = 98.8; Total Carb (g) = 20.6; Net Carb (g) = 20.6; Fat (g) = 0.6; Protein = 2.9

● Dried Hickorynuts ☞ serving size: 1 cup = 120 g; Calories = 788.4; Total Carb (g) = 21.9; Net Carb (g) = 14.2; Fat (g) = 77.2; Protein = 15.3

● Dried Japanese Chestnuts ☞ serving size: 1 cup = 155 g; Calories = 558; Total Carb (g) = 126.2; Net Carb (g) = 126.2; Fat (g) = 1.9; Protein = 8.1

● Dried Lotus Seeds ☞ serving size: 1 cup = 32 g; Calories = 106.2; Total Carb (g) = 20.6; Net Carb (g) = 20.6; Fat (g) = 0.6; Protein = 4.9

● Dried Pilinuts ☞ serving size: 1 cup = 120 g; Calories = 862.8; Total Carb (g) = 4.8; Net Carb (g) = 4.8; Fat (g) = 95.5; Protein = 13

● Dried Pine Nuts ☞ serving size: 1 oz = 28.4 g; Calories = 178.6; Total Carb (g) = 5.5; Net Carb (g) = 2.4; Fat (g) = 17.3; Protein = 3.3

● Dried Pumpkin And Squash Seeds ☞ serving size: 1 cup = 129 g; Calories = 721.1; Total Carb (g) = 13.8; Net Carb (g) = 6.1; Fat (g) = 63.3; Protein = 39

● Dried Sunflower Seeds ☞ serving size: 1 cup, with hulls, edible yield = 46 g; Calories = 268.6; Total Carb (g) = 9.2; Net Carb (g) = 5.2; Fat (g) = 23.7; Protein = 9.6

● Dry Roasted Almonds ☞ serving size: 1 cup whole kernels = 138 g; Calories = 825.2; Total Carb (g) = 29; Net Carb (g) = 14; Fat (g) = 72.5; Protein = 28.9

● Dry Roasted Hazelnuts ☞ serving size: 1 oz = 28.4 g; Calories = 183.5; Total Carb (g) = 5; Net Carb (g) = 2.3; Fat (g) = 17.7; Protein = 4.3

● Dry Roasted Macadamia Nuts ☞ serving size: 1 cup, whole or halves = 132 g; Calories = 947.8; Total Carb (g) = 17.7; Net Carb (g) = 7.1; Fat (g) = 100.4; Protein = 10.3

● Dry Roasted Peanuts ☞ serving size: 1 cup = 146 g; Calories = 857; Total Carb (g) = 31; Net Carb (g) = 18.8; Fat (g) = 72.5; Protein = 35.6

● Dry Roasted Pecans ☞ serving size: 1 oz = 28.4 g; Calories = 201.6; Total Carb (g) = 3.9; Net Carb (g) = 1.2; Fat (g) = 21.1; Protein = 2.7

● Dry Roasted Pistachio Nuts ☞ serving size: 1 cup = 123 g; Calories = 703.6; Total Carb (g) = 34.8; Net Carb (g) = 22.1; Fat (g) = 56.4; Protein = 25.9

● Dry Roasted Sunflower Seeds ☞ serving size: 1 cup = 128 g; Calories = 745; Total Carb (g) = 30.8; Net Carb (g) = 16.6; Fat (g) = 63.7; Protein = 24.7

● Dry Roasted Sunflower Seeds (With Salt) ☞ serving size: 1 cup = 128 g; Calories = 698.9; Total Carb (g) = 19.6; Net Carb (g) = 8.1; Fat (g) = 63.7; Protein = 24.7

● Dry-Roasted Cashews ☞ serving size: 1 cup, halves and whole = 137 g; Calories = 786.4; Total Carb (g) = 44.8; Net Carb (g) = 40.7; Fat (g) = 63.5; Protein = 21

● Dry-Roasted Mixed Nuts (Salted) ☞ serving size: 1 cup = 131 g; Calories = 795.2; Total Carb (g) = 29.4; Net Carb (g) = 21; Fat (g) = 70.1; Protein = 25.6

● Flax Seeds ☞ serving size: 1 tbsp, whole = 10.3 g; Calories = 55; Total Carb (g) = 3; Net Carb (g) = 0.2; Fat (g) = 4.3; Protein = 1.9

● Ginko Nuts ☞ serving size: 1 oz = 28.4 g; Calories = 51.7; Total Carb (g) = 10.7; Net Carb (g) = 10.7; Fat (g) = 0.5; Protein = 1.2

● Hazelnuts ☞ serving size: 1 cup, chopped = 115 g; Calories = 722.2; Total Carb (g) = 19.2; Net Carb (g) = 8.1; Fat (g) = 69.9; Protein = 17.2

● Hemp Seeds ☞ serving size: 3 tbsp = 30 g; Calories = 165.9; Total Carb (g) = 2.6; Net Carb (g) = 1.4; Fat (g) = 14.6; Protein = 9.5

● Lotus Seeds ☞ serving size: 1 oz = 28.4 g; Calories = 25.3; Total Carb (g) = 4.9; Net Carb (g) = 4.9; Fat (g) = 0.2; Protein = 1.2

● Macadamia Nuts ☞ serving size: 1 cup, whole or halves = 134 g; Calories = 962.1; Total Carb (g) = 18.5; Net Carb (g) = 7; Fat (g) = 101.5; Protein = 10.6

● Mixed Nuts Honey Roasted ☞ serving size: 1 cup = 142 g; Calories = 822.2; Total Carb (g) = 47.3; Net Carb (g) = 38.9; Fat (g) = 66; Protein = 21.8

● Mixed Nuts Nfs ☞ serving size: 1 cup = 142 g; Calories = 859.1; Total Carb (g) = 29.9; Net Carb (g) = 19.1; Fat (g) = 76.1; Protein = 27.8

● Mixed Nuts Unroasted ☞ serving size: 1 cup = 142 g; Calories = 860.5; Total Carb (g) = 32.9; Net Carb (g) = 22.1; Fat (g) = 76.9; Protein = 24.1

● Mixed Nuts With Peanuts Unsalted ☞ serving size: 1 cup = 142 g; Calories = 866.2; Total Carb (g) = 30.1; Net Carb (g) = 19.3; Fat (g) = 76.8; Protein = 28

● Mixed Nuts Without Peanuts Salted ☞ serving size: 1 cup = 142

g; Calories = 866.2; Total Carb (g) = 31.6; Net Carb (g) = 21.3; Fat (g) = 78.2; Protein = 23.2

● Mixed Nuts Without Peanuts Unsalted ☞ serving size: 1 cup = 142 g; Calories = 873.3; Total Carb (g) = 31.9; Net Carb (g) = 21.4; Fat (g) = 78.9; Protein = 23.3

● Mixed Seeds ☞ serving size: 1 cup = 145 g; Calories = 841; Total Carb (g) = 31.5; Net Carb (g) = 17; Fat (g) = 71.9; Protein = 31.8

● Nuts Acorn Flour Full Fat ☞ serving size: 1 oz = 28.4 g; Calories = 142.3; Total Carb (g) = 15.5; Net Carb (g) = 15.5; Fat (g) = 8.6; Protein = 2.1

● Nuts Acorns Raw ☞ serving size: 1 oz = 28.4 g; Calories = 109.9; Total Carb (g) = 11.6; Net Carb (g) = 11.6; Fat (g) = 6.8; Protein = 1.8

● Nuts Almond Butter Plain With Salt Added ☞ serving size: 1 tbsp = 16 g; Calories = 98.2; Total Carb (g) = 3; Net Carb (g) = 1.4; Fat (g) = 8.9; Protein = 3.4

● Nuts Almonds Blanched ☞ serving size: 1 cup whole kernels = 145 g; Calories = 855.5; Total Carb (g) = 27.1; Net Carb (g) = 12.7; Fat (g) = 76.2; Protein = 31

● Nuts Almonds Dry Roasted With Salt Added ☞ serving size: 1 cup whole kernels = 138 g; Calories = 825.2; Total Carb (g) = 29; Net Carb (g) = 14; Fat (g) = 72.5; Protein = 28.9

● Nuts Almonds Honey Roasted Unblanched ☞ serving size: 1 cup whole kernels = 144 g; Calories = 855.4; Total Carb (g) = 40.2; Net Carb (g) = 20.5; Fat (g) = 71.9; Protein = 26.2

● Nuts Almonds Oil Roasted Lightly Salted ☞ serving size: 1 cup whole kernels = 157 g; Calories = 953; Total Carb (g) = 27.8; Net Carb (g) = 11.3; Fat (g) = 86.6; Protein = 33.3

● Nuts Almonds Oil Roasted With Salt Added ☞ serving size: 1 cup whole kernels = 157 g; Calories = 953; Total Carb (g) = 27.8; Net Carb (g) = 11.3; Fat (g) = 86.6; Protein = 33.3

● Nuts Almonds Oil Roasted With Salt Added Smoke Flavor ☞ serving size: 1 oz (28 almonds) = 28 g; Calories = 170; Total Carb (g) = 5; Net Carb (g) = 2; Fat (g) = 15.7; Protein = 6

● Nuts Almonds Oil Roasted Without Salt Added ☞ serving size: 1 cup whole kernels = 157 g; Calories = 953; Total Carb (g) = 27.8; Net Carb (g) = 11.3; Fat (g) = 86.6; Protein = 33.3

● Nuts Cashew Butter Plain With Salt Added ☞ serving size: 1 tbsp = 16 g; Calories = 97.4; Total Carb (g) = 4.9; Net Carb (g) = 4.4; Fat (g) = 8.5; Protein = 1.9

● Nuts Cashew Nuts Dry Roasted With Salt Added ☞ serving size: 1 cup, halves and whole = 137 g; Calories = 786.4; Total Carb (g) = 44.8; Net Carb (g) = 40.7; Fat (g) = 63.5; Protein = 21

● Nuts Cashew Nuts Oil Roasted With Salt Added ☞ serving size: 1 cup, whole = 129 g; Calories = 749.5; Total Carb (g) = 38.9; Net Carb (g) = 34.7; Fat (g) = 61.6; Protein = 21.7

● Nuts Chestnuts European Dried Peeled ☞ serving size: 1 oz = 28.4 g; Calories = 104.8; Total Carb (g) = 22.3; Net Carb (g) = 22.3; Fat (g) = 1.1; Protein = 1.4

● Nuts Chestnuts European Dried Unpeeled ☞ serving size: 1 oz = 28.4 g; Calories = 106.2; Total Carb (g) = 22; Net Carb (g) = 18.6; Fat (g) = 1.3; Protein = 1.8

● Nuts Chestnuts European Raw Unpeeled ☞ serving size: 1 cup = 145 g; Calories = 308.9; Total Carb (g) = 66; Net Carb (g) = 54.3; Fat (g) = 3.3; Protein = 3.5

● Nuts Chestnuts Japanese Raw ☞ serving size: 1 oz = 28.4 g; Calories = 43.7; Total Carb (g) = 9.9; Net Carb (g) = 9.9; Fat (g) = 0.2; Protein = 0.6

● Nuts Chestnuts Japanese Roasted ☞ serving size: 1 oz = 28.4 g; Calories = 57.1; Total Carb (g) = 12.8; Net Carb (g) = 12.8; Fat (g) = 0.2; Protein = 0.8

● Nuts Coconut Cream Canned Sweetened ☞ serving size: 1 tbsp = 19 g; Calories = 67.8; Total Carb (g) = 10.1; Net Carb (g) = 10.1; Fat (g) = 3.1; Protein = 0.2

● Nuts Coconut Cream Raw (Liquid Expressed From Grated Meat) ☞ serving size: 1 tbsp = 15 g; Calories = 49.5; Total Carb (g) = 1; Net Carb (g) = 0.7; Fat (g) = 5.2; Protein = 0.5

● Nuts Coconut Meat Dried (Desiccated) Creamed ☞ serving size: 1 oz = 28.4 g; Calories = 194.3; Total Carb (g) = 6.1; Net Carb (g) = 6.1; Fat (g) = 19.6; Protein = 1.5

● Nuts Coconut Meat Dried (Desiccated) Sweetened Flaked Canned ☞ serving size: 1 cup = 77 g; Calories = 341.1; Total Carb (g) = 31.5; Net Carb (g) = 28; Fat (g) = 24.4; Protein = 2.6

● Nuts Coconut Meat Dried (Desiccated) Sweetened Flaked Packaged ☞ serving size: 1 cup = 85 g; Calories = 387.6; Total Carb (g) = 44.1; Net Carb (g) = 35.7; Fat (g) = 23.8; Protein = 2.7

● Nuts Coconut Meat Raw ☞ serving size: 1 cup, shredded = 80 g; Calories = 283.2; Total Carb (g) = 12.2; Net Carb (g) = 5; Fat (g) = 26.8; Protein = 2.7

● Nuts Coconut Milk Frozen (Liquid Expressed From Grated Meat And Water) ☞ serving size: 1 cup = 240 g; Calories = 484.8; Total Carb (g) = 13.4; Net Carb (g) = 13.4; Fat (g) = 49.9; Protein = 3.9

● Nuts Coconut Milk Raw (Liquid Expressed From Grated Meat And Water) ☞ serving size: 1 cup = 240 g; Calories = 552; Total Carb (g) = 13.3; Net Carb (g) = 8; Fat (g) = 57.2; Protein = 5.5

● Nuts Formulated Wheat-Based All Flavors Except Macadamia Without Salt ☞ serving size: 1 oz = 28.4 g; Calories = 183.7; Total Carb (g) = 5.9; Net Carb (g) = 4.4; Fat (g) = 17.7; Protein = 3.7

● Nuts Formulated Wheat-Based Unflavored With Salt Added ☞ serving size: 1 oz = 28.4 g; Calories = 176.6; Total Carb (g) = 6.7; Net Carb (g) = 5.3; Fat (g) = 16.4; Protein = 3.9

● Nuts Ginkgo Nuts Canned ☞ serving size: 1 cup (78 kernels) = 155 g; Calories = 172.1; Total Carb (g) = 34.3; Net Carb (g) = 19.8; Fat (g) = 2.5; Protein = 3.6

● Nuts Hazelnuts Or Filberts Blanched ☞ serving size: 1 oz = 28.4 g; Calories = 178.6; Total Carb (g) = 4.8; Net Carb (g) = 1.7; Fat (g) = 17.4; Protein = 3.9

● Nuts Macadamia Nuts Dry Roasted With Salt Added ☞ serving size: 1 cup, whole or halves = 132 g; Calories = 945.1; Total Carb (g) = 16.9; Net Carb (g) = 6.4; Fat (g) = 100.4; Protein = 10.3

● Nuts Mixed Nuts Dry Roasted With Peanuts Salt Added Chosen Roaster ☞ serving size: 1 cup = 132 g; Calories = 802.6; Total Carb (g) = 32.5; Net Carb (g) = 23.1; Fat (g) = 70.2; Protein = 23.8

● Nuts Mixed Nuts Dry Roasted With Peanuts Salt Added Planters Pistachio Blend ☞ serving size: 1 cup = 147 g; Calories = 840.8; Total Carb (g) = 33.9; Net Carb (g) = 22; Fat (g) = 69.9; Protein = 34.2

● Nuts Mixed Nuts Dry Roasted With Peanuts With Salt Added ☞ serving size: 1 cup = 137 g; Calories = 813.8; Total Carb (g) = 34.7; Net Carb (g) = 22.4; Fat (g) = 70.5; Protein = 23.7

● Nuts Mixed Nuts Oil Roasted With Peanuts Lightly Salted ☞ serving size: 1 oz = 28.4 g; Calories = 172.4; Total Carb (g) = 6; Net Carb (g) = 4; Fat (g) = 15.3; Protein = 5.7

● Nuts Mixed Nuts Oil Roasted With Peanuts With Salt Added ☞ serving size: 1 cup = 134 g; Calories = 813.4; Total Carb (g) = 28.2; Net Carb (g) = 18.8; Fat (g) = 72.3; Protein = 26.9

● Nuts Mixed Nuts Oil Roasted With Peanuts Without Salt Added ☞ serving size: 1 cup = 134 g; Calories = 813.4; Total Carb (g) = 28.2; Net Carb (g) = 18.8; Fat (g) = 72.3; Protein = 26.9

● Nuts Mixed Nuts Oil Roasted Without Peanuts Lightly Salted ☞ serving size: 1 oz = 28.4 g; Calories = 172.4; Total Carb (g) = 7.1; Net Carb (g) = 5.1; Fat (g) = 14.2; Protein = 5.1

● Nuts Mixed Nuts Oil Roasted Without Peanuts With Salt Added ☞ serving size: 1 cup = 144 g; Calories = 885.6; Total Carb (g) = 32.1; Net Carb (g) = 24.2; Fat (g) = 80.9; Protein = 22.4

● Nuts Mixed Nuts Oil Roasted Without Peanuts Without Salt Added ☞ serving size: 1 cup = 144 g; Calories = 885.6; Total Carb (g) = 32.1; Net Carb (g) = 24.2; Fat (g) = 80.9; Protein = 22.4

● Nuts Nfs ☞ serving size: 1 cup = 142 g; Calories = 859.1; Total Carb (g) = 29.9; Net Carb (g) = 19.1; Fat (g) = 76.1; Protein = 27.8

● Nuts Pecans Dry Roasted With Salt Added ☞ serving size: 1 oz = 28.4 g; Calories = 201.6; Total Carb (g) = 3.9; Net Carb (g) = 1.2; Fat (g) = 21.1; Protein = 2.7

● Nuts Pecans Oil Roasted With Salt Added ☞ serving size: 1 cup = 110 g; Calories = 786.5; Total Carb (g) = 14.3; Net Carb (g) = 3.9; Fat (g) = 82.8; Protein = 10.1

● Nuts Pecans Oil Roasted Without Salt Added ☞ serving size: 1 cup = 110 g; Calories = 786.5; Total Carb (g) = 14.3; Net Carb (g) = 3.9; Fat (g) = 82.8; Protein = 10.1

● Nuts Pistachio Nuts Dry Roasted With Salt Added ☞ serving size: 1 cup = 123 g; Calories = 699.9; Total Carb (g) = 33.9; Net Carb (g) = 21.2; Fat (g) = 56.4; Protein = 25.9

● Nuts Walnuts Dry Roasted With Salt Added ☞ serving size: 1 oz = 28 g; Calories = 180; Total Carb (g) = 5; Net Carb (g) = 3; Fat (g) = 17; Protein = 4

● Nuts Walnuts Glazed ☞ serving size: 1 oz = 28 g; Calories = 140; Total Carb (g) = 13.3; Net Carb (g) = 12.3; Fat (g) = 10; Protein = 2.3

● Oil Roasted Cashews ☞ serving size: 1 cup, whole = 129 g; Calories = 748.2; Total Carb (g) = 38.5; Net Carb (g) = 34.3; Fat (g) = 61.6; Protein = 21.7

● Peanut Butter And Chocolate Spread ☞ serving size: 1 tablespoon = 16 g; Calories = 79.7; Total Carb (g) = 6.8; Net Carb (g) = 6.4; Fat (g) = 5.5; Protein = 1.9

● Peanut Butter And Jelly ☞ serving size: 1 tablespoon = 16 g; Calories = 69.1; Total Carb (g) = 7.4; Net Carb (g) = 6.9; Fat (g) = 4.1; Protein = 1.8

● Peanut Butter Lower Sodium And Lower Sugar ☞ serving size: 1 tablespoon = 16 g; Calories = 99.8; Total Carb (g) = 2.9; Net Carb (g) = 1.9; Fat (g) = 8.5; Protein = 3.8

● Peanuts Dry Roasted Lightly Salted ☞ serving size: 1 peanut, without shell = 1 g; Calories = 5.8; Total Carb (g) = 0.2; Net Carb (g) = 0.1; Fat (g) = 0.5; Protein = 0.2

● Pecans ☞ serving size: 1 cup, chopped = 109 g; Calories = 753.2; Total Carb (g) = 15.1; Net Carb (g) = 4.6; Fat (g) = 78.5; Protein = 10

● Pecans Honey Roasted ☞ serving size: 1 nut = 2 g; Calories = 12.7; Total Carb (g) = 0.6; Net Carb (g) = 0.5; Fat (g) = 1.2; Protein = 0.1

● Pecans Salted ☞ serving size: 1 nut = 2 g; Calories = 13.8; Total Carb (g) = 0.3; Net Carb (g) = 0.1; Fat (g) = 1.4; Protein = 0.2

● Pecans Unsalted ☞ serving size: 1 nut = 2 g; Calories = 13.9; Total Carb (g) = 0.3; Net Carb (g) = 0.1; Fat (g) = 1.5; Protein = 0.2

● Pine Nuts (Dried) ☞ serving size: 1 cup = 135 g; Calories = 908.6; Total Carb (g) = 17.7; Net Carb (g) = 12.7; Fat (g) = 92.3; Protein = 18.5

● Pistachio Nuts ☞ serving size: 1 cup = 123 g; Calories = 688.8; Total Carb (g) = 33.4; Net Carb (g) = 20.4; Fat (g) = 55.7; Protein = 24.8

● Pistachio Nuts Lightly Salted ☞ serving size: 1 nut = 1 g; Calories = 5.8; Total Carb (g) = 0.3; Net Carb (g) = 0.2; Fat (g) = 0.5; Protein = 0.2

● Pistachio Nuts Salted ☞ serving size: 1 nut = 1 g; Calories = 5.8; Total Carb (g) = 0.3; Net Carb (g) = 0.2; Fat (g) = 0.5; Protein = 0.2

● Pistachio Nuts Unsalted ☞ serving size: 1 nut = 1 g; Calories = 5.8; Total Carb (g) = 0.3; Net Carb (g) = 0.2; Fat (g) = 0.5; Protein = 0.2

● Pumpkin Seeds Salted ☞ serving size: 1 cup, without shell = 144 g; Calories = 816.5; Total Carb (g) = 20.9; Net Carb (g) = 11.7; Fat (g) = 69.8; Protein = 42.5

● Raw Sesame Butter (Tahini) ☞ serving size: 1 tbsp = 15 g; Calories = 85.5; Total Carb (g) = 3.9; Net Carb (g) = 2.5; Fat (g) = 7.2; Protein = 2.7

● Roasted Chestnuts ☞ serving size: 1 cup = 143 g; Calories = 350.4; Total Carb (g) = 75.7; Net Carb (g) = 68.4; Fat (g) = 3.2; Protein = 4.5

● Roasted Chinese Chestnuts ☞ serving size: 1 oz = 28.4 g; Calories = 67.9; Total Carb (g) = 14.9; Net Carb (g) = 14.9; Fat (g) = 0.3; Protein = 1.3

● Roasted Squash And Pumpkin Seeds (Salted) ☞ serving size: 1 cup = 118 g; Calories = 677.3; Total Carb (g) = 17.4; Net Carb (g) = 9.7; Fat (g) = 57.9; Protein = 35.2

● Roasted Squash And Pumpkin Seeds (Unsalted) ☞ serving size: 1 cup = 118 g; Calories = 677.3; Total Carb (g) = 17.4; Net Carb (g) = 9.7; Fat (g) = 57.9; Protein = 35.2

● Roasted Squash And Pumpkin Seeds (With Shells) ☞ serving size: 1 cup = 64 g; Calories = 285.4; Total Carb (g) = 34.4; Net Carb (g) = 22.6; Fat (g) = 12.4; Protein = 11.9

● Safflower Seeds ☞ serving size: 1 oz = 28.4 g; Calories = 146.8; Total Carb (g) = 9.7; Net Carb (g) = 9.7; Fat (g) = 10.9; Protein = 4.6

● Seeds Breadfruit Seeds Raw ☞ serving size: 1 oz = 28.4 g; Calories = 54.2; Total Carb (g) = 8.3; Net Carb (g) = 6.8; Fat (g) = 1.6; Protein = 2.1

● Seeds Breadfruit Seeds Roasted ☞ serving size: 1 oz = 28.4 g; Calories = 58.8; Total Carb (g) = 11.4; Net Carb (g) = 9.7; Fat (g) = 0.8; Protein = 1.8

● Seeds Breadnut Tree Seeds Dried ☞ serving size: 1 cup = 160 g; Calories = 587.2; Total Carb (g) = 127; Net Carb (g) = 103.2; Fat (g) = 2.7; Protein = 13.8

● Seeds Breadnut Tree Seeds Raw ☞ serving size: 1 oz (8-14 seeds) = 28.4 g; Calories = 61.6; Total Carb (g) = 13.1; Net Carb (g) = 13.1; Fat (g) = 0.3; Protein = 1.7

● Seeds Cottonseed Flour Low Fat (Glandless) ☞ serving size: 1 oz = 28.4 g; Calories = 94.3; Total Carb (g) = 10.3; Net Carb (g) = 10.3; Fat (g) = 0.4; Protein = 14.2

● Seeds Cottonseed Flour Partially Defatted (Glandless) ☞ serving size: 1 cup = 94 g; Calories = 337.5; Total Carb (g) = 38.1; Net Carb (g) = 35.3; Fat (g) = 5.8; Protein = 38.5

● Seeds Cottonseed Kernels Roasted (Glandless) ☞ serving size: 1 cup = 149 g; Calories = 753.9; Total Carb (g) = 32.6; Net Carb (g) = 24.4; Fat (g) = 54.1; Protein = 48.6

● Seeds Cottonseed Meal Partially Defatted (Glandless) ☞ serving size: 1 oz = 28.4 g; Calories = 104.2; Total Carb (g) = 10.9; Net Carb (g) = 10.9; Fat (g) = 1.4; Protein = 13.9

● Seeds Pumpkin And Squash Seeds Whole Roasted With Salt Added ☞ serving size: 1 cup = 64 g; Calories = 285.4; Total Carb (g) = 34.4; Net Carb (g) = 22.6; Fat (g) = 12.4; Protein = 11.9

● Seeds Safflower Seed Meal Partially Defatted ☞ serving size: 1 oz = 28.4 g; Calories = 97.1; Total Carb (g) = 13.8; Net Carb (g) = 13.8; Fat (g) = 0.7; Protein = 10.1

● Seeds Sesame Butter Paste ☞ serving size: 1 tbsp = 16 g; Calories = 93.8; Total Carb (g) = 3.9; Net Carb (g) = 3; Fat (g) = 8.1; Protein = 2.9

● Seeds Sesame Butter Tahini From Unroasted Kernels (Non-Chemically Removed Seed Coat) ☞ serving size: 1 tbsp = 14 g; Calories = 85; Total Carb (g) = 2.5; Net Carb (g) = 1.2; Fat (g) = 7.9; Protein = 2.5

● Seeds Sesame Butter Tahini Type Of Kernels Unspecified ☞ serving size: 1 tbsp = 15 g; Calories = 88.8; Total Carb (g) = 3.2; Net Carb (g) = 2.5; Fat (g) = 8; Protein = 2.6

● Seeds Sesame Flour High-Fat ☞ serving size: 1 oz = 28.4 g; Calories = 149.4; Total Carb (g) = 7.6; Net Carb (g) = 7.6; Fat (g) = 10.5; Protein = 8.7

● Seeds Sesame Flour Low-Fat ☞ serving size: 1 oz = 28.4 g; Calories = 94.6; Total Carb (g) = 10.1; Net Carb (g) = 10.1; Fat (g) = 0.5; Protein = 14.2

● Seeds Sesame Flour Partially Defatted ☞ serving size: 1 oz = 28.4 g; Calories = 108.5; Total Carb (g) = 10; Net Carb (g) = 10; Fat (g) = 3.4; Protein = 11.5

● Seeds Sesame Meal Partially Defatted ☞ serving size: 1 oz = 28.4 g; Calories = 161; Total Carb (g) = 7.4; Net Carb (g) = 7.4; Fat (g) = 13.6; Protein = 4.8

● Seeds Sesame Seed Kernels Dried (Decorticated) ☞ serving size: 1 cup = 150 g; Calories = 946.5; Total Carb (g) = 17.6; Net Carb (g) = 0.2; Fat (g) = 91.8; Protein = 30.7

● Seeds Sesame Seed Kernels Toasted With Salt Added (Decorticated) ☞ serving size: 1 cup = 128 g; Calories = 725.8; Total Carb (g) = 33.3; Net Carb (g) = 11.7; Fat (g) = 61.4; Protein = 21.7

● Seeds Sesame Seed Kernels Toasted Without Salt Added (Decorticated) ☞ serving size: 1 cup = 128 g; Calories = 725.8; Total Carb (g) = 33.3; Net Carb (g) = 11.7; Fat (g) = 61.4; Protein = 21.7

● Seeds Sesame Seeds Whole Dried ☞ serving size: 1 cup = 144 g; Calories = 825.1; Total Carb (g) = 33.8; Net Carb (g) = 16.8; Fat (g) = 71.5; Protein = 25.5

● Seeds Sisymbrium Sp. Seeds Whole Dried ☞ serving size: 1 cup = 74 g; Calories = 235.3; Total Carb (g) = 43.1; Net Carb (g) = 43.1; Fat (g) = 3.4; Protein = 9

● Seeds Sunflower Seed Butter With Salt Added ☞ serving size: 1 tbsp = 16 g; Calories = 98.7; Total Carb (g) = 3.7; Net Carb (g) = 2.8; Fat (g) = 8.8; Protein = 2.8

● Seeds Sunflower Seed Butter Without Salt ☞ serving size: 1 tbsp = 16 g; Calories = 98.7; Total Carb (g) = 3.7; Net Carb (g) = 2.8; Fat (g) = 8.8; Protein = 2.8

● Seeds Sunflower Seed Flour Partially Defatted ☞ serving size: 1 cup = 64 g; Calories = 208.6; Total Carb (g) = 22.9; Net Carb (g) = 19.6; Fat (g) = 1; Protein = 30.8

● Seeds Sunflower Seed Kernels Dry Roasted With Salt Added ☞ serving size: 1 cup = 128 g; Calories = 745; Total Carb (g) = 30.8; Net Carb (g) = 19.3; Fat (g) = 63.7; Protein = 24.7

● Seeds Sunflower Seed Kernels Oil Roasted With Salt Added ☞ serving size: 1 cup = 135 g; Calories = 799.2; Total Carb (g) = 30.9; Net Carb (g) = 16.6; Fat (g) = 69.3; Protein = 27.1

● Seeds Sunflower Seed Kernels Oil Roasted Without Salt ☞ serving size: 1 cup = 135 g; Calories = 799.2; Total Carb (g) = 30.9; Net Carb (g) = 16.6; Fat (g) = 69.3; Protein = 27.1

● Seeds Sunflower Seed Kernels Toasted With Salt Added ☞ serving size: 1 cup = 134 g; Calories = 829.5; Total Carb (g) = 27.6; Net Carb (g) = 12.2; Fat (g) = 76.1; Protein = 23.1

● Seeds Sunflower Seed Kernels Toasted Without Salt ☞ serving size: 1 cup = 134 g; Calories = 829.5; Total Carb (g) = 27.6; Net Carb (g) = 12.2; Fat (g) = 76.1; Protein = 23.1

● Seeds Watermelon Seed Kernels Dried ☞ serving size: 1 cup = 108 g; Calories = 601.6; Total Carb (g) = 16.5; Net Carb (g) = 16.5; Fat (g) = 51.2; Protein = 30.6

● Sesame Butter (Tahini) ☞ serving size: 1 tbsp = 15 g; Calories = 89.3; Total Carb (g) = 3.2; Net Carb (g) = 1.8; Fat (g) = 8.1; Protein = 2.6

● Sesame Seeds (Toasted) ☞ serving size: 1 oz = 28.4 g; Calories =

160.5; Total Carb (g) = 7.3; Net Carb (g) = 3.3; Fat (g) = 13.6; Protein = 4.8

● Shredded Coconut Meat ☞ serving size: 1 cup, shredded = 93 g; Calories = 465.9; Total Carb (g) = 44.3; Net Carb (g) = 40.2; Fat (g) = 33; Protein = 2.7

● Sunflower Seeds Flavored ☞ serving size: 1 cup, without shell = 144 g; Calories = 816.5; Total Carb (g) = 37.3; Net Carb (g) = 22.1; Fat (g) = 68.5; Protein = 26.6

● Sunflower Seeds Plain Salted ☞ serving size: 1 cup, without shell = 144 g; Calories = 828; Total Carb (g) = 34.2; Net Carb (g) = 18.4; Fat (g) = 70.9; Protein = 27.5

● Trail Mix Nfs ☞ serving size: 1 cup = 140 g; Calories = 632.8; Total Carb (g) = 71.5; Net Carb (g) = 62.7; Fat (g) = 37.5; Protein = 15.2

● Trail Mix With Chocolate ☞ serving size: 1 cup = 140 g; Calories = 701.4; Total Carb (g) = 67.6; Net Carb (g) = 59.4; Fat (g) = 45.1; Protein = 16.3

● Trail Mix With Nuts ☞ serving size: 1 cup = 140 g; Calories = 840; Total Carb (g) = 29.7; Net Carb (g) = 18.3; Fat (g) = 74; Protein = 28.1

● Trail Mix With Nuts And Fruit ☞ serving size: 1 cup = 140 g; Calories = 632.8; Total Carb (g) = 71.5; Net Carb (g) = 62.7; Fat (g) = 37.5; Protein = 15.2

● Trail Mix With Pretzels Cereal Or Granola ☞ serving size: 1 cup = 140 g; Calories = 662.2; Total Carb (g) = 70.9; Net Carb (g) = 62.5; Fat (g) = 38.6; Protein = 18.3

● Walnuts ☞ serving size: 1 cup, chopped = 117 g; Calories = 765.2; Total Carb (g) = 16; Net Carb (g) = 8.2; Fat (g) = 76.3; Protein = 17.8

● Walnuts Honey Roasted ☞ serving size: 1 nut = 2 g; Calories = 12.2; Total Carb (g) = 0.6; Net Carb (g) = 0.5; Fat (g) = 1.1; Protein = 0.2

23

PREPARED MEALS

🦪 Almond Chicken ☞ serving size: 1 cup = 242 g; Calories = 476.7; Total Carb (g) = 11.8; Net Carb (g) = 8.9; Fat (g) = 31.9; Protein = 38.9

🦪 Banquet Salisbury Steak With Gravy Family Size Frozen Unprepared ☞ serving size: 1 patty = 72 g; Calories = 111.6; Total Carb (g) = 5; Net Carb (g) = 4.3; Fat (g) = 8; Protein = 5

🦪 Beans String Green Cooked Szechuan-Style ☞ serving size: 1 cup = 185 g; Calories = 175.8; Total Carb (g) = 15.2; Net Carb (g) = 10.1; Fat (g) = 12.3; Protein = 4.4

🦪 Beef And Broccoli ☞ serving size: 1 cup = 217 g; Calories = 336.4; Total Carb (g) = 11.5; Net Carb (g) = 8.5; Fat (g) = 22.7; Protein = 22.9

🦪 Beef And Noodles With Soy-Based Sauce ☞ serving size: 1 cup = 249 g; Calories = 425.8; Total Carb (g) = 18.8; Net Carb (g) = 17.3; Fat (g) = 24.7; Protein = 32.8

🦪 Beef And Rice With Soy-Based Sauce ☞ serving size: 1 cup = 244 g; Calories = 429.4; Total Carb (g) = 19.5; Net Carb (g) = 18.3; Fat (g) = 24.7; Protein = 33.1

🦪 Beef And Vegetables Excluding Carrots Broccoli And Dark-

Green Leafy; No Potatoes Soy-Based Sauce ☞ serving size: 1 cup = 217 g; Calories = 310.3; Total Carb (g) = 9.5; Net Carb (g) = 7.6; Fat (g) = 19.6; Protein = 26

🥩 Beef And Vegetables Including Carrots Broccoli And/or Dark-Green Leafy; No Potatoes Soy-Based Sauce ☞ serving size: 1 cup = 217 g; Calories = 306; Total Carb (g) = 10.4; Net Carb (g) = 7.5; Fat (g) = 18.9; Protein = 25.3

🥩 Beef Chow Mein Or Chop Suey No Noodles ☞ serving size: 1 cup = 220 g; Calories = 180.4; Total Carb (g) = 8.5; Net Carb (g) = 6.7; Fat (g) = 5.7; Protein = 23.7

🥩 Beef Chow Mein Or Chop Suey With Noodles ☞ serving size: 1 cup = 220 g; Calories = 286; Total Carb (g) = 27; Net Carb (g) = 24.4; Fat (g) = 9.2; Protein = 23

🥩 Beef Corned Beef Hash With Potato Canned ☞ serving size: 1 cup = 236 g; Calories = 387; Total Carb (g) = 21.9; Net Carb (g) = 19.3; Fat (g) = 24.2; Protein = 20.6

🥩 Beef Egg Foo Yung ☞ serving size: 1 patty = 86 g; Calories = 125.6; Total Carb (g) = 3.9; Net Carb (g) = 3.7; Fat (g) = 6.8; Protein = 11.9

🥩 Beef Enchilada Chili Gravy Rice Refried Beans Frozen Meal ☞ serving size: 1 meal (15 oz) = 425 g; Calories = 527; Total Carb (g) = 70.9; Net Carb (g) = 62; Fat (g) = 17.5; Protein = 21.4

🥩 Beef Enchilada Dinner NFS Frozen Meal ☞ serving size: 1 meal (15 oz) = 425 g; Calories = 527; Total Carb (g) = 70.9; Net Carb (g) = 62; Fat (g) = 17.5; Protein = 21.4

🥩 Beef Macaroni With Tomato Sauce Frozen Entree Reduced Fat ☞ serving size: 1 serving = 269 g; Calories = 304; Total Carb (g) = 48.4; Net Carb (g) = 44.6; Fat (g) = 5.3; Protein = 15.8

🥩 Beef Noodles And Vegetables Excluding Carrots Broccoli And Dark-Green Leafy; Soy-Based Sauce ☞ serving size: 1 cup = 217 g;

Calories = 301.6; Total Carb (g) = 16.2; Net Carb (g) = 14.3; Fat (g) = 16.8; Protein = 22.8

● Beef Noodles And Vegetables Including Carrots Broccoli And/or Dark-Green Leafy; Soy-Based Sauce ☞ serving size: 1 cup = 217 g; Calories = 297.3; Total Carb (g) = 16.7; Net Carb (g) = 13.9; Fat (g) = 16.2; Protein = 22.2

● Beef Pot Pie Frozen Entree Prepared ☞ serving size: 1 pie, cooked (average weight) = 268 g; Calories = 589.6; Total Carb (g) = 59.1; Net Carb (g) = 57; Fat (g) = 30.5; Protein = 19.4

● Beef Potatoes And Vegetables Excluding Carrots Broccoli And Dark-Green Leafy; Soy-Based Sauce ☞ serving size: 1 cup = 252 g; Calories = 365.4; Total Carb (g) = 14.7; Net Carb (g) = 12.5; Fat (g) = 21.9; Protein = 29.4

● Beef Potatoes And Vegetables Including Carrots Broccoli And/or Dark-Green Leafy; Soy-Based Sauce ☞ serving size: 1 cup = 252 g; Calories = 367.9; Total Carb (g) = 15.2; Net Carb (g) = 12.2; Fat (g) = 21.9; Protein = 29.4

● Beef Rice And Vegetables Excluding Carrots Broccoli And Dark-Green Leafy; Soy-Based Sauce ☞ serving size: 1 cup = 217 g; Calories = 310.3; Total Carb (g) = 16.9; Net Carb (g) = 15.2; Fat (g) = 17; Protein = 23.4

● Beef Rice And Vegetables Including Carrots Broccoli And/or Dark-Green Leafy; Soy-Based Sauce ☞ serving size: 1 cup = 217 g; Calories = 303.8; Total Carb (g) = 17.4; Net Carb (g) = 14.8; Fat (g) = 16.5; Protein = 22.8

● Beef Stew Canned Entree ☞ serving size: 1 cup (1 serving) = 196 g; Calories = 194; Total Carb (g) = 15.4; Net Carb (g) = 13.6; Fat (g) = 10.8; Protein = 8.6

● Beef Taco Filling: Beef Cheese Tomato Taco Sauce ☞ serving size: 1 cup = 204 g; Calories = 367.2; Total Carb (g) = 13.1; Net Carb (g) = 11.3; Fat (g) = 22.9; Protein = 26.4

🌰 Beef Tofu And Vegetables Excluding Carrots Broccoli And Dark-Green Leafy; No Potatoes Soy-Based Sauce ☞ serving size: 1 cup = 217 g; Calories = 247.4; Total Carb (g) = 9.7; Net Carb (g) = 7.8; Fat (g) = 17; Protein = 16.1

🌰 Beef Tofu And Vegetables Including Carrots Broccoli And/or Dark-Green Leafy; No Potatoes Soy-Based Sauce ☞ serving size: 1 cup = 217 g; Calories = 243; Total Carb (g) = 10.6; Net Carb (g) = 7.7; Fat (g) = 16.4; Protein = 15.7

🌰 Beef With Soy-Based Sauce ☞ serving size: 1 cup = 244 g; Calories = 449; Total Carb (g) = 8.2; Net Carb (g) = 7; Fat (g) = 29.8; Protein = 38.6

🌰 Beef With Sweet And Sour Sauce ☞ serving size: 1 cup = 252 g; Calories = 461.2; Total Carb (g) = 41; Net Carb (g) = 39; Fat (g) = 20.8; Protein = 29.2

🌰 Bibimbap Korean ☞ serving size: 1 cup = 162 g; Calories = 128; Total Carb (g) = 13.5; Net Carb (g) = 11.9; Fat (g) = 4.6; Protein = 8.7

🌰 Biryani With Chicken ☞ serving size: 1 cup = 196 g; Calories = 199.9; Total Carb (g) = 26.3; Net Carb (g) = 24.5; Fat (g) = 4.6; Protein = 13.8

🌰 Biryani With Meat ☞ serving size: 1 cup = 196 g; Calories = 282.2; Total Carb (g) = 23.7; Net Carb (g) = 21.9; Fat (g) = 13.3; Protein = 16.5

🌰 Biryani With Vegetables ☞ serving size: 1 cup = 172 g; Calories = 204.7; Total Carb (g) = 30.8; Net Carb (g) = 28.4; Fat (g) = 7.5; Protein = 4.1

🌰 Bread Stuffing Made With Egg ☞ serving size: 1 cup = 170 g; Calories = 326.4; Total Carb (g) = 30.2; Net Carb (g) = 28.8; Fat (g) = 20.2; Protein = 5.6

🌰 Burrito Bean And Cheese Frozen ☞ serving size: 1 burrito = 129 g; Calories = 285.1; Total Carb (g) = 43.9; Net Carb (g) = 39.5; Fat (g) = 8.1; Protein = 9.1

🍢 Burrito Beef And Bean Frozen ☞ serving size: 1 burrito frozen = 139 g; Calories = 332.2; Total Carb (g) = 42.9; Net Carb (g) = 37; Fat (g) = 13.4; Protein = 10.1

🍢 Burrito Beef And Bean Microwaved ☞ serving size: 1 burrito cooked = 116 g; Calories = 345.7; Total Carb (g) = 45.2; Net Carb (g) = 37.2; Fat (g) = 13.9; Protein = 10.1

🍢 Burrito With Beans And Rice Meatless ☞ serving size: 1 small burrito = 182 g; Calories = 384; Total Carb (g) = 39.1; Net Carb (g) = 33.1; Fat (g) = 18; Protein = 17

🍢 Burrito With Beans Meatless ☞ serving size: 1 small burrito = 170 g; Calories = 368.9; Total Carb (g) = 35.8; Net Carb (g) = 29.8; Fat (g) = 18; Protein = 16.6

🍢 Burrito With Beans Rice And Sour Cream Meatless ☞ serving size: 1 small burrito = 208 g; Calories = 436.8; Total Carb (g) = 40.4; Net Carb (g) = 34.3; Fat (g) = 23; Protein = 17.6

🍢 Burrito With Chicken ☞ serving size: 1 small burrito = 142 g; Calories = 343.6; Total Carb (g) = 23.5; Net Carb (g) = 21.5; Fat (g) = 17.1; Protein = 24

🍢 Burrito With Chicken And Beans ☞ serving size: 1 small burrito = 153 g; Calories = 348.8; Total Carb (g) = 29.2; Net Carb (g) = 25.3; Fat (g) = 17.1; Protein = 19.8

🍢 Burrito With Chicken And Sour Cream ☞ serving size: 1 small burrito = 162 g; Calories = 380.7; Total Carb (g) = 23.8; Net Carb (g) = 22; Fat (g) = 21.4; Protein = 23.6

🍢 Burrito With Chicken Beans And Rice ☞ serving size: 1 small burrito = 165 g; Calories = 364.7; Total Carb (g) = 32.5; Net Carb (g) = 28.6; Fat (g) = 17.2; Protein = 20.1

🍢 Burrito With Chicken Beans And Sour Cream ☞ serving size: 1 small burrito = 179 g; Calories = 401; Total Carb (g) = 30.4; Net Carb (g) = 26.5; Fat (g) = 22.2; Protein = 20.4

🫓 Burrito With Chicken Beans Rice And Sour Cream ☞ serving size: 1 small burrito = 191 g; Calories = 416.4; Total Carb (g) = 33.8; Net Carb (g) = 29.7; Fat (g) = 22.2; Protein = 20.8

🫓 Burrito With Meat ☞ serving size: 1 small burrito = 161 g; Calories = 389.6; Total Carb (g) = 23.3; Net Carb (g) = 21.3; Fat (g) = 23.3; Protein = 21

🫓 Burrito With Meat And Beans ☞ serving size: 1 small burrito = 166 g; Calories = 380.1; Total Carb (g) = 29.6; Net Carb (g) = 25.6; Fat (g) = 20.7; Protein = 18.9

🫓 Burrito With Meat And Sour Cream ☞ serving size: 1 small burrito = 187 g; Calories = 441.3; Total Carb (g) = 24.5; Net Carb (g) = 22.4; Fat (g) = 28.3; Protein = 21.6

🫓 Burrito With Meat Beans And Rice ☞ serving size: 1 small burrito = 177 g; Calories = 394.7; Total Carb (g) = 32.8; Net Carb (g) = 28.7; Fat (g) = 20.6; Protein = 19.1

🫓 Burrito With Meat Beans And Sour Cream ☞ serving size: 1 small burrito = 192 g; Calories = 432; Total Carb (g) = 30.8; Net Carb (g) = 26.8; Fat (g) = 25.7; Protein = 19.5

🫓 Burrito With Meat Beans And Sour Cream From Fast Food ☞ serving size: 1 small burrito = 192 g; Calories = 401.3; Total Carb (g) = 51.4; Net Carb (g) = 44.5; Fat (g) = 15.1; Protein = 16.4

🫓 Burrito With Meat Beans Rice And Sour Cream ☞ serving size: 1 small burrito = 203 g; Calories = 444.6; Total Carb (g) = 34; Net Carb (g) = 30; Fat (g) = 25.6; Protein = 19.8

🫓 Cake Made With Glutinous Rice ☞ serving size: 1 oz = 28 g; Calories = 77.3; Total Carb (g) = 15.1; Net Carb (g) = 14.7; Fat (g) = 1.8; Protein = 0.6

🫓 Cake Made With Glutinous Rice And Dried Beans ☞ serving size: 1 piece = 16 g; Calories = 29.9; Total Carb (g) = 6; Net Carb (g) = 5.5; Fat (g) = 0.1; Protein = 1.3

🍰 Cake Or Pancake Made With Rice Flour And/or Dried Beans ☞ serving size: 1 idli (2-1/4" dia) = 38 g; Calories = 48.6; Total Carb (g) = 9.5; Net Carb (g) = 7.3; Fat (g) = 0.1; Protein = 2.4

🍰 Cannelloni Cheese- And Spinach-Filled No Sauce ☞ serving size: 1 cannelloni = 74 g; Calories = 116.9; Total Carb (g) = 12.9; Net Carb (g) = 12; Fat (g) = 5; Protein = 5.1

🍰 Cannelloni Cheese-Filled With Tomato Sauce Diet Frozen Meal ☞ serving size: 1 meal (9.125 oz) = 259 g; Calories = 297.9; Total Carb (g) = 28.1; Net Carb (g) = 26.3; Fat (g) = 12.4; Protein = 18.3

🍰 Cheese Enchilada Frozen Meal ☞ serving size: 1 meal (10 oz) = 284 g; Calories = 536.8; Total Carb (g) = 58.7; Net Carb (g) = 49.1; Fat (g) = 24; Protein = 23.5

🍰 Cheese Quiche Meatless ☞ serving size: 1 piece (1/8 of 9" dia) = 192 g; Calories = 698.9; Total Carb (g) = 25.5; Net Carb (g) = 24; Fat (g) = 56.3; Protein = 23.5

🍰 Cheese Turnover Puerto Rican Style ☞ serving size: 1 turnover = 21 g; Calories = 88.2; Total Carb (g) = 7.7; Net Carb (g) = 7.5; Fat (g) = 5.4; Protein = 2

🍰 Chicken Burritos Diet Frozen Meal ☞ serving size: 1 meal (10 oz) = 284 g; Calories = 499.8; Total Carb (g) = 67.5; Net Carb (g) = 61.8; Fat (g) = 13.1; Protein = 27.3

🍰 Chicken Chow Mein With Rice Diet Frozen Meal ☞ serving size: 1 lean cuisine meal (11.25 oz) = 319 g; Calories = 290.3; Total Carb (g) = 37.8; Net Carb (g) = 35.9; Fat (g) = 6.3; Protein = 19.3

🍰 Chicken Egg Foo Yung ☞ serving size: 1 patty = 86 g; Calories = 116.1; Total Carb (g) = 3.9; Net Carb (g) = 3.7; Fat (g) = 6.2; Protein = 11

🍰 Chicken Enchilada Diet Frozen Meal ☞ serving size: 1 meal (8.5 oz) = 241 g; Calories = 351.9; Total Carb (g) = 28.9; Net Carb (g) = 26; Fat (g) = 15.2; Protein = 25.6

🍰 Chicken Fajitas Diet Frozen Meal ☞ serving size: 1 meal (6.75 oz)

= 191 g; Calories = 234.9; Total Carb (g) = 29.9; Net Carb (g) = 27.1; Fat
(g) = 5; Protein = 17.1

🍗 Chicken In Orange Sauce With Almond Rice Diet Frozen Meal
☞ serving size: 1 meal (8 oz) = 227 g; Calories = 301.9; Total Carb (g)
= 36.4; Net Carb (g) = 35.5; Fat (g) = 5; Protein = 25.7

🍗 Chicken In Soy-Based Sauce Rice And Vegetables Frozen Meal
☞ serving size: 1 meal (9 oz) = 255 g; Calories = 278; Total Carb (g) =
46; Net Carb (g) = 43.4; Fat (g) = 2.2; Protein = 17.1

🍗 Chicken Nuggets Dark And White Meat Precooked Frozen Not
Reheated ☞ serving size: 1 serving = 87 g; Calories = 233.2; Total
Carb (g) = 14; Net Carb (g) = 12.6; Fat (g) = 15.1; Protein = 10.5

🍗 Chicken Nuggets White Meat Precooked Frozen Not Reheated
☞ serving size: 1 serving = 82 g; Calories = 214; Total Carb (g) = 13.3;
Net Carb (g) = 12.7; Fat (g) = 12.6; Protein = 11.8

🍗 Chicken Or Turkey And Noodles With Soy-Based Sauce ☞
serving size: 1 cup = 224 g; Calories = 347.2; Total Carb (g) = 17.1; Net
Carb (g) = 15.7; Fat (g) = 19.9; Protein = 25.9

🍗 Chicken Or Turkey And Rice With Soy-Based Sauce ☞ serving
size: 1 cup = 244 g; Calories = 390.4; Total Carb (g) = 19.6; Net Carb
(g) = 18.4; Fat (g) = 22.1; Protein = 29.1

🍗 Chicken Or Turkey And Vegetables Excluding Carrots Broccoli
And Dark-Green Leafy; No Potatoes Soy-Based Sauce ☞ serving
size: 1 cup = 217 g; Calories = 279.9; Total Carb (g) = 9.6; Net Carb (g)
= 7.7; Fat (g) = 17.6; Protein = 22.9

🍗 Chicken Or Turkey Chow Mein Or Chop Suey No Noodles ☞
serving size: 1 cup = 220 g; Calories = 182.6; Total Carb (g) = 8.5; Net
Carb (g) = 6.7; Fat (g) = 7.1; Protein = 21.5

🍗 Chicken Or Turkey Chow Mein Or Chop Suey With Noodles ☞
serving size: 1 cup = 220 g; Calories = 288.2; Total Carb (g) = 27; Net
Carb (g) = 24.4; Fat (g) = 10.4; Protein = 21.1

🌑 Chicken Or Turkey Rice And Vegetables Excluding Carrots Broccoli And Dark-Green Leafy; Soy-Based Sauce ☞ serving size: 1 cup = 217 g; Calories = 282.1; Total Carb (g) = 17; Net Carb (g) = 15.3; Fat (g) = 15.3; Protein = 20.7

🌑 Chicken Or Turkey Rice And Vegetables Including Carrots Broccoli And/or Dark-Green Leafy; Soy-Based Sauce ☞ serving size: 1 cup = 217 g; Calories = 277.8; Total Carb (g) = 17.5; Net Carb (g) = 14.9; Fat (g) = 14.8; Protein = 20.2

🌑 Chicken Or Turkey With Teriyaki ☞ serving size: 1 cup = 244 g; Calories = 397.7; Total Carb (g) = 4; Net Carb (g) = 4; Fat (g) = 14.5; Protein = 62.8

🌑 Chicken Pot Pie Frozen Entree Prepared ☞ serving size: 1 pie = 302 g; Calories = 616.1; Total Carb (g) = 58; Net Carb (g) = 54.7; Fat (g) = 35.8; Protein = 15.4

🌑 Chicken Tenders Breaded Frozen Prepared ☞ serving size: 1 piece = 21 g; Calories = 50.4; Total Carb (g) = 3.1; Net Carb (g) = 2.8; Fat (g) = 2.9; Protein = 3.1

🌑 Chicken Thighs Frozen Breaded Reheated ☞ serving size: 1 thigh with bone and breading = 133 g; Calories = 444.2; Total Carb (g) = 18.9; Net Carb (g) = 18.8; Fat (g) = 29.9; Protein = 24.8

🌑 Chilaquiles Tortilla Casserole With Salsa And Cheese No Egg ☞ serving size: 1 cup = 232 g; Calories = 693.7; Total Carb (g) = 67.2; Net Carb (g) = 59.8; Fat (g) = 40.4; Protein = 16.9

🌑 Chilaquiles Tortilla Casserole With Salsa Cheese And Egg ☞ serving size: 1 cup = 232 g; Calories = 677.4; Total Carb (g) = 57.3; Net Carb (g) = 51.1; Fat (g) = 41.4; Protein = 19.9

🌑 Chiles Rellenos Cheese-Filled ☞ serving size: 1 chili = 143 g; Calories = 313.2; Total Carb (g) = 9.1; Net Carb (g) = 7.5; Fat (g) = 24.1; Protein = 15.6

🌑 Chiles Rellenos Filled With Meat And Cheese ☞ serving size: 1

chili = 143 g; Calories = 293.2; Total Carb (g) = 10.3; Net Carb (g) = 8.6; Fat (g) = 21.2; Protein = 15.8

🦐 Chili Con Carne With Beans Canned Entree ☞ serving size: 1 cup = 242 g; Calories = 258.9; Total Carb (g) = 31.7; Net Carb (g) = 23.7; Fat (g) = 8.4; Protein = 14

🦐 Chili No Beans Canned Entree ☞ serving size: 1 cup = 240 g; Calories = 283.2; Total Carb (g) = 14.6; Net Carb (g) = 13.4; Fat (g) = 17; Protein = 18.1

🦐 Chili With Beans Microwavable Bowls ☞ serving size: 1 cup = 244 g; Calories = 244; Total Carb (g) = 26.6; Net Carb (g) = 19.5; Fat (g) = 9; Protein = 14.3

🦐 Chimichanga Meatless ☞ serving size: 1 small chimichanga = 128 g; Calories = 288; Total Carb (g) = 34.5; Net Carb (g) = 29.5; Fat (g) = 12.9; Protein = 9.1

🦐 Chimichanga Meatless With Sour Cream ☞ serving size: 1 small chimichanga = 136 g; Calories = 303.3; Total Carb (g) = 33.9; Net Carb (g) = 29.1; Fat (g) = 14.8; Protein = 9.1

🦐 Chimichanga With Chicken ☞ serving size: 1 small chimichanga = 97 g; Calories = 263.8; Total Carb (g) = 28.7; Net Carb (g) = 25.3; Fat (g) = 12.3; Protein = 9.8

🦐 Chimichanga With Chicken And Sour Cream ☞ serving size: 1 small chimichanga = 108 g; Calories = 287.3; Total Carb (g) = 29.2; Net Carb (g) = 25.7; Fat (g) = 14.6; Protein = 10.1

🦐 Chimichanga With Meat ☞ serving size: 1 small chimichanga = 105 g; Calories = 273; Total Carb (g) = 29.2; Net Carb (g) = 25.7; Fat (g) = 13.2; Protein = 9.6

🦐 Chimichanga With Meat And Sour Cream ☞ serving size: 1 small chimichanga = 92 g; Calories = 259.4; Total Carb (g) = 25.1; Net Carb (g) = 22.9; Fat (g) = 14.1; Protein = 8.3

🦐 Chow Fun Noodles With Meat And Vegetables ☞ serving size: 1

cup = 152 g; Calories = 155; Total Carb (g) = 17.5; Net Carb (g) = 16.1; Fat (g) = 4.2; Protein = 10.8

🦞 Chow Fun Noodles With Vegetables Meatless ☞ serving size: 1 cup = 152 g; Calories = 112.5; Total Carb (g) = 22; Net Carb (g) = 20.3; Fat (g) = 1.5; Protein = 2.4

🦞 Chow Mein Or Chop Suey Meatless With Noodles ☞ serving size: 1 cup = 220 g; Calories = 257.4; Total Carb (g) = 38.1; Net Carb (g) = 34.5; Fat (g) = 8.9; Protein = 5.5

🦞 Chow Mein Or Chop Suey Ns As To Type Of Meat No Noodles ☞ serving size: 1 cup = 220 g; Calories = 182.6; Total Carb (g) = 8.5; Net Carb (g) = 6.7; Fat (g) = 7.1; Protein = 21.5

🦞 Chow Mein Or Chop Suey Ns As To Type Of Meat With Noodles ☞ serving size: 1 cup = 220 g; Calories = 288.2; Total Carb (g) = 27; Net Carb (g) = 24.4; Fat (g) = 10.4; Protein = 21.1

🦞 Chow Mein Or Chop Suey Various Types Of Meat With Noodles ☞ serving size: 1 cup = 220 g; Calories = 297; Total Carb (g) = 27; Net Carb (g) = 24.4; Fat (g) = 10.7; Protein = 22

🦞 Congee With Meat Poultry And/or Seafood ☞ serving size: 1 cup = 249 g; Calories = 132; Total Carb (g) = 15.2; Net Carb (g) = 15; Fat (g) = 2.3; Protein = 12

🦞 Congee With Meat Poultry And/or Seafood And Vegetables ☞ serving size: 1 cup = 249 g; Calories = 129.5; Total Carb (g) = 15.2; Net Carb (g) = 14.4; Fat (g) = 2.3; Protein = 11.5

🦞 Congee With Vegetables ☞ serving size: 1 cup = 249 g; Calories = 87.2; Total Carb (g) = 19.2; Net Carb (g) = 18.4; Fat (g) = 0.3; Protein = 1.9

🦞 Corn Dogs Frozen Prepared ☞ serving size: 1 corndog = 78 g; Calories = 195; Total Carb (g) = 21; Net Carb (g) = 20.3; Fat (g) = 9.4; Protein = 6.7

🦞 Cornmeal Dressing With Chicken Or Turkey And Vegetables ☞

serving size: 1 cup = 161 g; Calories = 380; Total Carb (g) = 30.9; Net Carb (g) = 28.9; Fat (g) = 23.1; Protein = 12.2

🍃 Crepe Filled With Meat Poultry Or Seafood No Sauce ☞ serving size: 1 crepe with filling, any size = 125 g; Calories = 242.5; Total Carb (g) = 13.9; Net Carb (g) = 12.9; Fat (g) = 13.2; Protein = 17.1

🍃 Crepe Filled With Meat Poultry Or Seafood With Sauce ☞ serving size: 1 crepe with filling, any size = 155 g; Calories = 285.2; Total Carb (g) = 12.4; Net Carb (g) = 11.6; Fat (g) = 17.1; Protein = 20.3

🍃 Dirty Rice ☞ serving size: 1 cup = 198 g; Calories = 221.8; Total Carb (g) = 34.2; Net Carb (g) = 33.1; Fat (g) = 4.4; Protein = 10.2

🍃 Dosa (Indian) With Filling ☞ serving size: 1 small = 113 g; Calories = 206.8; Total Carb (g) = 34.8; Net Carb (g) = 32.4; Fat (g) = 4.7; Protein = 6.2

🍃 Dressing With Chicken Or Turkey And Vegetables ☞ serving size: 1 cup = 161 g; Calories = 349.4; Total Carb (g) = 33.8; Net Carb (g) = 31.3; Fat (g) = 18; Protein = 12.9

🍃 Dressing With Meat And Vegetables ☞ serving size: 1 cup = 161 g; Calories = 420.2; Total Carb (g) = 33; Net Carb (g) = 30.8; Fat (g) = 27.1; Protein = 10.8

🍃 Dressing With Oysters ☞ serving size: 1 cup = 161 g; Calories = 304.3; Total Carb (g) = 29.6; Net Carb (g) = 27.4; Fat (g) = 17.4; Protein = 7.7

🍃 Dukboki Or Tteokbokki Korean ☞ serving size: 1 cup = 250 g; Calories = 330; Total Carb (g) = 49.7; Net Carb (g) = 47.2; Fat (g) = 10.2; Protein = 9.8

🍃 Dumpling Fried Puerto Rican Style ☞ serving size: 1 small dumpling = 16 g; Calories = 59.4; Total Carb (g) = 5.5; Net Carb (g) = 5.3; Fat (g) = 3.8; Protein = 0.9

🍃 Dumpling Meat-Filled ☞ serving size: 1 dumpling, any size = 97

g; Calories = 348.2; Total Carb (g) = 24.6; Net Carb (g) = 23.7; Fat (g) = 22.1; Protein = 12.2

🍃 Dumpling Potato- Or Cheese-Filled Frozen ☞ serving size: 3 pieces pierogies = 114 g; Calories = 222.3; Total Carb (g) = 33.8; Net Carb (g) = 32.8; Fat (g) = 7; Protein = 6

🍃 Dumpling Vegetable ☞ serving size: 1 dumpling, any size = 97 g; Calories = 159.1; Total Carb (g) = 26.6; Net Carb (g) = 24.9; Fat (g) = 3.7; Protein = 4.9

🍃 Egg Foo Yung Nfs ☞ serving size: 1 patty = 86 g; Calories = 105.8; Total Carb (g) = 4.3; Net Carb (g) = 4.1; Fat (g) = 5.1; Protein = 10

🍃 Egg Roll Meatless ☞ serving size: 1 miniature egg roll = 13 g; Calories = 35; Total Carb (g) = 3.9; Net Carb (g) = 3.6; Fat (g) = 1.8; Protein = 0.7

🍃 Egg Roll With Beef And/or Pork ☞ serving size: 1 miniature roll = 13 g; Calories = 36; Total Carb (g) = 3.6; Net Carb (g) = 3.4; Fat (g) = 1.9; Protein = 1.2

🍃 Egg Roll With Chicken Or Turkey ☞ serving size: 1 miniature egg roll = 13 g; Calories = 32.9; Total Carb (g) = 3.5; Net Carb (g) = 3.2; Fat (g) = 1.5; Protein = 1.3

🍃 Egg Roll With Shrimp ☞ serving size: 1 miniature egg roll = 13 g; Calories = 35; Total Carb (g) = 3.9; Net Carb (g) = 3.6; Fat (g) = 1.8; Protein = 0.7

🍃 Egg Rolls Chicken Refrigerated Heated ☞ serving size: 1 roll = 80 g; Calories = 157.6; Total Carb (g) = 22.8; Net Carb (g) = 20.9; Fat (g) = 3.6; Protein = 8.4

🍃 Egg Rolls Pork Refrigerated Heated ☞ serving size: 1 roll = 85 g; Calories = 193; Total Carb (g) = 24.2; Net Carb (g) = 24.2; Fat (g) = 7; Protein = 8.5

🍃 Egg Rolls Vegetable Frozen Prepared ☞ serving size: 1 egg roll =

68 g; Calories = 145.5; Total Carb (g) = 21.6; Net Carb (g) = 20; Fat (g) = 4.7; Protein = 4.1

🌶 Empanada Mexican Turnover Filled With Cheese And Vegetables ☞ serving size: 1 small/appetizer = 81 g; Calories = 258.4; Total Carb (g) = 27.9; Net Carb (g) = 26.6; Fat (g) = 13.4; Protein = 7

🌶 Empanada Mexican Turnover Filled With Chicken And Vegetables ☞ serving size: 1 small/appetizer = 81 g; Calories = 230.9; Total Carb (g) = 26.9; Net Carb (g) = 25.7; Fat (g) = 10.3; Protein = 7.8

🌶 Enchilada Just Cheese Meatless No Beans Green-Chile Or Enchilada Sauce ☞ serving size: 1 enchilada, any size = 111 g; Calories = 209.8; Total Carb (g) = 14.5; Net Carb (g) = 12.3; Fat (g) = 13.6; Protein = 8.7

🌶 Enchilada Just Cheese Meatless No Beans Red-Chile Or Enchilada Sauce ☞ serving size: 1 enchilada, any size = 119 g; Calories = 198.7; Total Carb (g) = 15.3; Net Carb (g) = 13.1; Fat (g) = 12; Protein = 8.7

🌶 Enchilada With Beans Green-Chile Or Enchilada Sauce ☞ serving size: 1 enchilada, any size = 132 g; Calories = 195.4; Total Carb (g) = 22; Net Carb (g) = 17.4; Fat (g) = 9.7; Protein = 6.6

🌶 Enchilada With Beans Meatless Red-Chile Or Enchilada Sauce ☞ serving size: 1 enchilada, any size = 141 g; Calories = 184.7; Total Carb (g) = 23; Net Carb (g) = 18.3; Fat (g) = 8.2; Protein = 6.7

🌶 Enchilada With Chicken And Beans Green-Chile Or Enchilada Sauce ☞ serving size: 1 enchilada, any size = 132 g; Calories = 196.7; Total Carb (g) = 19.4; Net Carb (g) = 15.7; Fat (g) = 9.9; Protein = 9.1

🌶 Enchilada With Chicken And Beans Red-Chile Or Enchilada Sauce ☞ serving size: 1 enchilada, any size = 132 g; Calories = 172.9; Total Carb (g) = 19; Net Carb (g) = 15.6; Fat (g) = 7.7; Protein = 8.6

🌶 Enchilada With Chicken Green-Chile Or Enchilada Sauce ☞

serving size: 1 enchilada, any size = 114 g; Calories = 171; Total Carb (g) = 14.1; Net Carb (g) = 11.8; Fat (g) = 8.7; Protein = 10.3

🦪 Enchilada With Chicken Red-Chile Or Enchilada Sauce ☞ serving size: 1 enchilada, any size = 123 g; Calories = 159.9; Total Carb (g) = 15; Net Carb (g) = 12.8; Fat (g) = 7.2; Protein = 10.4

🦪 Enchilada With Meat And Beans Green-Chile Or Enchilada Sauce ☞ serving size: 1 enchilada, any size = 123 g; Calories = 193.1; Total Carb (g) = 18.1; Net Carb (g) = 14.6; Fat (g) = 10; Protein = 8.9

🦪 Enchilada With Meat And Beans Red-Chile Or Enchilada Sauce ☞ serving size: 1 enchilada, any size = 132 g; Calories = 183.5; Total Carb (g) = 19; Net Carb (g) = 15.6; Fat (g) = 8.5; Protein = 9

🦪 Enchilada With Meat Green-Chile Or Enchilada Sauce ☞ serving size: 1 enchilada, any size = 114 g; Calories = 191.5; Total Carb (g) = 14.1; Net Carb (g) = 11.8; Fat (g) = 10.4; Protein = 11.2

🦪 Enchilada With Meat Red-Chile Or Enchilada Sauce ☞ serving size: 1 enchilada, any size = 122 g; Calories = 179.3; Total Carb (g) = 14.9; Net Carb (g) = 12.7; Fat (g) = 8.7; Protein = 11.3

🦪 Fajita With Vegetables ☞ serving size: 1 fajita = 141 g; Calories = 227; Total Carb (g) = 22.4; Net Carb (g) = 19.7; Fat (g) = 12.1; Protein = 7.7

🦪 Fish And Vegetables Excluding Carrots Broccoli And Dark-Green Leafy; No Potatoes Soy-Based Sauce ☞ serving size: 1 cup = 217 g; Calories = 221.3; Total Carb (g) = 9.5; Net Carb (g) = 7.5; Fat (g) = 13.2; Protein = 17.2

🦪 Fish And Vegetables Including Carrots Broccoli And/or Dark-Green Leafy; No Potatoes Soy-Based Sauce ☞ serving size: 1 cup = 217 g; Calories = 219.2; Total Carb (g) = 10.3; Net Carb (g) = 7.5; Fat (g) = 12.7; Protein = 16.7

🦪 Flavored Pasta ☞ serving size: 1 cup = 185 g; Calories = 161; Total Carb (g) = 26.7; Net Carb (g) = 26; Fat (g) = 4.1; Protein = 4.6

🍀 Flavored Rice And Pasta Mixture ☞ serving size: 1 cup, beef flavor = 184 g; Calories = 219; Total Carb (g) = 35; Net Carb (g) = 34.5; Fat (g) = 6.6; Protein = 4.9

🍀 Flavored Rice And Pasta Mixture Reduced Sodium ☞ serving size: 1 cup = 196 g; Calories = 219.5; Total Carb (g) = 34.3; Net Carb (g) = 33; Fat (g) = 6.8; Protein = 5.1

🍀 Flavored Rice Brown And Wild ☞ serving size: 1 cup = 217 g; Calories = 230; Total Carb (g) = 41.8; Net Carb (g) = 39.2; Fat (g) = 4.7; Protein = 6

🍀 Flavored Rice Mixture ☞ serving size: 1 cup = 218 g; Calories = 276.9; Total Carb (g) = 44.1; Net Carb (g) = 43.2; Fat (g) = 8.9; Protein = 4.2

🍀 Flavored Rice Mixture With Cheese ☞ serving size: 1 cup = 230 g; Calories = 285.2; Total Carb (g) = 58; Net Carb (g) = 56.6; Fat (g) = 2.8; Protein = 6.9

🍀 Fried Rice Puerto Rican Style ☞ serving size: 1 cup = 173 g; Calories = 205.9; Total Carb (g) = 14.8; Net Carb (g) = 13.7; Fat (g) = 5.8; Protein = 22.1

🍀 Fried Stuffed Potatoes Puerto Rican Style ☞ serving size: 1 fritter (4" x 2-1/4" x 3/4") = 95 g; Calories = 177.7; Total Carb (g) = 15.4; Net Carb (g) = 13.6; Fat (g) = 11.2; Protein = 4.6

🍀 Gnocchi Cheese ☞ serving size: 1 cup = 70 g; Calories = 124.6; Total Carb (g) = 6.6; Net Carb (g) = 6.5; Fat (g) = 8.3; Protein = 5.9

🍀 Gnocchi Potato ☞ serving size: 1 cup = 188 g; Calories = 250; Total Carb (g) = 32.1; Net Carb (g) = 30.2; Fat (g) = 11.7; Protein = 4.4

🍀 Gordita Sope Or Chalupa With Beans ☞ serving size: 1 small = 150 g; Calories = 313.5; Total Carb (g) = 38.4; Net Carb (g) = 32.1; Fat (g) = 14; Protein = 9.8

🍀 Gordita Sope Or Chalupa With Beans And Sour Cream ☞

serving size: 1 small = 165 g; Calories = 343.2; Total Carb (g) = 39.1; Net Carb (g) = 32.9; Fat (g) = 16.9; Protein = 10.2

🌑 Gordita Sope Or Chalupa With Chicken ☞ serving size: 1 small = 115 g; Calories = 285.2; Total Carb (g) = 28.1; Net Carb (g) = 25.1; Fat (g) = 14; Protein = 12.5

🌑 Gordita Sope Or Chalupa With Chicken And Sour Cream ☞ serving size: 1 small = 124 g; Calories = 300.1; Total Carb (g) = 27.4; Net Carb (g) = 24.6; Fat (g) = 16.1; Protein = 12.2

🌑 Gordita Sope Or Chalupa With Meat ☞ serving size: 1 small = 115 g; Calories = 287.5; Total Carb (g) = 27.5; Net Carb (g) = 24.4; Fat (g) = 15; Protein = 11.2

🌑 Gordita Sope Or Chalupa With Meat And Sour Cream ☞ serving size: 1 small = 132 g; Calories = 326; Total Carb (g) = 29.1; Net Carb (g) = 25.8; Fat (g) = 18.3; Protein = 11.9

🌑 Grape Leaves Stuffed With Rice ☞ serving size: 1 roll = 56 g; Calories = 91.3; Total Carb (g) = 7.8; Net Carb (g) = 6.1; Fat (g) = 6.5; Protein = 1.3

🌑 Ground Beef With Tomato Sauce And Taco Seasonings On A Cornbread Crust ☞ serving size: 1 cup = 179 g; Calories = 347.3; Total Carb (g) = 36.7; Net Carb (g) = 32; Fat (g) = 14.6; Protein = 17.1

🌑 Hopping John ☞ serving size: 1 cup = 224 g; Calories = 282.2; Total Carb (g) = 45.2; Net Carb (g) = 38.4; Fat (g) = 4.1; Protein = 15.8

🌑 Hot Pockets Croissant Pockets Chicken Broccoli And Cheddar Stuffed Sandwich Frozen ☞ serving size: 1 serving (1 hot pocket) = 127 g; Calories = 298.5; Total Carb (g) = 38.6; Net Carb (g) = 37.2; Fat (g) = 10.9; Protein = 11.3

🌑 Hot Pockets Ham N Cheese Stuffed Sandwich Frozen ☞ serving size: 1 serving (1 hot pocket) = 127 g; Calories = 342.9; Total Carb (g) = 31.4; Net Carb (g) = 29.5; Fat (g) = 19.1; Protein = 11.6

🌑 Hot Pockets Meatballs & Mozzarella Stuffed Sandwich Frozen

☞ serving size: 1 hot pocket (1 nlea serving) = 127 g; Calories = 320; Total Carb (g) = 39; Net Carb (g) = 36.2; Fat (g) = 13; Protein = 11.8

🥩 Hungry Man Salisbury Steak With Gravy Frozen Unprepared ☞ serving size: 1 patty = 64 g; Calories = 87; Total Carb (g) = 4.5; Net Carb (g) = 3.6; Fat (g) = 5.5; Protein = 5.1

🥩 Jalapeno Pepper Stuffed With Cheese Breaded Or Battered Fried ☞ serving size: 1 jalapeno pepper = 25 g; Calories = 60; Total Carb (g) = 4.1; Net Carb (g) = 3.5; Fat (g) = 3.9; Protein = 2.3

🥩 Jambalaya With Meat And Rice ☞ serving size: 1 cup = 244 g; Calories = 434.3; Total Carb (g) = 20.8; Net Carb (g) = 19.1; Fat (g) = 23.1; Protein = 35.4

🥩 Jimmy Dean Sausage Egg And Cheese Breakfast Biscuit Frozen Unprepared ☞ serving size: 1 biscuit = 128 g; Calories = 419.8; Total Carb (g) = 27; Net Carb (g) = 24.4; Fat (g) = 29.3; Protein = 11.9

🥩 Kishke Stuffed Derma ☞ serving size: 1 cubic inch, cooked = 18 g; Calories = 82.8; Total Carb (g) = 6.3; Net Carb (g) = 6; Fat (g) = 5.9; Protein = 0.9

🥩 Knish Cheese ☞ serving size: 1 knish = 60 g; Calories = 205.2; Total Carb (g) = 18.7; Net Carb (g) = 18; Fat (g) = 11.7; Protein = 6.1

🥩 Knish Meat ☞ serving size: 1 knish = 50 g; Calories = 174.5; Total Carb (g) = 12.8; Net Carb (g) = 12.3; Fat (g) = 10.6; Protein = 6.6

🥩 Knish Potato ☞ serving size: 1 knish = 61 g; Calories = 212.9; Total Carb (g) = 20.6; Net Carb (g) = 19.7; Fat (g) = 12.4; Protein = 4.6

🥩 Kung Pao Beef ☞ serving size: 1 cup = 162 g; Calories = 353.2; Total Carb (g) = 8.1; Net Carb (g) = 6.3; Fat (g) = 23.4; Protein = 29.7

🥩 Kung Pao Pork ☞ serving size: 1 cup = 162 g; Calories = 358; Total Carb (g) = 8.1; Net Carb (g) = 6.3; Fat (g) = 23.9; Protein = 28

🥩 Kung Pao Shrimp ☞ serving size: 1 cup = 162 g; Calories = 283.5; Total Carb (g) = 9.3; Net Carb (g) = 7.5; Fat (g) = 17.4; Protein = 23.3

Lasagna Cheese Frozen Prepared ☞ serving size: 1 cup 1 serving = 225 g; Calories = 292.5; Total Carb (g) = 31.1; Net Carb (g) = 27.3; Fat (g) = 12; Protein = 14.7

Lasagna Cheese Frozen Unprepared ☞ serving size: 1 cup 1 serving = 237 g; Calories = 343.7; Total Carb (g) = 51.2; Net Carb (g) = 47.2; Fat (g) = 10; Protein = 12

Lasagna Meatless Spinach Noodles ☞ serving size: 1 piece (1/6 of 8" square, approx 2-1/2" x 4") = 227 g; Calories = 385.9; Total Carb (g) = 26.2; Net Carb (g) = 23; Fat (g) = 19.5; Protein = 26.1

Lasagna Meatless Whole Wheat Noodles ☞ serving size: 1 piece (1/6 of 8" square, approx 2-1/2" x 4") = 227 g; Calories = 406.3; Total Carb (g) = 30.1; Net Carb (g) = 26; Fat (g) = 20.3; Protein = 27.3

Lasagna Meatless With Vegetables ☞ serving size: 1 piece (1/6 of 8" square, approx 2-1/2" x 4") = 227 g; Calories = 401.8; Total Carb (g) = 30.6; Net Carb (g) = 27.8; Fat (g) = 19.1; Protein = 26.6

Lasagna Vegetable Frozen Baked ☞ serving size: 1 serving = 227 g; Calories = 315.5; Total Carb (g) = 32.2; Net Carb (g) = 27.9; Fat (g) = 13.7; Protein = 15.6

Lasagna With Cheese And Meat Sauce Diet Frozen Meal ☞ serving size: 1 weight watchers meal (11 oz) = 312 g; Calories = 368.2; Total Carb (g) = 39.2; Net Carb (g) = 35.8; Fat (g) = 13.1; Protein = 23.7

Lasagna With Cheese And Sauce Diet Frozen Meal ☞ serving size: 1 meal (11 oz) = 312 g; Calories = 427.4; Total Carb (g) = 55; Net Carb (g) = 50.4; Fat (g) = 15.6; Protein = 17.8

Lasagna With Chicken Or Turkey ☞ serving size: 1 piece (1/6 of 8" square, approx 2-1/2" x 4") = 206 g; Calories = 401.7; Total Carb (g) = 26.7; Net Carb (g) = 24.7; Fat (g) = 19.4; Protein = 29.5

Lasagna With Chicken Or Turkey And Spinach ☞ serving size: 1 piece (1/6 of 8" square, approx 2-1/2" x 4") = 206 g; Calories = 393.5; Total Carb (g) = 26.3; Net Carb (g) = 24; Fat (g) = 18.9; Protein = 28.9

🥬 Lasagna With Meat ☞ serving size: 1 piece (1/6 of 8" square, approx 2-1/2" x 4") = 206 g; Calories = 286.3; Total Carb (g) = 33.3; Net Carb (g) = 30; Fat (g) = 10.2; Protein = 15.4

🥬 Lasagna With Meat & Sauce Frozen Entree ☞ serving size: 1 piece side = 134 g; Calories = 166.2; Total Carb (g) = 19.3; Net Carb (g) = 17.4; Fat (g) = 5.9; Protein = 8.9

🥬 Lasagna With Meat & Sauce Low-Fat Frozen Entree ☞ serving size: 1 package = 309 g; Calories = 312.1; Total Carb (g) = 41.7; Net Carb (g) = 37.7; Fat (g) = 6.9; Protein = 21

🥬 Lasagna With Meat And Spinach ☞ serving size: 1 piece (1/6 of 8" square, approx 2-1/2" x 4") = 206 g; Calories = 405.8; Total Carb (g) = 26.3; Net Carb (g) = 24; Fat (g) = 20.3; Protein = 28.6

🥬 Lasagna With Meat Home Recipe ☞ serving size: 1 piece (1/6 of 8" square, approx 2-1/2" x 4") = 206 g; Calories = 403.8; Total Carb (g) = 25.1; Net Carb (g) = 23; Fat (g) = 20.4; Protein = 29.3

🥬 Lasagna With Meat Sauce Frozen Prepared ☞ serving size: 1 piece side = 123 g; Calories = 166.1; Total Carb (g) = 18.9; Net Carb (g) = 16.8; Fat (g) = 6.1; Protein = 9

🥬 Lasagna With Meat Spinach Noodles ☞ serving size: 1 piece (1/6 of 8" square, approx 2-1/2" x 4") = 206 g; Calories = 399.6; Total Carb (g) = 22.8; Net Carb (g) = 20.3; Fat (g) = 21.1; Protein = 28.6

🥬 Lasagna With Meat Whole Wheat Noodles ☞ serving size: 1 piece (1/6 of 8" square, approx 2-1/2" x 4") = 206 g; Calories = 407.9; Total Carb (g) = 26.2; Net Carb (g) = 23; Fat (g) = 21.2; Protein = 29.2

🥬 Lean Pockets Ham N Cheddar ☞ serving size: 1 hot pocket (1 nlea serving) = 127 g; Calories = 292.1; Total Carb (g) = 41.3; Net Carb (g) = 39.1; Fat (g) = 8.3; Protein = 13.1

🥬 Lean Pockets Meatballs & Mozzarella ☞ serving size: 1 each = 128 g; Calories = 307.2; Total Carb (g) = 41.3; Net Carb (g) = 38.8; Fat (g) = 9.9; Protein = 13.4

🌿 Lefse (Norwegian) ☞ serving size: 1 lefse, any size = 80 g; Calories = 172.8; Total Carb (g) = 28.8; Net Carb (g) = 27.2; Fat (g) = 4.9; Protein = 3.4

🌿 Linguini With Vegetables And Seafood In White Wine Sauce Diet Frozen Meal ☞ serving size: 1 meal (9.5 oz) = 269 g; Calories = 306.7; Total Carb (g) = 31.9; Net Carb (g) = 29; Fat (g) = 10.1; Protein = 21.6

🌿 Lo Mein With Beef ☞ serving size: 1 cup = 200 g; Calories = 258; Total Carb (g) = 32.4; Net Carb (g) = 30.4; Fat (g) = 5.5; Protein = 19.5

🌿 Lo Mein With Chicken ☞ serving size: 1 cup = 200 g; Calories = 260; Total Carb (g) = 32.3; Net Carb (g) = 30.3; Fat (g) = 6.3; Protein = 18.3

🌿 Lo Mein With Pork ☞ serving size: 1 cup = 200 g; Calories = 276; Total Carb (g) = 32.4; Net Carb (g) = 30.4; Fat (g) = 7.6; Protein = 19

🌿 Lo Mein With Shrimp ☞ serving size: 1 cup = 200 g; Calories = 242; Total Carb (g) = 32.5; Net Carb (g) = 30.5; Fat (g) = 4.4; Protein = 17.1

🌿 Macaroni And Cheese Box Mix With Cheese Sauce Prepared ☞ serving size: 1 cup prepared = 189 g; Calories = 310; Total Carb (g) = 43.7; Net Carb (g) = 41.4; Fat (g) = 9.4; Protein = 12.6

🌿 Macaroni And Cheese Box Mix With Cheese Sauce Unprepared ☞ serving size: 1 serving (3.5 oz) = 25 g; Calories = 83.5; Total Carb (g) = 11.7; Net Carb (g) = 11.2; Fat (g) = 2.7; Protein = 3.2

🌿 Macaroni And Cheese Canned Entree ☞ serving size: 1 serving = 244 g; Calories = 200.1; Total Carb (g) = 28.1; Net Carb (g) = 26.9; Fat (g) = 6; Protein = 8.3

🌿 Macaroni And Cheese Canned Microwavable ☞ serving size: 7 (1/2) oz 1 serving = 213 g; Calories = 285.4; Total Carb (g) = 29.7; Net Carb (g) = 28.9; Fat (g) = 12.8; Protein = 12.7

🌿 Macaroni And Cheese Diet Frozen Meal ☞ serving size: 1 meal

(9 oz) = 255 g; Calories = 331.5; Total Carb (g) = 43.9; Net Carb (g) = 41.8; Fat (g) = 10.1; Protein = 15.3

🐟 Macaroni And Cheese Dinner With Dry Sauce Mix Boxed Uncooked ☞ serving size: 1 serving (makes about 1 cup prepared) = 70 g; Calories = 265.3; Total Carb (g) = 49.1; Net Carb (g) = 46.8; Fat (g) = 3.4; Protein = 9.7

🐟 Macaroni And Cheese Dry Mix Prepared With 2% Milk And 80% Stick Margarine From Dry Mix ☞ serving size: 1 cup = 198 g; Calories = 376.2; Total Carb (g) = 47.4; Net Carb (g) = 45; Fat (g) = 16.4; Protein = 9.7

🐟 Macaroni And Cheese Frozen Entree ☞ serving size: 1 cup = 137 g; Calories = 204.1; Total Carb (g) = 23.7; Net Carb (g) = 22.2; Fat (g) = 8.8; Protein = 7.7

🐟 Macaroni Or Noodles Creamed With Cheese ☞ serving size: 1 cup = 230 g; Calories = 361.1; Total Carb (g) = 50.1; Net Carb (g) = 47.1; Fat (g) = 12.6; Protein = 11.3

🐟 Macaroni Or Noodles Creamed With Cheese And Tuna ☞ serving size: 1 cup = 230 g; Calories = 328.9; Total Carb (g) = 39.4; Net Carb (g) = 37.1; Fat (g) = 10.4; Protein = 18.6

🐟 Macaroni Or Noodles With Cheese ☞ serving size: 1 cup = 230 g; Calories = 508.3; Total Carb (g) = 53.3; Net Carb (g) = 50.5; Fat (g) = 23.6; Protein = 19.7

🐟 Macaroni Or Noodles With Cheese And Chicken Or Turkey ☞ serving size: 1 cup = 230 g; Calories = 404.8; Total Carb (g) = 34.1; Net Carb (g) = 32.5; Fat (g) = 17.3; Protein = 28.8

🐟 Macaroni Or Noodles With Cheese And Egg ☞ serving size: 1 cup = 230 g; Calories = 430.1; Total Carb (g) = 43.6; Net Carb (g) = 41.8; Fat (g) = 22.1; Protein = 14.3

🐟 Macaroni Or Noodles With Cheese And Frankfurters Or Hot

Dogs ☞ serving size: 1 cup = 230 g; Calories = 487.6; Total Carb (g) = 43.1; Net Carb (g) = 41.3; Fat (g) = 28.6; Protein = 14.4

● Macaroni Or Noodles With Cheese And Meat ☞ serving size: 1 cup = 230 g; Calories = 480.7; Total Carb (g) = 34.8; Net Carb (g) = 33.2; Fat (g) = 25.4; Protein = 27.1

● Macaroni Or Noodles With Cheese And Meat Prepared From Hamburger Helper Mix ☞ serving size: 1 cup = 230 g; Calories = 331.2; Total Carb (g) = 23.6; Net Carb (g) = 23; Fat (g) = 17.4; Protein = 18.9

● Macaroni Or Noodles With Cheese And Tomato ☞ serving size: 1 cup = 230 g; Calories = 335.8; Total Carb (g) = 43; Net Carb (g) = 40.5; Fat (g) = 14.7; Protein = 9

● Macaroni Or Noodles With Cheese And Tuna ☞ serving size: 1 cup = 230 g; Calories = 372.6; Total Carb (g) = 41.8; Net Carb (g) = 40; Fat (g) = 15.3; Protein = 17.6

● Macaroni Or Noodles With Cheese Easy Mac Type ☞ serving size: 1 cup = 230 g; Calories = 253; Total Carb (g) = 46.2; Net Carb (g) = 45.1; Fat (g) = 4.3; Protein = 7.5

● Macaroni Or Noodles With Cheese Made From Packaged Mix ☞ serving size: 1 cup = 230 g; Calories = 407.1; Total Carb (g) = 50.9; Net Carb (g) = 48.6; Fat (g) = 18.1; Protein = 10.7

● Macaroni Or Noodles With Cheese Made From Reduced Fat Packaged Mix ☞ serving size: 1 cup = 230 g; Calories = 296.7; Total Carb (g) = 39.7; Net Carb (g) = 38.3; Fat (g) = 10.9; Protein = 10.5

● Macaroni Or Noodles With Cheese Made From Reduced Fat Packaged Mix Unprepared ☞ serving size: 1 serving (3.5 oz) = 99 g; Calories = 294; Total Carb (g) = 51.5; Net Carb (g) = 49.6; Fat (g) = 4; Protein = 13

● Macaroni Or Noodles With Cheese Microwaveable Unprepared

☞ serving size: 1 serving 1 pouch = 61 g; Calories = 236.7; Total Carb (g) = 43.2; Net Carb (g) = 42.2; Fat (g) = 4; Protein = 7

🍮 Macaroni Or Pasta Salad Made With Any Type Of Fat Free Dressing ☞ serving size: 1 cup = 204 g; Calories = 273.4; Total Carb (g) = 54.1; Net Carb (g) = 50.7; Fat (g) = 2.3; Protein = 8.7

🍮 Macaroni Or Pasta Salad Made With Creamy Dressing ☞ serving size: 1 cup = 204 g; Calories = 316.2; Total Carb (g) = 41; Net Carb (g) = 37.5; Fat (g) = 13.5; Protein = 7.8

🍮 Macaroni Or Pasta Salad Made With Italian Dressing ☞ serving size: 1 cup = 204 g; Calories = 269.3; Total Carb (g) = 42.6; Net Carb (g) = 39.1; Fat (g) = 7.6; Protein = 7.6

🍮 Macaroni Or Pasta Salad Made With Light Creamy Dressing ☞ serving size: 1 cup = 204 g; Calories = 248.9; Total Carb (g) = 41.2; Net Carb (g) = 37.7; Fat (g) = 5.9; Protein = 7.8

🍮 Macaroni Or Pasta Salad Made With Light Italian Dressing ☞ serving size: 1 cup = 204 g; Calories = 234.6; Total Carb (g) = 42; Net Carb (g) = 38.5; Fat (g) = 4; Protein = 7.5

🍮 Macaroni Or Pasta Salad Made With Light Mayonnaise ☞ serving size: 1 cup = 204 g; Calories = 324.4; Total Carb (g) = 52.4; Net Carb (g) = 49.5; Fat (g) = 8.5; Protein = 8.8

🍮 Macaroni Or Pasta Salad Made With Light Mayonnaise-Type Salad Dressing ☞ serving size: 1 cup = 204 g; Calories = 324.4; Total Carb (g) = 52.4; Net Carb (g) = 49.5; Fat (g) = 8.5; Protein = 8.8

🍮 Macaroni Or Pasta Salad Made With Mayonnaise ☞ serving size: 1 cup = 204 g; Calories = 450.8; Total Carb (g) = 50.3; Net Carb (g) = 47.4; Fat (g) = 23.5; Protein = 9.1

🍮 Macaroni Or Pasta Salad Made With Mayonnaise-Type Salad Dressing ☞ serving size: 1 cup = 204 g; Calories = 326.4; Total Carb (g) = 54.2; Net Carb (g) = 51.4; Fat (g) = 8.2; Protein = 8.9

🍮 Macaroni Or Pasta Salad With Cheese ☞ serving size: 1 cup =

204 g; Calories = 499.8; Total Carb (g) = 44.6; Net Carb (g) = 41.9; Fat (g) = 29.3; Protein = 14

🐚 Macaroni Or Pasta Salad With Chicken ☞ serving size: 1 cup = 204 g; Calories = 434.5; Total Carb (g) = 42.7; Net Carb (g) = 40.3; Fat (g) = 21.9; Protein = 16

🐚 Macaroni Or Pasta Salad With Crab Meat ☞ serving size: 1 cup = 204 g; Calories = 408; Total Carb (g) = 42.7; Net Carb (g) = 40.3; Fat (g) = 20.2; Protein = 13.2

🐚 Macaroni Or Pasta Salad With Egg ☞ serving size: 1 cup = 204 g; Calories = 438.6; Total Carb (g) = 46; Net Carb (g) = 43.3; Fat (g) = 23.3; Protein = 10.6

🐚 Macaroni Or Pasta Salad With Meat ☞ serving size: 1 cup = 204 g; Calories = 430.4; Total Carb (g) = 42.5; Net Carb (g) = 40; Fat (g) = 21.6; Protein = 15.6

🐚 Macaroni Or Pasta Salad With Shrimp ☞ serving size: 1 cup = 204 g; Calories = 416.2; Total Carb (g) = 43; Net Carb (g) = 40.6; Fat (g) = 20.5; Protein = 13.8

🐚 Macaroni Or Pasta Salad With Tuna ☞ serving size: 1 cup = 204 g; Calories = 410; Total Carb (g) = 42.6; Net Carb (g) = 40.1; Fat (g) = 20.2; Protein = 13.8

🐚 Macaroni Or Pasta Salad With Tuna And Egg ☞ serving size: 1 cup = 204 g; Calories = 401.9; Total Carb (g) = 39.5; Net Carb (g) = 37.2; Fat (g) = 20.3; Protein = 14.7

🐚 Macaroni With Tuna Puerto Rican Style ☞ serving size: 1 cup = 225 g; Calories = 330.8; Total Carb (g) = 40.7; Net Carb (g) = 38.7; Fat (g) = 10.7; Protein = 17.5

🐚 Manicotti Cheese-Filled No Sauce ☞ serving size: 1 manicotti = 127 g; Calories = 269.2; Total Carb (g) = 23.9; Net Carb (g) = 23.1; Fat (g) = 12.6; Protein = 14.4

🐚 Manicotti Cheese-Filled With Meat Sauce ☞ serving size: 1

manicotti = 143 g; Calories = 234.5; Total Carb (g) = 20.1; Net Carb (g) = 18.9; Fat (g) = 11; Protein = 13.5

🍢 Manicotti Cheese-Filled With Tomato Sauce Diet Frozen Meal ☞ serving size: 1 meal (9.25 oz) = 262 g; Calories = 322.3; Total Carb (g) = 29.2; Net Carb (g) = 27.4; Fat (g) = 14.6; Protein = 18.8

🍢 Manicotti Cheese-Filled With Tomato Sauce Meatless ☞ serving size: 1 manicotti = 143 g; Calories = 224.5; Total Carb (g) = 21.5; Net Carb (g) = 20.2; Fat (g) = 10.1; Protein = 11.9

🍢 Manicotti Vegetable- And Cheese-Filled With Tomato Sauce Meatless ☞ serving size: 1 manicotti = 143 g; Calories = 195.9; Total Carb (g) = 21.5; Net Carb (g) = 19.9; Fat (g) = 7.9; Protein = 10.1

🍢 Meat Pie Puerto Rican Style ☞ serving size: 1 pie (9" dia) = 1110 g; Calories = 5272.5; Total Carb (g) = 281.5; Net Carb (g) = 269.3; Fat (g) = 377.3; Protein = 174.3

🍢 Meat Turnover Puerto Rican Style ☞ serving size: 1 turnover = 28 g; Calories = 71.7; Total Carb (g) = 6.1; Net Carb (g) = 5.8; Fat (g) = 3.7; Protein = 3.3

🍢 Mexican Casserole Made With Ground Beef Beans Tomato Sauce Cheese Taco Seasonings And Corn Chips ☞ serving size: 1 cup = 144 g; Calories = 337; Total Carb (g) = 25.1; Net Carb (g) = 20.6; Fat (g) = 18.2; Protein = 19.1

🍢 Mexican Casserole Made With Ground Beef Tomato Sauce Cheese Taco Seasonings And Corn Chips ☞ serving size: 1 cup = 144 g; Calories = 385.9; Total Carb (g) = 20.9; Net Carb (g) = 18.6; Fat (g) = 24.6; Protein = 21.1

🍢 Moo Goo Gai Pan ☞ serving size: 1 cup = 216 g; Calories = 159.8; Total Carb (g) = 13.8; Net Carb (g) = 10.8; Fat (g) = 5.2; Protein = 15.7

🍢 Moo Shu Pork Without Chinese Pancake ☞ serving size: 1 cup = 151 g; Calories = 228; Total Carb (g) = 6.4; Net Carb (g) = 5.1; Fat (g) = 15.7; Protein = 15.9

🍢 Nachos With Cheese And Sour Cream ☞ serving size: 1 nacho = 7 g; Calories = 15.6; Total Carb (g) = 1.5; Net Carb (g) = 1.3; Fat (g) = 0.8; Protein = 0.6

🍢 Nachos With Chicken And Cheese ☞ serving size: 1 nacho = 7 g; Calories = 14.6; Total Carb (g) = 1.2; Net Carb (g) = 1; Fat (g) = 0.7; Protein = 1

🍢 Nachos With Chicken Cheese And Sour Cream ☞ serving size: 1 nacho = 7 g; Calories = 14.6; Total Carb (g) = 1.1; Net Carb (g) = 0.9; Fat (g) = 0.7; Protein = 0.9

🍢 Nachos With Chili ☞ serving size: 1 nacho = 7 g; Calories = 17.6; Total Carb (g) = 1.6; Net Carb (g) = 1.4; Fat (g) = 1; Protein = 0.7

🍢 Nachos With Meat And Cheese ☞ serving size: 1 nacho = 7 g; Calories = 16.5; Total Carb (g) = 1.3; Net Carb (g) = 1; Fat (g) = 0.9; Protein = 0.9

🍢 Nachos With Meat Cheese And Sour Cream ☞ serving size: 1 nacho = 7 g; Calories = 15.1; Total Carb (g) = 1.4; Net Carb (g) = 1.2; Fat (g) = 0.9; Protein = 0.4

🍢 Noodle Pudding ☞ serving size: 1 cup = 144 g; Calories = 301; Total Carb (g) = 44.6; Net Carb (g) = 42.4; Fat (g) = 10.6; Protein = 8.6

🍢 Noodles With Vegetables In Tomato-Based Sauce Diet Frozen Meal ☞ serving size: 1 meal (10 oz) = 284 g; Calories = 187.4; Total Carb (g) = 30.2; Net Carb (g) = 25.4; Fat (g) = 4.4; Protein = 9.3

🍢 Pad Thai Meatless ☞ serving size: 1 cup = 200 g; Calories = 328; Total Carb (g) = 32.6; Net Carb (g) = 29.2; Fat (g) = 18.2; Protein = 11.5

🍢 Pad Thai Nfs ☞ serving size: 1 cup = 200 g; Calories = 306; Total Carb (g) = 28.6; Net Carb (g) = 26.2; Fat (g) = 14.8; Protein = 16.2

🍢 Pad Thai With Chicken ☞ serving size: 1 cup = 200 g; Calories = 306; Total Carb (g) = 28.6; Net Carb (g) = 26.2; Fat (g) = 14.8; Protein = 16.2

🍤 Pad Thai With Meat ☞ serving size: 1 cup = 200 g; Calories = 316; Total Carb (g) = 29.4; Net Carb (g) = 27; Fat (g) = 15.6; Protein = 16.3

🍤 Pad Thai With Seafood ☞ serving size: 1 cup = 200 g; Calories = 290; Total Carb (g) = 30; Net Carb (g) = 27.6; Fat (g) = 13.4; Protein = 13.6

🍤 Paella Nfs ☞ serving size: 1 cup = 240 g; Calories = 400.8; Total Carb (g) = 37.9; Net Carb (g) = 36.5; Fat (g) = 17; Protein = 22.9

🍤 Paella With Meat Valenciana Style ☞ serving size: 1 cup, with bone (yield after bone removed) = 137 g; Calories = 369.9; Total Carb (g) = 22.9; Net Carb (g) = 22.3; Fat (g) = 17.2; Protein = 29.7

🍤 Paella With Seafood ☞ serving size: 1 cup = 240 g; Calories = 340.8; Total Carb (g) = 39.4; Net Carb (g) = 37.5; Fat (g) = 11.2; Protein = 19.3

🍤 Pasta Meat-Filled With Gravy Canned ☞ serving size: 1 cup = 250 g; Calories = 327.5; Total Carb (g) = 51.1; Net Carb (g) = 49.1; Fat (g) = 7.7; Protein = 12

🍤 Pasta Mix Classic Beef Unprepared ☞ serving size: 1 package = 122 g; Calories = 431.9; Total Carb (g) = 88.1; Net Carb (g) = 85.6; Fat (g) = 2.2; Protein = 15

🍤 Pasta Mix Classic Cheeseburger Macaroni Unprepared ☞ serving size: 1 package = 123 g; Calories = 429.3; Total Carb (g) = 88; Net Carb (g) = 84.6; Fat (g) = 2.3; Protein = 14.3

🍤 Pasta Mix Italian Four Cheese Lasagna Unprepared ☞ serving size: 1 package = 117 g; Calories = 415.4; Total Carb (g) = 82.2; Net Carb (g) = 79.2; Fat (g) = 3.2; Protein = 14.7

🍤 Pasta Mix Italian Lasagna Unprepared ☞ serving size: 1 package = 141 g; Calories = 502; Total Carb (g) = 104; Net Carb (g) = 100.1; Fat (g) = 2.8; Protein = 15.4

🍤 Pasta Whole Grain With Cream Sauce And Added Vegetables

Home Recipe ☞ serving size: 1 cup = 250 g; Calories = 335; Total Carb (g) = 41.3; Net Carb (g) = 35.8; Fat (g) = 16.1; Protein = 10.6

🍝 Pasta Whole Grain With Cream Sauce And Added Vegetables Ready-To-Heat ☞ serving size: 1 cup = 250 g; Calories = 367.5; Total Carb (g) = 40.4; Net Carb (g) = 35.2; Fat (g) = 20.3; Protein = 10.4

🍝 Pasta Whole Grain With Cream Sauce And Added Vegetables Restaurant ☞ serving size: 1 cup = 250 g; Calories = 460; Total Carb (g) = 38.1; Net Carb (g) = 33.1; Fat (g) = 32; Protein = 9.8

🍝 Pasta Whole Grain With Cream Sauce And Meat Home Recipe ☞ serving size: 1 cup = 250 g; Calories = 395; Total Carb (g) = 40; Net Carb (g) = 35; Fat (g) = 20.7; Protein = 16.2

🍝 Pasta Whole Grain With Cream Sauce And Meat Ready-To-Heat ☞ serving size: 1 cup = 250 g; Calories = 427.5; Total Carb (g) = 39.1; Net Carb (g) = 34.1; Fat (g) = 24.8; Protein = 15.8

🍝 Pasta Whole Grain With Cream Sauce And Meat Restaurant ☞ serving size: 1 cup = 250 g; Calories = 517.5; Total Carb (g) = 36.9; Net Carb (g) = 32.1; Fat (g) = 36.2; Protein = 14.9

🍝 Pasta Whole Grain With Cream Sauce And Poultry Home Recipe ☞ serving size: 1 cup = 250 g; Calories = 375; Total Carb (g) = 40; Net Carb (g) = 35; Fat (g) = 18.5; Protein = 16.6

🍝 Pasta Whole Grain With Cream Sauce And Poultry Ready-To-Heat ☞ serving size: 1 cup = 250 g; Calories = 407.5; Total Carb (g) = 39.1; Net Carb (g) = 34.1; Fat (g) = 22.6; Protein = 16.3

🍝 Pasta Whole Grain With Cream Sauce And Poultry Restaurant ☞ serving size: 1 cup = 250 g; Calories = 497.5; Total Carb (g) = 36.9; Net Carb (g) = 32.1; Fat (g) = 34.2; Protein = 15.3

🍝 Pasta Whole Grain With Cream Sauce And Seafood Home Recipe ☞ serving size: 1 cup = 250 g; Calories = 365; Total Carb (g) = 40.6; Net Carb (g) = 35.6; Fat (g) = 17.2; Protein = 15.4

🍝 Pasta Whole Grain With Cream Sauce And Seafood Ready-To-

Heat ☞ serving size: 1 cup = 250 g; Calories = 397.5; Total Carb (g) = 39.7; Net Carb (g) = 34.7; Fat (g) = 21.4; Protein = 15.1

🍝 Pasta Whole Grain With Cream Sauce And Seafood Restaurant ☞ serving size: 1 cup = 250 g; Calories = 487.5; Total Carb (g) = 37.5; Net Carb (g) = 32.8; Fat (g) = 33; Protein = 14.3

🍝 Pasta Whole Grain With Cream Sauce Home Recipe ☞ serving size: 1 cup = 250 g; Calories = 370; Total Carb (g) = 40.2; Net Carb (g) = 35.2; Fat (g) = 20.3; Protein = 11

🍝 Pasta Whole Grain With Cream Sauce Meat And Added Vegetables Home Recipe ☞ serving size: 1 cup = 250 g; Calories = 367.5; Total Carb (g) = 40.9; Net Carb (g) = 35.4; Fat (g) = 17.3; Protein = 15.9

🍝 Pasta Whole Grain With Cream Sauce Meat And Added Vegetables Ready-To-Heat ☞ serving size: 1 cup = 250 g; Calories = 400; Total Carb (g) = 40; Net Carb (g) = 34.7; Fat (g) = 21.5; Protein = 15.5

🍝 Pasta Whole Grain With Cream Sauce Meat And Added Vegetables Restaurant ☞ serving size: 1 cup = 250 g; Calories = 490; Total Carb (g) = 37.7; Net Carb (g) = 32.7; Fat (g) = 33.1; Protein = 14.6

🍝 Pasta Whole Grain With Cream Sauce Poultry And Added Vegetables Home Recipe ☞ serving size: 1 cup = 250 g; Calories = 347.5; Total Carb (g) = 40.9; Net Carb (g) = 35.4; Fat (g) = 15.1; Protein = 16.3

🍝 Pasta Whole Grain With Cream Sauce Poultry And Added Vegetables Ready-To-Heat ☞ serving size: 1 cup = 250 g; Calories = 380; Total Carb (g) = 40; Net Carb (g) = 34.7; Fat (g) = 19.3; Protein = 16

🍝 Pasta Whole Grain With Cream Sauce Poultry And Added Vegetables Restaurant ☞ serving size: 1 cup = 250 g; Calories = 472.5; Total Carb (g) = 37.7; Net Carb (g) = 32.7; Fat (g) = 31; Protein = 15.1

🍝 Pasta Whole Grain With Cream Sauce Ready-To-Heat ☞ serving size: 1 cup = 250 g; Calories = 402.5; Total Carb (g) = 39.3; Net Carb (g) = 34.3; Fat (g) = 24.4; Protein = 10.8

🍝 Pasta Whole Grain With Cream Sauce Restaurant ☞ serving size: 1 cup = 250 g; Calories = 492.5; Total Carb (g) = 37.1; Net Carb (g) = 32.3; Fat (g) = 35.8; Protein = 10.2

🍝 Pasta Whole Grain With Cream Sauce Seafood And Added Vegetables Home Recipe ☞ serving size: 1 cup = 250 g; Calories = 335; Total Carb (g) = 41.5; Net Carb (g) = 36; Fat (g) = 13.9; Protein = 15.1

🍝 Pasta Whole Grain With Cream Sauce Seafood And Added Vegetables Ready-To-Heat ☞ serving size: 1 cup = 250 g; Calories = 370; Total Carb (g) = 40.6; Net Carb (g) = 35.4; Fat (g) = 18.1; Protein = 14.8

🍝 Pasta Whole Grain With Cream Sauce Seafood And Added Vegetables Restaurant ☞ serving size: 1 cup = 250 g; Calories = 462.5; Total Carb (g) = 38.4; Net Carb (g) = 33.4; Fat (g) = 29.9; Protein = 14

🍝 Pasta Whole Grain With Tomato-Based Sauce And Added Vegetables Home Recipe ☞ serving size: 1 cup = 250 g; Calories = 245; Total Carb (g) = 47.3; Net Carb (g) = 40.3; Fat (g) = 3.8; Protein = 9.4

🍝 Pasta Whole Grain With Tomato-Based Sauce And Added Vegetables Ready-To-Heat ☞ serving size: 1 cup = 250 g; Calories = 280; Total Carb (g) = 46.2; Net Carb (g) = 39.2; Fat (g) = 8.3; Protein = 9.2

🍝 Pasta Whole Grain With Tomato-Based Sauce And Added Vegetables Restaurant ☞ serving size: 1 cup = 250 g; Calories = 380; Total Carb (g) = 43.8; Net Carb (g) = 37.3; Fat (g) = 20.7; Protein = 8.8

🍝 Pasta Whole Grain With Tomato-Based Sauce And Meat Home Recipe ☞ serving size: 1 cup = 250 g; Calories = 300; Total Carb (g) = 46.3; Net Carb (g) = 39.5; Fat (g) = 7.6; Protein = 14.9

🍝 Pasta Whole Grain With Tomato-Based Sauce And Meat Ready-To-Heat ☞ serving size: 1 cup = 250 g; Calories = 335; Total Carb (g) = 45.3; Net Carb (g) = 38.5; Fat (g) = 12; Protein = 14.6

🖤 Pasta Whole Grain With Tomato-Based Sauce And Meat Restaurant ☞ serving size: 1 cup = 250 g; Calories = 430; Total Carb (g) = 42.8; Net Carb (g) = 36.6; Fat (g) = 24.2; Protein = 13.8

🖤 Pasta Whole Grain With Tomato-Based Sauce And Poultry Home Recipe ☞ serving size: 1 cup = 250 g; Calories = 280; Total Carb (g) = 46.3; Net Carb (g) = 39.5; Fat (g) = 5.4; Protein = 15.4

🖤 Pasta Whole Grain With Tomato-Based Sauce And Poultry Ready-To-Heat ☞ serving size: 1 cup = 250 g; Calories = 315; Total Carb (g) = 45.3; Net Carb (g) = 38.5; Fat (g) = 9.8; Protein = 15

🖤 Pasta Whole Grain With Tomato-Based Sauce And Poultry Restaurant ☞ serving size: 1 cup = 250 g; Calories = 412.5; Total Carb (g) = 42.8; Net Carb (g) = 36.6; Fat (g) = 22.1; Protein = 14.2

🖤 Pasta Whole Grain With Tomato-Based Sauce And Seafood Home Recipe ☞ serving size: 1 cup = 250 g; Calories = 270; Total Carb (g) = 46.9; Net Carb (g) = 40.2; Fat (g) = 4.1; Protein = 14.2

🖤 Pasta Whole Grain With Tomato-Based Sauce And Seafood Ready-To-Heat ☞ serving size: 1 cup = 250 g; Calories = 302.5; Total Carb (g) = 45.9; Net Carb (g) = 39.2; Fat (g) = 8.6; Protein = 13.9

🖤 Pasta Whole Grain With Tomato-Based Sauce And Seafood Restaurant ☞ serving size: 1 cup = 250 g; Calories = 402.5; Total Carb (g) = 43.5; Net Carb (g) = 37.2; Fat (g) = 21; Protein = 13.1

🖤 Pasta Whole Grain With Tomato-Based Sauce Home Recipe ☞ serving size: 1 cup = 250 g; Calories = 252.5; Total Carb (g) = 47.9; Net Carb (g) = 40.7; Fat (g) = 4.2; Protein = 9.5

🖤 Pasta Whole Grain With Tomato-Based Sauce Meat And Added Vegetables Home Recipe ☞ serving size: 1 cup = 250 g; Calories = 295; Total Carb (g) = 45.7; Net Carb (g) = 39; Fat (g) = 7.3; Protein = 14.9

🖤 Pasta Whole Grain With Tomato-Based Sauce Meat And Added Vegetables Ready-To-Heat ☞ serving size: 1 cup = 250 g; Calories =

327.5; Total Carb (g) = 44.7; Net Carb (g) = 38.2; Fat (g) = 11.7; Protein = 14.6

🌿 Pasta Whole Grain With Tomato-Based Sauce Meat And Added Vegetables Restaurant ☞ serving size: 1 cup = 250 g; Calories = 425; Total Carb (g) = 42.3; Net Carb (g) = 36.1; Fat (g) = 23.9; Protein = 13.8

🌿 Pasta Whole Grain With Tomato-Based Sauce Poultry And Added Vegetables Home Recipe ☞ serving size: 1 cup = 250 g; Calories = 275; Total Carb (g) = 45.7; Net Carb (g) = 39; Fat (g) = 5.1; Protein = 15.4

🌿 Pasta Whole Grain With Tomato-Based Sauce Poultry And Added Vegetables Ready-To-Heat ☞ serving size: 1 cup = 250 g; Calories = 310; Total Carb (g) = 44.7; Net Carb (g) = 38.2; Fat (g) = 9.5; Protein = 15

🌿 Pasta Whole Grain With Tomato-Based Sauce Poultry And Added Vegetables Restaurant ☞ serving size: 1 cup = 250 g; Calories = 407.5; Total Carb (g) = 42.3; Net Carb (g) = 36.1; Fat (g) = 21.9; Protein = 14.2

🌿 Pasta Whole Grain With Tomato-Based Sauce Ready-To-Heat ☞ serving size: 1 cup = 250 g; Calories = 287.5; Total Carb (g) = 46.9; Net Carb (g) = 39.9; Fat (g) = 8.6; Protein = 9.2

🌿 Pasta Whole Grain With Tomato-Based Sauce Restaurant ☞ serving size: 1 cup = 250 g; Calories = 387.5; Total Carb (g) = 44.4; Net Carb (g) = 37.7; Fat (g) = 21; Protein = 8.8

🌿 Pasta Whole Grain With Tomato-Based Sauce Seafood And Added Vegetables Home Recipe ☞ serving size: 1 cup = 250 g; Calories = 262.5; Total Carb (g) = 46.4; Net Carb (g) = 39.6; Fat (g) = 3.8; Protein = 14.2

🌿 Pasta Whole Grain With Tomato-Based Sauce Seafood And Added Vegetables Ready-To-Heat ☞ serving size: 1 cup = 250 g; Calories = 297.5; Total Carb (g) = 45.4; Net Carb (g) = 38.9; Fat (g) = 8.3; Protein = 13.9

🍝 Pasta Whole Grain With Tomato-Based Sauce Seafood And Added Vegetables Restaurant ☞ serving size: 1 cup = 250 g; Calories = 395; Total Carb (g) = 42.9; Net Carb (g) = 36.7; Fat (g) = 20.7; Protein = 13.1

🍝 Pasta With Cream Sauce And Added Vegetables From Home Recipe ☞ serving size: 1 cup = 250 g; Calories = 347.5; Total Carb (g) = 42.3; Net Carb (g) = 39.6; Fat (g) = 15.1; Protein = 10.4

🍝 Pasta With Cream Sauce And Added Vegetables Ready-To-Heat ☞ serving size: 1 cup = 250 g; Calories = 380; Total Carb (g) = 41.4; Net Carb (g) = 38.7; Fat (g) = 19.3; Protein = 10.2

🍝 Pasta With Cream Sauce And Added Vegetables Restaurant ☞ serving size: 1 cup = 250 g; Calories = 472.5; Total Carb (g) = 39.1; Net Carb (g) = 36.6; Fat (g) = 31.1; Protein = 9.6

🍝 Pasta With Cream Sauce And Meat Home Recipe ☞ serving size: 1 cup = 250 g; Calories = 407.5; Total Carb (g) = 41; Net Carb (g) = 38.7; Fat (g) = 19.7; Protein = 15.9

🍝 Pasta With Cream Sauce And Meat Ready-To-Heat ☞ serving size: 1 cup = 250 g; Calories = 440; Total Carb (g) = 40.1; Net Carb (g) = 37.8; Fat (g) = 23.8; Protein = 15.6

🍝 Pasta With Cream Sauce And Meat Restaurant ☞ serving size: 1 cup = 250 g; Calories = 527.5; Total Carb (g) = 37.8; Net Carb (g) = 35.6; Fat (g) = 35.3; Protein = 14.7

🍝 Pasta With Cream Sauce And Poultry Home Recipe ☞ serving size: 1 cup = 250 g; Calories = 387.5; Total Carb (g) = 41; Net Carb (g) = 38.7; Fat (g) = 17.5; Protein = 16.4

🍝 Pasta With Cream Sauce And Poultry Ready-To-Heat ☞ serving size: 1 cup = 250 g; Calories = 420; Total Carb (g) = 40.1; Net Carb (g) = 37.8; Fat (g) = 21.6; Protein = 16

🍝 Pasta With Cream Sauce And Poultry Restaurant ☞ serving size:

1 cup = 250 g; Calories = 510; Total Carb (g) = 37.8; Net Carb (g) = 35.6; Fat (g) = 33.2; Protein = 15.1

🍝 Pasta With Cream Sauce And Seafood Home Recipe ☞ serving size: 1 cup = 250 g; Calories = 375; Total Carb (g) = 41.7; Net Carb (g) = 39.4; Fat (g) = 16.2; Protein = 15.2

🍝 Pasta With Cream Sauce And Seafood Ready-To-Heat ☞ serving size: 1 cup = 250 g; Calories = 407.5; Total Carb (g) = 40.7; Net Carb (g) = 38.5; Fat (g) = 20.4; Protein = 14.9

🍝 Pasta With Cream Sauce And Seafood Restaurant ☞ serving size: 1 cup = 250 g; Calories = 497.5; Total Carb (g) = 38.4; Net Carb (g) = 36.2; Fat (g) = 32.1; Protein = 14

🍝 Pasta With Cream Sauce Home Recipe ☞ serving size: 1 cup = 250 g; Calories = 382.5; Total Carb (g) = 41.2; Net Carb (g) = 39; Fat (g) = 19.3; Protein = 10.8

🍝 Pasta With Cream Sauce Meat And Added Vegetables Home Recipe ☞ serving size: 1 cup = 250 g; Calories = 380; Total Carb (g) = 41.9; Net Carb (g) = 39.2; Fat (g) = 16.3; Protein = 15.6

🍝 Pasta With Cream Sauce Meat And Added Vegetables Ready-To-Heat ☞ serving size: 1 cup = 250 g; Calories = 410; Total Carb (g) = 41; Net Carb (g) = 38.5; Fat (g) = 20.5; Protein = 15.3

🍝 Pasta With Cream Sauce Meat And Added Vegetables Restaurant ☞ serving size: 1 cup = 250 g; Calories = 502.5; Total Carb (g) = 38.7; Net Carb (g) = 36.2; Fat (g) = 32.2; Protein = 14.4

🍝 Pasta With Cream Sauce Poultry And Added Vegetables Home Recipe ☞ serving size: 1 cup = 250 g; Calories = 360; Total Carb (g) = 41.9; Net Carb (g) = 39.2; Fat (g) = 14.1; Protein = 16.1

🍝 Pasta With Cream Sauce Poultry And Added Vegetables Ready-To-Heat ☞ serving size: 1 cup = 250 g; Calories = 392.5; Total Carb (g) = 41; Net Carb (g) = 38.5; Fat (g) = 18.3; Protein = 15.7

🍝 Pasta With Cream Sauce Poultry And Added Vegetables Restaurant ☞ serving size: 1 cup = 250 g; Calories = 482.5; Total Carb (g) = 38.7; Net Carb (g) = 36.2; Fat (g) = 30.1; Protein = 14.8

🍝 Pasta With Cream Sauce Ready-To-Heat ☞ serving size: 1 cup = 250 g; Calories = 415; Total Carb (g) = 40.3; Net Carb (g) = 38.1; Fat (g) = 23.4; Protein = 10.5

🍝 Pasta With Cream Sauce Restaurant ☞ serving size: 1 cup = 250 g; Calories = 505; Total Carb (g) = 38; Net Carb (g) = 35.8; Fat (g) = 34.9; Protein = 9.9

🍝 Pasta With Cream Sauce Seafood And Added Vegetables Home Recipe ☞ serving size: 1 cup = 250 g; Calories = 347.5; Total Carb (g) = 42.6; Net Carb (g) = 39.8; Fat (g) = 12.9; Protein = 14.9

🍝 Pasta With Cream Sauce Seafood And Added Vegetables Ready-To-Heat ☞ serving size: 1 cup = 250 g; Calories = 380; Total Carb (g) = 41.7; Net Carb (g) = 39.2; Fat (g) = 17.1; Protein = 14.6

🍝 Pasta With Cream Sauce Seafood And Added Vegetables Restaurant ☞ serving size: 1 cup = 250 g; Calories = 472.5; Total Carb (g) = 39.3; Net Carb (g) = 36.8; Fat (g) = 29; Protein = 13.7

🍝 Pasta With Sauce And Meat From School Lunch ☞ serving size: 1 cup = 250 g; Calories = 292.5; Total Carb (g) = 43.8; Net Carb (g) = 37.3; Fat (g) = 7.8; Protein = 14.9

🍝 Pasta With Sauce Meatless School Lunch ☞ serving size: 1 cup = 250 g; Calories = 255; Total Carb (g) = 48.6; Net Carb (g) = 41.4; Fat (g) = 4; Protein = 9.5

🍝 Pasta With Sauce Nfs ☞ serving size: 1 cup = 250 g; Calories = 312.5; Total Carb (g) = 47.3; Net Carb (g) = 43.3; Fat (g) = 6.6; Protein = 14.7

🍝 Pasta With Sliced Franks In Tomato Sauce Canned Entree ☞ serving size: 1 serving (1 cup) = 252 g; Calories = 226.8; Total Carb (g) = 32; Net Carb (g) = 28; Fat (g) = 6; Protein = 11

🍝 Pasta With Tomato Sauce No Meat Canned ☞ serving size: 1

serving (1 nlea serving) = 252 g; Calories = 178.9; Total Carb (g) = 35.1; Net Carb (g) = 32.9; Fat (g) = 1.8; Protein = 5.6

🍝 Pasta With Tomato-Based Sauce And Added Vegetables Home Recipe ☞ serving size: 1 cup = 250 g; Calories = 257.5; Total Carb (g) = 48.3; Net Carb (g) = 43.8; Fat (g) = 2.8; Protein = 9.2

🍝 Pasta With Tomato-Based Sauce And Added Vegetables Ready-To-Heat ☞ serving size: 1 cup = 250 g; Calories = 292.5; Total Carb (g) = 47.2; Net Carb (g) = 43; Fat (g) = 7.3; Protein = 9

🍝 Pasta With Tomato-Based Sauce And Added Vegetables Restaurant ☞ serving size: 1 cup = 250 g; Calories = 390; Total Carb (g) = 44.7; Net Carb (g) = 40.7; Fat (g) = 19.7; Protein = 8.5

🍝 Pasta With Tomato-Based Sauce And Beans Or Lentils ☞ serving size: 1 cup = 227 g; Calories = 283.8; Total Carb (g) = 47.1; Net Carb (g) = 40.3; Fat (g) = 5.3; Protein = 11.9

🍝 Pasta With Tomato-Based Sauce And Cheese ☞ serving size: 1 cup = 250 g; Calories = 295; Total Carb (g) = 36.6; Net Carb (g) = 32.3; Fat (g) = 12.1; Protein = 9.3

🍝 Pasta With Tomato-Based Sauce And Meat Home Recipe ☞ serving size: 1 cup = 250 g; Calories = 312.5; Total Carb (g) = 47.3; Net Carb (g) = 43.3; Fat (g) = 6.6; Protein = 14.7

🍝 Pasta With Tomato-Based Sauce And Meat Ready-To-Heat ☞ serving size: 1 cup = 250 g; Calories = 345; Total Carb (g) = 46.3; Net Carb (g) = 42.3; Fat (g) = 11; Protein = 14.3

🍝 Pasta With Tomato-Based Sauce And Meat Restaurant ☞ serving size: 1 cup = 250 g; Calories = 442.5; Total Carb (g) = 43.8; Net Carb (g) = 40; Fat (g) = 23.3; Protein = 13.6

🍝 Pasta With Tomato-Based Sauce And Poultry Home Recipe ☞ serving size: 1 cup = 250 g; Calories = 292.5; Total Carb (g) = 47.3; Net Carb (g) = 43.3; Fat (g) = 4.4; Protein = 15.1

🍝 Pasta With Tomato-Based Sauce And Poultry Ready-To-Heat ☞

serving size: 1 cup = 250 g; Calories = 327.5; Total Carb (g) = 46.3; Net Carb (g) = 42.3; Fat (g) = 8.8; Protein = 14.8

🍝 Pasta With Tomato-Based Sauce And Poultry Restaurant ☞ serving size: 1 cup = 250 g; Calories = 422.5; Total Carb (g) = 43.8; Net Carb (g) = 40; Fat (g) = 21.2; Protein = 14

🍝 Pasta With Tomato-Based Sauce And Seafood Home Recipe ☞ serving size: 1 cup = 250 g; Calories = 280; Total Carb (g) = 47.9; Net Carb (g) = 43.9; Fat (g) = 3.1; Protein = 13.9

🍝 Pasta With Tomato-Based Sauce And Seafood Ready-To-Heat ☞ serving size: 1 cup = 250 g; Calories = 315; Total Carb (g) = 46.9; Net Carb (g) = 42.9; Fat (g) = 7.6; Protein = 13.6

🍝 Pasta With Tomato-Based Sauce And Seafood Restaurant ☞ serving size: 1 cup = 250 g; Calories = 412.5; Total Carb (g) = 44.4; Net Carb (g) = 40.7; Fat (g) = 20.1; Protein = 12.9

🍝 Pasta With Tomato-Based Sauce Cheese And Meat ☞ serving size: 1 cannelloni = 86 g; Calories = 128.1; Total Carb (g) = 10.8; Net Carb (g) = 10.2; Fat (g) = 6.3; Protein = 7

🍝 Pasta With Tomato-Based Sauce Home Recipe ☞ serving size: 1 cup = 250 g; Calories = 265; Total Carb (g) = 49; Net Carb (g) = 44.5; Fat (g) = 3.2; Protein = 9.2

🍝 Pasta With Tomato-Based Sauce Meat And Added Vegetables Home Recipe ☞ serving size: 1 cup = 250 g; Calories = 307.5; Total Carb (g) = 46.7; Net Carb (g) = 42.7; Fat (g) = 6.3; Protein = 14.7

🍝 Pasta With Tomato-Based Sauce Meat And Added Vegetables Ready-To-Heat ☞ serving size: 1 cup = 250 g; Calories = 340; Total Carb (g) = 45.7; Net Carb (g) = 41.7; Fat (g) = 10.7; Protein = 14.3

🍝 Pasta With Tomato-Based Sauce Meat And Added Vegetables Restaurant ☞ serving size: 1 cup = 250 g; Calories = 435; Total Carb (g) = 43.3; Net Carb (g) = 39.5; Fat (g) = 23; Protein = 13.6

🍝 Pasta With Tomato-Based Sauce Poultry And Added Vegetables

Home Recipe ☞ serving size: 1 cup = 250 g; Calories = 287.5; Total Carb (g) = 46.7; Net Carb (g) = 42.7; Fat (g) = 4.1; Protein = 15.1

🍝 Pasta With Tomato-Based Sauce Poultry And Added Vegetables Ready-To-Heat ☞ serving size: 1 cup = 250 g; Calories = 320; Total Carb (g) = 45.7; Net Carb (g) = 41.7; Fat (g) = 8.5; Protein = 14.8

🍝 Pasta With Tomato-Based Sauce Poultry And Added Vegetables Restaurant ☞ serving size: 1 cup = 250 g; Calories = 417.5; Total Carb (g) = 43.3; Net Carb (g) = 39.5; Fat (g) = 20.9; Protein = 14

🍝 Pasta With Tomato-Based Sauce Ready-To-Heat ☞ serving size: 1 cup = 250 g; Calories = 300; Total Carb (g) = 47.9; Net Carb (g) = 43.4; Fat (g) = 7.6; Protein = 9

🍝 Pasta With Tomato-Based Sauce Restaurant ☞ serving size: 1 cup = 250 g; Calories = 397.5; Total Carb (g) = 45.4; Net Carb (g) = 41.1; Fat (g) = 20.1; Protein = 8.5

🍝 Pasta With Tomato-Based Sauce Seafood And Added Vegetables Home Recipe ☞ serving size: 1 cup = 250 g; Calories = 275; Total Carb (g) = 47.4; Net Carb (g) = 43.4; Fat (g) = 2.8; Protein = 13.9

🍝 Pasta With Tomato-Based Sauce Seafood And Added Vegetables Ready-To-Heat ☞ serving size: 1 cup = 250 g; Calories = 310; Total Carb (g) = 46.4; Net Carb (g) = 42.4; Fat (g) = 7.3; Protein = 13.6

🍝 Pasta With Tomato-Based Sauce Seafood And Added Vegetables Restaurant ☞ serving size: 1 cup = 250 g; Calories = 407.5; Total Carb (g) = 43.9; Net Carb (g) = 40.1; Fat (g) = 19.8; Protein = 12.9

🍝 Pasta With Vegetables No Sauce Or Dressing ☞ serving size: 1 cup = 150 g; Calories = 214.5; Total Carb (g) = 34.8; Net Carb (g) = 31.2; Fat (g) = 5.2; Protein = 6.7

🍝 Pastry Egg And Cheese Filled ☞ serving size: 1 kolache = 142 g; Calories = 487.1; Total Carb (g) = 61.6; Net Carb (g) = 59.3; Fat (g) = 21.6; Protein = 11.4

🍝 Pastry Filled With Potatoes And Peas Fried ☞ serving size: 1

miniature samosa = 9 g; Calories = 27.7; Total Carb (g) = 2.9; Net Carb (g) = 2.8; Fat (g) = 1.6; Protein = 0.4

🍃 Pastry Meat / Poultry-Filled ☞ serving size: 1 kolache = 85 g; Calories = 287.3; Total Carb (g) = 26; Net Carb (g) = 25.1; Fat (g) = 16; Protein = 9.6

🍃 Pizza Rolls Frozen Unprepared ☞ serving size: 1 serving 6 rolls = 80 g; Calories = 262.4; Total Carb (g) = 40.6; Net Carb (g) = 39.6; Fat (g) = 8; Protein = 7

🍃 Pork And Onions With Soy-Based Sauce ☞ serving size: 1 cup = 256 g; Calories = 376.3; Total Carb (g) = 14; Net Carb (g) = 11.9; Fat (g) = 23.1; Protein = 28.2

🍃 Pork And Vegetables Excluding Carrots Broccoli And Dark-Green Leafy; No Potatoes Soy-Based Sauce ☞ serving size: 1 cup = 217 g; Calories = 314.7; Total Carb (g) = 9.5; Net Carb (g) = 7.6; Fat (g) = 20.1; Protein = 24.5

🍃 Pork And Vegetables Hawaiian Style ☞ serving size: 1 cup = 252 g; Calories = 226.8; Total Carb (g) = 19.2; Net Carb (g) = 14.7; Fat (g) = 9.1; Protein = 18.9

🍃 Pork And Vegetables Including Carrots Broccoli And/or Dark-Green Leafy; No Potatoes Soy-Based Sauce ☞ serving size: 1 cup = 217 g; Calories = 308.1; Total Carb (g) = 10.4; Net Carb (g) = 7.5; Fat (g) = 19.3; Protein = 23.8

🍃 Pork And Watercress With Soy-Based Sauce ☞ serving size: 1 cup = 162 g; Calories = 231.7; Total Carb (g) = 5.7; Net Carb (g) = 4.9; Fat (g) = 15.2; Protein = 18.5

🍃 Pork Chow Mein Or Chop Suey No Noodles ☞ serving size: 1 cup = 220 g; Calories = 215.6; Total Carb (g) = 8.5; Net Carb (g) = 6.7; Fat (g) = 9.5; Protein = 22.8

🍃 Pork Chow Mein Or Chop Suey With Noodles ☞ serving size: 1

cup = 220 g; Calories = 316.8; Total Carb (g) = 27; Net Carb (g) = 24.4; Fat (g) = 12.5; Protein = 22.2

● Pork Egg Foo Yung ☞ serving size: 1 patty = 86 g; Calories = 126.4; Total Carb (g) = 3.9; Net Carb (g) = 3.7; Fat (g) = 6.9; Protein = 11.4

● Pork Or Ham With Soy-Based Sauce ☞ serving size: 1 cup = 244 g; Calories = 456.3; Total Carb (g) = 8.2; Net Carb (g) = 7; Fat (g) = 30.6; Protein = 36.2

● Pork Rice And Vegetables Excluding Carrots Broccoli And Dark-Green Leafy; Soy-Based Sauce ☞ serving size: 1 cup = 217 g; Calories = 312.5; Total Carb (g) = 16.9; Net Carb (g) = 15.2; Fat (g) = 17.5; Protein = 22

● Pork Rice And Vegetables Including Carrots Broccoli And/or Dark-Green Leafy; Soy-Based Sauce ☞ serving size: 1 cup = 217 g; Calories = 308.1; Total Carb (g) = 17.4; Net Carb (g) = 14.8; Fat (g) = 16.9; Protein = 21.5

● Pork Tofu And Vegetables Excluding Carrots Broccoli And Dark-Green Leafy; No Potatoes Soy-Based Sauce ☞ serving size: 1 cup = 217 g; Calories = 247.4; Total Carb (g) = 9.7; Net Carb (g) = 7.8; Fat (g) = 17.2; Protein = 15.4

● Pork Tofu And Vegetables Including Carrots Broccoli And/or Dark-Green Leafy; No Potatoes Soy-Base Sauce ☞ serving size: 1 cup = 217 g; Calories = 245.2; Total Carb (g) = 10.6; Net Carb (g) = 7.7; Fat (g) = 16.6; Protein = 15

● Potato And Ham Fritters Puerto Rican Style ☞ serving size: 1 fritter (2-3/4" x 2-1/2" x 1") = 70 g; Calories = 137.2; Total Carb (g) = 8.7; Net Carb (g) = 7.7; Fat (g) = 9.6; Protein = 4.2

● Potato From Puerto Rican Beef Stew With Gravy ☞ serving size: 1 small = 122 g; Calories = 90.3; Total Carb (g) = 17.8; Net Carb (g) = 16.2; Fat (g) = 1.1; Protein = 3

● Potato From Puerto Rican Chicken Fricassee With Sauce ☞

serving size: 1 small = 123 g; Calories = 88.6; Total Carb (g) = 18; Net Carb (g) = 16.5; Fat (g) = 1.3; Protein = 1.7

🥔 Potato From Puerto Rican Style Stuffed Pot Roast With Gravy ☞ serving size: 1 small = 103 g; Calories = 76.2; Total Carb (g) = 15; Net Carb (g) = 13.7; Fat (g) = 0.9; Protein = 2.5

🥔 Potato Mashed From Dry Mix Made With Milk ☞ serving size: 1 cup = 250 g; Calories = 282.5; Total Carb (g) = 31.9; Net Carb (g) = 29.6; Fat (g) = 15.7; Protein = 5.1

🥔 Potato Mashed From Dry Mix Made With Milk With Cheese ☞ serving size: 1 cup = 250 g; Calories = 360; Total Carb (g) = 29.3; Net Carb (g) = 27.3; Fat (g) = 22.9; Protein = 10.7

🥔 Potato Mashed From Dry Mix Made With Milk With Gravy ☞ serving size: 1 cup = 250 g; Calories = 250; Total Carb (g) = 28.2; Net Carb (g) = 26.2; Fat (g) = 13.9; Protein = 4.5

🥔 Potato Mashed From Dry Mix Nfs ☞ serving size: 1 cup = 250 g; Calories = 282.5; Total Carb (g) = 31.9; Net Carb (g) = 29.6; Fat (g) = 15.7; Protein = 5.1

🥔 Potato Mashed From Fast Food With Gravy ☞ serving size: 1 cup = 250 g; Calories = 202.5; Total Carb (g) = 32; Net Carb (g) = 29.2; Fat (g) = 7; Protein = 3.7

🥔 Potato Mashed From Fresh Made With Milk ☞ serving size: 1 cup = 250 g; Calories = 277.5; Total Carb (g) = 44.2; Net Carb (g) = 41.2; Fat (g) = 9.5; Protein = 5.4

🥔 Potato Mashed From Fresh Made With Milk With Cheese ☞ serving size: 1 cup = 250 g; Calories = 357.5; Total Carb (g) = 40.3; Net Carb (g) = 37.8; Fat (g) = 17.4; Protein = 10.9

🥔 Potato Mashed From Fresh Made With Milk With Gravy ☞ serving size: 1 cup = 250 g; Calories = 247.5; Total Carb (g) = 38; Net Carb (g) = 35.5; Fat (g) = 8.9; Protein = 4.7

🥔 Potato Mashed From Fresh Nfs ☞ serving size: 1 cup = 250 g;

Calories = 277.5; Total Carb (g) = 44.2; Net Carb (g) = 41.2; Fat (g) = 9.5; Protein = 5.4

🥔 Potato Mashed From Restaurant ☞ serving size: 1 cup = 250 g; Calories = 335; Total Carb (g) = 42.1; Net Carb (g) = 39.4; Fat (g) = 17.1; Protein = 5.2

🥔 Potato Mashed From Restaurant With Gravy ☞ serving size: 1 cup = 250 g; Calories = 292.5; Total Carb (g) = 36.4; Net Carb (g) = 34.1; Fat (g) = 15; Protein = 4.5

🥔 Potato Mashed From School Lunch ☞ serving size: 1 cup = 250 g; Calories = 190; Total Carb (g) = 32.9; Net Carb (g) = 30.4; Fat (g) = 4.4; Protein = 5.4

🥔 Potato Mashed Nfs ☞ serving size: 1 cup = 250 g; Calories = 277.5; Total Carb (g) = 44.2; Net Carb (g) = 41.2; Fat (g) = 9.5; Protein = 5.4

🥔 Potato Mashed Ready-To-Heat With Cheese ☞ serving size: 1 cup = 250 g; Calories = 345; Total Carb (g) = 30.5; Net Carb (g) = 26.3; Fat (g) = 20.1; Protein = 10.5

🥔 Potato Mashed Ready-To-Heat With Gravy ☞ serving size: 1 cup = 250 g; Calories = 235; Total Carb (g) = 29.2; Net Carb (g) = 25.5; Fat (g) = 11.3; Protein = 4.3

🥔 Potato Pancake ☞ serving size: 1 miniature/bite size pancake = 10 g; Calories = 19.2; Total Carb (g) = 2.1; Net Carb (g) = 1.8; Fat (g) = 1.1; Protein = 0.5

🥔 Potato Pudding ☞ serving size: 1 cup = 228 g; Calories = 287.3; Total Carb (g) = 24.3; Net Carb (g) = 22.5; Fat (g) = 17.6; Protein = 8.1

🥔 Potato Salad From Restaurant ☞ serving size: 1 cup = 275 g; Calories = 475.8; Total Carb (g) = 44.6; Net Carb (g) = 40.2; Fat (g) = 31.6; Protein = 4.2

🥔 Potato Salad German Style ☞ serving size: 1 cup = 175 g; Calories = 182; Total Carb (g) = 28.7; Net Carb (g) = 25.9; Fat (g) = 5.6; Protein = 4.3

🍠 Potato Salad Made With Any Type Of Fat Free Dressing ☞ serving size: 1 cup = 275 g; Calories = 222.8; Total Carb (g) = 49.3; Net Carb (g) = 44.4; Fat (g) = 1.6; Protein = 3.8

🍠 Potato Salad Made With Creamy Dressing ☞ serving size: 1 cup = 275 g; Calories = 385; Total Carb (g) = 46.2; Net Carb (g) = 42.1; Fat (g) = 20.7; Protein = 4.4

🍠 Potato Salad Made With Italian Dressing ☞ serving size: 1 cup = 275 g; Calories = 297; Total Carb (g) = 49.1; Net Carb (g) = 45; Fat (g) = 9.8; Protein = 4

🍠 Potato Salad Made With Light Creamy Dressing ☞ serving size: 1 cup = 275 g; Calories = 261.3; Total Carb (g) = 46.6; Net Carb (g) = 42.5; Fat (g) = 6.8; Protein = 4.5

🍠 Potato Salad Made With Light Italian Dressing ☞ serving size: 1 cup = 275 g; Calories = 233.8; Total Carb (g) = 48.1; Net Carb (g) = 44; Fat (g) = 3.3; Protein = 4

🍠 Potato Salad Made With Light Mayonnaise ☞ serving size: 1 cup = 275 g; Calories = 288.8; Total Carb (g) = 46.7; Net Carb (g) = 42.5; Fat (g) = 10; Protein = 3.9

🍠 Potato Salad Made With Light Mayonnaise-Type Salad Dressing ☞ serving size: 1 cup = 275 g; Calories = 288.8; Total Carb (g) = 46.7; Net Carb (g) = 42.5; Fat (g) = 10; Protein = 3.9

🍠 Potato Salad Made With Mayonnaise ☞ serving size: 1 cup = 275 g; Calories = 462; Total Carb (g) = 43.5; Net Carb (g) = 39.3; Fat (g) = 30.6; Protein = 4.2

🍠 Potato Salad Made With Mayonnaise-Type Salad Dressing ☞ serving size: 1 cup = 275 g; Calories = 294.3; Total Carb (g) = 49.1; Net Carb (g) = 45; Fat (g) = 9.6; Protein = 4

🍠 Potato Salad With Egg ☞ serving size: 1/2 cup = 125 g; Calories = 196.3; Total Carb (g) = 20.2; Net Carb (g) = 18.6; Fat (g) = 11.8; Protein = 2.5

🦪 Potato Salad With Egg From Restaurant ☞ serving size: 1 cup = 275 g; Calories = 470.3; Total Carb (g) = 39.6; Net Carb (g) = 35.8; Fat (g) = 31.3; Protein = 7.9

🦪 Potato Salad With Egg Made With Any Type Of Fat Free Dressing ☞ serving size: 1 cup = 275 g; Calories = 244.8; Total Carb (g) = 44; Net Carb (g) = 39.6; Fat (g) = 4.8; Protein = 7.3

🦪 Potato Salad With Egg Made With Creamy Dressing ☞ serving size: 1 cup = 275 g; Calories = 390.5; Total Carb (g) = 40.9; Net Carb (g) = 37.4; Fat (g) = 21.8; Protein = 8.1

🦪 Potato Salad With Egg Made With Italian Dressing ☞ serving size: 1 cup = 275 g; Calories = 313.5; Total Carb (g) = 43.5; Net Carb (g) = 39.9; Fat (g) = 12.2; Protein = 7.7

🦪 Potato Salad With Egg Made With Light Creamy Dressing ☞ serving size: 1 cup = 275 g; Calories = 280.5; Total Carb (g) = 41.3; Net Carb (g) = 37.7; Fat (g) = 9.5; Protein = 8.1

🦪 Potato Salad With Egg Made With Light Italian Dressing ☞ serving size: 1 cup = 275 g; Calories = 258.5; Total Carb (g) = 42.6; Net Carb (g) = 39; Fat (g) = 6.5; Protein = 7.7

🦪 Potato Salad With Egg Made With Light Mayonnaise ☞ serving size: 1 cup = 275 g; Calories = 305.3; Total Carb (g) = 41.6; Net Carb (g) = 38; Fat (g) = 12.3; Protein = 7.5

🦪 Potato Salad With Egg Made With Light Mayonnaise-Type Salad Dressing ☞ serving size: 1 cup = 275 g; Calories = 305.3; Total Carb (g) = 41.6; Net Carb (g) = 38; Fat (g) = 12.3; Protein = 7.5

🦪 Potato Salad With Egg Made With Mayonnaise-Type Salad Dressing ☞ serving size: 1 cup = 275 g; Calories = 308; Total Carb (g) = 43.7; Net Carb (g) = 40.2; Fat (g) = 11.9; Protein = 7.6

🦪 Potato Scalloped From Dry Mix ☞ serving size: 1 cup = 250 g; Calories = 417.5; Total Carb (g) = 34.2; Net Carb (g) = 32.2; Fat (g) = 23.8; Protein = 17

🥔 Potato Scalloped From Dry Mix With Meat ☞ serving size: 1 cup = 250 g; Calories = 417.5; Total Carb (g) = 33.3; Net Carb (g) = 31.6; Fat (g) = 23.9; Protein = 17.9

🥔 Potato Scalloped From Fast Food Or Restaurant ☞ serving size: 1 cup = 250 g; Calories = 502.5; Total Carb (g) = 33.1; Net Carb (g) = 31.3; Fat (g) = 34.4; Protein = 16.4

🥔 Potato Scalloped From Fresh ☞ serving size: 1 cup = 250 g; Calories = 415; Total Carb (g) = 34.1; Net Carb (g) = 32.1; Fat (g) = 23.5; Protein = 17.5

🥔 Potato Scalloped From Fresh With Meat ☞ serving size: 1 cup = 250 g; Calories = 432.5; Total Carb (g) = 32.8; Net Carb (g) = 31; Fat (g) = 25.8; Protein = 18.2

🥔 Potato Scalloped Nfs ☞ serving size: 1 cup = 250 g; Calories = 415; Total Carb (g) = 34.1; Net Carb (g) = 32.1; Fat (g) = 23.5; Protein = 17.5

🥔 Potato Scalloped Ready-To-Heat ☞ serving size: 1 cup = 250 g; Calories = 437.5; Total Carb (g) = 33.6; Net Carb (g) = 31.8; Fat (g) = 26.7; Protein = 16.7

🥔 Potato Scalloped Ready-To-Heat With Meat ☞ serving size: 1 cup = 250 g; Calories = 452.5; Total Carb (g) = 32.4; Net Carb (g) = 30.6; Fat (g) = 28.7; Protein = 17.4

🥔 Potsticker Or Wonton Pork And Vegetable Frozen Unprepared ☞ serving size: 5 pieces 1 serving = 145 g; Calories = 197.2; Total Carb (g) = 19.3; Net Carb (g) = 17.2; Fat (g) = 8; Protein = 12

🥔 Puffs Fried Crab Meat And Cream Cheese Filled ☞ serving size: 1 puff = 23 g; Calories = 72.5; Total Carb (g) = 8.1; Net Carb (g) = 7.8; Fat (g) = 3.5; Protein = 2.1

🥔 Pulled Pork In Barbecue Sauce ☞ serving size: 1 cup = 249 g; Calories = 418.3; Total Carb (g) = 46.7; Net Carb (g) = 43.7; Fat (g) = 11; Protein = 32.8

🥔 Pupusa Bean-Filled ☞ serving size: 1 pupusa (about 5" dia) = 126

g; Calories = 228.1; Total Carb (g) = 37.5; Net Carb (g) = 33.1; Fat (g) = 6.1; Protein = 7.2

🦪 Quesadilla Just Cheese From Fast Food ☞ serving size: 1 slice or wedge = 18 g; Calories = 62.3; Total Carb (g) = 5.4; Net Carb (g) = 5; Fat (g) = 3.4; Protein = 2.4

🦪 Quesadilla Just Cheese Meatless ☞ serving size: 1 slice or wedge = 18 g; Calories = 61.7; Total Carb (g) = 5.9; Net Carb (g) = 5.5; Fat (g) = 3.2; Protein = 2.3

🦪 Quesadilla With Meat ☞ serving size: 1 slice or wedge = 20 g; Calories = 65.2; Total Carb (g) = 5.9; Net Carb (g) = 5.5; Fat (g) = 3.3; Protein = 2.9

🦪 Quesadilla With Vegetables ☞ serving size: 1 slice or wedge = 20 g; Calories = 61.4; Total Carb (g) = 5.9; Net Carb (g) = 5.5; Fat (g) = 3.2; Protein = 2.3

🦪 Quesadilla With Vegetables And Chicken ☞ serving size: 1 slice or wedge = 20 g; Calories = 63; Total Carb (g) = 5.9; Net Carb (g) = 5.5; Fat (g) = 3.2; Protein = 2.5

🦪 Quesadilla With Vegetables And Meat ☞ serving size: 1 slice or wedge = 20 g; Calories = 63.4; Total Carb (g) = 5.9; Net Carb (g) = 5.5; Fat (g) = 3.2; Protein = 2.6

🦪 Quiche With Meat Poultry Or Fish ☞ serving size: 1 piece (1/8 of 9" dia) = 192 g; Calories = 741.1; Total Carb (g) = 22.5; Net Carb (g) = 21.2; Fat (g) = 58.9; Protein = 30.3

🦪 Ravioli Cheese And Spinach Filled With Tomato Sauce ☞ serving size: 1 piece = 38 g; Calories = 44.5; Total Carb (g) = 6.2; Net Carb (g) = 5.7; Fat (g) = 1.3; Protein = 2.1

🦪 Ravioli Cheese And Spinach-Filled No Sauce ☞ serving size: 1 piece = 15 g; Calories = 22.7; Total Carb (g) = 3; Net Carb (g) = 2.9; Fat (g) = 0.7; Protein = 1

🦪 Ravioli Cheese And Spinach-Filled With Cream Sauce ☞

serving size: 1 piece = 38 g; Calories = 55.1; Total Carb (g) = 5.8; Net Carb (g) = 5.5; Fat (g) = 2.6; Protein = 2.2

🦐 Ravioli Cheese With Tomato Sauce Frozen Not Prepared Includes Regular And Light Entrees ☞ serving size: 1 cup = 159 g; Calories = 176.5; Total Carb (g) = 27.5; Net Carb (g) = 25.3; Fat (g) = 4.2; Protein = 7.2

🦐 Ravioli Cheese-Filled Canned ☞ serving size: 1 cup = 242 g; Calories = 186.3; Total Carb (g) = 33; Net Carb (g) = 29.9; Fat (g) = 3.5; Protein = 6

🦐 Ravioli Cheese-Filled No Sauce ☞ serving size: 1 piece = 15 g; Calories = 26.6; Total Carb (g) = 3.1; Net Carb (g) = 2.9; Fat (g) = 1; Protein = 1.3

🦐 Ravioli Cheese-Filled With Cream Sauce ☞ serving size: 1 piece = 38 g; Calories = 61.9; Total Carb (g) = 5.8; Net Carb (g) = 5.6; Fat (g) = 3.1; Protein = 2.5

🦐 Ravioli Cheese-Filled With Meat Sauce ☞ serving size: 1 piece = 35 g; Calories = 48.7; Total Carb (g) = 4.7; Net Carb (g) = 4.5; Fat (g) = 2.2; Protein = 2.4

🦐 Ravioli Cheese-Filled With Tomato Sauce ☞ serving size: 1 piece = 38 g; Calories = 37.2; Total Carb (g) = 5.8; Net Carb (g) = 5.3; Fat (g) = 0.9; Protein = 1.5

🦐 Ravioli Cheese-Filled With Tomato Sauce Diet Frozen Meal ☞ serving size: 1 meal (9 oz) = 255 g; Calories = 285.6; Total Carb (g) = 31; Net Carb (g) = 28.5; Fat (g) = 10.5; Protein = 17.6

🦐 Ravioli Meat-Filled No Sauce ☞ serving size: 1 piece = 15 g; Calories = 28.4; Total Carb (g) = 2.6; Net Carb (g) = 2.5; Fat (g) = 1.1; Protein = 1.9

🦐 Ravioli Meat-Filled With Cream Sauce ☞ serving size: 1 piece = 35 g; Calories = 61.3; Total Carb (g) = 4.7; Net Carb (g) = 4.6; Fat (g) = 3; Protein = 3.5

Ravioli Meat-Filled With Tomato Sauce Or Meat Sauce ☞ serving size: 1 piece = 35 g; Calories = 51.8; Total Carb (g) = 5; Net Carb (g) = 4.7; Fat (g) = 2.1; Protein = 3

Ravioli Meat-Filled With Tomato Sauce Or Meat Sauce Canned ☞ serving size: 1 cup = 262 g; Calories = 254.1; Total Carb (g) = 34.7; Net Carb (g) = 30.8; Fat (g) = 8.9; Protein = 8.5

Ravioli Ns As To Filling No Sauce ☞ serving size: 1 piece = 15 g; Calories = 27.9; Total Carb (g) = 2.9; Net Carb (g) = 2.8; Fat (g) = 1.1; Protein = 1.6

Ravioli Ns As To Filling With Cream Sauce ☞ serving size: 1 piece = 38 g; Calories = 64.6; Total Carb (g) = 5.6; Net Carb (g) = 5.4; Fat (g) = 3.2; Protein = 3.2

Ravioli Ns As To Filling With Tomato Sauce ☞ serving size: 1 piece = 38 g; Calories = 52.8; Total Carb (g) = 5.4; Net Carb (g) = 5; Fat (g) = 2.3; Protein = 2.7

Red Beans And Rice ☞ serving size: 1 cup = 224 g; Calories = 407.7; Total Carb (g) = 42.4; Net Carb (g) = 35.9; Fat (g) = 20.3; Protein = 14.6

Rice And Vermicelli Mix Beef Flavor Prepared With 80% Margarine ☞ serving size: 1 cup = 247 g; Calories = 318.6; Total Carb (g) = 54.4; Net Carb (g) = 52.9; Fat (g) = 7.9; Protein = 7

Rice And Vermicelli Mix Beef Flavor Unprepared ☞ serving size: 1/ 3 cup = 61 g; Calories = 219; Total Carb (g) = 46.4; Net Carb (g) = 45.4; Fat (g) = 0.8; Protein = 6.6

Rice And Vermicelli Mix Chicken Flavor Prepared With 80% Margarine ☞ serving size: 1 cup = 233 g; Calories = 316.9; Total Carb (g) = 54.9; Net Carb (g) = 53.2; Fat (g) = 8; Protein = 6.2

Rice And Vermicelli Mix Chicken Flavor Unprepared ☞ serving size: 1/ 3 cup = 56 g; Calories = 199.4; Total Carb (g) = 42.6; Net Carb (g) = 41.9; Fat (g) = 0.6; Protein = 6

Rice And Vermicelli Mix Rice Pilaf Flavor Prepared With 80% Margarine ☞ serving size: 1 cup = 238 g; Calories = 352.2; Total Carb (g) = 61.1; Net Carb (g) = 59.7; Fat (g) = 8.8; Protein = 7

Rice And Vermicelli Mix Rice Pilaf Flavor Unprepared ☞ serving size: 1/ 3 cup = 68 g; Calories = 244.1; Total Carb (g) = 51.9; Net Carb (g) = 51.1; Fat (g) = 0.9; Protein = 7.1

Rice Bowl With Chicken Frozen Entree Prepared (Includes Fried Teriyaki And Sweet And Sour Varieties) ☞ serving size: 1 bowl = 340 g; Calories = 428.4; Total Carb (g) = 76.4; Net Carb (g) = 74; Fat (g) = 5.3; Protein = 19.2

Rice Brown With Beans ☞ serving size: 1 cup = 239 g; Calories = 360.9; Total Carb (g) = 54.3; Net Carb (g) = 43.8; Fat (g) = 11.4; Protein = 11.5

Rice Brown With Beans And Tomatoes ☞ serving size: 1 cup = 239 g; Calories = 291.6; Total Carb (g) = 44.4; Net Carb (g) = 35.3; Fat (g) = 9.1; Protein = 9.5

Rice Brown With Carrots And Dark Green Vegetables Fat Added In Cooking ☞ serving size: 1 cup = 189 g; Calories = 223; Total Carb (g) = 40.3; Net Carb (g) = 36.7; Fat (g) = 4.9; Protein = 4.6

Rice Brown With Carrots And Dark Green Vegetables Fat Not Added In Cooking ☞ serving size: 1 cup = 186 g; Calories = 193.4; Total Carb (g) = 40.4; Net Carb (g) = 36.9; Fat (g) = 1.5; Protein = 4.6

Rice Brown With Carrots And Dark Green Vegetables Ns As To Fat Added In Cooking ☞ serving size: 1 cup = 189 g; Calories = 223; Total Carb (g) = 40.3; Net Carb (g) = 36.7; Fat (g) = 4.9; Protein = 4.6

Rice Brown With Carrots And Tomatoes And/or Tomato-Based Sauce Fat Added In Cooking ☞ serving size: 1 cup = 229 g; Calories = 254.2; Total Carb (g) = 45.9; Net Carb (g) = 42; Fat (g) = 5.7; Protein = 5

Rice Brown With Carrots And Tomatoes And/or Tomato-Based

Sauce Fat Not Added In Cooking ☞ serving size: 1 cup = 225 g; Calories = 218.3; Total Carb (g) = 45.9; Net Carb (g) = 41.8; Fat (g) = 1.8; Protein = 5

🍚 Rice Brown With Carrots And Tomatoes And/or Tomato-Based Sauce Ns As To Fat Added In Cooking ☞ serving size: 1 cup = 229 g; Calories = 254.2; Total Carb (g) = 45.9; Net Carb (g) = 42; Fat (g) = 5.7; Protein = 5

🍚 Rice Brown With Carrots Dark Green Vegetables And Tomatoes And/or Tomato-Based Sauce Fat Added In Cooking ☞ serving size: 1 cup = 186 g; Calories = 210.2; Total Carb (g) = 38; Net Carb (g) = 34.6; Fat (g) = 4.7; Protein = 4.3

🍚 Rice Brown With Carrots Dark Green Vegetables And Tomatoes And/or Tomato-Based Sauce Fat Not Added In Cooking ☞ serving size: 1 cup = 220 g; Calories = 220; Total Carb (g) = 45.7; Net Carb (g) = 41.8; Fat (g) = 1.8; Protein = 5.2

🍚 Rice Brown With Carrots Dark Green Vegetables And Tomatoes And/or Tomato-Based Sauce Ns As To Fat Added In Cooking ☞ serving size: 1 cup = 224 g; Calories = 253.1; Total Carb (g) = 45.7; Net Carb (g) = 41.7; Fat (g) = 5.6; Protein = 5.2

🍚 Rice Brown With Carrots Fat Added In Cooking ☞ serving size: 1 cup = 189 g; Calories = 223; Total Carb (g) = 40.5; Net Carb (g) = 36.9; Fat (g) = 4.9; Protein = 4.3

🍚 Rice Brown With Carrots Fat Not Added In Cooking ☞ serving size: 1 cup = 186 g; Calories = 193.4; Total Carb (g) = 40.6; Net Carb (g) = 37.1; Fat (g) = 1.5; Protein = 4.3

🍚 Rice Brown With Carrots Ns As To Fat Added In Cooking ☞ serving size: 1 cup = 189 g; Calories = 223; Total Carb (g) = 40.5; Net Carb (g) = 36.9; Fat (g) = 4.9; Protein = 4.3

🍚 Rice Brown With Cheese And/or Cream Based Sauce Fat Added In Cooking ☞ serving size: 1 cup = 282 g; Calories = 439.9; Total Carb (g) = 54.4; Net Carb (g) = 51.3; Fat (g) = 18.6; Protein = 13.7

🦐 Rice Brown With Cheese And/or Cream Based Sauce Fat Not Added In Cooking ☞ serving size: 1 cup = 277 g; Calories = 398.9; Total Carb (g) = 54.3; Net Carb (g) = 51; Fat (g) = 14; Protein = 13.7

🦐 Rice Brown With Cheese And/or Cream Based Sauce Ns As To Fat Added In Cooking ☞ serving size: 1 cup = 282 g; Calories = 439.9; Total Carb (g) = 54.4; Net Carb (g) = 51.3; Fat (g) = 18.6; Protein = 13.7

🦐 Rice Brown With Corn Fat Added In Cooking ☞ serving size: 1 cup = 191 g; Calories = 248.3; Total Carb (g) = 45.9; Net Carb (g) = 42.7; Fat (g) = 5.4; Protein = 5.4

🦐 Rice Brown With Corn Fat Not Added In Cooking ☞ serving size: 1 cup = 188 g; Calories = 220; Total Carb (g) = 46; Net Carb (g) = 42.6; Fat (g) = 2; Protein = 5.4

🦐 Rice Brown With Corn Ns As To Fat Added In Cooking ☞ serving size: 1 cup = 191 g; Calories = 248.3; Total Carb (g) = 45.9; Net Carb (g) = 42.7; Fat (g) = 5.4; Protein = 5.4

🦐 Rice Brown With Dark Green Vegetables And Tomatoes And/or Tomato-Based Sauce Fat Added In Cooking ☞ serving size: 1 cup = 229 g; Calories = 254.2; Total Carb (g) = 45.6; Net Carb (g) = 41.5; Fat (g) = 5.7; Protein = 5.4

🦐 Rice Brown With Dark Green Vegetables And Tomatoes And/or Tomato-Based Sauce Fat Not Added In Cooking ☞ serving size: 1 cup = 229 g; Calories = 222.1; Total Carb (g) = 46.4; Net Carb (g) = 42.3; Fat (g) = 1.8; Protein = 5.5

🦐 Rice Brown With Dark Green Vegetables And Tomatoes And/or Tomato-Based Sauce Ns As To Fat Added In Cooking ☞ serving size: 1 cup = 229 g; Calories = 254.2; Total Carb (g) = 45.6; Net Carb (g) = 41.5; Fat (g) = 5.7; Protein = 5.4

🦐 Rice Brown With Dark Green Vegetables Fat Added In Cooking ☞ serving size: 1 cup = 189 g; Calories = 223; Total Carb (g) = 40.1; Net Carb (g) = 36.5; Fat (g) = 5; Protein = 4.9

Rice Brown With Dark Green Vegetables Fat Not Added In Cooking ☞ serving size: 1 cup = 186 g; Calories = 193.4; Total Carb (g) = 40.2; Net Carb (g) = 36.5; Fat (g) = 1.6; Protein = 4.9

Rice Brown With Dark Green Vegetables Ns As To Fat Added In Cooking ☞ serving size: 1 cup = 189 g; Calories = 223; Total Carb (g) = 40.1; Net Carb (g) = 36.5; Fat (g) = 5; Protein = 4.9

Rice Brown With Gravy Fat Added In Cooking ☞ serving size: 1 cup = 237 g; Calories = 270.2; Total Carb (g) = 45.8; Net Carb (g) = 43.2; Fat (g) = 7.2; Protein = 5

Rice Brown With Gravy Fat Not Added In Cooking ☞ serving size: 1 cup = 237 g; Calories = 239.4; Total Carb (g) = 46.6; Net Carb (g) = 43.7; Fat (g) = 3.4; Protein = 5.1

Rice Brown With Gravy Ns As To Fat Added In Cooking ☞ serving size: 1 cup = 237 g; Calories = 270.2; Total Carb (g) = 45.8; Net Carb (g) = 43.2; Fat (g) = 7.2; Protein = 5

Rice Brown With Other Vegetables Fat Added In Cooking ☞ serving size: 1 cup = 190 g; Calories = 224.2; Total Carb (g) = 40.9; Net Carb (g) = 37.8; Fat (g) = 4.9; Protein = 4.6

Rice Brown With Other Vegetables Fat Not Added In Cooking ☞ serving size: 1 cup = 186 g; Calories = 193.4; Total Carb (g) = 40.7; Net Carb (g) = 37.7; Fat (g) = 1.5; Protein = 4.5

Rice Brown With Other Vegetables Ns As To Fat Added In Cooking ☞ serving size: 1 cup = 190 g; Calories = 224.2; Total Carb (g) = 40.9; Net Carb (g) = 37.8; Fat (g) = 4.9; Protein = 4.6

Rice Brown With Peas And Carrots Fat Added In Cooking ☞ serving size: 1 cup = 190 g; Calories = 228; Total Carb (g) = 41.4; Net Carb (g) = 37.8; Fat (g) = 5; Protein = 5.2

Rice Brown With Peas And Carrots Fat Not Added In Cooking ☞ serving size: 1 cup = 187 g; Calories = 198.2; Total Carb (g) = 41.5; Net Carb (g) = 37.9; Fat (g) = 1.6; Protein = 5.2

Rice Brown With Peas And Carrots Ns As To Fat Added In Cooking ☞ serving size: 1 cup = 190 g; Calories = 228; Total Carb (g) = 41.4; Net Carb (g) = 37.8; Fat (g) = 5; Protein = 5.2

Rice Brown With Peas Fat Added In Cooking ☞ serving size: 1 cup = 190 g; Calories = 243.2; Total Carb (g) = 43.6; Net Carb (g) = 39; Fat (g) = 4.9; Protein = 6.1

Rice Brown With Peas Fat Not Added In Cooking ☞ serving size: 1 cup = 187 g; Calories = 213.2; Total Carb (g) = 43.7; Net Carb (g) = 39.2; Fat (g) = 1.5; Protein = 6.2

Rice Brown With Peas Ns As To Fat Added In Cooking ☞ serving size: 1 cup = 190 g; Calories = 243.2; Total Carb (g) = 43.6; Net Carb (g) = 39; Fat (g) = 4.9; Protein = 6.1

Rice Brown With Soy-Based Sauce Fat Added In Cooking ☞ serving size: 1 cup = 237 g; Calories = 267.8; Total Carb (g) = 49; Net Carb (g) = 46.4; Fat (g) = 5.7; Protein = 5.1

Rice Brown With Soy-Based Sauce Fat Not Added In Cooking ☞ serving size: 1 cup = 237 g; Calories = 239.4; Total Carb (g) = 49.8; Net Carb (g) = 47; Fat (g) = 1.8; Protein = 5.2

Rice Brown With Soy-Based Sauce Ns As To Fat Added In Cooking ☞ serving size: 1 cup = 237 g; Calories = 267.8; Total Carb (g) = 49; Net Carb (g) = 46.4; Fat (g) = 5.7; Protein = 5.1

Rice Brown With Tomatoes And/or Tomato Based Sauce Fat Added In Cooking ☞ serving size: 1 cup = 243 g; Calories = 252.7; Total Carb (g) = 45.6; Net Carb (g) = 41.5; Fat (g) = 5.8; Protein = 5.2

Rice Brown With Tomatoes And/or Tomato Based Sauce Fat Not Added In Cooking ☞ serving size: 1 cup = 243 g; Calories = 223.6; Total Carb (g) = 46.4; Net Carb (g) = 42.2; Fat (g) = 1.9; Protein = 5.3

Rice Brown With Tomatoes And/or Tomato Based Sauce Ns As To Fat Added In Cooking ☞ serving size: 1 cup = 243 g; Calories =

252.7; Total Carb (g) = 45.6; Net Carb (g) = 41.5; Fat (g) = 5.8; Protein = 5.2

🍴 Rice Brown With Vegetables And Gravy Fat Added In Cooking ☞ serving size: 1 cup = 292 g; Calories = 306.6; Total Carb (g) = 53.2; Net Carb (g) = 48.2; Fat (g) = 7.4; Protein = 6.5

🍴 Rice Brown With Vegetables And Gravy Fat Not Added In Cooking ☞ serving size: 1 cup = 288 g; Calories = 270.7; Total Carb (g) = 53.2; Net Carb (g) = 48.3; Fat (g) = 3.5; Protein = 6.6

🍴 Rice Brown With Vegetables And Gravy Ns As To Fat Added In Cooking ☞ serving size: 1 cup = 292 g; Calories = 306.6; Total Carb (g) = 53.2; Net Carb (g) = 48.2; Fat (g) = 7.4; Protein = 6.5

🍴 Rice Brown With Vegetables Cheese And/or Cream Based Sauce Fat Added In Cooking ☞ serving size: 1 cup = 293 g; Calories = 410.2; Total Carb (g) = 53.3; Net Carb (g) = 48.3; Fat (g) = 15.9; Protein = 13.2

🍴 Rice Brown With Vegetables Cheese And/or Cream Based Sauce Fat Not Added In Cooking ☞ serving size: 1 cup = 289 g; Calories = 375.7; Total Carb (g) = 53.3; Net Carb (g) = 48.4; Fat (g) = 12.1; Protein = 13.2

🍴 Rice Brown With Vegetables Cheese And/or Cream Based Sauce Ns As To Fat Added In Cooking ☞ serving size: 1 cup = 293 g; Calories = 410.2; Total Carb (g) = 53.3; Net Carb (g) = 48.3; Fat (g) = 15.9; Protein = 13.2

🍴 Rice Brown With Vegetables Soy-Based Sauce Fat Added In Cooking ☞ serving size: 1 cup = 290 g; Calories = 304.5; Total Carb (g) = 56; Net Carb (g) = 51.1; Fat (g) = 5.8; Protein = 6.6

🍴 Rice Brown With Vegetables Soy-Based Sauce Fat Not Added In Cooking ☞ serving size: 1 cup = 286 g; Calories = 268.8; Total Carb (g) = 56; Net Carb (g) = 50.9; Fat (g) = 1.9; Protein = 6.6

🍴 Rice Brown With Vegetables Soy-Based Sauce Ns As To Fat

Added In Cooking ☞ serving size: 1 cup = 290 g; Calories = 304.5; Total Carb (g) = 56; Net Carb (g) = 51.1; Fat (g) = 5.8; Protein = 6.6

🍚 Rice Cooked With Coconut Milk ☞ serving size: 1 cup = 200 g; Calories = 534; Total Carb (g) = 53.1; Net Carb (g) = 49.3; Fat (g) = 34.5; Protein = 7.1

🍚 Rice Croquette ☞ serving size: 1 croquette (1-1/2" dia, 2" high) = 62 g; Calories = 95.5; Total Carb (g) = 12.4; Net Carb (g) = 11.8; Fat (g) = 4.1; Protein = 2.1

🍚 Rice Dessert Or Salad With Fruit ☞ serving size: 1 cup = 155 g; Calories = 240.3; Total Carb (g) = 33.7; Net Carb (g) = 32.5; Fat (g) = 11.3; Protein = 2.5

🍚 Rice Dressing ☞ serving size: 1 cup = 167 g; Calories = 183.7; Total Carb (g) = 29.5; Net Carb (g) = 28.5; Fat (g) = 5.6; Protein = 3.3

🍚 Rice Fried With Beef ☞ serving size: 1 cup = 198 g; Calories = 352.4; Total Carb (g) = 55.2; Net Carb (g) = 53.4; Fat (g) = 7.7; Protein = 15.9

🍚 Rice Fried With Chicken ☞ serving size: 1 cup = 198 g; Calories = 342.5; Total Carb (g) = 55.2; Net Carb (g) = 53.4; Fat (g) = 6.9; Protein = 14.8

🍚 Rice Fried With Pork ☞ serving size: 1 cup = 198 g; Calories = 354.4; Total Carb (g) = 55.2; Net Carb (g) = 53.4; Fat (g) = 7.8; Protein = 15.3

🍚 Rice Fried With Shrimp ☞ serving size: 1 cup = 198 g; Calories = 328.7; Total Carb (g) = 55.6; Net Carb (g) = 53.9; Fat (g) = 5.5; Protein = 13.6

🍚 Rice Meal Fritter Puerto Rican Style ☞ serving size: 1 cruller (3" x 2" x 1/2") = 30 g; Calories = 93.3; Total Carb (g) = 11; Net Carb (g) = 10.7; Fat (g) = 4.2; Protein = 2.7

🍚 Rice Mix Cheese Flavor Dry Mix Unprepared ☞ serving size: 1/4 cup dry rice mix = 57 g; Calories = 206.3; Total Carb (g) = 42.1; Net Carb (g) = 41.1; Fat (g) = 2; Protein = 5

● Rice Mix White And Wild Flavored Unprepared ☞ serving size: 2 oz (1/4 c dry rice mix and 4 tsp seasoning mix) = 57 g; Calories = 80.9; Total Carb (g) = 15; Net Carb (g) = 14.5; Fat (g) = 1.5; Protein = 2

● Rice White With Carrots And Dark Green Vegetables Fat Added In Cooking ☞ serving size: 1 cup = 172 g; Calories = 209.8; Total Carb (g) = 38.7; Net Carb (g) = 36.8; Fat (g) = 4.1; Protein = 4

● Rice White With Carrots And Dark Green Vegetables Fat Not Added In Cooking ☞ serving size: 1 cup = 172 g; Calories = 182.3; Total Carb (g) = 39.6; Net Carb (g) = 37.7; Fat (g) = 0.5; Protein = 4.1

● Rice White With Carrots And Dark Green Vegetables Ns As To Fat Added In Cooking ☞ serving size: 1 cup = 172 g; Calories = 209.8; Total Carb (g) = 38.7; Net Carb (g) = 36.8; Fat (g) = 4.1; Protein = 4

● Rice White With Carrots And Tomatoes And/or Tomato-Based Sauce Fat Added In Cooking ☞ serving size: 1 cup = 172 g; Calories = 196.1; Total Carb (g) = 36; Net Carb (g) = 34.4; Fat (g) = 3.9; Protein = 3.6

● Rice White With Carrots And Tomatoes And/or Tomato-Based Sauce Fat Not Added In Cooking ☞ serving size: 1 cup = 172 g; Calories = 168.6; Total Carb (g) = 36.7; Net Carb (g) = 35; Fat (g) = 0.5; Protein = 3.7

● Rice White With Carrots And Tomatoes And/or Tomato-Based Sauce Ns As To Fat Added In Cooking ☞ serving size: 1 cup = 172 g; Calories = 196.1; Total Carb (g) = 36; Net Carb (g) = 34.4; Fat (g) = 3.9; Protein = 3.6

● Rice White With Carrots Dark Green Vegetables And Tomatoes And/or Tomato-Based Sauce Fat Added In Cooking ☞ serving size: 1 cup = 172 g; Calories = 201.2; Total Carb (g) = 36.8; Net Carb (g) = 35.1; Fat (g) = 3.9; Protein = 3.8

🍚 Rice White With Carrots Dark Green Vegetables And Tomatoes And/or Tomato-Based Sauce Fat Not Added In Cooking ☞ serving size: 1 cup = 172 g; Calories = 173.7; Total Carb (g) = 37.6; Net Carb (g) = 35.8; Fat (g) = 0.5; Protein = 3.9

🍚 Rice White With Carrots Dark Green Vegetables And Tomatoes And/or Tomato-Based Sauce Ns As To Fat Added In Cooking ☞ serving size: 1 cup = 172 g; Calories = 201.2; Total Carb (g) = 36.8; Net Carb (g) = 35.1; Fat (g) = 3.9; Protein = 3.8

🍚 Rice White With Carrots Fat Added In Cooking ☞ serving size: 1 cup = 160 g; Calories = 196.8; Total Carb (g) = 36.2; Net Carb (g) = 34.6; Fat (g) = 3.8; Protein = 3.5

🍚 Rice White With Carrots Fat Not Added In Cooking ☞ serving size: 1 cup = 160 g; Calories = 169.6; Total Carb (g) = 37; Net Carb (g) = 35.4; Fat (g) = 0.4; Protein = 3.5

🍚 Rice White With Carrots Ns As To Fat Added In Cooking ☞ serving size: 1 cup = 160 g; Calories = 196.8; Total Carb (g) = 36.2; Net Carb (g) = 34.6; Fat (g) = 3.8; Protein = 3.5

🍚 Rice White With Cheese And/or Cream Based Sauce Fat Added In Cooking ☞ serving size: 1 cup = 204 g; Calories = 338.6; Total Carb (g) = 40.8; Net Carb (g) = 40.2; Fat (g) = 14.2; Protein = 10.5

🍚 Rice White With Cheese And/or Cream Based Sauce Fat Not Added In Cooking ☞ serving size: 1 cup = 204 g; Calories = 310.1; Total Carb (g) = 41.6; Net Carb (g) = 41; Fat (g) = 10.7; Protein = 10.7

🍚 Rice White With Cheese And/or Cream Based Sauce Ns As To Fat Added In Cooking ☞ serving size: 1 cup = 204 g; Calories = 338.6; Total Carb (g) = 40.8; Net Carb (g) = 40.2; Fat (g) = 14.2; Protein = 10.5

🍚 Rice White With Corn Fat Added In Cooking ☞ serving size: 1 cup = 161 g; Calories = 220.6; Total Carb (g) = 41.3; Net Carb (g) = 39.9; Fat (g) = 4.3; Protein = 4.5

🦪 Rice White With Corn Fat Not Added In Cooking ☞ serving size: 1 cup = 161 g; Calories = 194.8; Total Carb (g) = 42.2; Net Carb (g) = 40.7; Fat (g) = 1; Protein = 4.6

🦪 Rice White With Corn Ns As To Fat Added In Cooking ☞ serving size: 1 cup = 161 g; Calories = 220.6; Total Carb (g) = 41.3; Net Carb (g) = 39.9; Fat (g) = 4.3; Protein = 4.5

🦪 Rice White With Dark Green Vegetables And Tomatoes And/or Tomato-Based Sauce Fat Added In Cooking ☞ serving size: 1 cup = 172 g; Calories = 196.1; Total Carb (g) = 35.8; Net Carb (g) = 34.1; Fat (g) = 3.9; Protein = 3.9

🦪 Rice White With Dark Green Vegetables And Tomatoes And/or Tomato-Based Sauce Fat Not Added In Cooking ☞ serving size: 1 cup = 172 g; Calories = 168.6; Total Carb (g) = 36.5; Net Carb (g) = 34.8; Fat (g) = 0.5; Protein = 4

🦪 Rice White With Dark Green Vegetables And Tomatoes And/or Tomato-Based Sauce Ns As To Fat Added In Cooking ☞ serving size: 1 cup = 172 g; Calories = 196.1; Total Carb (g) = 35.8; Net Carb (g) = 34.1; Fat (g) = 3.9; Protein = 3.9

🦪 Rice White With Dark Green Vegetables Fat Added In Cooking ☞ serving size: 1 cup = 172 g; Calories = 209.8; Total Carb (g) = 38.5; Net Carb (g) = 36.6; Fat (g) = 4.2; Protein = 4.4

🦪 Rice White With Dark Green Vegetables Fat Not Added In Cooking ☞ serving size: 1 cup = 172 g; Calories = 182.3; Total Carb (g) = 39.3; Net Carb (g) = 37.4; Fat (g) = 0.5; Protein = 4.5

🦪 Rice White With Dark Green Vegetables Ns As To Fat Added In Cooking ☞ serving size: 1 cup = 172 g; Calories = 209.8; Total Carb (g) = 38.5; Net Carb (g) = 36.6; Fat (g) = 4.2; Protein = 4.4

🦪 Rice White With Gravy Fat Added In Cooking ☞ serving size: 1 cup = 237 g; Calories = 277.3; Total Carb (g) = 47.5; Net Carb (g) = 46.8; Fat (g) = 6.9; Protein = 4.7

Rice White With Gravy Fat Not Added In Cooking ☞ serving size: 1 cup = 237 g; Calories = 241.7; Total Carb (g) = 48.4; Net Carb (g) = 47.7; Fat (g) = 2.5; Protein = 4.8

Rice White With Gravy Ns As To Fat Added In Cooking ☞ serving size: 1 cup = 237 g; Calories = 277.3; Total Carb (g) = 47.5; Net Carb (g) = 46.8; Fat (g) = 6.9; Protein = 4.7

Rice White With Lentils Fat Added In Cooking ☞ serving size: 1 cup = 207 g; Calories = 308.4; Total Carb (g) = 44.5; Net Carb (g) = 36; Fat (g) = 9.8; Protein = 11.4

Rice White With Lentils Fat Not Added In Cooking ☞ serving size: 1 cup = 198 g; Calories = 227.7; Total Carb (g) = 44.5; Net Carb (g) = 36; Fat (g) = 0.7; Protein = 11.4

Rice White With Lentils Ns As To Fat Added In Cooking ☞ serving size: 1 cup = 207 g; Calories = 308.4; Total Carb (g) = 44.5; Net Carb (g) = 36; Fat (g) = 9.8; Protein = 11.4

Rice White With Other Vegetables Fat Added In Cooking ☞ serving size: 1 cup = 172 g; Calories = 211.6; Total Carb (g) = 39; Net Carb (g) = 37.8; Fat (g) = 4.1; Protein = 4

Rice White With Other Vegetables Fat Not Added In Cooking ☞ serving size: 1 cup = 172 g; Calories = 182.3; Total Carb (g) = 39.9; Net Carb (g) = 38.7; Fat (g) = 0.5; Protein = 4

Rice White With Other Vegetables Ns As To Fat Added In Cooking ☞ serving size: 1 cup = 172 g; Calories = 211.6; Total Carb (g) = 39; Net Carb (g) = 37.8; Fat (g) = 4.1; Protein = 4

Rice White With Peas And Carrots Fat Added In Cooking ☞ serving size: 1 cup = 160 g; Calories = 200; Total Carb (g) = 36.8; Net Carb (g) = 35.1; Fat (g) = 3.8; Protein = 4.4

Rice White With Peas And Carrots Fat Not Added In Cooking ☞ serving size: 1 cup = 160 g; Calories = 174.4; Total Carb (g) = 37.6; Net Carb (g) = 35.8; Fat (g) = 0.5; Protein = 4.5

 Rice White With Peas And Carrots Ns As To Fat Added In Cooking ☞ serving size: 1 cup = 160 g; Calories = 200; Total Carb (g) = 36.8; Net Carb (g) = 35.1; Fat (g) = 3.8; Protein = 4.4

 Rice White With Peas Fat Added In Cooking ☞ serving size: 1 cup = 160 g; Calories = 214.4; Total Carb (g) = 39; Net Carb (g) = 36.4; Fat (g) = 3.8; Protein = 5.3

 Rice White With Peas Fat Not Added In Cooking ☞ serving size: 1 cup = 160 g; Calories = 188.8; Total Carb (g) = 39.8; Net Carb (g) = 37.1; Fat (g) = 0.4; Protein = 5.4

 Rice White With Peas Ns As To Fat Added In Cooking ☞ serving size: 1 cup = 160 g; Calories = 214.4; Total Carb (g) = 39; Net Carb (g) = 36.4; Fat (g) = 3.8; Protein = 5.3

 Rice White With Soy-Based Sauce Fat Added In Cooking ☞ serving size: 1 cup = 237 g; Calories = 274.9; Total Carb (g) = 51.2; Net Carb (g) = 50.5; Fat (g) = 5.1; Protein = 4.8

 Rice White With Soy-Based Sauce Fat Not Added In Cooking ☞ serving size: 1 cup = 237 g; Calories = 241.7; Total Carb (g) = 52.2; Net Carb (g) = 51.5; Fat (g) = 0.7; Protein = 4.9

 Rice White With Soy-Based Sauce Ns As To Fat Added In Cooking ☞ serving size: 1 cup = 237 g; Calories = 274.9; Total Carb (g) = 51.2; Net Carb (g) = 50.5; Fat (g) = 5.1; Protein = 4.8

 Rice White With Tomatoes And/or Tomato-Based Sauce Fat Added In Cooking ☞ serving size: 1 cup = 209 g; Calories = 221.5; Total Carb (g) = 40.6; Net Carb (g) = 38.7; Fat (g) = 4.5; Protein = 4.2

 Rice White With Tomatoes And/or Tomato-Based Sauce Fat Not Added In Cooking ☞ serving size: 1 cup = 206 g; Calories = 187.5; Total Carb (g) = 40.8; Net Carb (g) = 38.9; Fat (g) = 0.6; Protein = 4.2

 Rice White With Tomatoes And/or Tomato-Based Sauce Ns As To Fat Added In Cooking ☞ serving size: 1 cup = 209 g; Calories =

221.5; Total Carb (g) = 40.6; Net Carb (g) = 38.7; Fat (g) = 4.5; Protein = 4.2

🍃 Rice White With Vegetables And Gravy Fat Added In Cooking ☞ serving size: 1 cup = 260 g; Calories = 275.6; Total Carb (g) = 48.5; Net Carb (g) = 45.7; Fat (g) = 6.1; Protein = 5.6

🍃 Rice White With Vegetables And Gravy Fat Not Added In Cooking ☞ serving size: 1 cup = 256 g; Calories = 243.2; Total Carb (g) = 48.5; Net Carb (g) = 45.7; Fat (g) = 2.2; Protein = 5.6

🍃 Rice White With Vegetables And Gravy Ns As To Fat Added In Cooking ☞ serving size: 1 cup = 260 g; Calories = 275.6; Total Carb (g) = 48.5; Net Carb (g) = 45.7; Fat (g) = 6.1; Protein = 5.6

🍃 Rice White With Vegetables Cheese And/or Cream Based Sauce Fat Added In Cooking ☞ serving size: 1 cup = 262 g; Calories = 382.5; Total Carb (g) = 48.8; Net Carb (g) = 46; Fat (g) = 14.7; Protein = 12.3

🍃 Rice White With Vegetables Cheese And/or Cream Based Sauce Fat Not Added In Cooking ☞ serving size: 1 cup = 258 g; Calories = 345.7; Total Carb (g) = 48.8; Net Carb (g) = 46; Fat (g) = 10.8; Protein = 12.3

🍃 Rice White With Vegetables Cheese And/or Cream Based Sauce Ns As To Fat Added In Cooking ☞ serving size: 1 cup = 261 g; Calories = 381.1; Total Carb (g) = 48.7; Net Carb (g) = 45.8; Fat (g) = 14.7; Protein = 12.3

🍃 Rice White With Vegetables Soy-Based Sauce Fat Added In Cooking ☞ serving size: 1 cup = 258 g; Calories = 273.5; Total Carb (g) = 51.4; Net Carb (g) = 48.5; Fat (g) = 4.5; Protein = 5.7

🍃 Rice White With Vegetables Soy-Based Sauce Fat Not Added In Cooking ☞ serving size: 1 cup = 255 g; Calories = 239.7; Total Carb (g) = 51.5; Net Carb (g) = 48.7; Fat (g) = 0.6; Protein = 5.7

🍃 Rice White With Vegetables Soy-Based Sauce Ns As To Fat

Added In Cooking ☞ serving size: 1 cup = 258 g; Calories = 273.5; Total Carb (g) = 51.4; Net Carb (g) = 48.5; Fat (g) = 4.5; Protein = 5.7

🍚 Rice With Beans ☞ serving size: 1 cup = 239 g; Calories = 372.8; Total Carb (g) = 56.1; Net Carb (g) = 46.1; Fat (g) = 11.6; Protein = 12

🍚 Rice With Beans And Beef ☞ serving size: 1 cup = 239 g; Calories = 413.5; Total Carb (g) = 47.2; Net Carb (g) = 38.8; Fat (g) = 16.1; Protein = 19.7

🍚 Rice With Beans And Chicken ☞ serving size: 1 cup = 239 g; Calories = 377.6; Total Carb (g) = 47.3; Net Carb (g) = 38.9; Fat (g) = 12.1; Protein = 20.1

🍚 Rice With Beans And Pork ☞ serving size: 1 cup = 239 g; Calories = 403.9; Total Carb (g) = 47.2; Net Carb (g) = 38.8; Fat (g) = 15; Protein = 20.1

🍚 Rice With Beans And Tomatoes ☞ serving size: 1 cup = 239 g; Calories = 296.4; Total Carb (g) = 45.1; Net Carb (g) = 36.5; Fat (g) = 9; Protein = 9.6

🍚 Rice With Broccoli Cheese Sauce Frozen Side Dish ☞ serving size: 1 side dish (4.5 oz) = 128 g; Calories = 152.3; Total Carb (g) = 21.9; Net Carb (g) = 19.9; Fat (g) = 5.3; Protein = 4.7

🍚 Rice With Chicken Puerto Rican Style ☞ serving size: 1 cup, with bone (yield after bone removed) = 157 g; Calories = 466.3; Total Carb (g) = 49.4; Net Carb (g) = 48.1; Fat (g) = 22; Protein = 15.9

🍚 Rice With Green Beans Water Chestnuts In Sherry Mushroom Sauce Frozen Side Dish ☞ serving size: 1 side dish (10 oz) = 284 g; Calories = 275.5; Total Carb (g) = 41.6; Net Carb (g) = 37.9; Fat (g) = 9.2; Protein = 7.4

🍚 Rice With Onions Puerto Rican Style ☞ serving size: 1 cup = 165 g; Calories = 285.5; Total Carb (g) = 31.1; Net Carb (g) = 29; Fat (g) = 16.1; Protein = 5.7

Rice With Raisins ☞ serving size: 1 cup = 185 g; Calories = 299.7; Total Carb (g) = 59.4; Net Carb (g) = 58.1; Fat (g) = 4.9; Protein = 4.9

Rice With Spanish Sausage Puerto Rican Style ☞ serving size: 1 cup = 180 g; Calories = 567; Total Carb (g) = 58.1; Net Carb (g) = 56.6; Fat (g) = 28.7; Protein = 17.2

Rice With Squid Puerto Rican Style ☞ serving size: 1 cup = 160 g; Calories = 414.4; Total Carb (g) = 47; Net Carb (g) = 45.4; Fat (g) = 18.4; Protein = 14.3

Rice With Stewed Beans Puerto Rican Style ☞ serving size: 1 cup = 188 g; Calories = 257.6; Total Carb (g) = 43.3; Net Carb (g) = 40.5; Fat (g) = 6.1; Protein = 6.9

Rice With Vienna Sausage Puerto Rican Style ☞ serving size: 1 cup = 180 g; Calories = 482.4; Total Carb (g) = 60.4; Net Carb (g) = 59; Fat (g) = 20.7; Protein = 11.6

Rigatoni With Meat Sauce And Cheese Diet Frozen Meal ☞ serving size: 1 meal (9.75 oz) = 276 g; Calories = 251.2; Total Carb (g) = 23.9; Net Carb (g) = 20.9; Fat (g) = 10.2; Protein = 17.1

Roll With Meat And/or Shrimp Vegetables And Rice Paper Not Fried ☞ serving size: 1 roll (4-1/4" x 1-1/2" dia) = 71 g; Calories = 78.8; Total Carb (g) = 12.2; Net Carb (g) = 10.7; Fat (g) = 1.9; Protein = 3.9

Salisbury Steak With Gravy Frozen ☞ serving size: 1 patty = 63 g; Calories = 93.9; Total Carb (g) = 4.3; Net Carb (g) = 3.6; Fat (g) = 6.6; Protein = 4.4

Sausage Egg And Cheese Breakfast Biscuit ☞ serving size: 1 biscuit = 126 g; Calories = 408.2; Total Carb (g) = 27.2; Net Carb (g) = 24.7; Fat (g) = 27.9; Protein = 12

Seafood Paella Puerto Rican Style ☞ serving size: 1 cup = 230 g; Calories = 331.2; Total Carb (g) = 36.1; Net Carb (g) = 34; Fat (g) = 12.6; Protein = 17.5

Seaweed Prepared With Soy Sauce ☞ serving size: 1 cup = 96 g;

Calories = 41.3; Total Carb (g) = 7.2; Net Carb (g) = 6.6; Fat (g) = 0.5; Protein = 4

🦪 Shellfish Mixture And Vegetables Excluding Carrots Broccoli And Dark-Green Leafy; No Potatoes Soy-Based Sauce ☞ serving size: 1 cup = 217 g; Calories = 256.1; Total Carb (g) = 12.3; Net Carb (g) = 10.4; Fat (g) = 14.1; Protein = 20.8

🦪 Shellfish Mixture And Vegetables Including Carrots Broccoli And/or Dark-Green Leafy; No Potatoes Soy-Based Sauce ☞ serving size: 1 cup = 217 g; Calories = 253.9; Total Carb (g) = 13; Net Carb (g) = 10.2; Fat (g) = 13.6; Protein = 20.3

🦪 Shrimp And Noodles With Soy-Based Sauce ☞ serving size: 1 cup = 224 g; Calories = 311.4; Total Carb (g) = 18.4; Net Carb (g) = 17; Fat (g) = 15.9; Protein = 22.8

🦪 Shrimp And Vegetables Excluding Carrots Broccoli And Dark-Green Leafy; No Potatoes Soy-Based Sauce ☞ serving size: 1 cup = 217 g; Calories = 247.4; Total Carb (g) = 10.6; Net Carb (g) = 8.7; Fat (g) = 14.1; Protein = 20.3

🦪 Shrimp And Vegetables Including Carrots Broccoli And/or Dark-Green Leafy; No Potatoes Soy-Based Sauce ☞ serving size: 1 cup = 217 g; Calories = 245.2; Total Carb (g) = 11.4; Net Carb (g) = 8.6; Fat (g) = 13.6; Protein = 19.7

🦪 Shrimp Chow Mein Or Chop Suey No Noodles ☞ serving size: 1 cup = 220 g; Calories = 151.8; Total Carb (g) = 9.4; Net Carb (g) = 7.6; Fat (g) = 3.7; Protein = 19.4

🦪 Shrimp Chow Mein Or Chop Suey With Noodles ☞ serving size: 1 cup = 220 g; Calories = 259.6; Total Carb (g) = 27.4; Net Carb (g) = 25; Fat (g) = 7.3; Protein = 19.2

🦪 Shrimp Egg Foo Yung ☞ serving size: 1 cup = 175 g; Calories = 215.3; Total Carb (g) = 8.7; Net Carb (g) = 8.3; Fat (g) = 10.4; Protein = 20.4

🦐 Shrimp Teriyaki ☞ serving size: 1 cup = 201 g; Calories = 241.2; Total Carb (g) = 6.7; Net Carb (g) = 6.7; Fat (g) = 3.1; Protein = 43.5

🦐 Soft Taco With Chicken And Beans ☞ serving size: 1 small taco or tostada = 112 g; Calories = 222.9; Total Carb (g) = 25.4; Net Carb (g) = 21.8; Fat (g) = 9; Protein = 10.3

🦐 Soft Taco With Chicken Beans And Sour Cream ☞ serving size: 1 small taco or tostada = 127 g; Calories = 252.7; Total Carb (g) = 26; Net Carb (g) = 22.5; Fat (g) = 12; Protein = 10.6

🦐 Soft Taco With Fish ☞ serving size: 1 small taco or tostada = 94 g; Calories = 187.1; Total Carb (g) = 20; Net Carb (g) = 18.1; Fat (g) = 7.5; Protein = 9.6

🦐 Soft Taco With Meat ☞ serving size: 1 small taco or tostada = 103 g; Calories = 227.6; Total Carb (g) = 21; Net Carb (g) = 18.9; Fat (g) = 11; Protein = 11

🦐 Soft Taco With Meat And Beans ☞ serving size: 1 small taco or tostada = 117 g; Calories = 235.2; Total Carb (g) = 26.1; Net Carb (g) = 22.3; Fat (g) = 10.1; Protein = 10

🦐 Soft Taco With Meat And Sour Cream From Fast Food ☞ serving size: 1 small taco or tostada = 117 g; Calories = 234; Total Carb (g) = 22; Net Carb (g) = 18.9; Fat (g) = 11.7; Protein = 10.2

🦐 Soft Taco With Meat Beans And Sour Cream ☞ serving size: 1 small taco or tostada = 132 g; Calories = 266.6; Total Carb (g) = 26.9; Net Carb (g) = 23.2; Fat (g) = 13.2; Protein = 10.5

🦐 Somen Salad With Noodles Lettuce Egg Fish And Pork ☞ serving size: 1 cup = 160 g; Calories = 219.2; Total Carb (g) = 14.2; Net Carb (g) = 12.9; Fat (g) = 9.8; Protein = 18.1

🦐 Spaghetti And Meatballs Dinner NFS Frozen Meal ☞ serving size: 1 meal (12.5 oz) = 354 g; Calories = 396.5; Total Carb (g) = 52.5; Net Carb (g) = 48.3; Fat (g) = 11.8; Protein = 19.6

🦐 Spaghetti And Meatballs With Tomato Sauce Sliced Apples

Bread Frozen Meal ☞ serving size: 1 meal (11.5 oz) = 326 g; Calories = 423.8; Total Carb (g) = 53.3; Net Carb (g) = 47.8; Fat (g) = 12.1; Protein = 25.1

🍝 Spaghetti With Corned Beef Puerto Rican Style ☞ serving size: 1 cup = 215 g; Calories = 539.7; Total Carb (g) = 37.4; Net Carb (g) = 35; Fat (g) = 30.7; Protein = 27.6

🍝 Spaghetti With Meat And Mushroom Sauce Diet Frozen Meal ☞ serving size: 1 meal (11.5 oz) = 326 g; Calories = 374.9; Total Carb (g) = 53.8; Net Carb (g) = 49.2; Fat (g) = 9.1; Protein = 19.9

🍝 Spaghetti With Meat Sauce Diet Frozen Meal ☞ serving size: 1 meal (10.5 oz) = 298 g; Calories = 333.8; Total Carb (g) = 44.2; Net Carb (g) = 40.6; Fat (g) = 9.9; Protein = 16.5

🍝 Spaghetti With Meat Sauce Frozen Entree ☞ serving size: 1 serving = 283 g; Calories = 254.7; Total Carb (g) = 43.1; Net Carb (g) = 38; Fat (g) = 2.9; Protein = 14.3

🍝 Spaghetti With Meatballs In Tomato Sauce Canned ☞ serving size: 1 cup = 246 g; Calories = 246; Total Carb (g) = 28.2; Net Carb (g) = 21.5; Fat (g) = 10.1; Protein = 10.8

🍝 Spanakopitta ☞ serving size: 1 cubic inch = 12 g; Calories = 24.7; Total Carb (g) = 1.3; Net Carb (g) = 1.1; Fat (g) = 1.8; Protein = 0.9

🍝 Spanish Rice Fat Added In Cooking ☞ serving size: 1 cup = 243 g; Calories = 277; Total Carb (g) = 47.8; Net Carb (g) = 44.9; Fat (g) = 6.3; Protein = 7

🍝 Spanish Rice Fat Not Added In Cooking ☞ serving size: 1 cup = 243 g; Calories = 245.4; Total Carb (g) = 48.4; Net Carb (g) = 45.5; Fat (g) = 2.5; Protein = 7.1

🍝 Spanish Rice Mix Dry Mix Prepared (With Canola/vegetable Oil Blend Or Diced Tomatoes And Margarine) ☞ serving size: 1 cup = 198 g; Calories = 247.5; Total Carb (g) = 45; Net Carb (g) = 42.1; Fat (g) = 4.7; Protein = 6.5

🌾 Spanish Rice Mix Dry Mix Unprepared ☞ serving size: 1/2 cup = 70 g; Calories = 254.1; Total Carb (g) = 53.5; Net Carb (g) = 51.4; Fat (g) = 1.1; Protein = 7.4

🌾 Spanish Rice Ns As To Fat Added In Cooking ☞ serving size: 1 cup = 243 g; Calories = 277; Total Carb (g) = 47.8; Net Carb (g) = 44.9; Fat (g) = 6.2; Protein = 7

🌾 Spanish Rice With Ground Beef ☞ serving size: 1 cup = 230 g; Calories = 372.6; Total Carb (g) = 34; Net Carb (g) = 32; Fat (g) = 15.8; Protein = 22.3

🌾 Spinach Quiche Meatless ☞ serving size: 1 piece (1/8 of 9" dia) = 143 g; Calories = 423.3; Total Carb (g) = 16.4; Net Carb (g) = 14.7; Fat (g) = 33.6; Protein = 15

🌾 Steak Teriyaki ☞ serving size: 1 cup = 244 g; Calories = 483.1; Total Carb (g) = 4.7; Net Carb (g) = 4.7; Fat (g) = 20.1; Protein = 70.4

🌾 Stewed Potatoes ☞ serving size: 1 cup = 250 g; Calories = 285; Total Carb (g) = 49.8; Net Carb (g) = 46.3; Fat (g) = 8.1; Protein = 4.6

🌾 Stewed Potatoes Puerto Rican Style ☞ serving size: 1 small = 123 g; Calories = 140.2; Total Carb (g) = 23.1; Net Carb (g) = 20.8; Fat (g) = 4.5; Protein = 2.6

🌾 Stewed Potatoes With Tomatoes ☞ serving size: 1 cup = 250 g; Calories = 230; Total Carb (g) = 37.9; Net Carb (g) = 34.9; Fat (g) = 7.8; Protein = 3.9

🌾 Stewed Rice Puerto Rican Style ☞ serving size: 1 cup = 170 g; Calories = 377.4; Total Carb (g) = 56.9; Net Carb (g) = 55.7; Fat (g) = 13.1; Protein = 6.8

🌾 Stir Fried Beef And Vegetables In Soy Sauce ☞ serving size: 1 cup = 162 g; Calories = 150.7; Total Carb (g) = 6.9; Net Carb (g) = 5.4; Fat (g) = 6; Protein = 17.6

🌾 Stuffed Shells Cheese- And Spinach- Filled No Sauce ☞ serving size: 1 shell (jumbo) = 60 g; Calories = 112.8; Total Carb (g) = 12.9; Net Carb (g) = 12.3; Fat (g) = 4.1; Protein = 5.9

● Stuffed Shells Cheese-Filled No Sauce ☞ serving size: 1 shell (jumbo) = 60 g; Calories = 126; Total Carb (g) = 12.4; Net Carb (g) = 12; Fat (g) = 5.4; Protein = 6.5

● Stuffed Shells Cheese-Filled With Meat Sauce ☞ serving size: 1 shell (jumbo) = 85 g; Calories = 136.9; Total Carb (g) = 13.3; Net Carb (g) = 12.5; Fat (g) = 5.9; Protein = 7.6

● Stuffed Shells Cheese-Filled With Tomato Sauce Meatless ☞ serving size: 1 shell (jumbo) = 85 g; Calories = 126.7; Total Carb (g) = 13.5; Net Carb (g) = 12.7; Fat (g) = 5.2; Protein = 6.4

● Stuffed Shells With Chicken With Tomato Sauce ☞ serving size: 1 shell (jumbo) = 83 g; Calories = 112.9; Total Carb (g) = 13.3; Net Carb (g) = 12.4; Fat (g) = 2.7; Protein = 8.9

● Stuffed Shells With Fish And/or Shellfish With Tomato Sauce ☞ serving size: 1 shell (jumbo) = 83 g; Calories = 96.3; Total Carb (g) = 13.2; Net Carb (g) = 12.3; Fat (g) = 1.5; Protein = 7.3

● Sushi Nfs ☞ serving size: 1 piece = 30 g; Calories = 27.9; Total Carb (g) = 5.5; Net Carb (g) = 5.2; Fat (g) = 0.2; Protein = 0.9

● Sushi Roll Avocado ☞ serving size: 1 piece = 30 g; Calories = 27.6; Total Carb (g) = 5.3; Net Carb (g) = 4.9; Fat (g) = 0.4; Protein = 0.5

● Sushi Roll California ☞ serving size: 1 piece = 30 g; Calories = 27.9; Total Carb (g) = 5.5; Net Carb (g) = 5.2; Fat (g) = 0.2; Protein = 0.9

● Sushi Roll Eel ☞ serving size: 1 piece = 30 g; Calories = 38.1; Total Carb (g) = 4.6; Net Carb (g) = 4.4; Fat (g) = 1.1; Protein = 2.1

● Sushi Roll Salmon ☞ serving size: 1 piece = 30 g; Calories = 30.9; Total Carb (g) = 4.6; Net Carb (g) = 4.4; Fat (g) = 0.4; Protein = 2.1

● Sushi Roll Shrimp ☞ serving size: 1 piece = 30 g; Calories = 30; Total Carb (g) = 4.7; Net Carb (g) = 4.5; Fat (g) = 0.2; Protein = 2.1

🍣 Sushi Roll Tuna ☞ serving size: 1 piece = 30 g; Calories = 29.1; Total Carb (g) = 4.6; Net Carb (g) = 4.4; Fat (g) = 0.1; Protein = 2.2

🍣 Sushi Roll Vegetable ☞ serving size: 1 piece = 22 g; Calories = 20.2; Total Carb (g) = 3.9; Net Carb (g) = 3.6; Fat (g) = 0.3; Protein = 0.4

🍣 Sushi Topped With Crab ☞ serving size: 1 piece = 35 g; Calories = 33.3; Total Carb (g) = 6.5; Net Carb (g) = 6.2; Fat (g) = 0.1; Protein = 1.4

🍣 Sushi Topped With Eel ☞ serving size: 1 piece = 35 g; Calories = 49.7; Total Carb (g) = 4.7; Net Carb (g) = 4.5; Fat (g) = 1.8; Protein = 3.2

🍣 Sushi Topped With Egg ☞ serving size: 1 piece = 50 g; Calories = 58; Total Carb (g) = 5.4; Net Carb (g) = 5.2; Fat (g) = 2.3; Protein = 3.5

🍣 Sushi Topped With Salmon ☞ serving size: 1 piece = 35 g; Calories = 37.5; Total Carb (g) = 4.7; Net Carb (g) = 4.5; Fat (g) = 0.6; Protein = 3.1

🍣 Sushi Topped With Shrimp ☞ serving size: 1 piece = 35 g; Calories = 36.1; Total Carb (g) = 4.9; Net Carb (g) = 4.7; Fat (g) = 0.3; Protein = 3.2

🍣 Sushi Topped With Tuna ☞ serving size: 1 piece = 35 g; Calories = 35; Total Carb (g) = 4.7; Net Carb (g) = 4.5; Fat (g) = 0.1; Protein = 3.4

🍣 Sweet And Sour Pork ☞ serving size: 1 cup = 226 g; Calories = 438.4; Total Carb (g) = 40.9; Net Carb (g) = 38.9; Fat (g) = 18.8; Protein = 26.2

🍣 Sweet And Sour Pork With Rice ☞ serving size: 1 cup = 244 g; Calories = 449; Total Carb (g) = 48.8; Net Carb (g) = 46.8; Fat (g) = 17.1; Protein = 24.8

🍣 Sweet And Sour Shrimp ☞ serving size: 1 cup = 176 g; Calories = 295.7; Total Carb (g) = 27.8; Net Carb (g) = 26.4; Fat (g) = 15; Protein = 12.6

🦪 Sweet Bread Dough Filled With Meat Steamed ☞ serving size: 1 manapua = 93 g; Calories = 253; Total Carb (g) = 36.6; Net Carb (g) = 35.5; Fat (g) = 7; Protein = 10.2

🦪 Tabbouleh ☞ serving size: 1 cup = 160 g; Calories = 196.8; Total Carb (g) = 15.5; Net Carb (g) = 12.6; Fat (g) = 15; Protein = 2.6

🦪 Taco Or Tostada Salad Meatless ☞ serving size: 1 small taco salad = 234 g; Calories = 376.7; Total Carb (g) = 45.1; Net Carb (g) = 36.2; Fat (g) = 17.2; Protein = 12.4

🦪 Taco Or Tostada Salad Meatless With Sour Cream ☞ serving size: 1 small taco salad = 266 g; Calories = 441.6; Total Carb (g) = 46.5; Net Carb (g) = 37.7; Fat (g) = 23.4; Protein = 13.2

🦪 Taco Or Tostada Salad With Chicken ☞ serving size: 1 small taco salad = 240 g; Calories = 398.4; Total Carb (g) = 39; Net Carb (g) = 32; Fat (g) = 19.2; Protein = 18.8

🦪 Taco Or Tostada Salad With Chicken And Sour Cream ☞ serving size: 1 small taco salad = 273 g; Calories = 464.1; Total Carb (g) = 40.6; Net Carb (g) = 33.7; Fat (g) = 25.5; Protein = 19.7

🦪 Taco Or Tostada Salad With Meat ☞ serving size: 1 small taco salad = 237 g; Calories = 421.9; Total Carb (g) = 39; Net Carb (g) = 32.1; Fat (g) = 22; Protein = 17.7

🦪 Taco Or Tostada Salad With Meat And Sour Cream ☞ serving size: 1 small taco salad = 264 g; Calories = 475.2; Total Carb (g) = 39.7; Net Carb (g) = 32.8; Fat (g) = 27.8; Protein = 18.1

🦪 Taco Or Tostada With Beans ☞ serving size: 1 small taco or tostada = 125 g; Calories = 252.5; Total Carb (g) = 29.2; Net Carb (g) = 23.4; Fat (g) = 11.9; Protein = 8

🦪 Taco Or Tostada With Beans And Sour Cream ☞ serving size: 1 small taco or tostada = 140 g; Calories = 281.4; Total Carb (g) = 29.7; Net Carb (g) = 23.9; Fat (g) = 14.9; Protein = 8.3

🦪 Taco Or Tostada With Chicken ☞ serving size: 1 small taco or tostada = 80 g; Calories = 204; Total Carb (g) = 16.4; Net Carb (g) = 14.3; Fat (g) = 11; Protein = 10.2

🍃 Taco Or Tostada With Chicken And Beans ☞ serving size: 1 small taco or tostada = 103 g; Calories = 229.7; Total Carb (g) = 22.9; Net Carb (g) = 18.9; Fat (g) = 11.6; Protein = 9.2

🍃 Taco Or Tostada With Chicken And Sour Cream ☞ serving size: 1 small taco or tostada = 96 g; Calories = 235.2; Total Carb (g) = 17.2; Net Carb (g) = 15; Fat (g) = 14.1; Protein = 10.6

🍃 Taco Or Tostada With Chicken Beans And Sour Cream ☞ serving size: 1 small taco or tostada = 118 g; Calories = 258.4; Total Carb (g) = 23.4; Net Carb (g) = 19.5; Fat (g) = 14.5; Protein = 9.5

🍃 Taco Or Tostada With Fish ☞ serving size: 1 miniature taco = 20 g; Calories = 45.8; Total Carb (g) = 4.1; Net Carb (g) = 3.6; Fat (g) = 2.4; Protein = 2

🍃 Taco Or Tostada With Meat ☞ serving size: 1 miniature taco = 22 g; Calories = 54.1; Total Carb (g) = 4.2; Net Carb (g) = 3.7; Fat (g) = 3.2; Protein = 2.3

🍃 Taco Or Tostada With Meat And Beans ☞ serving size: 1 small taco or tostada = 109 g; Calories = 242; Total Carb (g) = 23.6; Net Carb (g) = 19.5; Fat (g) = 12.7; Protein = 8.9

🍃 Taco Or Tostada With Meat And Beans From Fast Food ☞ serving size: 1 small taco or tostada = 109 g; Calories = 238.7; Total Carb (g) = 21.4; Net Carb (g) = 17.1; Fat (g) = 13.2; Protein = 9.4

🍃 Taco Or Tostada With Meat And Sour Cream ☞ serving size: 1 small taco or tostada = 109 g; Calories = 264.9; Total Carb (g) = 19; Net Carb (g) = 16.5; Fat (g) = 16.6; Protein = 10.3

🍃 Taco Or Tostada With Meat Beans And Sour Cream ☞ serving size: 1 small taco or tostada = 124 g; Calories = 272.8; Total Carb (g) = 24.3; Net Carb (g) = 20.2; Fat (g) = 15.8; Protein = 9.3

🍃 Taco With Crab Meat Puerto Rican Style ☞ serving size: 1 taco

(4-1/2" dia) = 121 g; Calories = 263.8; Total Carb (g) = 20.1; Net Carb (g) = 18.7; Fat (g) = 13.7; Protein = 14.6

🌿 Tamal In A Leaf Puerto Rican Style ☞ serving size: 1 tamal (6" x 2" x 1/2") = 41 g; Calories = 62.7; Total Carb (g) = 4.8; Net Carb (g) = 4.2; Fat (g) = 3.4; Protein = 3.9

🌿 Tamale Casserole Puerto Rican Style ☞ serving size: 1 cup = 237 g; Calories = 372.1; Total Carb (g) = 26.2; Net Carb (g) = 22.6; Fat (g) = 22.9; Protein = 16.5

🌿 Tamale Casserole With Meat ☞ serving size: 1 cup = 244 g; Calories = 390.4; Total Carb (g) = 37.7; Net Carb (g) = 33.5; Fat (g) = 20.1; Protein = 15.4

🌿 Tamale Meatless With Sauce Puerto Rican Or Caribbean Style ☞ serving size: 1 tamale = 72 g; Calories = 324.7; Total Carb (g) = 6.7; Net Carb (g) = 5.5; Fat (g) = 33.2; Protein = 1.1

🌿 Tamale Plain Meatless No Sauce Puerto Rican Style Or Carribean Style ☞ serving size: 1 tamale = 36 g; Calories = 77.8; Total Carb (g) = 4.2; Net Carb (g) = 3.6; Fat (g) = 6.8; Protein = 0.7

🌿 Tamale With Chicken ☞ serving size: 1 small tamale = 84 g; Calories = 185.6; Total Carb (g) = 12.6; Net Carb (g) = 11.5; Fat (g) = 12.1; Protein = 7.2

🌿 Taquito Or Flauta With Cheese ☞ serving size: 1 small taquito = 36 g; Calories = 96.8; Total Carb (g) = 12; Net Carb (g) = 10.3; Fat (g) = 4; Protein = 3.7

🌿 Taquitos Frozen Beef And Cheese Oven-Heated ☞ serving size: 1 piece = 42 g; Calories = 120.5; Total Carb (g) = 14.1; Net Carb (g) = 12.9; Fat (g) = 5.4; Protein = 4

🌿 Taquitos Frozen Chicken And Cheese Oven-Heated ☞ serving size: 1 piece = 42 g; Calories = 119.3; Total Carb (g) = 14.1; Net Carb (g) = 12.9; Fat (g) = 5.3; Protein = 3.9

🌿 Tofu And Vegetables Excluding Carrots Broccoli And Dark-

Green Leafy; No Potatoes With Soy-Based Sauce ☞ serving size: 1 cup = 217 g; Calories = 195.3; Total Carb (g) = 9.6; Net Carb (g) = 7.7; Fat (g) = 14.8; Protein = 8.9

🍲 Tofu And Vegetables Including Carrots Broccoli And/or Dark-Green Leafy; No Potatoes With Soy-Based Sauce ☞ serving size: 1 cup = 217 g; Calories = 193.1; Total Carb (g) = 10.4; Net Carb (g) = 7.6; Fat (g) = 14.3; Protein = 8.8

🍲 Tortellini Cheese-Filled Meatless With Tomato Sauce ☞ serving size: 1 cup = 250 g; Calories = 372.5; Total Carb (g) = 56.8; Net Carb (g) = 52.8; Fat (g) = 9.3; Protein = 15.5

🍲 Tortellini Cheese-Filled Meatless With Tomato Sauce Canned ☞ serving size: 1 cup = 247 g; Calories = 224.8; Total Carb (g) = 39.1; Net Carb (g) = 37.1; Fat (g) = 3.7; Protein = 8.7

🍲 Tortellini Cheese-Filled Meatless With Vegetables And Vinai-grette Dressing ☞ serving size: 1 cup = 169 g; Calories = 375.2; Total Carb (g) = 25.5; Net Carb (g) = 22.7; Fat (g) = 25.4; Protein = 11.2

🍲 Tortellini Cheese-Filled Meatless With Vinaigrette Dressing ☞ serving size: 1 cup = 169 g; Calories = 332.9; Total Carb (g) = 29.7; Net Carb (g) = 28.7; Fat (g) = 18.2; Protein = 11.9

🍲 Tortellini Cheese-Filled No Sauce ☞ serving size: 1 cup = 150 g; Calories = 354; Total Carb (g) = 54.2; Net Carb (g) = 52; Fat (g) = 8.3; Protein = 15.6

🍲 Tortellini Cheese-Filled With Cream Sauce ☞ serving size: 1 cup = 250 g; Calories = 390; Total Carb (g) = 39; Net Carb (g) = 37.8; Fat (g) = 18.5; Protein = 16

🍲 Tortellini Meat-Filled No Sauce ☞ serving size: 1 cup = 190 g; Calories = 362.9; Total Carb (g) = 33.9; Net Carb (g) = 32.8; Fat (g) = 14.3; Protein = 22.7

🍲 Tortellini Meat-Filled With Tomato Sauce ☞ serving size: 1 cup

= 210 g; Calories = 281.4; Total Carb (g) = 33.3; Net Carb (g) = 31.2; Fat (g) = 10.4; Protein = 13.4

🍲 Tortellini Meat-Filled With Tomato Sauce Canned ☞ serving size: 1 cup = 233 g; Calories = 212; Total Carb (g) = 35.7; Net Carb (g) = 33.4; Fat (g) = 4.4; Protein = 8.2

🍲 Tortellini Pasta With Cheese Filling Fresh-Refrigerated As Purchased ☞ serving size: 3/4 cup = 81 g; Calories = 248.7; Total Carb (g) = 38.1; Net Carb (g) = 36.5; Fat (g) = 5.9; Protein = 10.9

🍲 Tortellini Spinach-Filled No Sauce ☞ serving size: 1 cup = 122 g; Calories = 228.1; Total Carb (g) = 25.9; Net Carb (g) = 24.8; Fat (g) = 8.7; Protein = 10.6

🍲 Tortellini Spinach-Filled With Tomato Sauce ☞ serving size: 1 cup = 200 g; Calories = 240; Total Carb (g) = 32.4; Net Carb (g) = 30; Fat (g) = 8.6; Protein = 8.8

🍲 Turkey Pot Pie Frozen Entree ☞ serving size: 1 package yields = 397 g; Calories = 698.7; Total Carb (g) = 70.3; Net Carb (g) = 65.9; Fat (g) = 34.9; Protein = 25.8

🍲 Turkey Stuffing Mashed Potatoes W/gravy Assorted Vegetables Frozen Microwaved ☞ serving size: 1 serving = 385 g; Calories = 492.8; Total Carb (g) = 62.8; Net Carb (g) = 57.8; Fat (g) = 15; Protein = 26.8

🍲 Turnover Cheese-Filled Tomato-Based Sauce ☞ serving size: 1 hot pockets four cheese pizza = 128 g; Calories = 345.6; Total Carb (g) = 40.2; Net Carb (g) = 37.9; Fat (g) = 13.9; Protein = 15.1

🍲 Turnover Cheese-Filled Tomato-Based Sauce Frozen Unprepared ☞ serving size: 1 serving 4.5 oz = 127 g; Calories = 298.5; Total Carb (g) = 34.7; Net Carb (g) = 32.6; Fat (g) = 12; Protein = 13

🍲 Turnover Chicken With Gravy ☞ serving size: 1 turnover = 112 g; Calories = 312.5; Total Carb (g) = 22.6; Net Carb (g) = 21.8; Fat (g) = 20.1; Protein = 10.6

🦪 Turnover Chicken- Or Turkey- And Vegetable-Filled Reduced Fat Frozen ☞ serving size: 1 piece turnover 1 serving = 127 g; Calories = 213.4; Total Carb (g) = 27.6; Net Carb (g) = 23.7; Fat (g) = 7; Protein = 10

🦪 Turnover Filled With Egg Meat And Cheese Frozen ☞ serving size: 1 piece turnover 1 serving = 127 g; Calories = 289.6; Total Carb (g) = 26.3; Net Carb (g) = 25.2; Fat (g) = 16; Protein = 10

🦪 Turnover Filled With Ground Beef And Cabbage ☞ serving size: 1 bierock = 215 g; Calories = 509.6; Total Carb (g) = 63.9; Net Carb (g) = 60.2; Fat (g) = 17.7; Protein = 22.1

🦪 Turnover Filled With Meat And Vegetable No Potatoes No Gravy ☞ serving size: 1 turnover = 88 g; Calories = 268.4; Total Carb (g) = 20.2; Net Carb (g) = 19; Fat (g) = 16.6; Protein = 9.4

🦪 Turnover Meat- And Bean-Filled No Gravy ☞ serving size: 1 turnover = 88 g; Calories = 305.4; Total Carb (g) = 22.8; Net Carb (g) = 21.4; Fat (g) = 18.7; Protein = 11

🦪 Turnover Meat- And Cheese-Filled No Gravy ☞ serving size: 1 turnover = 96 g; Calories = 231.4; Total Carb (g) = 29.3; Net Carb (g) = 27.9; Fat (g) = 8.8; Protein = 8.8

🦪 Turnover Meat- And Cheese-Filled Tomato-Based Sauce ☞ serving size: 1 turnover = 73 g; Calories = 184.7; Total Carb (g) = 22.2; Net Carb (g) = 20.6; Fat (g) = 7.6; Protein = 6.8

🦪 Turnover Meat- And Cheese-Filled Tomato-Based Sauce Reduced Fat Frozen ☞ serving size: 1 piece turnover 1 serving = 127 g; Calories = 273.1; Total Carb (g) = 40.5; Net Carb (g) = 39.5; Fat (g) = 7; Protein = 12

🦪 Turnover Meat- Potato- And Vegetable-Filled No Gravy ☞ serving size: 1 turnover = 88 g; Calories = 257; Total Carb (g) = 20.1; Net Carb (g) = 19.1; Fat (g) = 15.6; Protein = 8.8

🦪 Turnover Meat-Filled No Gravy ☞ serving size: 1 turnover = 88 g; Calories = 326.5; Total Carb (g) = 23; Net Carb (g) = 22.1; Fat (g) = 20.8; Protein = 11.3

🔥 Turnover Meat-Filled With Gravy ☞ serving size: 1 turnover = 152 g; Calories = 378.5; Total Carb (g) = 27.3; Net Carb (g) = 26.3; Fat (g) = 23.5; Protein = 14.3

🔥 Vada Fried Dumpling ☞ serving size: 1 vada = 29 g; Calories = 76.9; Total Carb (g) = 9.7; Net Carb (g) = 8; Fat (g) = 2.8; Protein = 3.7

🔥 Veal Lasagna Diet Frozen Meal ☞ serving size: 1 meal (10.25 oz) = 291 g; Calories = 259; Total Carb (g) = 30.9; Net Carb (g) = 27.2; Fat (g) = 6.6; Protein = 19.3

🔥 Vegetable Combination Excluding Carrots Broccoli And Dark-Green Leafy; Cooked With Soy-Based Sauce ☞ serving size: 1 cup = 185 g; Calories = 198; Total Carb (g) = 12.2; Net Carb (g) = 9.6; Fat (g) = 16.3; Protein = 3.3

🔥 Vegetable Combination Including Carrots Broccoli And/or Dark-Green Leafy; Cooked With Soy-Based Sauce ☞ serving size: 1 cup = 185 g; Calories = 194.3; Total Carb (g) = 13; Net Carb (g) = 9.5; Fat (g) = 15.4; Protein = 3.3

🔥 Vegetables And Cheese In Pastry ☞ serving size: 1 pastry = 103 g; Calories = 324.5; Total Carb (g) = 20.3; Net Carb (g) = 17.5; Fat (g) = 24.3; Protein = 8.1

🔥 Vegetables In Pastry ☞ serving size: 1 pastry = 103 g; Calories = 316.2; Total Carb (g) = 21.8; Net Carb (g) = 18.6; Fat (g) = 23.5; Protein = 6.7

🔥 Wonton Fried Filled With Meat Poultry Or Seafood ☞ serving size: 1 wonton, any size = 19 g; Calories = 36.3; Total Carb (g) = 2.7; Net Carb (g) = 2.4; Fat (g) = 2.1; Protein = 1.7

🔥 Wonton Fried Filled With Meat Poultry Or Seafood And Vegetable ☞ serving size: 1 wonton, any size = 19 g; Calories = 36.3; Total Carb (g) = 2.7; Net Carb (g) = 2.4; Fat (g) = 2.1; Protein = 1.7

Wonton Fried Meatless ☞ serving size: 1 wonton, any size = 19 g; Calories = 36.3; Total Carb (g) = 2.7; Net Carb (g) = 2.4; Fat (g) = 2.1; Protein = 1.7

Yat Ga Mein With Meat Fish Or Poultry ☞ serving size: 1 cup = 205 g; Calories = 276.8; Total Carb (g) = 25.2; Net Carb (g) = 22.7; Fat (g) = 10; Protein = 20.6

Yellow Rice With Seasoning Dry Packet Mix Unprepared ☞ serving size: 1 serving (2 oz) = 57 g; Calories = 195.5; Total Carb (g) = 42.6; Net Carb (g) = 41.5; Fat (g) = 1; Protein = 4

Zucchini Lasagna Diet Frozen Meal ☞ serving size: 1 lean cuisine meal (11 oz) = 312 g; Calories = 308.9; Total Carb (g) = 39.8; Net Carb (g) = 35.8; Fat (g) = 10; Protein = 16.7

24

RESTAURANT FOODS

📖 Applebees 9 Oz House Sirloin Steak ☞ serving size: 1 serving = 157 g; Calories = 296.7; Total Carb (g) = 0; Net Carb (g) = 0; Fat (g) = 14.3; Protein = 42.2

📖 Applebees Chicken Tenders From Kids Menu ☞ serving size: 1 piece = 35 g; Calories = 103.6; Total Carb (g) = 6.4; Net Carb (g) = 6; Fat (g) = 5.7; Protein = 6.7

📖 Applebees Chicken Tenders Platter ☞ serving size: 1 serving = 209 g; Calories = 620.7; Total Carb (g) = 37.6; Net Carb (g) = 35.5; Fat (g) = 33.9; Protein = 41

📖 Applebees Chili ☞ serving size: 1 cup = 136 g; Calories = 213.5; Total Carb (g) = 6.2; Net Carb (g) = 4.3; Fat (g) = 13.3; Protein = 17.1

📖 Applebees Coleslaw ☞ serving size: 1 serving = 76 g; Calories = 91.2; Total Carb (g) = 10; Net Carb (g) = 7.9; Fat (g) = 5.4; Protein = 0.6

📖 Applebees Double Crunch Shrimp ☞ serving size: 1 serving = 206 g; Calories = 665.4; Total Carb (g) = 53.5; Net Carb (g) = 48.1; Fat (g) = 38.9; Protein = 25.4

📖 Applebees Fish Hand Battered ☞ serving size: 1 serving = 250 g;

Calories = 505; Total Carb (g) = 41.6; Net Carb (g) = 39.4; Fat (g) = 22.9; Protein = 33.1

📖 Applebees French Fries ☞ serving size: 1 serving = 164 g; Calories = 475.6; Total Carb (g) = 64.8; Net Carb (g) = 58.4; Fat (g) = 21.6; Protein = 5.4

📖 Applebees Kraft Macaroni & Cheese From Kids Menu ☞ serving size: 1 cup = 124 g; Calories = 177.3; Total Carb (g) = 26.1; Net Carb (g) = 24.5; Fat (g) = 5.4; Protein = 6.2

📖 Applebees Mozzarella Sticks ☞ serving size: 1 piece = 32 g; Calories = 101.1; Total Carb (g) = 7.3; Net Carb (g) = 6.7; Fat (g) = 5.9; Protein = 4.8

📖 Carrabbas Italian Grill Cheese Ravioli With Marinara Sauce ☞ serving size: 1 serving varied from 8 to 10 ravioli per serving = 365 g; Calories = 569.4; Total Carb (g) = 64.3; Net Carb (g) = 59.2; Fat (g) = 21.9; Protein = 29.1

📖 Carrabbas Italian Grill Chicken Parmesan Without Cavatappi Pasta ☞ serving size: 1 serving = 339 g; Calories = 698.3; Total Carb (g) = 26.4; Net Carb (g) = 23.4; Fat (g) = 37.1; Protein = 64.4

📖 Carrabbas Italian Grill Lasagne ☞ serving size: 1 serving = 437 g; Calories = 834.7; Total Carb (g) = 54; Net Carb (g) = 48.3; Fat (g) = 48.3; Protein = 45.8

📖 Carrabbas Italian Grill Spaghetti With Meat Sauce ☞ serving size: 1 serving = 537 g; Calories = 655.1; Total Carb (g) = 84.4; Net Carb (g) = 76.3; Fat (g) = 21.1; Protein = 31.5

📖 Carrabbas Italian Grill Spaghetti With Pomodoro Sauce ☞ serving size: 1 serving = 489 g; Calories = 508.6; Total Carb (g) = 91.1; Net Carb (g) = 82.8; Fat (g) = 8.6; Protein = 16.7

📖 Cracker Barrel Chicken Tenderloin Platter Fried ☞ serving size: 1 serving = 175 g; Calories = 512.8; Total Carb (g) = 35.5; Net Carb (g) = 34.3; Fat (g) = 27.1; Protein = 31.6

📖 Cracker Barrel Chicken Tenderloin Platter Fried From Kids Menu ☞ serving size: 1 serving = 103 g; Calories = 302.8; Total Carb (g) = 20.9; Net Carb (g) = 19.8; Fat (g) = 15.9; Protein = 19.2

📖 Cracker Barrel Coleslaw ☞ serving size: 1 serving = 167 g; Calories = 292.3; Total Carb (g) = 21.7; Net Carb (g) = 19.1; Fat (g) = 22.1; Protein = 1.5

📖 Cracker Barrel Country Fried Shrimp Platter ☞ serving size: 1 serving = 149 g; Calories = 427.6; Total Carb (g) = 31.9; Net Carb (g) = 31.4; Fat (g) = 25; Protein = 18.8

📖 Cracker Barrel Farm Raised Catfish Platter ☞ serving size: 1 serving = 178 g; Calories = 473.5; Total Carb (g) = 9.5; Net Carb (g) = 6.6; Fat (g) = 30.4; Protein = 40.8

📖 Cracker Barrel Grilled Sirloin Steak ☞ serving size: 1 steak = 151 g; Calories = 306.5; Total Carb (g) = 0; Net Carb (g) = 0; Fat (g) = 12.9; Protein = 47.6

📖 Cracker Barrel Macaroni N Cheese ☞ serving size: 1 serving = 175 g; Calories = 339.5; Total Carb (g) = 27.3; Net Carb (g) = 25.4; Fat (g) = 20.6; Protein = 11.4

📖 Cracker Barrel Macaroni N Cheese Plate From Kids Menu ☞ serving size: 1 serving = 257 g; Calories = 493.4; Total Carb (g) = 40; Net Carb (g) = 38.2; Fat (g) = 29.6; Protein = 16.6

📖 Cracker Barrel Onion Rings Thick-Cut ☞ serving size: 1 serving = 261 g; Calories = 853.5; Total Carb (g) = 106.9; Net Carb (g) = 101.1; Fat (g) = 41.8; Protein = 12.5

📖 Cracker Barrel Steak Fries ☞ serving size: 1 serving = 198 g; Calories = 504.9; Total Carb (g) = 61.1; Net Carb (g) = 54.2; Fat (g) = 26.1; Protein = 6.5

📖 Dennys Chicken Nuggets Star Shaped From Kids Menu ☞ serving size: 1 serving 4 pieces in serving = 67 g; Calories = 252.6; Total Carb (g) = 9.1; Net Carb (g) = 8.6; Fat (g) = 19.1; Protein = 10.9

Dennys Chicken Strips ☞ serving size: 1 serving = 194 g; Calories = 572.3; Total Carb (g) = 42.7; Net Carb (g) = 40.6; Fat (g) = 28.1; Protein = 37.2

Dennys Coleslaw ☞ serving size: 1 serving = 91 g; Calories = 166.5; Total Carb (g) = 9.9; Net Carb (g) = 8.7; Fat (g) = 13.7; Protein = 0.9

Dennys Fish Fillet Battered Or Breaded Fried ☞ serving size: 1 serving = 201 g; Calories = 470.3; Total Carb (g) = 35; Net Carb (g) = 33; Fat (g) = 24.4; Protein = 27.6

Dennys French Fries ☞ serving size: 1 serving = 165 g; Calories = 465.3; Total Carb (g) = 58.1; Net Carb (g) = 52.3; Fat (g) = 23.3; Protein = 5.6

Dennys Golden Fried Shrimp ☞ serving size: 1 piece = 16 g; Calories = 51; Total Carb (g) = 3.4; Net Carb (g) = 3.1; Fat (g) = 3.2; Protein = 2.2

Dennys Hash Browns ☞ serving size: 1 serving = 124 g; Calories = 244.3; Total Carb (g) = 33; Net Carb (g) = 29.6; Fat (g) = 11.2; Protein = 3.1

Dennys Macaroni & Cheese From Kids Menu ☞ serving size: 1 serving = 180 g; Calories = 270; Total Carb (g) = 38.1; Net Carb (g) = 35.9; Fat (g) = 8.9; Protein = 9.3

Dennys Mozzarella Cheese Sticks ☞ serving size: 1 serving = 228 g; Calories = 738.7; Total Carb (g) = 62.1; Net Carb (g) = 58.4; Fat (g) = 40.7; Protein = 30.9

Dennys Onion Rings ☞ serving size: 1 serving = 166 g; Calories = 639.1; Total Carb (g) = 68.1; Net Carb (g) = 64.2; Fat (g) = 36.9; Protein = 8.8

Dennys Spaghetti And Meatballs ☞ serving size: 1 serving = 565 g; Calories = 960.5; Total Carb (g) = 87.6; Net Carb (g) = 79.2; Fat (g) = 48.1; Protein = 44.3

Dennys Top Sirloin Steak ☞ serving size: 1 steak = 107 g; Calories = 194.7; Total Carb (g) = 0.2; Net Carb (g) = 0.2; Fat (g) = 7.9; Protein = 30.9

French Fries ☞ serving size: 10 strip = 69 g; Calories = 111.1; Total Carb (g) = 19; Net Carb (g) = 17.4; Fat (g) = 3.5; Protein = 1.7

Fried Onion Rings ☞ serving size: 1 serving = 350 g; Calories = 1246; Total Carb (g) = 140.6; Net Carb (g) = 129.8; Fat (g) = 68.6; Protein = 16

Hash Browns ☞ serving size: 1 cup = 156 g; Calories = 413.4; Total Carb (g) = 54.8; Net Carb (g) = 49.8; Fat (g) = 19.5; Protein = 4.7

Olive Garden Cheese Ravioli With Marinara Sauce ☞ serving size: 1 serving varied from 7-9 ravioli per serving = 454 g; Calories = 721.9; Total Carb (g) = 89.2; Net Carb (g) = 84.2; Fat (g) = 25.5; Protein = 33.8

Olive Garden Chicken Parmigiana Without Pasta ☞ serving size: 1 serving = 304 g; Calories = 641.4; Total Carb (g) = 37.3; Net Carb (g) = 34.6; Fat (g) = 34.1; Protein = 46.6

Olive Garden Lasagna Classico ☞ serving size: 1 serving = 422 g; Calories = 776.5; Total Carb (g) = 43.6; Net Carb (g) = 36.8; Fat (g) = 45.7; Protein = 47.6

Olive Garden Spaghetti With Meat Sauce ☞ serving size: 1 serving = 525 g; Calories = 635.3; Total Carb (g) = 90.3; Net Carb (g) = 81.3; Fat (g) = 17.2; Protein = 30.5

Olive Garden Spaghetti With Pomodoro Sauce ☞ serving size: 1 serving = 478 g; Calories = 487.6; Total Carb (g) = 81.9; Net Carb (g) = 73.8; Fat (g) = 8.8; Protein = 20.4

On The Border Cheese Enchilada ☞ serving size: 1 serving serving size varied from 1 to 3 enchiladas = 250 g; Calories = 677.5; Total Carb (g) = 40.5; Net Carb (g) = 36; Fat (g) = 44.4; Protein = 29.2

On The Border Cheese Quesadilla ☞ serving size: 1 serving 1

quesadilla = 203 g; Calories = 799.8; Total Carb (g) = 49.2; Net Carb (g) = 44.8; Fat (g) = 51.8; Protein = 34.3

On The Border Mexican Rice ☞ serving size: 1 cup = 114 g; Calories = 222.3; Total Carb (g) = 38.9; Net Carb (g) = 37.7; Fat (g) = 5.5; Protein = 4.1

On The Border Refried Beans ☞ serving size: 1 cup = 135 g; Calories = 194.4; Total Carb (g) = 23.7; Net Carb (g) = 12.6; Fat (g) = 6.8; Protein = 9.9

On The Border Soft Taco With Ground Beef Cheese And Lettuce ☞ serving size: 1 serving varied from 2-3 tacos per serving = 324 g; Calories = 742; Total Carb (g) = 62.5; Net Carb (g) = 56.6; Fat (g) = 35.8; Protein = 42.7

Onion Rings ☞ serving size: 1 cup = 48 g; Calories = 132.5; Total Carb (g) = 16.2; Net Carb (g) = 15.2; Fat (g) = 6.9; Protein = 2

Restaurant Chinese Beef And Vegetables ☞ serving size: 1 order = 574 g; Calories = 602.7; Total Carb (g) = 41.8; Net Carb (g) = 33.2; Fat (g) = 30.4; Protein = 40.6

Restaurant Chinese Chicken And Vegetables ☞ serving size: 1 order = 693 g; Calories = 658.4; Total Carb (g) = 37.3; Net Carb (g) = 31.1; Fat (g) = 31.6; Protein = 56.7

Restaurant Chinese Chicken Chow Mein ☞ serving size: 1 order = 604 g; Calories = 513.4; Total Carb (g) = 50.1; Net Carb (g) = 44; Fat (g) = 16.9; Protein = 40.8

Restaurant Chinese Egg Rolls Assorted ☞ serving size: 1 piece = 89 g; Calories = 222.5; Total Carb (g) = 24.3; Net Carb (g) = 22; Fat (g) = 10.6; Protein = 7.4

Restaurant Chinese Fried Rice Without Meat ☞ serving size: 1 cup = 137 g; Calories = 238.4; Total Carb (g) = 44.9; Net Carb (g) = 43.4; Fat (g) = 4.1; Protein = 5.6

Restaurant Chinese General Tsos Chicken ☞ serving size: 1

order = 535 g; Calories = 1578.3; Total Carb (g) = 128.4; Net Carb (g) = 123.5; Fat (g) = 87.5; Protein = 69

Restaurant Chinese Kung Pao Chicken ☞ serving size: 1 order = 604 g; Calories = 779.2; Total Carb (g) = 41.5; Net Carb (g) = 32.4; Fat (g) = 42.2; Protein = 59

Restaurant Chinese Lemon Chicken ☞ serving size: 1 order = 623 g; Calories = 1570; Total Carb (g) = 128.4; Net Carb (g) = 122.2; Fat (g) = 84.4; Protein = 74

Restaurant Chinese Orange Chicken ☞ serving size: 1 order = 648 g; Calories = 1697.8; Total Carb (g) = 145.5; Net Carb (g) = 140.4; Fat (g) = 82.2; Protein = 93.7

Restaurant Chinese Sesame Chicken ☞ serving size: 1 order = 547 g; Calories = 1602.7; Total Carb (g) = 147; Net Carb (g) = 143.2; Fat (g) = 78; Protein = 78.4

Restaurant Chinese Shrimp And Vegetables ☞ serving size: 1 order = 601 g; Calories = 468.8; Total Carb (g) = 27.2; Net Carb (g) = 18.8; Fat (g) = 24.3; Protein = 35.5

Restaurant Chinese Sweet And Sour Chicken ☞ serving size: 1 order = 706 g; Calories = 1765; Total Carb (g) = 168.5; Net Carb (g) = 161.4; Fat (g) = 89.3; Protein = 71.3

Restaurant Chinese Sweet And Sour Pork ☞ serving size: 1 order = 609 g; Calories = 1644.3; Total Carb (g) = 142.1; Net Carb (g) = 136.1; Fat (g) = 95.4; Protein = 54.3

Restaurant Chinese Vegetable Chow Mein Without Meat Or Noodles ☞ serving size: 1 order = 777 g; Calories = 334.1; Total Carb (g) = 44.6; Net Carb (g) = 35.3; Fat (g) = 13.1; Protein = 10.4

Restaurant Chinese Vegetable Lo Mein Without Meat ☞ serving size: 1 order = 741 g; Calories = 896.6; Total Carb (g) = 149.4; Net Carb (g) = 139.8; Fat (g) = 17.4; Protein = 35.4

Restaurant Family Style Chicken Fingers From Kids Menu ☞

serving size: 1 serving = 114 g; Calories = 350; Total Carb (g) = 21.4; Net Carb (g) = 20.1; Fat (g) = 19.9; Protein = 21.3

Restaurant Family Style Chicken Tenders ☞ serving size: 1 serving = 201 g; Calories = 607; Total Carb (g) = 38.8; Net Carb (g) = 37; Fat (g) = 33.4; Protein = 38

Restaurant Family Style Chili With Meat And Beans ☞ serving size: 1 cup = 136 g; Calories = 213.5; Total Carb (g) = 6.2; Net Carb (g) = 4.3; Fat (g) = 13.3; Protein = 17.1

Restaurant Family Style Coleslaw ☞ serving size: 1 serving = 108 g; Calories = 171.7; Total Carb (g) = 13.3; Net Carb (g) = 11.3; Fat (g) = 12.7; Protein = 1

Restaurant Family Style Fish Fillet Battered Or Breaded Fried ☞ serving size: 1 serving = 226 g; Calories = 494.9; Total Carb (g) = 38.2; Net Carb (g) = 36.1; Fat (g) = 24.4; Protein = 30.5

Restaurant Family Style French Fries ☞ serving size: 1 serving = 170 g; Calories = 491.3; Total Carb (g) = 63.2; Net Carb (g) = 56.6; Fat (g) = 23.9; Protein = 5.9

Restaurant Family Style Fried Mozzarella Sticks ☞ serving size: 1 serving = 245 g; Calories = 796.3; Total Carb (g) = 61.6; Net Carb (g) = 56.7; Fat (g) = 44.9; Protein = 36.1

Restaurant Family Style Hash Browns ☞ serving size: 1 cup = 94 g; Calories = 185.2; Total Carb (g) = 25; Net Carb (g) = 22.5; Fat (g) = 8.5; Protein = 2.3

Restaurant Family Style Macaroni & Cheese From Kids Menu ☞ serving size: 1 cup = 136 g; Calories = 205.4; Total Carb (g) = 25.6; Net Carb (g) = 24.1; Fat (g) = 8.2; Protein = 7.4

Restaurant Family Style Onion Rings ☞ serving size: 1 serving = 259 g; Calories = 922; Total Carb (g) = 105.5; Net Carb (g) = 98.7; Fat (g) = 49.9; Protein = 12.7

Restaurant Family Style Shrimp Breaded And Fried ☞ serving

size: 1 serving = 169 g; Calories = 520.5; Total Carb (g) = 37.7; Net Carb (g) = 35.1; Fat (g) = 31.6; Protein = 21.4

🏮 Restaurant Family Style Sirloin Steak ☞ serving size: 1 serving = 166 g; Calories = 323.7; Total Carb (g) = 0; Net Carb (g) = 0; Fat (g) = 14.1; Protein = 49.5

🏮 Restaurant Family Style Spaghetti And Meatballs ☞ serving size: 1 cup = 134 g; Calories = 227.8; Total Carb (g) = 20.8; Net Carb (g) = 18.8; Fat (g) = 11.4; Protein = 10.5

🏮 Restaurant Italian Cheese Ravioli With Marinara Sauce ☞ serving size: 1 serving serving size varied by diameter and count of raviloi = 427 g; Calories = 657.6; Total Carb (g) = 79; Net Carb (g) = 73.9; Fat (g) = 24.3; Protein = 30.2

🏮 Restaurant Italian Chicken Parmesan Without Pasta ☞ serving size: 1 serving = 301 g; Calories = 614; Total Carb (g) = 32.9; Net Carb (g) = 30.2; Fat (g) = 32; Protein = 48.7

🏮 Restaurant Italian Lasagna With Meat ☞ serving size: 1 serving = 457 g; Calories = 845.5; Total Carb (g) = 51.9; Net Carb (g) = 45.1; Fat (g) = 48.9; Protein = 49.5

🏮 Restaurant Italian Spaghetti With Meat Sauce ☞ serving size: 1 serving = 554 g; Calories = 670.3; Total Carb (g) = 90.9; Net Carb (g) = 82; Fat (g) = 19.9; Protein = 32.1

🏮 Restaurant Italian Spaghetti With Pomodoro Sauce (No Meat) ☞ serving size: 1 serving = 510 g; Calories = 530.4; Total Carb (g) = 90.6; Net Carb (g) = 82; Fat (g) = 9.6; Protein = 19.9

🏮 Restaurant Latino Arepa (Unleavened Cornmeal Bread) ☞ serving size: 1 piece = 98 g; Calories = 214.6; Total Carb (g) = 36.4; Net Carb (g) = 33.9; Fat (g) = 5.3; Protein = 5.4

🏮 Restaurant Latino Arroz Con Frijoles Negros (Rice And Black Beans) ☞ serving size: 1 serving = 461 g; Calories = 696.1; Total Carb (g) = 112.5; Net Carb (g) = 96.8; Fat (g) = 17.8; Protein = 21.4

Restaurant Latino Arroz Con Grandules (Rice And Pigeonpeas) ☞ serving size: 1 serving = 653 g; Calories = 1188.5; Total Carb (g) = 200.8; Net Carb (g) = 191.7; Fat (g) = 32.5; Protein = 22.9

Restaurant Latino Arroz Con Habichuelas Colorados (Rice And Red Beans) ☞ serving size: 1 serving = 590 g; Calories = 837.8; Total Carb (g) = 140.1; Net Carb (g) = 124.7; Fat (g) = 20.4; Protein = 23.4

Restaurant Latino Arroz Con Leche (Rice Pudding) ☞ serving size: 1 serving = 283 g; Calories = 413.2; Total Carb (g) = 70.5; Net Carb (g) = 69.1; Fat (g) = 10.4; Protein = 9.1

Restaurant Latino Black Bean Soup ☞ serving size: 1 cup = 246 g; Calories = 253.4; Total Carb (g) = 36.4; Net Carb (g) = 24.3; Fat (g) = 6.3; Protein = 12.6

Restaurant Latino Bunuelos (Fried Yeast Bread) ☞ serving size: 1 piece = 70 g; Calories = 323.4; Total Carb (g) = 34; Net Carb (g) = 33; Fat (g) = 18.4; Protein = 5.6

Restaurant Latino Chicken And Rice Entree Prepared ☞ serving size: 1 cup = 141 g; Calories = 245.3; Total Carb (g) = 28.2; Net Carb (g) = 26.6; Fat (g) = 7.1; Protein = 17

Restaurant Latino Empanadas Beef Prepared ☞ serving size: 1 piece = 89 g; Calories = 298.2; Total Carb (g) = 27.8; Net Carb (g) = 26; Fat (g) = 16.4; Protein = 10.1

Restaurant Latino Pupusas Con Frijoles (Pupusas Bean) ☞ serving size: 1 piece = 126 g; Calories = 288.5; Total Carb (g) = 39.7; Net Carb (g) = 32.4; Fat (g) = 11.4; Protein = 7

Restaurant Latino Pupusas Con Queso (Pupusas Cheese) ☞ serving size: 1 piece = 117 g; Calories = 299.5; Total Carb (g) = 26.2; Net Carb (g) = 22.8; Fat (g) = 15.5; Protein = 13.7

Restaurant Latino Pupusas Del Cerdo (Pupusas Pork) ☞ serving size: 1 piece = 122 g; Calories = 283; Total Carb (g) = 28.1; Net Carb (g) = 24.9; Fat (g) = 12.7; Protein = 14

Restaurant Latino Tamale Corn ☞ serving size: 1 piece = 166 g; Calories = 308.8; Total Carb (g) = 44.3; Net Carb (g) = 39; Fat (g) = 12; Protein = 5.8

Restaurant Latino Tamale Pork ☞ serving size: 1 piece = 142 g; Calories = 247.1; Total Carb (g) = 22.4; Net Carb (g) = 19; Fat (g) = 12.8; Protein = 10.4

Restaurant Latino Tripe Soup ☞ serving size: 1 cup = 200 g; Calories = 148; Total Carb (g) = 8.1; Net Carb (g) = 8.1; Fat (g) = 5.2; Protein = 17.2

Restaurant Mexican Cheese Enchilada ☞ serving size: 1 serving serving size varied from 1 to 3 enchiladas = 244 g; Calories = 666.1; Total Carb (g) = 37.7; Net Carb (g) = 33.1; Fat (g) = 45.1; Protein = 27.4

Restaurant Mexican Cheese Quesadilla ☞ serving size: 1 serving serving size varied on diameter and count of quesadila = 205 g; Calories = 754.4; Total Carb (g) = 49.4; Net Carb (g) = 45.9; Fat (g) = 47.3; Protein = 32.7

Restaurant Mexican Cheese Tamales ☞ serving size: 1 serving serving size varied from 1 to 3 tamales = 302 g; Calories = 652.3; Total Carb (g) = 54.3; Net Carb (g) = 47.6; Fat (g) = 36.2; Protein = 27.2

Restaurant Mexican Refried Beans ☞ serving size: 1 cup = 148 g; Calories = 230.9; Total Carb (g) = 24.9; Net Carb (g) = 13; Fat (g) = 10; Protein = 10.2

Restaurant Mexican Soft Taco With Ground Beef Cheese And Lettuce ☞ serving size: 1 serving varied from 1 to 3 tacos per serving = 281 g; Calories = 615.4; Total Carb (g) = 50.4; Net Carb (g) = 46.1; Fat (g) = 30.4; Protein = 35.3

Restaurant Mexican Spanish Rice ☞ serving size: 1 cup = 116 g; Calories = 214.6; Total Carb (g) = 36.2; Net Carb (g) = 34.8; Fat (g) = 6.1; Protein = 3.8

TGI Fridays Chicken Fingers ☞ serving size: 1 serving = 225 g;

Calories = 731.3; Total Carb (g) = 37.9; Net Carb (g) = 36.1; Fat (g) = 45.7; Protein = 42

TGI Fridays Chicken Fingers From Kids Menu ☞ serving size: 1 piece = 41 g; Calories = 135.3; Total Carb (g) = 7.3; Net Carb (g) = 6.9; Fat (g) = 8.5; Protein = 7.4

TGI Fridays Classic Sirloin Steak (10 Oz) ☞ serving size: 1 serving = 176 g; Calories = 345; Total Carb (g) = 0.8; Net Carb (g) = 0.8; Fat (g) = 13.8; Protein = 54.6

TGI Fridays French Fries ☞ serving size: 1 serving = 184 g; Calories = 544.6; Total Carb (g) = 67.9; Net Carb (g) = 60.4; Fat (g) = 27.3; Protein = 6.9

TGI Fridays Fridays Shrimp Breaded ☞ serving size: 1 serving = 175 g; Calories = 528.5; Total Carb (g) = 36.5; Net Carb (g) = 36.5; Fat (g) = 33.3; Protein = 20.8

TGI Fridays Fried Mozzarella ☞ serving size: 1 piece = 35 g; Calories = 116.6; Total Carb (g) = 8.9; Net Carb (g) = 8.1; Fat (g) = 6.6; Protein = 5.5

TGI Fridays Macaroni & Cheese From Kids Menu ☞ serving size: 1 cup = 144 g; Calories = 174.2; Total Carb (g) = 25.1; Net Carb (g) = 23.6; Fat (g) = 5; Protein = 7.2

25

SNACKS

🍪 Bean Chips ☞ serving size: 1 chip = 3 g; Calories = 13.5; Total Carb (g) = 1.6; Net Carb (g) = 1.3; Fat (g) = 0.7; Protein = 0.4

🍪 Breadsticks Hard Reduced Sodium ☞ serving size: 1 snack size stick = 2 g; Calories = 8.6; Total Carb (g) = 1.4; Net Carb (g) = 1.4; Fat (g) = 0.2; Protein = 0.2

🍪 Breadsticks Hard Whole Wheat ☞ serving size: 1 snack size stick = 2 g; Calories = 8.2; Total Carb (g) = 1.4; Net Carb (g) = 1.2; Fat (g) = 0.2; Protein = 0.3

🍪 Breakfast Bar Cereal Crust With Fruit Filling Lowfat ☞ serving size: 1 bar = 37 g; Calories = 139.5; Total Carb (g) = 27; Net Carb (g) = 26.2; Fat (g) = 2.8; Protein = 1.6

🍪 Breakfast Bar Corn Flake Crust With Fruit ☞ serving size: 1 oz = 28.4 g; Calories = 106.8; Total Carb (g) = 20.7; Net Carb (g) = 20.1; Fat (g) = 2.1; Protein = 1.3

🍪 Breakfast Bar Nfs ☞ serving size: 1 bar = 43 g; Calories = 162.1; Total Carb (g) = 31.4; Net Carb (g) = 30.4; Fat (g) = 3.2; Protein = 1.9

Breakfast Bars Oats Sugar Raisins Coconut (Include Granola Bar) ☞ serving size: 1 bar = 43 g; Calories = 199.5; Total Carb (g) = 28.7; Net Carb (g) = 27.4; Fat (g) = 7.6; Protein = 4.2

Cereal Or Granola Bar With Rice Cereal ☞ serving size: 1 bar = 28 g; Calories = 115.9; Total Carb (g) = 22.5; Net Carb (g) = 22.5; Fat (g) = 2.5; Protein = 1

Cheese Flavored Corn Snacks ☞ serving size: 1 piece = 2 g; Calories = 11.2; Total Carb (g) = 1.1; Net Carb (g) = 1; Fat (g) = 0.7; Protein = 0.1

Cheese Flavored Corn Snacks (Cheetos) ☞ serving size: 1 piece = 2 g; Calories = 11.2; Total Carb (g) = 1.1; Net Carb (g) = 1; Fat (g) = 0.7; Protein = 0.1

Cheese Puffs And Twists Corn Based Baked Low Fat ☞ serving size: 1 oz = 28.4 g; Calories = 122.7; Total Carb (g) = 20.6; Net Carb (g) = 19.5; Fat (g) = 3.4; Protein = 2.4

Corn Chips Flavored ☞ serving size: 1 chip = 1 g; Calories = 5.4; Total Carb (g) = 0.6; Net Carb (g) = 0.5; Fat (g) = 0.3; Protein = 0.1

Corn Chips Flavored (Fritos) ☞ serving size: 1 chip = 1 g; Calories = 5.4; Total Carb (g) = 0.6; Net Carb (g) = 0.5; Fat (g) = 0.3; Protein = 0.1

Corn Chips Plain ☞ serving size: 1 chip = 1 g; Calories = 5.3; Total Carb (g) = 0.6; Net Carb (g) = 0.5; Fat (g) = 0.3; Protein = 0.1

Corn Chips Plain (Fritos) ☞ serving size: 1 chip = 1 g; Calories = 5.4; Total Carb (g) = 0.6; Net Carb (g) = 0.5; Fat (g) = 0.3; Protein = 0.1

Corn Chips Reduced Sodium ☞ serving size: 1 chip = 1 g; Calories = 5.5; Total Carb (g) = 0.6; Net Carb (g) = 0.5; Fat (g) = 0.3; Protein = 0.1

Crackers Breakfast Biscuit ☞ serving size: 1 biscuit, nfs = 15 g; Calories = 64.1; Total Carb (g) = 10.7; Net Carb (g) = 9.6; Fat (g) = 2.3; Protein = 1.1

Crackers Flatbread ☞ serving size: 1 flatbread = 10 g; Calories = 41.2; Total Carb (g) = 7.5; Net Carb (g) = 6.5; Fat (g) = 0.8; Protein = 1

Crackers Rice And Nuts ☞ serving size: 1 cracker = 3 g; Calories = 12.9; Total Carb (g) = 2.3; Net Carb (g) = 2.3; Fat (g) = 0.3; Protein = 0.3

Crackers Saltine Reduced Sodium ☞ serving size: 1 cracker = 3 g; Calories = 12.5; Total Carb (g) = 2.2; Net Carb (g) = 2.1; Fat (g) = 0.3; Protein = 0.3

Crackers Sandwich Cheese Filled (Ritz) ☞ serving size: 1 sandwich = 7 g; Calories = 33.5; Total Carb (g) = 3.9; Net Carb (g) = 3.8; Fat (g) = 1.8; Protein = 0.5

Crackers Sandwich Peanut Butter Filled (Ritz) ☞ serving size: 1 sandwich = 7 g; Calories = 33.7; Total Carb (g) = 4; Net Carb (g) = 3.8; Fat (g) = 1.8; Protein = 0.5

Crackers Wheat ☞ serving size: 1 cracker = 3 g; Calories = 13.2; Total Carb (g) = 2.1; Net Carb (g) = 1.9; Fat (g) = 0.5; Protein = 0.3

Crackers Wheat Flavored (Wheat Thins) ☞ serving size: 1 cracker = 3 g; Calories = 13.2; Total Carb (g) = 2.1; Net Carb (g) = 1.9; Fat (g) = 0.5; Protein = 0.3

Crackers Wheat Plain (Wheat Thins) ☞ serving size: 1 cracker = 3 g; Calories = 13.2; Total Carb (g) = 2.1; Net Carb (g) = 1.9; Fat (g) = 0.5; Protein = 0.3

Crackers Woven Wheat ☞ serving size: 1 cracker = 5 g; Calories = 22.1; Total Carb (g) = 3.5; Net Carb (g) = 3.1; Fat (g) = 0.8; Protein = 0.5

Crackers Woven Wheat Flavored (Triscuit) ☞ serving size: 1 cracker = 5 g; Calories = 22.1; Total Carb (g) = 3.5; Net Carb (g) = 3.1; Fat (g) = 0.8; Protein = 0.5

Crackers Woven Wheat Plain (Triscuit) ☞ serving size: 1 cracker = 5 g; Calories = 22.1; Total Carb (g) = 3.5; Net Carb (g) = 3.1; Fat (g) = 0.8; Protein = 0.5

⚫ Extruded Corn Chips ☞ serving size: 1 cup, crushed = 88 g; Calories = 490.2; Total Carb (g) = 50.5; Net Carb (g) = 46.6; Fat (g) = 29.4; Protein = 5.8

⚫ Formulated Bar High Fiber Chewy Oats And Chocolate ☞ serving size: 1 bar = 40 g; Calories = 155.6; Total Carb (g) = 27.9; Net Carb (g) = 18.9; Fat (g) = 4; Protein = 2

⚫ Formulated Bar Luna Bar Nutz Over Chocolate ☞ serving size: 1 bar = 48 g; Calories = 193.4; Total Carb (g) = 25.2; Net Carb (g) = 23.1; Fat (g) = 5.9; Protein = 10

⚫ Formulated Bar Mars Snackfood Us Cocoavia Chocolate Almond Snack Bar ☞ serving size: 1 bar = 22 g; Calories = 76.3; Total Carb (g) = 11.4; Net Carb (g) = 10.2; Fat (g) = 3.1; Protein = 1.7

⚫ Formulated Bar Mars Snackfood Us Cocoavia Chocolate Blueberry Snack Bar ☞ serving size: 1 bar = 22 g; Calories = 71.5; Total Carb (g) = 12.7; Net Carb (g) = 11.7; Fat (g) = 2; Protein = 1.4

⚫ Formulated Bar Mars Snackfood Us Snickers Marathon Chewy Chocolate Peanut Bar ☞ serving size: 1 bar = 55 g; Calories = 217.8; Total Carb (g) = 26; Net Carb (g) = 24.6; Fat (g) = 7.2; Protein = 13.4

⚫ Formulated Bar Mars Snackfood Us Snickers Marathon Energy Bar All Flavors ☞ serving size: 1 bar = 55 g; Calories = 212.3; Total Carb (g) = 27.7; Net Carb (g) = 24; Fat (g) = 5.9; Protein = 12.1

⚫ Formulated Bar Mars Snackfood Us Snickers Marathon Honey Nut Oat Bar ☞ serving size: 1 bar = 55 g; Calories = 209.6; Total Carb (g) = 30.3; Net Carb (g) = 24.3; Fat (g) = 4.3; Protein = 12.4

⚫ Formulated Bar Mars Snackfood Us Snickers Marathon Multigrain Crunch Bar ☞ serving size: 1 bar = 55 g; Calories = 232.1; Total Carb (g) = 31.5; Net Carb (g) = 30; Fat (g) = 7.3; Protein = 10.2

⚫ Formulated Bar Mars Snackfood Us Snickers Marathon Protein Performance Bar Caramel Nut Rush ☞ serving size: 1 bar = 80 g;

Calories = 332; Total Carb (g) = 40.4; Net Carb (g) = 30.4; Fat (g) = 10; Protein = 20

● Formulated Bar Power Bar Chocolate ☞ serving size: 1 bar = 68 g; Calories = 246.8; Total Carb (g) = 47.4; Net Carb (g) = 43.5; Fat (g) = 2.1; Protein = 9.6

● Formulated Bar Slim-Fast Optima Meal Bar Milk Chocolate Peanut ☞ serving size: 1 bar = 55 g; Calories = 212.3; Total Carb (g) = 33.1; Net Carb (g) = 30.3; Fat (g) = 4.9; Protein = 8.9

● Formulated Bar Zone Perfect Classic Crunch Bar Mixed Flavors ☞ serving size: 1 bar = 50 g; Calories = 213; Total Carb (g) = 22.5; Net Carb (g) = 21.5; Fat (g) = 7; Protein = 15

● Granola Bar Soft Milk Chocolate Coated Peanut Butter ☞ serving size: 1 oz = 28.4 g; Calories = 152.2; Total Carb (g) = 15.4; Net Carb (g) = 14.3; Fat (g) = 8.9; Protein = 2.7

● Microwave Popcorn ☞ serving size: 1 oz = 28.4 g; Calories = 114.2; Total Carb (g) = 21.6; Net Carb (g) = 17.7; Fat (g) = 1.7; Protein = 3

● Milk And Cereal Bar ☞ serving size: 1 bar = 25 g; Calories = 103.3; Total Carb (g) = 18; Net Carb (g) = 17.9; Fat (g) = 2.8; Protein = 1.6

● Nutrition Bar (Clif Kids Organic Zbar) ☞ serving size: 1 bar = 36 g; Calories = 147.2; Total Carb (g) = 26.9; Net Carb (g) = 23.9; Fat (g) = 3.5; Protein = 2

● Nutrition Bar (Tiger's Milk) ☞ serving size: 1 bar = 35 g; Calories = 147.7; Total Carb (g) = 19.8; Net Carb (g) = 19; Fat (g) = 5; Protein = 5.9

● Nutrition Bar (Zone Perfect Classic Crunch) ☞ serving size: 1 bar = 50 g; Calories = 211; Total Carb (g) = 22.5; Net Carb (g) = 21.5; Fat (g) = 7; Protein = 15

● Nutrition Bar Or Meal Replacement Bar Nfs ☞ serving size: 1 bar = 34 g; Calories = 143.5; Total Carb (g) = 15.3; Net Carb (g) = 14.6; Fat (g) = 4.8; Protein = 10.2

◉ Popcorn Air-Popped Unbuttered ☞ serving size: 1 cup, popped = 8 g; Calories = 30.8; Total Carb (g) = 6.2; Net Carb (g) = 5.1; Fat (g) = 0.4; Protein = 1

◉ Popcorn Air-Popped With Added Butter Or Margarine ☞ serving size: 1 cup, popped = 11 g; Calories = 46.8; Total Carb (g) = 7.2; Net Carb (g) = 5.9; Fat (g) = 1.6; Protein = 1.2

◉ Popcorn Caramel Coated ☞ serving size: 1 cup = 35 g; Calories = 149.8; Total Carb (g) = 27.5; Net Carb (g) = 25.6; Fat (g) = 4.5; Protein = 1.3

◉ Popcorn Caramel Coated With Nuts ☞ serving size: 1 cup = 42 g; Calories = 166.7; Total Carb (g) = 33.6; Net Carb (g) = 32; Fat (g) = 3.3; Protein = 2.7

◉ Popcorn Chips Other Flavors ☞ serving size: 1 chip = 1 g; Calories = 4.4; Total Carb (g) = 0.7; Net Carb (g) = 0.7; Fat (g) = 0.1; Protein = 0.1

◉ Popcorn Chips Plain ☞ serving size: 1 chip = 1 g; Calories = 4.4; Total Carb (g) = 0.7; Net Carb (g) = 0.7; Fat (g) = 0.1; Protein = 0.1

◉ Popcorn Chips Sweet Flavors ☞ serving size: 1 chip = 1 g; Calories = 4.5; Total Carb (g) = 0.8; Net Carb (g) = 0.7; Fat (g) = 0.1; Protein = 0.1

◉ Popcorn Microwave Butter Flavored ☞ serving size: 1 regular microwave bag = 85 g; Calories = 457.3; Total Carb (g) = 47.6; Net Carb (g) = 39; Fat (g) = 26.4; Protein = 7.4

◉ Popcorn Microwave Butter Flavored Light ☞ serving size: 1 regular microwave bag = 85 g; Calories = 357.9; Total Carb (g) = 60.8; Net Carb (g) = 48.8; Fat (g) = 8; Protein = 10.6

◉ Popcorn Microwave Cheese Flavored ☞ serving size: 1 regular microwave bag = 85 g; Calories = 455.6; Total Carb (g) = 47.4; Net Carb (g) = 38.8; Fat (g) = 26.3; Protein = 7.4

◉ Popcorn Microwave Kettle Corn ☞ serving size: 1 regular

microwave bag = 85 g; Calories = 438.6; Total Carb (g) = 49.5; Net Carb (g) = 40.1; Fat (g) = 23; Protein = 8.4

🍿 Popcorn Microwave Kettle Corn Light ☞ serving size: 1 regular microwave bag = 85 g; Calories = 358.7; Total Carb (g) = 61.5; Net Carb (g) = 49.7; Fat (g) = 7.9; Protein = 10.5

🍿 Popcorn Microwave Low Fat And Sodium ☞ serving size: 1 oz = 28.4 g; Calories = 121.8; Total Carb (g) = 20.8; Net Carb (g) = 16.8; Fat (g) = 2.7; Protein = 3.6

🍿 Popcorn Microwave Low Sodium ☞ serving size: 1 regular microwave bag = 85 g; Calories = 421.6; Total Carb (g) = 49; Net Carb (g) = 40.6; Fat (g) = 23.7; Protein = 7.6

🍿 Popcorn Microwave Nfs ☞ serving size: 1 regular microwave bag = 85 g; Calories = 457.3; Total Carb (g) = 47.6; Net Carb (g) = 39; Fat (g) = 26.4; Protein = 7.4

🍿 Popcorn Microwave Other Flavored ☞ serving size: 1 regular microwave bag = 85 g; Calories = 455.6; Total Carb (g) = 47.4; Net Carb (g) = 38.8; Fat (g) = 26.3; Protein = 7.4

🍿 Popcorn Microwave Plain ☞ serving size: 1 regular microwave bag = 85 g; Calories = 457.3; Total Carb (g) = 47.6; Net Carb (g) = 39; Fat (g) = 26.4; Protein = 7.4

🍿 Popcorn Microwave Plain Light ☞ serving size: 1 regular microwave bag = 85 g; Calories = 357.9; Total Carb (g) = 60.8; Net Carb (g) = 48.8; Fat (g) = 8; Protein = 10.6

🍿 Popcorn Microwave Regular (Butter) Flavor Made With Palm Oil ☞ serving size: 1 cup = 7.9 g; Calories = 42.3; Total Carb (g) = 4.5; Net Carb (g) = 3.7; Fat (g) = 2.4; Protein = 0.7

🍿 Popcorn Microwave Unsalted ☞ serving size: 1 regular microwave bag = 85 g; Calories = 421.6; Total Carb (g) = 49; Net Carb (g) = 40.6; Fat (g) = 23.7; Protein = 7.6

🍿 Popcorn Movie Theater Unbuttered ☞ serving size: 1 kids size order = 66 g; Calories = 398; Total Carb (g) = 26.3; Net Carb (g) = 21.8; Fat (g) = 32.1; Protein = 4.1

Popcorn Movie Theater With Added Butter ☞ serving size: 1 kids size order = 84 g; Calories = 551; Total Carb (g) = 26.6; Net Carb (g) = 22.1; Fat (g) = 49.4; Protein = 4.2

Popcorn Nfs ☞ serving size: 1 regular microwave bag = 85 g; Calories = 457.3; Total Carb (g) = 47.6; Net Carb (g) = 39; Fat (g) = 26.4; Protein = 7.4

Popcorn Popped In Oil Unbuttered ☞ serving size: 1 cup, popped = 11 g; Calories = 54.8; Total Carb (g) = 6.4; Net Carb (g) = 5.3; Fat (g) = 3.1; Protein = 1

Popcorn Popped In Oil With Added Butter Or Margarine ☞ serving size: 1 cup, popped = 14 g; Calories = 72.8; Total Carb (g) = 6.9; Net Carb (g) = 5.7; Fat (g) = 4.9; Protein = 1.1

Popcorn Ready-To-Eat Packaged Butter Flavored ☞ serving size: 1 cup = 14 g; Calories = 74.2; Total Carb (g) = 7.5; Net Carb (g) = 6.1; Fat (g) = 4.6; Protein = 1.2

Popcorn Ready-To-Eat Packaged Butter Flavored Light ☞ serving size: 1 cup = 8 g; Calories = 34.8; Total Carb (g) = 5.4; Net Carb (g) = 4.4; Fat (g) = 1.2; Protein = 0.9

Popcorn Ready-To-Eat Packaged Cheese Flavored Light ☞ serving size: 1 cup = 8 g; Calories = 34.8; Total Carb (g) = 5.4; Net Carb (g) = 4.4; Fat (g) = 1.2; Protein = 0.9

Popcorn Ready-To-Eat Packaged Kettle Corn Light ☞ serving size: 1 cup = 8 g; Calories = 34.6; Total Carb (g) = 5.9; Net Carb (g) = 5.1; Fat (g) = 1; Protein = 0.7

Popcorn Ready-To-Eat Packaged Low Sodium ☞ serving size: 1 cup = 11 g; Calories = 53.5; Total Carb (g) = 6.8; Net Carb (g) = 5.5; Fat (g) = 2.6; Protein = 1.1

Popcorn Ready-To-Eat Packaged Nfs ☞ serving size: 1 cup = 14 g;

Calories = 74.2; Total Carb (g) = 7.5; Net Carb (g) = 6.1; Fat (g) = 4.6; Protein = 1.2

Popcorn Ready-To-Eat Packaged Plain ☞ serving size: 1 cup = 11 g; Calories = 53; Total Carb (g) = 6.7; Net Carb (g) = 5.5; Fat (g) = 2.6; Protein = 1.1

Popcorn Ready-To-Eat Packaged Plain Light ☞ serving size: 1 cup = 8 g; Calories = 35; Total Carb (g) = 5.5; Net Carb (g) = 4.4; Fat (g) = 1.2; Protein = 0.9

Popcorn Ready-To-Eat Packaged Unsalted ☞ serving size: 1 cup = 11 g; Calories = 53.5; Total Carb (g) = 6.8; Net Carb (g) = 5.5; Fat (g) = 2.6; Protein = 1.1

Popcorn Ready-To-Eat-Packaged Kettle Corn ☞ serving size: 1 cup = 14 g; Calories = 73.8; Total Carb (g) = 8.6; Net Carb (g) = 7.7; Fat (g) = 4.2; Protein = 0.8

Popcorn Sugar Syrup/caramel Fat-Free ☞ serving size: 1 oz = 28.4 g; Calories = 108.2; Total Carb (g) = 25.6; Net Carb (g) = 24.9; Fat (g) = 0.4; Protein = 0.6

Potato Chips Baked Flavored ☞ serving size: 1 chip = 2 g; Calories = 9.3; Total Carb (g) = 1.4; Net Carb (g) = 1.3; Fat (g) = 0.4; Protein = 0.1

Potato Chips Fat Free ☞ serving size: 1 chip = 1 g; Calories = 4.8; Total Carb (g) = 0.7; Net Carb (g) = 0.6; Fat (g) = 0.2; Protein = 0.1

Potato Chips Lightly Salted ☞ serving size: 1 chip = 2 g; Calories = 11.2; Total Carb (g) = 1.1; Net Carb (g) = 1; Fat (g) = 0.7; Protein = 0.1

Potato Chips Popped Flavored ☞ serving size: 1 chip = 1 g; Calories = 4.7; Total Carb (g) = 0.7; Net Carb (g) = 0.7; Fat (g) = 0.2; Protein = 0.1

Potato Chips Reduced Fat ☞ serving size: 1 chip = 2 g; Calories = 9.6; Total Carb (g) = 1.3; Net Carb (g) = 1.2; Fat (g) = 0.4; Protein = 0.1

Potato Chips Restructured Flavored ☞ serving size: 1 chip = 2 g; Calories = 10.8; Total Carb (g) = 1.1; Net Carb (g) = 1; Fat (g) = 0.7; Protein = 0.1

Potato Chips Restructured Lightly Salted ☞ serving size: 1 chip = 2 g; Calories = 11.2; Total Carb (g) = 1.1; Net Carb (g) = 1; Fat (g) = 0.7; Protein = 0.1

Potato Chips Restructured Plain ☞ serving size: 1 chip = 2 g; Calories = 10.9; Total Carb (g) = 1.1; Net Carb (g) = 1.1; Fat (g) = 0.7; Protein = 0.1

Potato Chips Unsalted ☞ serving size: 1 chip = 2 g; Calories = 10.7; Total Carb (g) = 1.2; Net Carb (g) = 1.1; Fat (g) = 0.6; Protein = 0.1

Potato Chips Without Salt Reduced Fat ☞ serving size: 1 oz = 28.4 g; Calories = 138.3; Total Carb (g) = 19.3; Net Carb (g) = 17.5; Fat (g) = 5.9; Protein = 2

Potato Sticks Flavored ☞ serving size: 10 sticks = 3 g; Calories = 15.5; Total Carb (g) = 1.6; Net Carb (g) = 1.5; Fat (g) = 1; Protein = 0.2

Potato Sticks Fry Shaped ☞ serving size: 10 sticks = 3 g; Calories = 15.5; Total Carb (g) = 1.6; Net Carb (g) = 1.5; Fat (g) = 1; Protein = 0.2

Pretzel Chips Hard Flavored ☞ serving size: 1 pretzel chip/crisp/thin = 3 g; Calories = 11.1; Total Carb (g) = 2.3; Net Carb (g) = 2.2; Fat (g) = 0.1; Protein = 0.3

Pretzel Chips Hard Gluten Free ☞ serving size: 1 pretzel chip/crisp/thin = 3 g; Calories = 11.4; Total Carb (g) = 2.3; Net Carb (g) = 2.2; Fat (g) = 0.2; Protein = 0.1

Pretzel Chips Hard Plain ☞ serving size: 1 pretzel chip/crisp/thin = 3 g; Calories = 11.3; Total Carb (g) = 2.4; Net Carb (g) = 2.3; Fat (g) = 0.1; Protein = 0.3

Pretzels Hard Coated Gluten Free ☞ serving size: 1 minia-ture/bite size = 4 g; Calories = 18; Total Carb (g) = 3; Net Carb (g) = 3; Fat (g) = 0.6; Protein = 0.2

Pretzels Hard Flavored ☞ serving size: 1 miniature/bite size = 2 g; Calories = 7.8; Total Carb (g) = 1.6; Net Carb (g) = 1.5; Fat (g) = 0.1; Protein = 0.2

Pretzels Hard Flavored Gluten Free ☞ serving size: 1 pretzel stick = 1 g; Calories = 3.9; Total Carb (g) = 0.8; Net Carb (g) = 0.7; Fat (g) = 0.1; Protein = 0

Pretzels Hard Multigrain ☞ serving size: 1 miniature/bite size = 2 g; Calories = 7.6; Total Carb (g) = 1.6; Net Carb (g) = 1.5; Fat (g) = 0.1; Protein = 0.2

Pretzels Hard Peanut Butter Filled ☞ serving size: 1 miniature/bite size = 3 g; Calories = 13.6; Total Carb (g) = 1.8; Net Carb (g) = 1.7; Fat (g) = 0.6; Protein = 0.4

Pretzels Hard Plain Lightly Salted ☞ serving size: 1 miniature/bite size = 2 g; Calories = 7.6; Total Carb (g) = 1.6; Net Carb (g) = 1.5; Fat (g) = 0.1; Protein = 0.2

Pretzels Hard White Chocolate Coated ☞ serving size: 1 miniature/bite size = 4 g; Calories = 17.7; Total Carb (g) = 3; Net Carb (g) = 2.9; Fat (g) = 0.6; Protein = 0.2

Pretzels Hard Yogurt Coated ☞ serving size: 1 miniature/bite size = 4 g; Calories = 17.4; Total Carb (g) = 3.1; Net Carb (g) = 3; Fat (g) = 0.5; Protein = 0.2

Pretzels Soft Filled With Cheese ☞ serving size: 1 medium/regular = 99 g; Calories = 334.6; Total Carb (g) = 61.9; Net Carb (g) = 60.4; Fat (g) = 5.2; Protein = 10.1

Pretzels Soft From Frozen Cinnamon Sugar Coated ☞ serving size: 1 medium/regular = 71 g; Calories = 263.4; Total Carb (g) = 52.6; Net Carb (g) = 51.1; Fat (g) = 4.3; Protein = 4.4

Pretzels Soft From Frozen Coated Or Flavored ☞ serving size: 1 medium/regular = 71 g; Calories = 259.2; Total Carb (g) = 46.9; Net Carb (g) = 45.8; Fat (g) = 5.5; Protein = 5.6

⬤ Pretzels Soft From Frozen Nfs ☞ serving size: 1 medium/regular = 71 g; Calories = 242.1; Total Carb (g) = 48.4; Net Carb (g) = 47.2; Fat (g) = 2.9; Protein = 5.7

⬤ Pretzels Soft From Frozen Salted ☞ serving size: 1 medium/regular = 71 g; Calories = 238.6; Total Carb (g) = 48.9; Net Carb (g) = 47.7; Fat (g) = 2.2; Protein = 5.8

⬤ Pretzels Soft From Frozen Topped With Cheese ☞ serving size: 1 medium/regular = 71 g; Calories = 240; Total Carb (g) = 44.4; Net Carb (g) = 43.3; Fat (g) = 3.8; Protein = 7.3

⬤ Pretzels Soft From Frozen Topped With Meat ☞ serving size: 1 medium/regular = 71 g; Calories = 249.2; Total Carb (g) = 38.1; Net Carb (g) = 37.2; Fat (g) = 7.1; Protein = 8.2

⬤ Pretzels Soft From School Lunch ☞ serving size: 1 medium/regular = 71 g; Calories = 240.7; Total Carb (g) = 50.2; Net Carb (g) = 47.6; Fat (g) = 2.2; Protein = 6.1

⬤ Pretzels Soft Gluten Free ☞ serving size: 1 medium/regular = 95 g; Calories = 282.2; Total Carb (g) = 54.4; Net Carb (g) = 50.6; Fat (g) = 5.5; Protein = 3.8

⬤ Pretzels Soft Gluten Free Cinnamon Sugar Coated ☞ serving size: 1 medium/regular = 95 g; Calories = 319.2; Total Carb (g) = 60.6; Net Carb (g) = 57; Fat (g) = 7.7; Protein = 3

⬤ Pretzels Soft Gluten Free Coated Or Flavored ☞ serving size: 1 medium/regular = 95 g; Calories = 309.7; Total Carb (g) = 51.5; Net Carb (g) = 47.9; Fat (g) = 9.9; Protein = 3.9

⬤ Pretzels Soft Multigrain ☞ serving size: 1 small = 62 g; Calories = 205.8; Total Carb (g) = 42.9; Net Carb (g) = 40.6; Fat (g) = 2; Protein = 5.3

⬤ Pretzels Soft Nfs ☞ serving size: 1 bite size/nugget = 14 g; Calories = 47.7; Total Carb (g) = 9.6; Net Carb (g) = 9.3; Fat (g) = 0.6; Protein = 1.1

● Pretzels Soft Ready-To-Eat Cinnamon Sugar Coated ☞ serving size: 1 bite size/nugget = 14 g; Calories = 51.9; Total Carb (g) = 10.4; Net Carb (g) = 10.1; Fat (g) = 0.9; Protein = 0.9

● Pretzels Soft Ready-To-Eat Coated Or Flavored ☞ serving size: 1 bite size/nugget = 14 g; Calories = 51.1; Total Carb (g) = 9.2; Net Carb (g) = 9; Fat (g) = 1.1; Protein = 1.1

● Pretzels Soft Ready-To-Eat Nfs ☞ serving size: 1 bite size/nugget = 14 g; Calories = 47.7; Total Carb (g) = 9.6; Net Carb (g) = 9.3; Fat (g) = 0.6; Protein = 1.1

● Pretzels Soft Ready-To-Eat Salted Buttered ☞ serving size: 1 bite size/nugget = 14 g; Calories = 47.7; Total Carb (g) = 9.6; Net Carb (g) = 9.3; Fat (g) = 0.6; Protein = 1.1

● Pretzels Soft Ready-To-Eat Salted No Butter ☞ serving size: 1 bite size/nugget = 14 g; Calories = 47; Total Carb (g) = 9.7; Net Carb (g) = 9.4; Fat (g) = 0.4; Protein = 1.1

● Pretzels Soft Ready-To-Eat Topped With Cheese ☞ serving size: 1 bite size/nugget = 14 g; Calories = 47.3; Total Carb (g) = 8.8; Net Carb (g) = 8.5; Fat (g) = 0.7; Protein = 1.4

● Pretzels Soft Ready-To-Eat Topped With Meat ☞ serving size: 1 bite size/nugget = 14 g; Calories = 49.1; Total Carb (g) = 7.5; Net Carb (g) = 7.3; Fat (g) = 1.4; Protein = 1.6

● Pretzels Soft Ready-To-Eat Unsalted Buttered ☞ serving size: 1 bite size/nugget = 14 g; Calories = 49; Total Carb (g) = 9.9; Net Carb (g) = 9.6; Fat (g) = 0.6; Protein = 1.1

● Rice And Wheat Cereal Bar ☞ serving size: 1 bar = 22 g; Calories = 90; Total Carb (g) = 16; Net Carb (g) = 15.6; Fat (g) = 2; Protein = 2

● Rice Cake Cracker (Include Hain Mini Rice Cakes) ☞ serving size: 1 cubic inch = 4.2 g; Calories = 16.5; Total Carb (g) = 3.4; Net Carb (g) = 3.2; Fat (g) = 0.2; Protein = 0.3

● Rice Paper ☞ serving size: 1 small paper (6-3/8" dia) = 5 g; Calo-

ries = 16.5; Total Carb (g) = 3.6; Net Carb (g) = 3.5; Fat (g) = 0.1; Protein = 0.3

Snack Mix ☞ serving size: 1 cup = 60 g; Calories = 300.6; Total Carb (g) = 37.6; Net Carb (g) = 35.6; Fat (g) = 15.4; Protein = 4.2

Snack Mix Plain (Chex Mix) ☞ serving size: 1 cup = 60 g; Calories = 256.8; Total Carb (g) = 45.4; Net Carb (g) = 41.9; Fat (g) = 6; Protein = 5.3

Snack Mixed Berry Bar ☞ serving size: 1 bar = 38 g; Calories = 145.5; Total Carb (g) = 22.4; Net Carb (g) = 19.4; Fat (g) = 4; Protein = 5

Snack Potato Chips Made From Dried Potatoes Plain ☞ serving size: 1 oz = 28 g; Calories = 152.6; Total Carb (g) = 15.5; Net Carb (g) = 14.7; Fat (g) = 9.9; Protein = 1.3

Snack Pretzel Hard Chocolate Coated ☞ serving size: 1 serving = 28 g; Calories = 130.8; Total Carb (g) = 19.6; Net Carb (g) = 18.6; Fat (g) = 4.9; Protein = 2

Snacks Bagel Chips Plain ☞ serving size: 1 oz = 28.4 g; Calories = 128.1; Total Carb (g) = 18.9; Net Carb (g) = 17.7; Fat (g) = 4.3; Protein = 3.5

Snacks Banana Chips ☞ serving size: 1 oz = 28.4 g; Calories = 147.4; Total Carb (g) = 16.6; Net Carb (g) = 14.4; Fat (g) = 9.5; Protein = 0.7

Snacks Beef Jerky Chopped And Formed ☞ serving size: 1 oz = 28.4 g; Calories = 116.4; Total Carb (g) = 3.1; Net Carb (g) = 2.6; Fat (g) = 7.3; Protein = 9.4

Snacks Beef Sticks Smoked ☞ serving size: 1 oz = 28.4 g; Calories = 156.2; Total Carb (g) = 1.5; Net Carb (g) = 1.5; Fat (g) = 14.1; Protein = 6.1

Snacks Brown Rice Chips ☞ serving size: 1 cake = 9 g; Calories = 34.6; Total Carb (g) = 7.3; Net Carb (g) = 7; Fat (g) = 0.3; Protein = 0.7

🍪 Snacks Candy Bits Yogurt Covered With Vitamin C ☞ serving size: 1 package = 20 g; Calories = 83; Total Carb (g) = 17.4; Net Carb (g) = 17.3; Fat (g) = 1.5; Protein = 0

🍪 Snacks Candy Rolls Yogurt-Covered Fruit Flavored With High Vitamin C ☞ serving size: 1 roll = 23 g; Calories = 82.6; Total Carb (g) = 17.2; Net Carb (g) = 16.4; Fat (g) = 1.5; Protein = 0.1

🍪 Snacks Clif Bar Mixed Flavors ☞ serving size: 1 bar = 68 g; Calories = 235.3; Total Carb (g) = 44.5; Net Carb (g) = 39.5; Fat (g) = 4; Protein = 10

🍪 Snacks Corn Cakes ☞ serving size: 1 cake = 9 g; Calories = 34.8; Total Carb (g) = 7.5; Net Carb (g) = 7.3; Fat (g) = 0.2; Protein = 0.7

🍪 Snacks Corn Cakes Very Low Sodium ☞ serving size: 1 cake = 9 g; Calories = 34.8; Total Carb (g) = 7.5; Net Carb (g) = 7.5; Fat (g) = 0.2; Protein = 0.7

🍪 Snacks Corn-Based Extruded Chips Barbecue-Flavor ☞ serving size: 1 oz = 28.4 g; Calories = 148.5; Total Carb (g) = 16; Net Carb (g) = 14.5; Fat (g) = 9.3; Protein = 2

🍪 Snacks Corn-Based Extruded Chips Barbecue-Flavor Made With Enriched Masa Flour ☞ serving size: 1 oz = 28.4 g; Calories = 148.5; Total Carb (g) = 16; Net Carb (g) = 16; Fat (g) = 9.3; Protein = 2

🍪 Snacks Corn-Based Extruded Chips Plain ☞ serving size: 1 oz = 28 g; Calories = 150.9; Total Carb (g) = 16; Net Carb (g) = 14.9; Fat (g) = 9.3; Protein = 1.7

🍪 Snacks Corn-Based Extruded Cones Plain ☞ serving size: 1 oz = 28.4 g; Calories = 144.8; Total Carb (g) = 17.9; Net Carb (g) = 17.6; Fat (g) = 7.6; Protein = 1.7

🍪 Snacks Corn-Based Extruded Onion-Flavor ☞ serving size: 1 oz = 28.4 g; Calories = 141.7; Total Carb (g) = 18.5; Net Carb (g) = 17.4; Fat (g) = 6.4; Protein = 2.2

Snacks Corn-Based Extruded Puffs Or Twists Cheese-Flavor ☞ serving size: 1 oz = 28.4 g; Calories = 161; Total Carb (g) = 15.5; Net Carb (g) = 15.3; Fat (g) = 10.4; Protein = 1.6

Snacks Corn-Based Extruded Puffs Or Twists Cheese-Flavor Unenriched ☞ serving size: 1 oz = 28.4 g; Calories = 158.5; Total Carb (g) = 15.4; Net Carb (g) = 14.7; Fat (g) = 10.2; Protein = 1.6

Snacks Cornnuts Barbecue-Flavor ☞ serving size: 1 oz = 28.4 g; Calories = 123.8; Total Carb (g) = 20.4; Net Carb (g) = 18; Fat (g) = 4.1; Protein = 2.6

Snacks Crisped Rice Bar Almond ☞ serving size: 1 bar (1 oz) = 28 g; Calories = 128.2; Total Carb (g) = 18.1; Net Carb (g) = 17.1; Fat (g) = 5.7; Protein = 2

Snacks Crisped Rice Bar Chocolate Chip ☞ serving size: 1 bar (1 oz) = 28 g; Calories = 113.1; Total Carb (g) = 20.4; Net Carb (g) = 19.8; Fat (g) = 3.8; Protein = 1.4

Snacks Farley Candy Farley Fruit Snacks With Vitamins A C And E ☞ serving size: 1 pouch = 26 g; Calories = 88.7; Total Carb (g) = 21; Net Carb (g) = 21; Fat (g) = 0; Protein = 1.1

Snacks Fritolay Sunchips Multigrain French Onion Flavor ☞ serving size: 1 oz = 28.4 g; Calories = 140.9; Total Carb (g) = 18.6; Net Carb (g) = 16.4; Fat (g) = 6.3; Protein = 2.5

Snacks Fritolay Sunchips Multigrain Snack Harvest Cheddar Flavor ☞ serving size: 1 oz = 28.4 g; Calories = 139.4; Total Carb (g) = 18.4; Net Carb (g) = 16.1; Fat (g) = 6.3; Protein = 2.3

Snacks Fritolay Sunchips Multigrain Snack Original Flavor ☞ serving size: 1 oz = 28.4 g; Calories = 139.4; Total Carb (g) = 19.1; Net Carb (g) = 16.6; Fat (g) = 6; Protein = 2.3

Snacks Fruit Leather Pieces With Vitamin C ☞ serving size: 1 serving = 21 g; Calories = 78.3; Total Carb (g) = 17.9; Net Carb (g) = 17.2; Fat (g) = 0.7; Protein = 0

Snacks General Mills Betty Crocker Fruit Roll Ups Berry Flavored With Vitamin C ☞ serving size: 2 rolls = 28 g; Calories = 104.4; Total Carb (g) = 23.9; Net Carb (g) = 23.9; Fat (g) = 1; Protein = 0

Snacks Granola Bar Chewy Reduced Sugar All Flavors ☞ serving size: 1 bar = 24 g; Calories = 98.9; Total Carb (g) = 16.7; Net Carb (g) = 15.9; Fat (g) = 3; Protein = 1.3

Snacks Granola Bar General Mills Nature Valley Chewy Trail Mix ☞ serving size: 1 bar = 35 g; Calories = 145.3; Total Carb (g) = 25.3; Net Carb (g) = 24; Fat (g) = 4; Protein = 2

Snacks Granola Bar General Mills Nature Valley Sweet&salty Nut Peanut ☞ serving size: 1 bar = 35 g; Calories = 170.5; Total Carb (g) = 21.4; Net Carb (g) = 20.4; Fat (g) = 8; Protein = 3.2

Snacks Granola Bar General Mills Nature Valley With Yogurt Coating ☞ serving size: 1 bar = 35 g; Calories = 148.1; Total Carb (g) = 26; Net Carb (g) = 24.5; Fat (g) = 4; Protein = 2

Snacks Granola Bar Kashi Golean Chewy Mixed Flavors ☞ serving size: 1 bar = 78 g; Calories = 304.2; Total Carb (g) = 49.5; Net Carb (g) = 43.5; Fat (g) = 6; Protein = 13

Snacks Granola Bar Kashi Golean Crunchy Mixed Flavors ☞ serving size: 1 bar = 47 g; Calories = 184.7; Total Carb (g) = 28; Net Carb (g) = 25.2; Fat (g) = 4.3; Protein = 8.4

Snacks Granola Bar Kashi Tlc Bar Chewy Mixed Flavors ☞ serving size: 1 bar = 35 g; Calories = 150.2; Total Carb (g) = 18.6; Net Carb (g) = 14.7; Fat (g) = 5.5; Protein = 6.5

Snacks Granola Bar Kashi Tlc Bar Crunchy Mixed Flavors ☞ serving size: 2 bar = 40 g; Calories = 178.4; Total Carb (g) = 25.1; Net Carb (g) = 21.1; Fat (g) = 6; Protein = 6

Snacks Granola Bar Quaker Chewy 90 Calorie Bar ☞ serving size: 1 bar = 24 g; Calories = 97.9; Total Carb (g) = 19; Net Carb (g) = 18; Fat (g) = 2; Protein = 1

⚫ Snacks Granola Bar Quaker Dipps All Flavors ☞ serving size: 1 bar = 31 g; Calories = 148.8; Total Carb (g) = 20.1; Net Carb (g) = 19.2; Fat (g) = 6.3; Protein = 2.3

⚫ Snacks Granola Bar With Coconut Chocolate Coated ☞ serving size: 1 oz = 28.4 g; Calories = 150.8; Total Carb (g) = 15.7; Net Carb (g) = 13.9; Fat (g) = 9.1; Protein = 1.5

⚫ Snacks Granola Bars Hard Almond ☞ serving size: 1 oz = 28.4 g; Calories = 140.6; Total Carb (g) = 17.6; Net Carb (g) = 16.2; Fat (g) = 7.2; Protein = 2.2

⚫ Snacks Granola Bars Hard Chocolate Chip ☞ serving size: 1 oz = 28.4 g; Calories = 124.4; Total Carb (g) = 20.5; Net Carb (g) = 19.2; Fat (g) = 4.6; Protein = 2.1

⚫ Snacks Granola Bars Hard Peanut Butter ☞ serving size: 1 oz = 28.4 g; Calories = 137.2; Total Carb (g) = 17.7; Net Carb (g) = 16.9; Fat (g) = 6.8; Protein = 2.8

⚫ Snacks Granola Bars Hard Plain ☞ serving size: 1 bar = 21 g; Calories = 98.9; Total Carb (g) = 13.5; Net Carb (g) = 12.4; Fat (g) = 4.2; Protein = 2.1

⚫ Snacks Granola Bars Quaker Oatmeal To Go All Flavors ☞ serving size: 1 bar = 60 g; Calories = 233.4; Total Carb (g) = 45.3; Net Carb (g) = 42.5; Fat (g) = 4; Protein = 4

⚫ Snacks Granola Bars Soft Almond Confectioners Coating ☞ serving size: 1 bar = 35 g; Calories = 159.3; Total Carb (g) = 21.1; Net Carb (g) = 19.5; Fat (g) = 7; Protein = 3

⚫ Snacks Granola Bars Soft Coated Milk Chocolate Coating Chocolate Chip ☞ serving size: 1 bar (1.25 oz) = 35 g; Calories = 163.1; Total Carb (g) = 22.3; Net Carb (g) = 21.1; Fat (g) = 8.7; Protein = 2

⚫ Snacks Granola Bars Soft Coated Milk Chocolate Coating Peanut Butter ☞ serving size: 1 oz = 28.4 g; Calories = 144.3; Total Carb (g) = 15.2; Net Carb (g) = 14.4; Fat (g) = 8.8; Protein = 2.9

Snacks Granola Bars Soft Uncoated Chocolate Chip ☞ serving size: 1 bar (1.5 oz) = 43 g; Calories = 179.7; Total Carb (g) = 30.2; Net Carb (g) = 28.6; Fat (g) = 7.1; Protein = 2.4

Snacks Granola Bars Soft Uncoated Chocolate Chip Graham And Marshmallow ☞ serving size: 1 bar (1 oz) = 28 g; Calories = 119.6; Total Carb (g) = 19.8; Net Carb (g) = 18.7; Fat (g) = 4.3; Protein = 1.7

Snacks Granola Bars Soft Uncoated Nut And Raisin ☞ serving size: 1 bar (1 oz) = 28 g; Calories = 127.1; Total Carb (g) = 17.8; Net Carb (g) = 16.2; Fat (g) = 5.7; Protein = 2.2

Snacks Granola Bars Soft Uncoated Peanut Butter ☞ serving size: 1 bar (1 oz) = 28 g; Calories = 119.3; Total Carb (g) = 18; Net Carb (g) = 16.8; Fat (g) = 4.4; Protein = 2.9

Snacks Granola Bars Soft Uncoated Peanut Butter And Chocolate Chip ☞ serving size: 1 bar (1 oz) = 28 g; Calories = 121; Total Carb (g) = 17.4; Net Carb (g) = 16.2; Fat (g) = 5.6; Protein = 2.7

Snacks Granola Bars Soft Uncoated Plain ☞ serving size: 1 bar (1 oz) = 28 g; Calories = 124; Total Carb (g) = 18.8; Net Carb (g) = 17.6; Fat (g) = 4.8; Protein = 2.1

Snacks Granola Bars Soft Uncoated Raisin ☞ serving size: 1 bar (1.5 oz) = 43 g; Calories = 192.6; Total Carb (g) = 28.6; Net Carb (g) = 26.8; Fat (g) = 7.7; Protein = 3.3

Snacks Granola Bites Mixed Flavors ☞ serving size: 1 package = 20 g; Calories = 90.2; Total Carb (g) = 13.3; Net Carb (g) = 12.1; Fat (g) = 3.5; Protein = 1.4

Snacks Kellogg Kelloggs Low Fat Granola Bar Crunchy Almond/brown Sugar ☞ serving size: 1 bar = 37 g; Calories = 144.3; Total Carb (g) = 28.9; Net Carb (g) = 26.6; Fat (g) = 2.7; Protein = 3

Snacks Kellogg Kelloggs Rice Krispies Treats Squares ☞ serving size: 1 serving = 22 g; Calories = 91.7; Total Carb (g) = 17.7; Net Carb (g) = 17.7; Fat (g) = 2; Protein = 0.8

🥄 Snacks Kraft Cornnuts Plain ☞ serving size: 1 oz = 28.4 g; Calories = 126.7; Total Carb (g) = 20.4; Net Carb (g) = 18.5; Fat (g) = 4.4; Protein = 2.4

🥄 Snacks M&m Mars Combos Snacks Cheddar Cheese Pretzel ☞ serving size: 1 oz = 28.4 g; Calories = 131.5; Total Carb (g) = 18.9; Net Carb (g) = 17.9; Fat (g) = 4.8; Protein = 2.8

🥄 Snacks M&m Mars Kudos Whole Grain Bar Chocolate Chip ☞ serving size: 1 bar = 28 g; Calories = 117.6; Total Carb (g) = 20.3; Net Carb (g) = 19.5; Fat (g) = 3.7; Protein = 1.3

🥄 Snacks M&m Mars Kudos Whole Grain Bar M&Ms Milk Chocolate ☞ serving size: 1 bar = 24 g; Calories = 99.6; Total Carb (g) = 17.5; Net Carb (g) = 17; Fat (g) = 2.9; Protein = 0.9

🥄 Snacks M&m Mars Kudos Whole Grain Bars Peanut Butter ☞ serving size: 1 bar = 28 g; Calories = 129.6; Total Carb (g) = 18.1; Net Carb (g) = 17.4; Fat (g) = 5.8; Protein = 1.7

🥄 Snacks Nutri-Grain Fruit And Nut Bar ☞ serving size: 1 bar = 32 g; Calories = 129; Total Carb (g) = 21.4; Net Carb (g) = 19; Fat (g) = 3.5; Protein = 3

🥄 Snacks Oriental Mix Rice-Based ☞ serving size: 1 oz = 28.4 g; Calories = 143.7; Total Carb (g) = 14.7; Net Carb (g) = 10.9; Fat (g) = 7.3; Protein = 4.9

🥄 Snacks Pita Chips Salted ☞ serving size: 1 oz = 28.4 g; Calories = 129.8; Total Carb (g) = 19.4; Net Carb (g) = 18.3; Fat (g) = 4.3; Protein = 3.4

🥄 Snacks Plantain Chips Salted ☞ serving size: 1 oz = 28.4 g; Calories = 150.8; Total Carb (g) = 18.1; Net Carb (g) = 17.1; Fat (g) = 8.4; Protein = 0.7

Snacks Popcorn Air-Popped ☞ serving size: 1 cup = 8 g; Calories = 31; Total Carb (g) = 6.2; Net Carb (g) = 5.1; Fat (g) = 0.4; Protein = 1

Snacks Popcorn Air-Popped (Unsalted) ☞ serving size: 1 cup = 8 g; Calories = 30.6; Total Carb (g) = 6.2; Net Carb (g) = 5; Fat (g) = 0.3; Protein = 1

Snacks Popcorn Cakes ☞ serving size: 1 cake = 10 g; Calories = 38.4; Total Carb (g) = 8; Net Carb (g) = 7.7; Fat (g) = 0.3; Protein = 1

Snacks Popcorn Caramel-Coated With Peanuts ☞ serving size: 1 oz (approx 2/3 cup) = 28.4 g; Calories = 113.6; Total Carb (g) = 22.9; Net Carb (g) = 21.8; Fat (g) = 2.2; Protein = 1.8

Snacks Popcorn Caramel-Coated Without Peanuts ☞ serving size: 1 oz = 28.4 g; Calories = 122.4; Total Carb (g) = 22.5; Net Carb (g) = 21; Fat (g) = 3.6; Protein = 1.1

Snacks Popcorn Cheese-Flavor ☞ serving size: 1 cup = 11 g; Calories = 57.9; Total Carb (g) = 5.7; Net Carb (g) = 4.6; Fat (g) = 3.7; Protein = 1

Snacks Popcorn Home-Prepared Oil-Popped Unsalted ☞ serving size: 1 cup = 8 g; Calories = 40; Total Carb (g) = 4.7; Net Carb (g) = 3.9; Fat (g) = 2.3; Protein = 0.7

Snacks Popcorn Microwave Low Fat ☞ serving size: 1 oz = 28.4 g; Calories = 120.4; Total Carb (g) = 20.5; Net Carb (g) = 16.4; Fat (g) = 2.7; Protein = 3.6

Snacks Popcorn Microwave Regular (Butter) Flavor Made With Partially Hydrogenated Oil ☞ serving size: 1 cup = 7.9 g; Calories = 44; Total Carb (g) = 4.4; Net Carb (g) = 3.6; Fat (g) = 2.7; Protein = 0.6

Snacks Popcorn Oil-Popped Microwave Regular Flavor No Trans Fat ☞ serving size: 1 cup = 11 g; Calories = 64.1; Total Carb (g) = 5; Net Carb (g) = 4.1; Fat (g) = 4.8; Protein = 0.8

Snacks Popcorn Oil-Popped White Popcorn Salt Added ☞

serving size: 1 cup = 11 g; Calories = 55; Total Carb (g) = 6.3; Net Carb (g) = 5.2; Fat (g) = 3.1; Protein = 1

🥫 Snacks Pork Skins Barbecue-Flavor ☞ serving size: 1 oz = 28.4 g; Calories = 152.8; Total Carb (g) = 0.5; Net Carb (g) = 0.5; Fat (g) = 9; Protein = 16.4

🥫 Snacks Pork Skins Plain ☞ serving size: 1 oz = 28.4 g; Calories = 154.5; Total Carb (g) = 0; Net Carb (g) = 0; Fat (g) = 8.9; Protein = 17.4

🥫 Snacks Potato Chips Barbecue-Flavor ☞ serving size: 1 oz = 28.4 g; Calories = 138.3; Total Carb (g) = 15.9; Net Carb (g) = 14.8; Fat (g) = 8.8; Protein = 1.9

🥫 Snacks Potato Chips Cheese-Flavor ☞ serving size: 1 oz = 28.4 g; Calories = 140.9; Total Carb (g) = 16.4; Net Carb (g) = 14.9; Fat (g) = 7.7; Protein = 2.4

🥫 Snacks Potato Chips Fat Free Salted ☞ serving size: 1 oz = 28.4 g; Calories = 107.6; Total Carb (g) = 23.8; Net Carb (g) = 21.7; Fat (g) = 0.2; Protein = 2.7

🥫 Snacks Potato Chips Fat-Free Made With Olestra ☞ serving size: 1 oz = 28.4 g; Calories = 77.8; Total Carb (g) = 18.5; Net Carb (g) = 16.5; Fat (g) = 0.2; Protein = 2.2

🥫 Snacks Potato Chips Lightly Salted ☞ serving size: pieces = 28 g; Calories = 156.8; Total Carb (g) = 15; Net Carb (g) = 13.8; Fat (g) = 9.9; Protein = 1.9

🥫 Snacks Potato Chips Made From Dried Potatoes (Preformed) Multigrain ☞ serving size: 1 oz = 28.4 g; Calories = 143.4; Total Carb (g) = 18.6; Net Carb (g) = 17.8; Fat (g) = 7; Protein = 1.5

🥫 Snacks Potato Chips Made From Dried Potatoes Cheese-Flavor ☞ serving size: 1 oz = 28.4 g; Calories = 156.5; Total Carb (g) = 14.4; Net Carb (g) = 13.4; Fat (g) = 10.5; Protein = 2

🥫 Snacks Potato Chips Made From Dried Potatoes Fat-Free Made

With Olestra ☞ serving size: 1 oz = 28.4 g; Calories = 71.9; Total Carb (g) = 15.9; Net Carb (g) = 13.8; Fat (g) = 0.3; Protein = 1.4

🥔 Snacks Potato Chips Made From Dried Potatoes Reduced Fat ☞ serving size: 1 oz = 28.4 g; Calories = 142.6; Total Carb (g) = 18.4; Net Carb (g) = 17.5; Fat (g) = 7.4; Protein = 1.3

🥔 Snacks Potato Chips Made From Dried Potatoes Sour-Cream And Onion-Flavor ☞ serving size: 1 oz = 28.4 g; Calories = 155.3; Total Carb (g) = 14.6; Net Carb (g) = 14.2; Fat (g) = 10.5; Protein = 1.9

🥔 Snacks Potato Chips Plain Made With Partially Hydrogenated Soybean Oil Salted ☞ serving size: 1 oz = 28.4 g; Calories = 152.2; Total Carb (g) = 15; Net Carb (g) = 13.7; Fat (g) = 9.8; Protein = 2

🥔 Snacks Potato Chips Plain Made With Partially Hydrogenated Soybean Oil Unsalted ☞ serving size: 1 oz = 28.4 g; Calories = 152.2; Total Carb (g) = 15; Net Carb (g) = 13.7; Fat (g) = 9.8; Protein = 2

🥔 Snacks Potato Chips Plain Salted ☞ serving size: 1 oz = 28 g; Calories = 149; Total Carb (g) = 15.1; Net Carb (g) = 14.2; Fat (g) = 9.5; Protein = 1.8

🥔 Snacks Potato Chips Plain Unsalted ☞ serving size: 1 oz = 28.4 g; Calories = 152.2; Total Carb (g) = 15; Net Carb (g) = 13.7; Fat (g) = 9.8; Protein = 2

🥔 Snacks Potato Chips Reduced Fat ☞ serving size: 1 oz = 28.4 g; Calories = 133.8; Total Carb (g) = 19; Net Carb (g) = 17.3; Fat (g) = 5.9; Protein = 2

🥔 Snacks Potato Chips Sour-Cream-And-Onion-Flavor ☞ serving size: 1 oz = 28.4 g; Calories = 150.8; Total Carb (g) = 14.6; Net Carb (g) = 13.2; Fat (g) = 9.6; Protein = 2.3

🥔 Snacks Potato Chips White Restructured Baked ☞ serving size: 1 cup = 34 g; Calories = 159.5; Total Carb (g) = 24.3; Net Carb (g) = 22.6; Fat (g) = 6.2; Protein = 1.7

Snacks Potato Sticks ☞ serving size: 1 oz = 28.4 g; Calories = 148.2; Total Carb (g) = 15.1; Net Carb (g) = 14.2; Fat (g) = 9.8; Protein = 1.9

Snacks Pretzels Hard Confectioners Coating Chocolate-Flavor ☞ serving size: 1 oz = 28.4 g; Calories = 129.8; Total Carb (g) = 20.1; Net Carb (g) = 19.5; Fat (g) = 4.7; Protein = 2.1

Snacks Pretzels Hard Plain Made With Enriched Flour Unsalted ☞ serving size: 1 oz = 28.4 g; Calories = 108.2; Total Carb (g) = 22.5; Net Carb (g) = 21.7; Fat (g) = 1; Protein = 2.6

Snacks Pretzels Hard Plain Made With Unenriched Flour Salted ☞ serving size: 1 oz = 28.4 g; Calories = 108.2; Total Carb (g) = 22.5; Net Carb (g) = 21.7; Fat (g) = 1; Protein = 2.6

Snacks Pretzels Hard Plain Made With Unenriched Flour Unsalted ☞ serving size: 1 oz = 28.4 g; Calories = 108.2; Total Carb (g) = 22.5; Net Carb (g) = 21.7; Fat (g) = 1; Protein = 2.6

Snacks Pretzels Hard Plain Salted ☞ serving size: 1 oz = 28.4 g; Calories = 109.1; Total Carb (g) = 22.8; Net Carb (g) = 21.9; Fat (g) = 0.8; Protein = 2.9

Snacks Pretzels Hard Whole-Wheat Including Both Salted And Unsalted ☞ serving size: 1 oz = 28.4 g; Calories = 102.8; Total Carb (g) = 23.1; Net Carb (g) = 20.9; Fat (g) = 0.7; Protein = 3.2

Snacks Rice Cakes Brown Rice Buckwheat ☞ serving size: 1 cake = 9 g; Calories = 34.2; Total Carb (g) = 7.2; Net Carb (g) = 6.9; Fat (g) = 0.3; Protein = 0.8

Snacks Rice Cakes Brown Rice Buckwheat Unsalted ☞ serving size: 1 cake = 9 g; Calories = 34.2; Total Carb (g) = 7.2; Net Carb (g) = 7.2; Fat (g) = 0.3; Protein = 0.8

Snacks Rice Cakes Brown Rice Corn ☞ serving size: 1 cake = 9 g; Calories = 34.7; Total Carb (g) = 7.3; Net Carb (g) = 7.1; Fat (g) = 0.3; Protein = 0.8

Snacks Rice Cakes Brown Rice Multigrain ☞ serving size: 1 cake = 9 g; Calories = 34.8; Total Carb (g) = 7.2; Net Carb (g) = 6.9; Fat (g) = 0.3; Protein = 0.8

Snacks Rice Cakes Brown Rice Multigrain Unsalted ☞ serving size: 1 cake = 9 g; Calories = 34.8; Total Carb (g) = 7.2; Net Carb (g) = 7.2; Fat (g) = 0.3; Protein = 0.8

Snacks Rice Cakes Brown Rice Plain Unsalted ☞ serving size: 1 cake = 9 g; Calories = 34.8; Total Carb (g) = 7.3; Net Carb (g) = 7; Fat (g) = 0.3; Protein = 0.7

Snacks Rice Cakes Brown Rice Rye ☞ serving size: 1 cake = 9 g; Calories = 34.7; Total Carb (g) = 7.2; Net Carb (g) = 6.8; Fat (g) = 0.3; Protein = 0.7

Snacks Rice Cakes Brown Rice Sesame Seed ☞ serving size: 1 cake = 9 g; Calories = 35.3; Total Carb (g) = 7.3; Net Carb (g) = 6.9; Fat (g) = 0.3; Protein = 0.7

Snacks Rice Cakes Brown Rice Sesame Seed Unsalted ☞ serving size: 1 cake = 9 g; Calories = 35.3; Total Carb (g) = 7.3; Net Carb (g) = 7.3; Fat (g) = 0.3; Protein = 0.7

Snacks Rice Cracker Brown Rice Plain ☞ serving size: 1 cake = 9 g; Calories = 34.8; Total Carb (g) = 7.3; Net Carb (g) = 7; Fat (g) = 0.3; Protein = 0.7

Snacks Sesame Sticks Wheat-Based Salted ☞ serving size: 1 oz = 28.4 g; Calories = 153.6; Total Carb (g) = 13.2; Net Carb (g) = 12.4; Fat (g) = 10.4; Protein = 3.1

Snacks Sesame Sticks Wheat-Based Unsalted ☞ serving size: 1 oz = 28.4 g; Calories = 153.6; Total Carb (g) = 13.2; Net Carb (g) = 13.2; Fat (g) = 10.4; Protein = 3.1

Snacks Sunkist Sunkist Fruit Roll Strawberry With Vitamins A C And E ☞ serving size: 1 roll = 21 g; Calories = 71.8; Total Carb (g) = 17.4; Net Carb (g) = 15.8; Fat (g) = 0.2; Protein = 0.1

Snacks Sweet Potato Chips Unsalted ☞ serving size: 1 oz = 28.4 g; Calories = 151.1; Total Carb (g) = 16.1; Net Carb (g) = 13.6; Fat (g) = 9.2; Protein = 0.8

Snacks Taro Chips ☞ serving size: 1 oz = 28.4 g; Calories = 141.4; Total Carb (g) = 19.3; Net Carb (g) = 17.3; Fat (g) = 7.1; Protein = 0.7

Snacks Tortilla Chips Light (Baked With Less Oil) ☞ serving size: 1 cup, crushed = 63 g; Calories = 293; Total Carb (g) = 46.2; Net Carb (g) = 42.7; Fat (g) = 9.6; Protein = 5.5

Snacks Tortilla Chips Low Fat Made With Olestra Nacho Cheese ☞ serving size: 1 oz = 28.4 g; Calories = 90.3; Total Carb (g) = 18.5; Net Carb (g) = 16.7; Fat (g) = 1; Protein = 2.4

Snacks Tortilla Chips Low Fat Unsalted ☞ serving size: 1 oz = 28.4 g; Calories = 118.1; Total Carb (g) = 22.8; Net Carb (g) = 21.2; Fat (g) = 1.6; Protein = 3.1

Snacks Tortilla Chips Nacho Cheese ☞ serving size: 1 oz = 28.4 g; Calories = 147.4; Total Carb (g) = 17.3; Net Carb (g) = 15.8; Fat (g) = 7.8; Protein = 2.1

Snacks Tortilla Chips Nacho-Flavor Made With Enriched Masa Flour ☞ serving size: 1 oz = 28.4 g; Calories = 145.1; Total Carb (g) = 17.7; Net Carb (g) = 16.2; Fat (g) = 7.3; Protein = 2.2

Snacks Tortilla Chips Nacho-Flavor Reduced Fat ☞ serving size: 1 oz = 28.4 g; Calories = 126.4; Total Carb (g) = 20.3; Net Carb (g) = 19; Fat (g) = 4.3; Protein = 2.5

Snacks Tortilla Chips Plain White Corn Salted ☞ serving size: 1 oz = 28.4 g; Calories = 134; Total Carb (g) = 19.3; Net Carb (g) = 17.7; Fat (g) = 5.9; Protein = 2

Snacks Tortilla Chips Ranch-Flavor ☞ serving size: 1 oz = 28.4 g; Calories = 142.3; Total Carb (g) = 17.8; Net Carb (g) = 16.7; Fat (g) = 7; Protein = 2

Snacks Tortilla Chips Taco-Flavor ☞ serving size: 1 oz = 28.4 g;

Calories = 136.3; Total Carb (g) = 17.9; Net Carb (g) = 16.4; Fat (g) = 6.9; Protein = 2.2

Snacks Tortilla Chips Unsalted White Corn ☞ serving size: 1 cup = 26 g; Calories = 130.8; Total Carb (g) = 17; Net Carb (g) = 15.6; Fat (g) = 6.1; Protein = 2

Snacks Trail Mix Regular ☞ serving size: 1 cup = 150 g; Calories = 693; Total Carb (g) = 67.4; Net Carb (g) = 67.4; Fat (g) = 44.1; Protein = 20.7

Snacks Trail Mix Regular Unsalted ☞ serving size: 1 cup = 150 g; Calories = 693; Total Carb (g) = 67.4; Net Carb (g) = 67.4; Fat (g) = 44.1; Protein = 20.7

Snacks Trail Mix Regular With Chocolate Chips Unsalted Nuts And Seeds ☞ serving size: 1 cup = 146 g; Calories = 706.6; Total Carb (g) = 65.6; Net Carb (g) = 65.6; Fat (g) = 46.6; Protein = 20.7

Snacks Trail Mix Tropical ☞ serving size: 1 cup = 140 g; Calories = 618.8; Total Carb (g) = 91.8; Net Carb (g) = 91.8; Fat (g) = 23.9; Protein = 8.8

Snacks Vegetable Chips Hain Celestial Group Terra Chips ☞ serving size: 1 oz = 28.4 g; Calories = 146.8; Total Carb (g) = 16.5; Net Carb (g) = 13.4; Fat (g) = 8.5; Protein = 1.2

Snacks Vegetable Chips Made From Garden Vegetables ☞ serving size: 1 oz = 28.4 g; Calories = 134.3; Total Carb (g) = 17.2; Net Carb (g) = 15.8; Fat (g) = 6.6; Protein = 1.5

Snacks Yucca (Cassava) Chips Salted ☞ serving size: 1 oz = 28.4 g; Calories = 146.3; Total Carb (g) = 19.7; Net Carb (g) = 18.6; Fat (g) = 7.4; Protein = 0.4

Snickers Marathon Double Chocolate Nut Bar ☞ serving size: 1 bar = 55 g; Calories = 207.4; Total Carb (g) = 28.4; Net Carb (g) = 22.6; Fat (g) = 4.9; Protein = 12.3

● Soft Pretzels ☞ serving size: 1 large = 143 g; Calories = 493.4; Total Carb (g) = 101.6; Net Carb (g) = 99.2; Fat (g) = 4.4; Protein = 11.7

● Soft Pretzels (Salted) ☞ serving size: 1 large = 143 g; Calories = 483.3; Total Carb (g) = 99.2; Net Carb (g) = 96.8; Fat (g) = 4.4; Protein = 11.7

● Soychips ☞ serving size: 1 oz = 28.4 g; Calories = 109.3; Total Carb (g) = 15.1; Net Carb (g) = 14.1; Fat (g) = 2.1; Protein = 7.5

● Sweet Potato Chips ☞ serving size: 1 chip = 2 g; Calories = 10.6; Total Carb (g) = 1.1; Net Carb (g) = 1; Fat (g) = 0.6; Protein = 0.1

● Tortilla Chips Cool Ranch Flavor (Doritos) ☞ serving size: 1 chip = 3 g; Calories = 14.1; Total Carb (g) = 2; Net Carb (g) = 1.9; Fat (g) = 0.6; Protein = 0.2

● Tortilla Chips Low Fat Baked Without Fat ☞ serving size: 1 oz = 28.4 g; Calories = 127.2; Total Carb (g) = 22.8; Net Carb (g) = 21.3; Fat (g) = 1.6; Protein = 3.1

● Tortilla Chips Popped ☞ serving size: 1 chip = 2 g; Calories = 8.8; Total Carb (g) = 1.5; Net Carb (g) = 1.4; Fat (g) = 0.2; Protein = 0.2

● Tortilla Chips Reduced Fat Flavored ☞ serving size: 1 chip = 2 g; Calories = 8.2; Total Carb (g) = 1.6; Net Carb (g) = 1.5; Fat (g) = 0.1; Protein = 0.2

● Tortilla Chips Reduced Fat Plain ☞ serving size: 1 chip = 2 g; Calories = 8.2; Total Carb (g) = 1.6; Net Carb (g) = 1.5; Fat (g) = 0.1; Protein = 0.2

● Tortilla Chips Reduced Sodium ☞ serving size: 1 chip = 2 g; Calories = 9.8; Total Carb (g) = 1.4; Net Carb (g) = 1.3; Fat (g) = 0.4; Protein = 0.2

● Tortilla Chips Yellow Plain Salted ☞ serving size: 1 oz = 28.4 g; Calories = 141.1; Total Carb (g) = 19.1; Net Carb (g) = 17.8; Fat (g) = 6.3; Protein = 1.9

Trail Mix ☞ serving size: 1 cup = 146 g; Calories = 706.6; Total Carb (g) = 65.6; Net Carb (g) = 58.3; Fat (g) = 46.6; Protein = 20.7

Vegetable Chips ☞ serving size: 1 chip = 2 g; Calories = 9.9; Total Carb (g) = 1.2; Net Carb (g) = 1; Fat (g) = 0.5; Protein = 0.1

26

SOUPS AND SAUCES

Alfredo Sauce ☞ serving size: 1 cup = 260 g; Calories = 382.2; Total Carb (g) = 2.6; Net Carb (g) = 2.6; Fat (g) = 39; Protein = 7

Alfredo Sauce With Added Vegetables ☞ serving size: 1 cup = 260 g; Calories = 306.8; Total Carb (g) = 5; Net Carb (g) = 4.2; Fat (g) = 30.1; Protein = 6.2

Alfredo Sauce With Meat ☞ serving size: 1 cup = 260 g; Calories = 436.8; Total Carb (g) = 2.1; Net Carb (g) = 2.1; Fat (g) = 39.9; Protein = 18.1

Alfredo Sauce With Meat And Added Vegetables ☞ serving size: 1 cup = 260 g; Calories = 377; Total Carb (g) = 4.1; Net Carb (g) = 3.3; Fat (g) = 32.6; Protein = 17.5

Alfredo Sauce With Poultry ☞ serving size: 1 cup = 260 g; Calories = 395.2; Total Carb (g) = 2.1; Net Carb (g) = 2.1; Fat (g) = 35.1; Protein = 19.1

Alfredo Sauce With Poultry And Added Vegetables ☞ serving size: 1 cup = 260 g; Calories = 332.8; Total Carb (g) = 4.1; Net Carb (g) = 3.3; Fat (g) = 27.8; Protein = 18.5

Alfredo Sauce With Seafood ☞ serving size: 1 cup = 260 g; Calories = 369.2; Total Carb (g) = 3.5; Net Carb (g) = 3.5; Fat (g) = 32.4; Protein = 16.5

Alfredo Sauce With Seafood And Added Vegetables ☞ serving size: 1 cup = 260 g; Calories = 309.4; Total Carb (g) = 5.5; Net Carb (g) = 4.7; Fat (g) = 25.1; Protein = 15.9

Artichoke Dip ☞ serving size: 1 tablespoon = 15 g; Calories = 49.5; Total Carb (g) = 0.8; Net Carb (g) = 0.7; Fat (g) = 5; Protein = 0.5

Asparagus Soup Cream Of Ns As To Made With Milk Or Water ☞ serving size: 1 cup = 248 g; Calories = 148.8; Total Carb (g) = 16.6; Net Carb (g) = 16.1; Fat (g) = 6.6; Protein = 6.3

Asparagus Soup Cream Of Prepared With Milk ☞ serving size: 1 cup = 248 g; Calories = 148.8; Total Carb (g) = 16.6; Net Carb (g) = 16.1; Fat (g) = 6.6; Protein = 6.3

Asparagus Soup Cream Of Prepared With Water ☞ serving size: 1 cup = 244 g; Calories = 85.4; Total Carb (g) = 10.6; Net Carb (g) = 10.1; Fat (g) = 4.1; Protein = 2.3

Bacon Soup Cream Of Prepared With Water ☞ serving size: 1 cup = 244 g; Calories = 112.2; Total Carb (g) = 8.9; Net Carb (g) = 8.9; Fat (g) = 7.2; Protein = 3

Barbecue Sauce ☞ serving size: 1 tbsp = 17 g; Calories = 29.2; Total Carb (g) = 6.9; Net Carb (g) = 6.8; Fat (g) = 0.1; Protein = 0.1

Barley Soup Sweet With Or Without Nuts Asian Style ☞ serving size: 1 cup = 244 g; Calories = 148.8; Total Carb (g) = 28.2; Net Carb (g) = 26.3; Fat (g) = 3.8; Protein = 2.5

Bean And Ham Soup Home Recipe ☞ serving size: 1 cup = 247 g; Calories = 202.5; Total Carb (g) = 20.5; Net Carb (g) = 15.6; Fat (g) = 4.9; Protein = 19

Bean Soup Home Recipe ☞ serving size: 1 cup = 247 g; Calories =

160.6; Total Carb (g) = 24.1; Net Carb (g) = 18.2; Fat (g) = 1.9; Protein = 12.6

Bean Soup Mixed Beans Home Recipe Canned Or Ready-To-Serve ☞ serving size: 1 cup = 238 g; Calories = 149.9; Total Carb (g) = 22.6; Net Carb (g) = 16; Fat (g) = 1.9; Protein = 11.3

Bean Soup Nfs ☞ serving size: 1 cup = 253 g; Calories = 172; Total Carb (g) = 22.5; Net Carb (g) = 14.7; Fat (g) = 5.9; Protein = 7.8

Bean Soup With Macaroni Home Recipe Canned Or Ready-To-Serve ☞ serving size: 1 cup = 253 g; Calories = 227.7; Total Carb (g) = 32.8; Net Carb (g) = 27; Fat (g) = 5.7; Protein = 12.2

Bean With Bacon Or Ham Soup Canned Or Ready-To-Serve ☞ serving size: 1 cup = 253 g; Calories = 172; Total Carb (g) = 22.5; Net Carb (g) = 14.7; Fat (g) = 5.9; Protein = 7.8

Beef And Rice Soup Puerto Rican Style ☞ serving size: 1 cup = 250 g; Calories = 147.5; Total Carb (g) = 15.6; Net Carb (g) = 13.3; Fat (g) = 3; Protein = 14.6

Beef Broth From Bouillon ☞ serving size: 1 cup (8 fl oz) = 241 g; Calories = 28.9; Total Carb (g) = 1.8; Net Carb (g) = 1.8; Fat (g) = 0; Protein = 5.4

Beef Broth With Tomato Home Recipe ☞ serving size: 1 cup = 237 g; Calories = 116.1; Total Carb (g) = 5; Net Carb (g) = 3.5; Fat (g) = 9.9; Protein = 2.8

Beef Noodle Soup Canned Or Ready-To-Serve ☞ serving size: 1 cup = 244 g; Calories = 83; Total Carb (g) = 8.9; Net Carb (g) = 8.1; Fat (g) = 3.1; Protein = 4.8

Beef Noodle Soup Home Recipe ☞ serving size: 1 cup = 244 g; Calories = 170.8; Total Carb (g) = 11.2; Net Carb (g) = 10.3; Fat (g) = 5.8; Protein = 17.5

Beef Noodle Soup Puerto Rican Style ☞ serving size: 1 cup = 250

g; Calories = 147.5; Total Carb (g) = 15.4; Net Carb (g) = 13.2; Fat (g) = 3.1; Protein = 14.7

Beef Stock ☞ serving size: 1 cup = 240 g; Calories = 31.2; Total Carb (g) = 2.9; Net Carb (g) = 2.9; Fat (g) = 0.2; Protein = 4.7

Beef Vegetable Soup Home Recipe Mexican Style ☞ serving size: 1 cup = 239 g; Calories = 167.3; Total Carb (g) = 11.7; Net Carb (g) = 9.1; Fat (g) = 5.3; Protein = 18.9

Beer Cheese Soup Made With Milk ☞ serving size: 1 cup = 245 g; Calories = 470.4; Total Carb (g) = 16.3; Net Carb (g) = 15.5; Fat (g) = 37.6; Protein = 15

Bird's Nest Soup ☞ serving size: 1 cup = 244 g; Calories = 112.2; Total Carb (g) = 7.4; Net Carb (g) = 7.4; Fat (g) = 3.1; Protein = 13.2

Black Bean Sauce ☞ serving size: 1 cup = 275 g; Calories = 599.5; Total Carb (g) = 36.1; Net Carb (g) = 27; Fat (g) = 46.5; Protein = 15.2

Black Bean Soup ☞ serving size: 1 cup = 247 g; Calories = 113.6; Total Carb (g) = 19; Net Carb (g) = 10.7; Fat (g) = 1.6; Protein = 6

Borscht ☞ serving size: 1 cup = 245 g; Calories = 100.5; Total Carb (g) = 13.3; Net Carb (g) = 10.6; Fat (g) = 4.3; Protein = 3.4

Broccoli Cheese Soup Prepared With Milk Home Recipe Canned Or Ready-To-Serve ☞ serving size: 1 cup = 239 g; Calories = 164.9; Total Carb (g) = 15; Net Carb (g) = 12.9; Fat (g) = 8.8; Protein = 6.4

Broccoli Soup Prepared With Milk Home Recipe Canned Or Ready-To-Serve ☞ serving size: 1 cup = 237 g; Calories = 163.5; Total Carb (g) = 14.9; Net Carb (g) = 12.8; Fat (g) = 8.7; Protein = 6.4

Broccoli Soup Prepared With Water Home Recipe Canned Or Ready-To-Serve ☞ serving size: 1 cup = 239 g; Calories = 105.2; Total Carb (g) = 9.3; Net Carb (g) = 7.2; Fat (g) = 6.4; Protein = 2.5

Brown Nut Gravy Meatless ☞ serving size: 1 tablespoon = 15 g;

Calories = 18.6; Total Carb (g) = 0.9; Net Carb (g) = 0.7; Fat (g) = 1.6; Protein = 0.3

🍲 Cabbage Soup Home Recipe Canned Or Ready-To-Serve ☞ serving size: 1 cup = 245 g; Calories = 93.1; Total Carb (g) = 15.3; Net Carb (g) = 12.4; Fat (g) = 2.1; Protein = 4.4

🍲 Cabbage With Meat Soup Home Recipe Canned Or Ready-To-Serve ☞ serving size: 1 cup = 245 g; Calories = 112.7; Total Carb (g) = 9.7; Net Carb (g) = 7.7; Fat (g) = 3.2; Protein = 11.8

🍲 Campbells Beef Barley Soup ☞ serving size: 1 cup = 206 g; Calories = 115.4; Total Carb (g) = 18.5; Net Carb (g) = 16.4; Fat (g) = 1.9; Protein = 6

🍲 Campbells Chunky Classic Chicken Noodle Soup ☞ serving size: 1 cup = 243 g; Calories = 114.2; Total Carb (g) = 13.2; Net Carb (g) = 10.7; Fat (g) = 3.2; Protein = 8.3

🍲 Campbells Chunky New England Clam Chowder ☞ serving size: 1 cup = 251 g; Calories = 203.3; Total Carb (g) = 22.6; Net Carb (g) = 19.6; Fat (g) = 9.7; Protein = 6.2

🍲 Campbells Chunky Soups Old Fashioned Vegetable Beef Soup ☞ serving size: 1 cup = 247 g; Calories = 121; Total Carb (g) = 15.4; Net Carb (g) = 12.2; Fat (g) = 3; Protein = 7.8

🍲 Campbells Cream Of Mushroom Soup Condensed ☞ serving size: 1/2 cup condensed = 129 g; Calories = 104.5; Total Carb (g) = 8.5; Net Carb (g) = 7.7; Fat (g) = 7.1; Protein = 1.7

🍲 Campbells Red And White Chicken Noodle Soup Condensed ☞ serving size: 1/2 cup = 123 g; Calories = 57.8; Total Carb (g) = 7.3; Net Carb (g) = 7.3; Fat (g) = 1.9; Protein = 2.9

🍲 Campbells Tomato Soup Condensed ☞ serving size: 1/2 cup condensed = 124 g; Calories = 88; Total Carb (g) = 18.9; Net Carb (g) = 17.5; Fat (g) = 0.6; Protein = 1.8

Canned Minestrone ☞ serving size: 1 cup = 240 g; Calories = 127.2; Total Carb (g) = 20.7; Net Carb (g) = 15; Fat (g) = 2.8; Protein = 5.1

Canned Pizza Sauce ☞ serving size: 1/4 cup = 63 g; Calories = 34; Total Carb (g) = 5.5; Net Carb (g) = 4.2; Fat (g) = 0.7; Protein = 1.4

Carrot Soup Cream Of Prepared With Milk Home Recipe Canned Or Ready-To-Serve ☞ serving size: 1 cup = 237 g; Calories = 75.8; Total Carb (g) = 11.9; Net Carb (g) = 9.5; Fat (g) = 1.8; Protein = 3.7

Carrot With Rice Soup Cream Of Prepared With Milk Home Recipe Canned Or Ready-To-Serve ☞ serving size: 1 cup = 245 g; Calories = 134.8; Total Carb (g) = 24.8; Net Carb (g) = 22.3; Fat (g) = 1.9; Protein = 4.8

Celery Soup Cream Of Prepared With Milk Home Recipe Canned Or Ready-To-Serve ☞ serving size: 1 cup = 248 g; Calories = 151.3; Total Carb (g) = 14.7; Net Carb (g) = 14; Fat (g) = 8.1; Protein = 5.7

Celery Soup Cream Of Prepared With Water Home Recipe Canned Or Ready-To-Serve ☞ serving size: 1 cup = 244 g; Calories = 90.3; Total Carb (g) = 8.7; Net Carb (g) = 8; Fat (g) = 5.5; Protein = 1.6

Cheddar Cheese Soup Home Recipe Canned Or Ready-To-Serve ☞ serving size: 1 cup = 251 g; Calories = 168.2; Total Carb (g) = 20.4; Net Carb (g) = 17.6; Fat (g) = 7.5; Protein = 5.1

Cheese Dip ☞ serving size: 1 tablespoon = 15 g; Calories = 24; Total Carb (g) = 1.2; Net Carb (g) = 1.1; Fat (g) = 2; Protein = 0.5

Cheese Fondue ☞ serving size: 1 tablespoon = 13 g; Calories = 35.9; Total Carb (g) = 0.3; Net Carb (g) = 0.3; Fat (g) = 2.8; Protein = 2.5

Cheese Sauce ☞ serving size: 1 cup = 243 g; Calories = 388.8; Total Carb (g) = 18.6; Net Carb (g) = 17.9; Fat (g) = 31.6; Protein = 7.9

Cheese Sauce Made With Lowfat Cheese ☞ serving size: 1 cup = 243 g; Calories = 303.8; Total Carb (g) = 17.1; Net Carb (g) = 16.9; Fat (g) = 18.8; Protein = 16.6

Chicken Or Turkey And Corn Hominy Soup Home Recipe Mexican Style ☞ serving size: 1 cup = 238 g; Calories = 178.5; Total Carb (g) = 12.2; Net Carb (g) = 11.2; Fat (g) = 5.8; Protein = 18.8

Chicken Or Turkey Broth With Tomato Home Recipe ☞ serving size: 1 cup = 237 g; Calories = 113.8; Total Carb (g) = 5.6; Net Carb (g) = 4.2; Fat (g) = 9.9; Protein = 2

Chicken Or Turkey Corn Soup With Noodles Home Recipe ☞ serving size: 1 cup = 251 g; Calories = 155.6; Total Carb (g) = 18.4; Net Carb (g) = 16.9; Fat (g) = 4.5; Protein = 11.7

Chicken Or Turkey Mushroom Soup Cream Of Prepared With Milk ☞ serving size: 1 cup = 248 g; Calories = 186; Total Carb (g) = 20.8; Net Carb (g) = 16.9; Fat (g) = 8.5; Protein = 6.1

Chicken Or Turkey Noodle Soup Canned Or Ready-To-Serve ☞ serving size: 1 cup = 241 g; Calories = 57.8; Total Carb (g) = 7.4; Net Carb (g) = 6.2; Fat (g) = 1.9; Protein = 2.9

Chicken Or Turkey Noodle Soup Cream Of Home Recipe Canned Or Ready-To-Serve ☞ serving size: 1 cup = 245 g; Calories = 120.1; Total Carb (g) = 13.4; Net Carb (g) = 12.4; Fat (g) = 4.4; Protein = 6.9

Chicken Or Turkey Noodle Soup Home Recipe ☞ serving size: 1 cup = 241 g; Calories = 147; Total Carb (g) = 11.9; Net Carb (g) = 10.9; Fat (g) = 5.3; Protein = 13.4

Chicken Or Turkey Rice Soup Canned Or Ready-To-Serve ☞ serving size: 1 cup = 241 g; Calories = 81.9; Total Carb (g) = 14; Net Carb (g) = 12.8; Fat (g) = 1.9; Protein = 2.2

Chicken Or Turkey Rice Soup Home Recipe ☞ serving size: 1 cup = 231 g; Calories = 143.2; Total Carb (g) = 13.1; Net Carb (g) = 12.4; Fat (g) = 4.6; Protein = 12.1

Chicken Or Turkey Rice Soup Reduced Sodium Canned

Prepared With Milk ☞ serving size: 1 cup = 245 g; Calories = 117.6; Total Carb (g) = 14.7; Net Carb (g) = 13.7; Fat (g) = 4; Protein = 6

🥣 Chicken Or Turkey Rice Soup Reduced Sodium Canned Prepared With Water Or Ready-To-Serve ☞ serving size: 1 cup = 241 g; Calories = 55.4; Total Carb (g) = 8.7; Net Carb (g) = 7.7; Fat (g) = 1.5; Protein = 1.9

🥣 Chicken Or Turkey Soup Cream Of Canned Reduced Sodium Made With Milk ☞ serving size: 1 cup = 248 g; Calories = 133.9; Total Carb (g) = 17.8; Net Carb (g) = 17.3; Fat (g) = 4.1; Protein = 6.3

🥣 Chicken Or Turkey Soup Cream Of Canned Reduced Sodium Made With Water ☞ serving size: 1 cup = 244 g; Calories = 70.8; Total Carb (g) = 11.8; Net Carb (g) = 11.3; Fat (g) = 1.6; Protein = 2.2

🥣 Chicken Or Turkey Soup Cream Of Canned Reduced Sodium Ns As To Made With Milk Or Water ☞ serving size: 1 cup = 244 g; Calories = 70.8; Total Carb (g) = 11.8; Net Carb (g) = 11.3; Fat (g) = 1.6; Protein = 2.2

🥣 Chicken Or Turkey Soup Cream Of Ns As To Prepared With Milk Or Water ☞ serving size: 1 cup = 244 g; Calories = 112.2; Total Carb (g) = 8.9; Net Carb (g) = 8.9; Fat (g) = 7.2; Protein = 3

🥣 Chicken Or Turkey Soup Cream Of Prepared With Milk ☞ serving size: 1 cup = 248 g; Calories = 173.6; Total Carb (g) = 14.9; Net Carb (g) = 14.9; Fat (g) = 9.7; Protein = 7

🥣 Chicken Or Turkey Soup Cream Of Prepared With Water ☞ serving size: 1 cup = 244 g; Calories = 112.2; Total Carb (g) = 8.9; Net Carb (g) = 8.9; Fat (g) = 7.2; Protein = 3

🥣 Chicken Or Turkey Soup With Vegetables And Fruit Asian Style ☞ serving size: 1 cup = 234 g; Calories = 91.3; Total Carb (g) = 4.9; Net Carb (g) = 4.4; Fat (g) = 2.9; Protein = 11.9

🥣 Chicken Or Turkey Soup With Vegetables Broccoli Carrots Celery Potatoes And Onions Asian Style ☞ serving size: 1 cup = 228 g; Calories = 111.7; Total Carb (g) = 5; Net Carb (g) = 3.6; Fat (g) = 5; Protein = 12.4

Chicken Or Turkey Vegetable Soup Home Recipe ☞ serving size: 1 cup = 239 g; Calories = 114.7; Total Carb (g) = 10; Net Carb (g) = 8.1; Fat (g) = 4.1; Protein = 10.9

Chicken Or Turkey Vegetable Soup With Rice Home Recipe Mexican Style ☞ serving size: 1 cup = 242 g; Calories = 186.3; Total Carb (g) = 19.2; Net Carb (g) = 16.6; Fat (g) = 5.3; Protein = 16.6

Chicken Rice Soup Puerto Rican Style ☞ serving size: 1 cup = 220 g; Calories = 169.4; Total Carb (g) = 18.9; Net Carb (g) = 17; Fat (g) = 3.5; Protein = 15.9

Chicken Soup With Noodles And Potatoes Puerto Rican Style ☞ serving size: 1 cup = 220 g; Calories = 162.8; Total Carb (g) = 19.1; Net Carb (g) = 17.1; Fat (g) = 3.2; Protein = 14.9

Chicken Stock ☞ serving size: 1 cup = 240 g; Calories = 86.4; Total Carb (g) = 8.5; Net Carb (g) = 8.5; Fat (g) = 2.9; Protein = 6.1

Chipotle Dip Light ☞ serving size: 1 tablespoon = 15 g; Calories = 29.1; Total Carb (g) = 2; Net Carb (g) = 2; Fat (g) = 2.3; Protein = 0.3

Chipotle Dip Regular ☞ serving size: 1 tablespoon = 15 g; Calories = 64.1; Total Carb (g) = 0.4; Net Carb (g) = 0.4; Fat (g) = 6.9; Protein = 0.3

Chipotle Dip Yogurt Based ☞ serving size: 1 tablespoon = 15 g; Calories = 28.4; Total Carb (g) = 0.5; Net Carb (g) = 0.5; Fat (g) = 2.4; Protein = 1.2

Chutney ☞ serving size: 1 tablespoon = 17 g; Calories = 25.5; Total Carb (g) = 6.3; Net Carb (g) = 5.9; Fat (g) = 0.1; Protein = 0.2

Clam Chowder New England Prepared With Milk ☞ serving size: 1 cup = 248 g; Calories = 151.3; Total Carb (g) = 18.7; Net Carb (g) = 18; Fat (g) = 5.1; Protein = 8

Clam Chowder Ns As To Manhattan Or New England Style ☞ serving size: 1 cup = 244 g; Calories = 148.8; Total Carb (g) = 18.4; Net Carb (g) = 17.7; Fat (g) = 5; Protein = 7.9

Cocktail Sauce ☞ serving size: 1 cup = 273 g; Calories = 338.5; Total Carb (g) = 77; Net Carb (g) = 72.1; Fat (g) = 2.9; Protein = 3.7

Codfish Rice And Vegetable Soup Puerto Rican Style ☞ serving size: 1 cup = 245 g; Calories = 166.6; Total Carb (g) = 18.6; Net Carb (g) = 17.6; Fat (g) = 4; Protein = 13

Codfish Soup With Noodles Puerto Rican Style ☞ serving size: 1 cup = 245 g; Calories = 176.4; Total Carb (g) = 18.4; Net Carb (g) = 16.9; Fat (g) = 5.1; Protein = 14

Corn Soup Cream Of Prepared With Milk ☞ serving size: 1 cup = 248 g; Calories = 104.2; Total Carb (g) = 16.9; Net Carb (g) = 14.9; Fat (g) = 2.8; Protein = 5.1

Corn Soup Cream Of Prepared With Water ☞ serving size: 1 cup = 244 g; Calories = 158.6; Total Carb (g) = 31.7; Net Carb (g) = 29.7; Fat (g) = 4.3; Protein = 3.1

Crab Soup Cream Of Prepared With Milk ☞ serving size: 1 cup = 248 g; Calories = 126.5; Total Carb (g) = 4.2; Net Carb (g) = 3.7; Fat (g) = 6.4; Protein = 12.5

Crab Soup Ns As To Tomato-Base Or Cream Style ☞ serving size: 1 cup = 244 g; Calories = 124.4; Total Carb (g) = 4.2; Net Carb (g) = 3.7; Fat (g) = 6.3; Protein = 12.3

Crab Soup Tomato-Base ☞ serving size: 1 cup = 244 g; Calories = 95.2; Total Carb (g) = 12.5; Net Carb (g) = 10.1; Fat (g) = 0.8; Protein = 10.4

Cream Of Asparagus Soup ☞ serving size: 1 cup (8 fl oz) = 244 g; Calories = 85.4; Total Carb (g) = 10.7; Net Carb (g) = 10.2; Fat (g) = 4.1; Protein = 2.3

Cream Of Chicken Soup ☞ serving size: 1 cup = 244 g; Calories = 117.1; Total Carb (g) = 9.3; Net Carb (g) = 9; Fat (g) = 7.4; Protein = 3.4

Cream Of Mushroom Soup ☞ serving size: 1 serving 1 cup = 248 g; Calories = 96.7; Total Carb (g) = 8.3; Net Carb (g) = 7.5; Fat (g) = 6.4; Protein = 1.6

Dark-Green Leafy Vegetable Soup Meatless Asian Style ☞ serving size: 1 cup = 226 g; Calories = 108.5; Total Carb (g) = 14.4; Net Carb (g) = 11.7; Fat (g) = 4.4; Protein = 3.5

Dark-Green Leafy Vegetable Soup With Meat Asian Style ☞ serving size: 1 cup = 228 g; Calories = 175.6; Total Carb (g) = 12.3; Net Carb (g) = 10; Fat (g) = 7.5; Protein = 14.7

Dill Dip Light ☞ serving size: 1 tablespoon = 15 g; Calories = 29.6; Total Carb (g) = 2; Net Carb (g) = 2; Fat (g) = 2.3; Protein = 0.3

Dill Dip Regular ☞ serving size: 1 tablespoon = 15 g; Calories = 64.4; Total Carb (g) = 0.5; Net Carb (g) = 0.4; Fat (g) = 6.9; Protein = 0.3

Dill Dip Yogurt Based ☞ serving size: 1 tablespoon = 15 g; Calories = 28.7; Total Carb (g) = 0.6; Net Carb (g) = 0.5; Fat (g) = 2.4; Protein = 1.2

Dip Bean Original Flavor ☞ serving size: 2 tbsp = 36 g; Calories = 42.8; Total Carb (g) = 5.7; Net Carb (g) = 4; Fat (g) = 1.3; Protein = 2

Dip Fritos Bean Original Flavor ☞ serving size: 2 tbsp - 36 g; Calories = 42.8; Total Carb (g) = 5.7; Net Carb (g) = 4; Fat (g) = 1.3; Protein = 2

Dip Nfs ☞ serving size: 1 tablespoon = 15 g; Calories = 65; Total Carb (g) = 0.5; Net Carb (g) = 0.5; Fat (g) = 6.9; Protein = 0.3

Dip Salsa Con Queso Cheese And Salsa- Medium ☞ serving size: 2 tbsp = 30 g; Calories = 42.9; Total Carb (g) = 3.3; Net Carb (g) = 3.1; Fat (g) = 2.9; Protein = 0.9

Dip Tostitos Salsa Con Queso Medium ☞ serving size: 2 tbsp = 30 g; Calories = 39.9; Total Carb (g) = 3.5; Net Carb (g) = 3.3; Fat (g) = 2.5; Protein = 0.9

Duck Sauce ☞ serving size: 1 cup = 290 g; Calories = 710.5; Total Carb (g) = 175.8; Net Carb (g) = 174; Fat (g) = 0.4; Protein = 1

Duck Soup ☞ serving size: 1 cup = 244 g; Calories = 183; Total Carb (g) = 2.7; Net Carb (g) = 2.5; Fat (g) = 7.8; Protein = 24.2

Eggplant Dip ☞ serving size: 1 tablespoon = 15 g; Calories = 25.1; Total Carb (g) = 1.7; Net Carb (g) = 1.1; Fat (g) = 2; Protein = 0.6

Enchilada Sauce Green ☞ serving size: 1 cup = 250 g; Calories = 70; Total Carb (g) = 13.8; Net Carb (g) = 10.3; Fat (g) = 1.5; Protein = 2.5

Fish And Vegetable Soup No Potatoes Mexican Style ☞ serving size: 1 cup = 250 g; Calories = 97.5; Total Carb (g) = 3.7; Net Carb (g) = 2.9; Fat (g) = 3.2; Protein = 12.9

Fish Broth ☞ serving size: 1 cup = 244 g; Calories = 39; Total Carb (g) = 1; Net Carb (g) = 1; Fat (g) = 1.5; Protein = 4.9

Fish Chowder ☞ serving size: 1 cup = 244 g; Calories = 275.7; Total Carb (g) = 14.9; Net Carb (g) = 12.9; Fat (g) = 15.2; Protein = 19.7

Fish Soup With Potatoes Mexican Style ☞ serving size: 1 cup = 241 g; Calories = 110.9; Total Carb (g) = 6.4; Net Carb (g) = 5.6; Fat (g) = 3.2; Protein = 13.2

Fish Stock ☞ serving size: 1 cup = 233 g; Calories = 37.3; Total Carb (g) = 0; Net Carb (g) = 0; Fat (g) = 1.9; Protein = 5.3

Flour And Water Gravy ☞ serving size: 1 cup = 240 g; Calories = 192; Total Carb (g) = 40.1; Net Carb (g) = 38.7; Fat (g) = 0.5; Protein = 5.4

Garbanzo Bean Or Chickpea Soup Home Recipe Canned Or Ready-To-Serve ☞ serving size: 1 cup = 253 g; Calories = 179.6; Total Carb (g) = 25.4; Net Carb (g) = 18.6; Fat (g) = 3.8; Protein = 11.8

Garlic Cooked ☞ serving size: 1 clove = 2 g; Calories = 3; Total Carb (g) = 0.7; Net Carb (g) = 0.6; Fat (g) = 0; Protein = 0.1

Garlic Egg Soup Puerto Rican Style ☞ serving size: 1 cup = 202 g; Calories = 163.6; Total Carb (g) = 11.2; Net Carb (g) = 10.6; Fat (g) = 9.7; Protein = 7.5

Garlic Sauce ☞ serving size: 1 cup = 228 g; Calories = 246.2; Total Carb (g) = 16.7; Net Carb (g) = 16.2; Fat (g) = 16.9; Protein = 7

Gazpacho ☞ serving size: 1 cup = 244 g; Calories = 90.3; Total Carb (g) = 9.4; Net Carb (g) = 6.7; Fat (g) = 5.7; Protein = 2.1

Gravy Au Jus Canned ☞ serving size: 1/4 cup = 59 g; Calories = 9.4; Total Carb (g) = 1.5; Net Carb (g) = 1.5; Fat (g) = 0.1; Protein = 0.7

Gravy Au Jus Dry ☞ serving size: 1 tsp = 3 g; Calories = 9.4; Total Carb (g) = 1.4; Net Carb (g) = 1.4; Fat (g) = 0.3; Protein = 0.3

Gravy Beef Canned Ready-To-Serve ☞ serving size: 1 cup = 233 g; Calories = 123.5; Total Carb (g) = 11.2; Net Carb (g) = 10.3; Fat (g) = 5.5; Protein = 8.7

Gravy Beef Or Meat Fat Free ☞ serving size: 1 cup = 227 g; Calories = 93.1; Total Carb (g) = 15; Net Carb (g) = 14.1; Fat (g) = 2.7; Protein = 2.3

Gravy Beef Or Meat Home Recipe ☞ serving size: 1 cup = 233 g; Calories = 247; Total Carb (g) = 5.7; Net Carb (g) = 5.5; Fat (g) = 22.9; Protein = 3.9

Gravy Brown Dry ☞ serving size: 1 tbsp = 6 g; Calories = 22; Total Carb (g) = 3.6; Net Carb (g) = 3.4; Fat (g) = 0.6; Protein = 0.6

Gravy Brown Instant Dry ☞ serving size: 1 serving = 6.7 g; Calories = 25.5; Total Carb (g) = 4; Net Carb (g) = 3.8; Fat (g) = 0.8; Protein = 0.6

Gravy Campbells Chicken ☞ serving size: 1/4 cup = 56 g; Calo-

ries = 28.6; Total Carb (g) = 3.3; Net Carb (g) = 3.3; Fat (g) = 1.5; Protein = 0.4

Gravy Chicken Canned Or Bottled Ready-To-Serve ☞ serving size: 1/4 cup = 57 g; Calories = 27.4; Total Carb (g) = 3; Net Carb (g) = 3; Fat (g) = 1.5; Protein = 0.4

Gravy Chicken Dry ☞ serving size: 1 tbsp = 8 g; Calories = 30.5; Total Carb (g) = 5; Net Carb (g) = 5; Fat (g) = 0.8; Protein = 0.9

Gravy Giblet ☞ serving size: 1 cup = 238 g; Calories = 145.2; Total Carb (g) = 11.1; Net Carb (g) = 10.7; Fat (g) = 6.4; Protein = 9.9

Gravy Heinz Home Style Classic Chicken ☞ serving size: 1/4 cup = 58 g; Calories = 26.7; Total Carb (g) = 2.9; Net Carb (g) = 2.9; Fat (g) = 1.5; Protein = 0.4

Gravy Heinz Home Style Savory Beef ☞ serving size: 1 serving 1/4 cup 2 oz = 57 g; Calories = 22.2; Total Carb (g) = 3.6; Net Carb (g) = 3.2; Fat (g) = 0.6; Protein = 0.6

Gravy Instant Beef Dry ☞ serving size: 1 serving = 6.7 g; Calories = 24.7; Total Carb (g) = 4.1; Net Carb (g) = 3.8; Fat (g) = 0.6; Protein = 0.7

Gravy Instant Turkey Dry ☞ serving size: 1 serving = 6.7 g; Calories = 27.4; Total Carb (g) = 3.9; Net Carb (g) = 3.6; Fat (g) = 1; Protein = 0.8

Gravy Meat Or Poultry Low Sodium Prepared ☞ serving size: 1 cup = 236 g; Calories = 125.1; Total Carb (g) = 14.5; Net Carb (g) = 13.8; Fat (g) = 5.7; Protein = 9

Gravy Meat Or Poultry With Wine ☞ serving size: 1 cup = 236 g; Calories = 87.3; Total Carb (g) = 9.1; Net Carb (g) = 8.7; Fat (g) = 4.1; Protein = 4

Gravy Meat With Fruit ☞ serving size: 1 cup = 238 g; Calories = 119; Total Carb (g) = 16.6; Net Carb (g) = 15.9; Fat (g) = 4.5; Protein = 4.2

🥣 Gravy Meat-Based From Puerto-Rican Style Beef Stew ☞ serving size: 1 cup = 208 g; Calories = 170.6; Total Carb (g) = 3.1; Net Carb (g) = 2.2; Fat (g) = 17.5; Protein = 0.6

🥣 Gravy Meat-Based From Puerto-Rican Style Stuffed Pot Roast ☞ serving size: 1 cup = 272 g; Calories = 666.4; Total Carb (g) = 0; Net Carb (g) = 0; Fat (g) = 74.3; Protein = 0

🥣 Gravy Mushroom ☞ serving size: 1 cup = 238 g; Calories = 64.3; Total Carb (g) = 12.7; Net Carb (g) = 11.7; Fat (g) = 0.8; Protein = 2

🥣 Gravy Mushroom Canned ☞ serving size: 1 cup = 238 g; Calories = 119; Total Carb (g) = 13; Net Carb (g) = 12.1; Fat (g) = 6.5; Protein = 3

🥣 Gravy Mushroom Dry Powder ☞ serving size: 1 cup (8 fl oz) = 21 g; Calories = 68.9; Total Carb (g) = 13.6; Net Carb (g) = 12.6; Fat (g) = 0.8; Protein = 2.1

🥣 Gravy Onion Dry Mix ☞ serving size: 1 cup (8 fl oz) = 24 g; Calories = 77.3; Total Carb (g) = 16.2; Net Carb (g) = 14.8; Fat (g) = 0.7; Protein = 2.2

🥣 Gravy Or Sauce Made With Soy Sauce Stock Or Bouillon Cornstarch ☞ serving size: 1 cup = 233 g; Calories = 104.9; Total Carb (g) = 22.9; Net Carb (g) = 22.7; Fat (g) = 0.7; Protein = 1.9

🥣 Gravy Or Sauce Poultry-Based From Puerto Rican-Style Chicken Fricasse ☞ serving size: 1 cup = 240 g; Calories = 508.8; Total Carb (g) = 12.6; Net Carb (g) = 9.5; Fat (g) = 51.6; Protein = 2.1

🥣 Gravy Pork Dry Powder ☞ serving size: 1 serving = 6.7 g; Calories = 24.6; Total Carb (g) = 4.3; Net Carb (g) = 4.1; Fat (g) = 0.6; Protein = 0.6

🥣 Gravy Poultry Fat Free ☞ serving size: 1 cup = 227 g; Calories = 102.2; Total Carb (g) = 14.3; Net Carb (g) = 13.4; Fat (g) = 3.7; Protein = 2.9

🥣 Gravy Poultry Home Recipe ☞ serving size: 1 cup = 238 g; Calo-

ries = 249.9; Total Carb (g) = 6.8; Net Carb (g) = 6.5; Fat (g) = 23.4; Protein = 2.8

Gravy Redeye ☞ serving size: 1 cup = 242 g; Calories = 106.5; Total Carb (g) = 0; Net Carb (g) = 0; Fat (g) = 11; Protein = 1.3

Gravy Turkey Canned Ready-To-Serve ☞ serving size: 1 cup = 238 g; Calories = 121.4; Total Carb (g) = 12.1; Net Carb (g) = 11.2; Fat (g) = 5; Protein = 6.2

Gravy Turkey Dry ☞ serving size: 1 serving = 7 g; Calories = 25.7; Total Carb (g) = 4.6; Net Carb (g) = 4.6; Fat (g) = 0.5; Protein = 0.7

Gravy Unspecified Type Dry ☞ serving size: 1 cup (8 fl oz) = 25 g; Calories = 86; Total Carb (g) = 14.5; Net Carb (g) = 14.5; Fat (g) = 2; Protein = 3.3

Guacamole Nfs ☞ serving size: 1 tablespoon = 15 g; Calories = 23.3; Total Carb (g) = 1.3; Net Carb (g) = 0.3; Fat (g) = 2.1; Protein = 0.3

Guacamole With Tomatoes ☞ serving size: 1 tablespoon = 15 g; Calories = 21.8; Total Carb (g) = 1.2; Net Carb (g) = 0.3; Fat (g) = 2; Protein = 0.3

Ham Noodle And Vegetable Soup Puerto Rican Style ☞ serving size: 1 cup = 250 g; Calories = 150; Total Carb (g) = 15.8; Net Carb (g) = 13.6; Fat (g) = 3.3; Protein = 14.7

Ham Rice And Potato Soup Puerto Rican Style ☞ serving size: 1 cup = 240 g; Calories = 134.4; Total Carb (g) = 19.1; Net Carb (g) = 17.6; Fat (g) = 2.5; Protein = 8.6

Hoisin Sauce ☞ serving size: 1 tbsp = 16 g; Calories = 35.2; Total Carb (g) = 7.1; Net Carb (g) = 6.6; Fat (g) = 0.5; Protein = 0.5

Hollandaise Sauce ☞ serving size: 1 cup = 257 g; Calories = 1295.3; Total Carb (g) = 3.9; Net Carb (g) = 3.9; Fat (g) = 139.4; Protein = 12

Honey Mustard Dip ☞ serving size: 1 tablespoon = 15 g; Calories

= 40.1; Total Carb (g) = 3.8; Net Carb (g) = 3.7; Fat (g) = 2.7; Protein = 0.3

🍲 Hot Sauce ☞ serving size: 1 tsp = 4.7 g; Calories = 0.5; Total Carb (g) = 0.1; Net Carb (g) = 0.1; Fat (g) = 0; Protein = 0

🍲 Hummus Flavored ☞ serving size: 1 tablespoon = 15 g; Calories = 38.7; Total Carb (g) = 2.9; Net Carb (g) = 2.1; Fat (g) = 2.7; Protein = 1.2

🍲 Hummus Plain ☞ serving size: 1 tablespoon = 15 g; Calories = 39; Total Carb (g) = 3; Net Carb (g) = 2.1; Fat (g) = 2.7; Protein = 1.2

🍲 Instant Soup Noodle ☞ serving size: 1 cup = 240 g; Calories = 60; Total Carb (g) = 10; Net Carb (g) = 9.5; Fat (g) = 1.1; Protein = 2.5

🍲 Instant Soup Noodle With Egg Shrimp Or Chicken ☞ serving size: 1 cup = 240 g; Calories = 160.8; Total Carb (g) = 22; Net Carb (g) = 21.1; Fat (g) = 6.4; Protein = 3.7

🍲 Italian Wedding Soup ☞ serving size: 1 cup = 244 g; Calories = 168.4; Total Carb (g) = 15.6; Net Carb (g) = 13.7; Fat (g) = 6.4; Protein = 12

🍲 Lamb Pasta And Vegetable Soup Puerto Rican Style ☞ serving size: 1 cup = 250 g; Calories = 225; Total Carb (g) = 15.1; Net Carb (g) = 12.6; Fat (g) = 13; Protein = 12

🍲 Layer Dip ☞ serving size: 1 tablespoon = 15 g; Calories = 21.8; Total Carb (g) = 1; Net Carb (g) = 0.7; Fat (g) = 1.7; Protein = 0.8

🍲 Leek Soup Cream Of Prepared With Milk ☞ serving size: 1 cup = 248 g; Calories = 171.1; Total Carb (g) = 18.9; Net Carb (g) = 18.4; Fat (g) = 7.7; Protein = 6.8

🍲 Lemon-Butter Sauce ☞ serving size: 1 cup = 228 g; Calories = 1420.4; Total Carb (g) = 2.2; Net Carb (g) = 1.7; Fat (g) = 160; Protein = 2.1

🍲 Lentil Soup Home Recipe Canned Or Ready-To-Serve ☞

serving size: 1 cup = 248 g; Calories = 158.7; Total Carb (g) = 22; Net Carb (g) = 14; Fat (g) = 4.1; Protein = 9.7

Lima Bean Soup Home Recipe Canned Or Ready-To-Serve ☞ serving size: 1 cup = 253 g; Calories = 146.7; Total Carb (g) = 21.6; Net Carb (g) = 14.7; Fat (g) = 2; Protein = 11.3

Lobster Bisque ☞ serving size: 1 cup = 248 g; Calories = 129; Total Carb (g) = 4.2; Net Carb (g) = 3.7; Fat (g) = 6.5; Protein = 13

Lobster Sauce ☞ serving size: 1 cup = 234 g; Calories = 341.6; Total Carb (g) = 9.9; Net Carb (g) = 9.6; Fat (g) = 24.4; Protein = 20.1

Low Sodium Minestrone ☞ serving size: 1 cup = 245 g; Calories = 122.5; Total Carb (g) = 22.1; Net Carb (g) = 16.2; Fat (g) = 2; Protein = 4.9

Manhattan Clam Chowder ☞ serving size: 1 cup (8 fl oz) = 240 g; Calories = 134.4; Total Carb (g) = 18.8; Net Carb (g) = 15.9; Fat (g) = 3.4; Protein = 7.3

Manhattan Clam Chowder (Prepared With Equal Part Water) ☞ serving size: 1 serving 1 cup = 249 g; Calories = 74.7; Total Carb (g) = 11.9; Net Carb (g) = 10.4; Fat (g) = 2.1; Protein = 2.1

Matzo Ball Soup ☞ serving size: 1 cup = 241 g; Calories = 144.6; Total Carb (g) = 18.7; Net Carb (g) = 17.5; Fat (g) = 4.9; Protein = 6.3

Meat And Corn Hominy Soup Home Recipe Mexican Style ☞ serving size: 1 cup = 238 g; Calories = 214.2; Total Carb (g) = 12.2; Net Carb (g) = 11.2; Fat (g) = 9.8; Protein = 17.8

Meatball Soup Home Recipe Mexican Style ☞ serving size: 1 cup = 237 g; Calories = 256; Total Carb (g) = 23.5; Net Carb (g) = 19.4; Fat (g) = 11; Protein = 16.2

Menudo Soup Canned Prepared With Water Or Ready-To-Serve ☞ serving size: 1 cup = 241 g; Calories = 96.4; Total Carb (g) = 10.1; Net Carb (g) = 6.2; Fat (g) = 3.4; Protein = 8.1

Menudo Soup Home Recipe ☞ serving size: 1 cup = 241 g; Calories = 118.1; Total Carb (g) = 8; Net Carb (g) = 6.8; Fat (g) = 3.9; Protein = 12.6

Mexican Style Chicken Broth Soup Stock ☞ serving size: 1 cup = 242 g; Calories = 118.6; Total Carb (g) = 18.7; Net Carb (g) = 15.3; Fat (g) = 3.1; Protein = 5.7

Milk Gravy Quick Gravy ☞ serving size: 1 cup = 250 g; Calories = 340; Total Carb (g) = 21.4; Net Carb (g) = 21.1; Fat (g) = 24; Protein = 9.7

Minestrone ☞ serving size: 1 cup (8 fl oz) = 241 g; Calories = 81.9; Total Carb (g) = 11.2; Net Carb (g) = 10.3; Fat (g) = 2.5; Protein = 4.3

Minestrone Soup Canned Prepared With Water Or Ready-To-Serve ☞ serving size: 1 cup = 241 g; Calories = 81.9; Total Carb (g) = 11.1; Net Carb (g) = 10.1; Fat (g) = 2.5; Protein = 4.2

Minestrone Soup Home Recipe ☞ serving size: 1 cup = 235 g; Calories = 143.4; Total Carb (g) = 22.8; Net Carb (g) = 18.5; Fat (g) = 2.6; Protein = 8.2

Miso Sauce ☞ serving size: 1 cup = 240 g; Calories = 372; Total Carb (g) = 66.9; Net Carb (g) = 61.1; Fat (g) = 6.5; Protein = 13.9

Mole Poblano Sauce ☞ serving size: 1 cup = 265 g; Calories = 376.3; Total Carb (g) = 30.6; Net Carb (g) = 23.2; Fat (g) = 27.3; Protein = 7.7

Mole Verde Sauce ☞ serving size: 1 cup = 265 g; Calories = 220; Total Carb (g) = 14.5; Net Carb (g) = 10; Fat (g) = 15.2; Protein = 11.3

Mushroom Barley Soup ☞ serving size: 1 cup (8 fl oz) = 244 g; Calories = 73.2; Total Carb (g) = 11.7; Net Carb (g) = 11; Fat (g) = 2.3; Protein = 1.9

Mushroom Soup Cream Of Canned Reduced Sodium Ns As To Made With Milk Or Water ☞ serving size: 1 cup = 246 g; Calories = 64; Total Carb (g) = 10.1; Net Carb (g) = 9.4; Fat (g) = 2.1; Protein = 1.5

Mushroom Soup Cream Of Canned Reduced Sodium Prepared With Milk ☞ serving size: 1 cup = 248 g; Calories = 126.5; Total Carb (g) = 16.1; Net Carb (g) = 15.3; Fat (g) = 4.6; Protein = 5.6

Mushroom Soup Cream Of Canned Reduced Sodium Prepared With Water ☞ serving size: 1 cup = 244 g; Calories = 63.4; Total Carb (g) = 10; Net Carb (g) = 9.3; Fat (g) = 2.1; Protein = 1.5

Mushroom Soup Cream Of Ns As To Made With Milk Or Water ☞ serving size: 1 cup = 246 g; Calories = 159.9; Total Carb (g) = 14.3; Net Carb (g) = 13.6; Fat (g) = 9; Protein = 5.7

Mushroom Soup Cream Of Prepared With Milk ☞ serving size: 1 cup = 248 g; Calories = 161.2; Total Carb (g) = 14.4; Net Carb (g) = 13.7; Fat (g) = 9.1; Protein = 5.7

Mushroom Soup Cream Of Prepared With Water ☞ serving size: 1 cup = 244 g; Calories = 97.6; Total Carb (g) = 8.4; Net Carb (g) = 7.4; Fat (g) = 6.5; Protein = 1.7

Mushroom Soup With Meat Broth Prepared With Water ☞ serving size: 1 cup = 244 g; Calories = 83; Total Carb (g) = 9.2; Net Carb (g) = 8.9; Fat (g) = 4; Protein = 3.1

Mushroom With Chicken Soup Cream Of Prepared With Milk ☞ serving size: 1 cup = 248 g; Calories = 186; Total Carb (g) = 20.8; Net Carb (g) = 16.9; Fat (g) = 8.5; Protein = 6.1

New England Clam Chowder ☞ serving size: 1 serving 1 cup = 248 g; Calories = 86.8; Total Carb (g) = 12.5; Net Carb (g) = 11.8; Fat (g) = 2.5; Protein = 3.8

Noodle And Potato Soup Puerto Rican Style ☞ serving size: 1 cup = 245 g; Calories = 71.1; Total Carb (g) = 15.9; Net Carb (g) = 13.9; Fat (g) = 0.3; Protein = 2.1

Noodle Soup Nfs ☞ serving size: 1 cup = 241 g; Calories = 161.5; Total Carb (g) = 22.1; Net Carb (g) = 21.1; Fat (g) = 6.5; Protein = 3.7

Noodle Soup With Fish Ball Shrimp And Dark Green Leafy

Vegetable ☞ serving size: 1 cup = 234 g; Calories = 173.2; Total Carb (g) = 23.9; Net Carb (g) = 22.3; Fat (g) = 3.7; Protein = 10.4

Noodle Soup With Vegetables Asian Style ☞ serving size: 1 cup = 228 g; Calories = 161.9; Total Carb (g) = 30; Net Carb (g) = 27.3; Fat (g) = 2.7; Protein = 4.4

Onion Dip Light ☞ serving size: 1 tablespoon = 15 g; Calories = 24.5; Total Carb (g) = 1.7; Net Carb (g) = 1.7; Fat (g) = 1.9; Protein = 0.3

Onion Dip Regular ☞ serving size: 1 tablespoon = 15 g; Calories = 51.8; Total Carb (g) = 0.5; Net Carb (g) = 0.5; Fat (g) = 5.4; Protein = 0.3

Onion Dip Yogurt Based ☞ serving size: 1 tablespoon = 15 g; Calories = 23.7; Total Carb (g) = 0.6; Net Carb (g) = 0.5; Fat (g) = 1.9; Protein = 1

Onion Soup Cream Of Prepared With Milk ☞ serving size: 1 cup = 248 g; Calories = 171.1; Total Carb (g) = 18.9; Net Carb (g) = 18.4; Fat (g) = 7.7; Protein = 6.8

Onion Soup French ☞ serving size: 1 cup = 241 g; Calories = 378.4; Total Carb (g) = 41.9; Net Carb (g) = 39; Fat (g) = 15.9; Protein = 17.9

Osyter Sauce ☞ serving size: 1 tbsp = 18 g; Calories = 9.2; Total Carb (g) = 2; Net Carb (g) = 1.9; Fat (g) = 0.1; Protein = 0.2

Oxtail Soup ☞ serving size: 1 cup = 244 g; Calories – 207.4; Total Carb (g) = 3.3; Net Carb (g) = 2.6; Fat (g) = 11.9; Protein = 20.5

Oyster Sauce ☞ serving size: 1 cup = 256 g; Calories = 325.1; Total Carb (g) = 19.9; Net Carb (g) = 19.4; Fat (g) = 20.8; Protein = 14.1

Oyster Stew ☞ serving size: 1 cup = 245 g; Calories = 196; Total Carb (g) = 10.3; Net Carb (g) = 10.3; Fat (g) = 12.6; Protein = 10.3

Pasta Sauce ☞ serving size: 1 serving 1/2 cup = 132 g; Calories = 66; Total Carb (g) = 9.8; Net Carb (g) = 7.4; Fat (g) = 2.1; Protein = 1.8

🥣 Pea Soup Prepared With Milk ☞ serving size: 1 cup = 254 g; Calories = 226.1; Total Carb (g) = 32.2; Net Carb (g) = 27.2; Fat (g) = 5.4; Protein = 12.6

🥣 Pepper Hot Chili Raw ☞ serving size: 1 piece = 11 g; Calories = 4.4; Total Carb (g) = 1; Net Carb (g) = 0.8; Fat (g) = 0; Protein = 0.2

🥣 Pepperpot Soup ☞ serving size: 1 cup = 241 g; Calories = 113.3; Total Carb (g) = 7.5; Net Carb (g) = 6.8; Fat (g) = 5.8; Protein = 8.4

🥣 Peppers Hot Cooked From Canned Fat Added In Cooking Ns As To Type Of Fat ☞ serving size: 1 cup, chopped = 141 g; Calories = 59.2; Total Carb (g) = 7.2; Net Carb (g) = 5.4; Fat (g) = 3.4; Protein = 1.3

🥣 Peppers Hot Cooked From Canned Fat Not Added In Cooking ☞ serving size: 1 cup, chopped = 136 g; Calories = 29.9; Total Carb (g) = 7.2; Net Carb (g) = 5.4; Fat (g) = 0.1; Protein = 1.3

🥣 Peppers Hot Cooked From Canned Ns As To Fat Added In Cooking ☞ serving size: 1 cup, chopped = 141 g; Calories = 59.2; Total Carb (g) = 7.2; Net Carb (g) = 5.4; Fat (g) = 3.4; Protein = 1.3

🥣 Peppers Hot Cooked From Fresh Fat Added In Cooking Ns As To Type Of Fat ☞ serving size: 1 cup, chopped = 141 g; Calories = 86; Total Carb (g) = 13.4; Net Carb (g) = 11.3; Fat (g) = 3.6; Protein = 2.9

🥣 Peppers Hot Cooked From Fresh Fat Not Added In Cooking ☞ serving size: 1 cup, chopped = 136 g; Calories = 55.8; Total Carb (g) = 13.3; Net Carb (g) = 11.2; Fat (g) = 0.3; Protein = 2.8

🥣 Peppers Hot Cooked From Fresh Ns As To Fat Added In Cooking ☞ serving size: 1 cup, chopped = 141 g; Calories = 86; Total Carb (g) = 13.4; Net Carb (g) = 11.3; Fat (g) = 3.6; Protein = 2.9

🥣 Peppers Hot Cooked From Frozen Fat Added In Cooking Ns As To Type Of Fat ☞ serving size: 1 cup, chopped = 141 g; Calories = 86; Total Carb (g) = 13.4; Net Carb (g) = 11.3; Fat (g) = 3.6; Protein = 2.9

🥣 Peppers Hot Cooked From Frozen Fat Not Added In Cooking ☞

serving size: 1 cup, chopped = 136 g; Calories = 55.8; Total Carb (g) = 13.3; Net Carb (g) = 11.2; Fat (g) = 0.3; Protein = 2.8

Peppers Hot Cooked From Frozen Ns As To Fat Added In Cooking ☞ serving size: 1 cup, chopped = 141 g; Calories = 86; Total Carb (g) = 13.4; Net Carb (g) = 11.3; Fat (g) = 3.6; Protein = 2.9

Peppers Hot Cooked Ns As To Form Fat Added In Cooking Ns As To Type Of Fat ☞ serving size: 1 cup, chopped = 141 g; Calories = 86; Total Carb (g) = 13.4; Net Carb (g) = 11.3; Fat (g) = 3.6; Protein = 2.9

Peppers Hot Cooked Ns As To Form Fat Not Added In Cooking ☞ serving size: 1 cup, chopped = 136 g; Calories = 55.8; Total Carb (g) = 13.3; Net Carb (g) = 11.2; Fat (g) = 0.3; Protein = 2.8

Peppers Hot Cooked Ns As To Form Ns As To Fat Added In Cooking ☞ serving size: 1 cup, chopped = 141 g; Calories = 86; Total Carb (g) = 13.4; Net Carb (g) = 11.3; Fat (g) = 3.6; Protein = 2.9

Pesto ☞ serving size: 1/4 cup = 63 g; Calories = 263.3; Total Carb (g) = 6.4; Net Carb (g) = 5.2; Fat (g) = 23.7; Protein = 6.2

Pesto Sauce ☞ serving size: 1 cup = 232 g; Calories = 1320.1; Total Carb (g) = 14.3; Net Carb (g) = 12; Fat (g) = 135.8; Protein = 19.7

Pho ☞ serving size: 1 cup = 244 g; Calories = 214.7; Total Carb (g) = 25.4; Net Carb (g) = 23.9; Fat (g) = 5.5; Protein = 15

Pigeon Pea Asopao Asopao De Gandules ☞ serving size: 1 cup = 178 g; Calories = 247.4; Total Carb (g) = 43.8; Net Carb (g) = 40.3; Fat (g) = 4.5; Protein = 7.6

Pimiento ☞ serving size: 1 cup = 192 g; Calories = 53.8; Total Carb (g) = 12; Net Carb (g) = 7.6; Fat (g) = 0.7; Protein = 2.6

Pinto Bean Soup Home Recipe Canned Or Ready-To-Serve ☞ serving size: 1 cup = 253 g; Calories = 359.3; Total Carb (g) = 59.7; Net Carb (g) = 45.1; Fat (g) = 2.7; Protein = 23.8

Plantain Soup Puerto Rican Style ☞ serving size: 1 cup = 245 g;

Calories = 98; Total Carb (g) = 17.5; Net Carb (g) = 16.3; Fat (g) = 1.2; Protein = 5.7

Plum Sauce Asian Style ☞ serving size: 1 cup = 311 g; Calories = 622; Total Carb (g) = 157.6; Net Carb (g) = 154.2; Fat (g) = 0.9; Protein = 2

Pork Vegetable Soup With Potato Pasta Or Rice Stew Type Chunky Style ☞ serving size: 1 cup = 240 g; Calories = 132; Total Carb (g) = 9.3; Net Carb (g) = 7.4; Fat (g) = 5; Protein = 12.5

Pork With Vegetable Excluding Carrots Broccoli And/or Dark-Green Leafy; Soup Asian Style ☞ serving size: 1 cup = 228 g; Calories = 123.1; Total Carb (g) = 4.4; Net Carb (g) = 3.1; Fat (g) = 5.6; Protein = 13.8

Portuguese Bean Soup Home Recipe Canned Or Ready-To-Serve ☞ serving size: 1 cup = 253 g; Calories = 275.8; Total Carb (g) = 37.4; Net Carb (g) = 29.3; Fat (g) = 7.7; Protein = 15.7

Potato And Cheese Soup ☞ serving size: 1 cup = 248 g; Calories = 183.5; Total Carb (g) = 21.2; Net Carb (g) = 18.8; Fat (g) = 8.3; Protein = 6.7

Potato Chowder ☞ serving size: 1 cup = 248 g; Calories = 228.2; Total Carb (g) = 21.7; Net Carb (g) = 20.2; Fat (g) = 11.9; Protein = 9.5

Potato Soup Cream Of Prepared With Milk ☞ serving size: 1 cup = 248 g; Calories = 153.8; Total Carb (g) = 21.9; Net Carb (g) = 20.4; Fat (g) = 4.9; Protein = 5.9

Potato Soup Instant Dry Mix ☞ serving size: 1 serving 1/3 cup = 39 g; Calories = 133.8; Total Carb (g) = 29.7; Net Carb (g) = 26.7; Fat (g) = 1.2; Protein = 3.6

Potato Soup Ns As To Made With Milk Or Water ☞ serving size: 1 cup = 244 g; Calories = 122; Total Carb (g) = 18.7; Net Carb (g) = 17; Fat (g) = 3.6; Protein = 3.9

Potato Soup Prepared With Water ☞ serving size: 1 cup = 244 g;

Calories = 92.7; Total Carb (g) = 15.8; Net Carb (g) = 14.1; Fat (g) = 2.3; Protein = 1.9

🥣 Puerto Rican Seasoning With Ham ☞ serving size: 1 cup = 240 g; Calories = 619.2; Total Carb (g) = 17.6; Net Carb (g) = 13.1; Fat (g) = 58.3; Protein = 9.7

🥣 Puerto Rican Seasoning With Ham And Tomato Sauce ☞ serving size: 1 cup = 240 g; Calories = 417.6; Total Carb (g) = 12.7; Net Carb (g) = 9.1; Fat (g) = 35.8; Protein = 12.3

🥣 Puerto Rican Seasoning Without Ham And Tomato Sauce ☞ serving size: 1 cup = 240 g; Calories = 295.2; Total Carb (g) = 17.4; Net Carb (g) = 13.3; Fat (g) = 25.3; Protein = 2.8

🥣 Ranch Dip Light ☞ serving size: 1 tablespoon = 15 g; Calories = 30; Total Carb (g) = 2.1; Net Carb (g) = 2.1; Fat (g) = 2.3; Protein = 0.4

🥣 Ranch Dip Regular ☞ serving size: 1 tablespoon = 15 g; Calories = 65; Total Carb (g) = 0.5; Net Carb (g) = 0.5; Fat (g) = 6.9; Protein = 0.3

🥣 Ranch Dip Yogurt Based ☞ serving size: 1 tablespoon = 15 g; Calories = 29.3; Total Carb (g) = 0.6; Net Carb (g) = 0.6; Fat (g) = 2.4; Protein = 1.3

🥣 Recaito ☞ serving size: 1 cup = 240 g; Calories = 55.2; Total Carb (g) = 8.8; Net Carb (g) = 2.1; Fat (g) = 1.3; Protein = 5.1

🥣 Rice And Potato Soup Puerto Rican Style ☞ serving size: 1 cup = 245 g; Calories = 183.8; Total Carb (g) = 30.9; Net Carb (g) = 29.7; Fat (g) = 5; Protein = 3.4

🥣 Rice Soup Nfs ☞ serving size: 1 cup = 241 g; Calories = 81.9; Total Carb (g) = 14; Net Carb (g) = 12.8; Fat (g) = 1.9; Protein = 2.2

🥣 Salmon Soup Cream Style ☞ serving size: 1 cup = 248 g; Calories = 146.3; Total Carb (g) = 4.2; Net Carb (g) = 3.7; Fat (g) = 8.3; Protein = 13.2

Salsa Pico De Gallo ☞ serving size: 1 cup = 240 g; Calories = 40.8; Total Carb (g) = 8.9; Net Carb (g) = 6.2; Fat (g) = 0.3; Protein = 1.7

Salsa Red Homemade ☞ serving size: 1 cup = 234 g; Calories = 131; Total Carb (g) = 10.1; Net Carb (g) = 5.9; Fat (g) = 10.2; Protein = 1.9

Sauce Barbecue Bulls-Eye Original ☞ serving size: 1 tbsp = 16 g; Calories = 27.2; Total Carb (g) = 6.4; Net Carb (g) = 6.2; Fat (g) = 0.1; Protein = 0.2

Sauce Barbecue Kc Masterpiece Original ☞ serving size: 1 tbsp = 18 g; Calories = 28.8; Total Carb (g) = 6.8; Net Carb (g) = 6.6; Fat (g) = 0.1; Protein = 0.2

Sauce Barbecue Kraft Original ☞ serving size: 1 tbsp = 16 g; Calories = 27.5; Total Carb (g) = 6.5; Net Carb (g) = 6.5; Fat (g) = 0.1; Protein = 0.1

Sauce Barbecue Open Pit Original ☞ serving size: 1 tbsp = 17 g; Calories = 22.4; Total Carb (g) = 5; Net Carb (g) = 4.9; Fat (g) = 0.2; Protein = 0.1

Sauce Barbecue Sweet Baby Rays Original ☞ serving size: 1 tbsp = 18 g; Calories = 34.6; Total Carb (g) = 8.3; Net Carb (g) = 8.1; Fat (g) = 0.1; Protein = 0.2

Sauce Cheese Ready-To-Serve ☞ serving size: 1/4 cup = 63 g; Calories = 109.6; Total Carb (g) = 4.3; Net Carb (g) = 4; Fat (g) = 8.4; Protein = 4.2

Sauce Chili Peppers Hot Immature Green Canned ☞ serving size: 1 tbsp = 15 g; Calories = 3; Total Carb (g) = 0.8; Net Carb (g) = 0.5; Fat (g) = 0; Protein = 0.1

Sauce Cocktail Ready-To-Serve ☞ serving size: 1/4 cup = 60 g; Calories = 76.8; Total Carb (g) = 16.9; Net Carb (g) = 15.9; Fat (g) = 0.6; Protein = 0.8

Sauce Duck Ready-To-Serve ☞ serving size: 2 tbsp = 33 g; Calories = 80.9; Total Carb (g) = 20; Net Carb (g) = 19.8; Fat (g) = 0; Protein = 0.1

Sauce Enchilada Red Mild Ready To Serve ☞ serving size: 1/4 cup = 56 g; Calories = 16.8; Total Carb (g) = 2.7; Net Carb (g) = 2.5; Fat (g) = 0.5; Protein = 0.4

Sauce Fish Ready-To-Serve ☞ serving size: 1 tbsp = 18 g; Calories = 6.3; Total Carb (g) = 0.7; Net Carb (g) = 0.7; Fat (g) = 0; Protein = 0.9

Sauce Homemade White Medium ☞ serving size: 1 cup = 250 g; Calories = 367.5; Total Carb (g) = 22.9; Net Carb (g) = 22.4; Fat (g) = 26.6; Protein = 9.6

Sauce Homemade White Thick ☞ serving size: 1 cup = 250 g; Calories = 465; Total Carb (g) = 29; Net Carb (g) = 28.3; Fat (g) = 34.6; Protein = 10

Sauce Horseradish ☞ serving size: 1 tsp = 5.6 g; Calories = 28.2; Total Carb (g) = 0.6; Net Carb (g) = 0.5; Fat (g) = 2.9; Protein = 0.1

Sauce Hot Chile Sriracha Cha! By Texas Pete ☞ serving size: 1 tsp = 6.9 g; Calories = 7.5; Total Carb (g) = 1.6; Net Carb (g) = 1.4; Fat (g) = 0.1; Protein = 0.1

Sauce Hot Chile Sriracha Tuong Ot Sriracha ☞ serving size: 1 tsp = 6.2 g; Calories = 4.9; Total Carb (g) = 1; Net Carb (g) = 0.9; Fat (g) = 0.1; Protein = 0.1

Sauce Pasta Spaghetti/marinara Ready-To-Serve Low Sodium ☞ serving size: 1 serving 1/2 cup = 128 g; Calories = 65.3; Total Carb (g) = 10.3; Net Carb (g) = 8; Fat (g) = 1.9; Protein = 1.8

Sauce Peanut Made From Coconut Water Sugar Peanuts ☞ serving size: 1 tbsp = 17 g; Calories = 30.4; Total Carb (g) = 4.8; Net Carb (g) = 4.7; Fat (g) = 1.1; Protein = 0.3

Sauce Peanut Made From Peanut Butter Water Soy Sauce ☞ serving size: 1 tbsp = 18 g; Calories = 46.3; Total Carb (g) = 4; Net Carb (g) = 3.6; Fat (g) = 2.9; Protein = 1.1

Sauce Peppers Hot Chili Mature Red Canned ☞ serving size: 1 tbsp = 15 g; Calories = 3.2; Total Carb (g) = 0.6; Net Carb (g) = 0.5; Fat (g) = 0.1; Protein = 0.1

Sauce Pesto Buitoni Pesto With Basil Ready-To-Serve Refrigerated ☞ serving size: 1/4 cup = 63 g; Calories = 263.3; Total Carb (g) = 6.4; Net Carb (g) = 5.2; Fat (g) = 23.7; Protein = 6.2

Sauce Pesto Classico Basil Pesto Ready-To-Serve ☞ serving size: 1/4 cup = 62 g; Calories = 230.6; Total Carb (g) = 4.3; Net Carb (g) = 3; Fat (g) = 22.6; Protein = 2.6

Sauce Pesto Mezzetta Napa Valley Bistro Basil Pesto Ready-To-Serve ☞ serving size: 1/4 cup = 60 g; Calories = 297.6; Total Carb (g) = 3.1; Net Carb (g) = 2.3; Fat (g) = 29.9; Protein = 4

Sauce Pesto Ready-To-Serve Shelf Stable ☞ serving size: 1/4 cup = 61 g; Calories = 259.9; Total Carb (g) = 3.8; Net Carb (g) = 2.7; Fat (g) = 25.9; Protein = 3.1

Sauce Plum Ready-To-Serve ☞ serving size: 1 tbsp = 19 g; Calories = 35; Total Carb (g) = 8.1; Net Carb (g) = 8; Fat (g) = 0.2; Protein = 0.2

Sauce Salsa Ready-To-Serve ☞ serving size: 2 tbsp = 36 g; Calories = 10.4; Total Carb (g) = 2.4; Net Carb (g) = 1.7; Fat (g) = 0.1; Protein = 0.6

Sauce Salsa Verde Ready-To-Serve ☞ serving size: 2 tbsp = 30 g; Calories = 11.4; Total Carb (g) = 1.9; Net Carb (g) = 1.3; Fat (g) = 0.3; Protein = 0.3

Sauce Sofrito Prepared From Recipe ☞ serving size: 1/2 cup = 103 g; Calories = 244.1; Total Carb (g) = 5.6; Net Carb (g) = 3.9; Fat (g) = 18.8; Protein = 13.2

Sauce Steak Tomato Based ☞ serving size: 2 tbsp = 34 g; Calories = 32.3; Total Carb (g) = 7.5; Net Carb (g) = 7; Fat (g) = 0.1; Protein = 0.4

Sauce Sweet And Sour Ready-To-Serve ☞ serving size: 2 tbsp =

35 g; Calories = 53.9; Total Carb (g) = 13.4; Net Carb (g) = 13.3; Fat (g) = 0; Protein = 0.1

Sauce Tartar Ready-To-Serve ☞ serving size: 2 tablespoons = 30 g; Calories = 63.3; Total Carb (g) = 4; Net Carb (g) = 3.8; Fat (g) = 5; Protein = 0.3

Sauce Teriyaki Ready-To-Serve ☞ serving size: 1 tbsp = 18 g; Calories = 16; Total Carb (g) = 2.8; Net Carb (g) = 2.8; Fat (g) = 0; Protein = 1.1

Sauce Tomato Chili Sauce Bottled With Salt ☞ serving size: 1 packet = 6 g; Calories = 5.5; Total Carb (g) = 1.2; Net Carb (g) = 1; Fat (g) = 0; Protein = 0.2

Seafood Dip ☞ serving size: 1 tablespoon = 15 g; Calories = 50.7; Total Carb (g) = 0.6; Net Carb (g) = 0.6; Fat (g) = 5; Protein = 0.9

Seafood Soup With Potatoes And Vegetables Excluding Carrots Broccoli And Dark-Green Leafy ☞ serving size: 1 cup = 244 g; Calories = 109.8; Total Carb (g) = 9.6; Net Carb (g) = 7.9; Fat (g) = 3; Protein = 11

Seafood Soup With Potatoes And Vegetables Including Carrots Broccoli And/or Dark-Green Leafy ☞ serving size: 1 cup = 244 g; Calories = 109.8; Total Carb (g) = 10; Net Carb (g) = 8.1; Fat (g) = 3; Protein = 10.8

Seafood Soup With Vegetables Excluding Carrots Broccoli And Dark-Green Leafy; No Potatoes ☞ serving size: 1 cup = 244 g; Calories = 102.5; Total Carb (g) = 6.9; Net Carb (g) = 5.5; Fat (g) = 3.2; Protein = 11.4

Seafood Soup With Vegetables Including Carrots Broccoli And/or Dark-Green Leafy; No Potatoes ☞ serving size: 1 cup = 244 g; Calories = 102.5; Total Carb (g) = 7.5; Net Carb (g) = 5.8; Fat (g) = 3.1; Protein = 11.1

🥣 Seaweed Soup ☞ serving size: 1 cup = 230 g; Calories = 80.5; Total Carb (g) = 5.5; Net Carb (g) = 5.1; Fat (g) = 3.1; Protein = 8.5

🥣 Shav Soup ☞ serving size: 1 cup = 240 g; Calories = 124.8; Total Carb (g) = 9.5; Net Carb (g) = 8.5; Fat (g) = 6.1; Protein = 7.4

🥣 Smart Soup French Lentil ☞ serving size: 10 oz 1 pouch = 283 g; Calories = 150; Total Carb (g) = 26.9; Net Carb (g) = 18.7; Fat (g) = 3; Protein = 8.2

🥣 Smart Soup Greek Minestrone ☞ serving size: 10 oz 1 pouch = 283 g; Calories = 113.2; Total Carb (g) = 23.8; Net Carb (g) = 16.1; Fat (g) = 1.5; Protein = 4.8

🥣 Smart Soup Indian Bean Masala ☞ serving size: 10 oz 1 pouch = 283 g; Calories = 161.3; Total Carb (g) = 29.7; Net Carb (g) = 22.4; Fat (g) = 2.5; Protein = 9.3

🥣 Smart Soup Moroccan Chick Pea ☞ serving size: 10 oz 1 pouch = 283 g; Calories = 144.3; Total Carb (g) = 27.5; Net Carb (g) = 18.7; Fat (g) = 3; Protein = 5.7

🥣 Smart Soup Santa Fe Corn Chowder ☞ serving size: 10 oz 1 pouch = 283 g; Calories = 155.7; Total Carb (g) = 31.7; Net Carb (g) = 26; Fat (g) = 2; Protein = 5.7

🥣 Smart Soup Thai Coconut Curry ☞ serving size: 10 oz 1 pouch = 283 g; Calories = 101.9; Total Carb (g) = 18.4; Net Carb (g) = 15.6; Fat (g) = 3; Protein = 2.3

🥣 Smart Soup Vietnamese Carrot Lemongrass ☞ serving size: 10 oz 1 pouch = 283 g; Calories = 124.5; Total Carb (g) = 23.2; Net Carb (g) = 19; Fat (g) = 3; Protein = 3.7

🥣 Sopa De Fideo Aguada Mexican Style Noodle Soup Home Recipe ☞ serving size: 1 cup = 242 g; Calories = 193.6; Total Carb (g) = 21.2; Net Carb (g) = 20.2; Fat (g) = 8.4; Protein = 8

🥣 Sopa De Tortilla Mexican Style Tortilla Soup Home Recipe ☞

serving size: 1 cup = 240 g; Calories = 280.8; Total Carb (g) = 18; Net Carb (g) = 16.5; Fat (g) = 18.3; Protein = 11.6

Sopa Seca De Arroz Home Recipe Mexican Style ☞ serving size: 1 cup = 218 g; Calories = 324.8; Total Carb (g) = 45.3; Net Carb (g) = 43.1; Fat (g) = 13.9; Protein = 5.1

Sopa Seca De Fideo Mexican Style Made With Dry Noodles Home Recipe ☞ serving size: 1 cup = 218 g; Calories = 300.8; Total Carb (g) = 36.2; Net Carb (g) = 33.3; Fat (g) = 14.9; Protein = 6.8

Sopa Seca Mexican Style Nfs ☞ serving size: 1 cup = 218 g; Calories = 305.2; Total Carb (g) = 39.8; Net Carb (g) = 37.4; Fat (g) = 13.9; Protein = 5.8

Soup Bean & Ham Canned Reduced Sodium Prepared With Water Or Ready-To-Serve ☞ serving size: 1 cup = 245 g; Calories = 198.5; Total Carb (g) = 33.5; Net Carb (g) = 23.7; Fat (g) = 2.5; Protein = 10.3

Soup Bean With Bacon Condensed Single Brand ☞ serving size: 1 serving 1/2 cup = 128 g; Calories = 149.8; Total Carb (g) = 23; Net Carb (g) = 17.2; Fat (g) = 2.7; Protein = 8.3

Soup Bean With Frankfurters Canned Condensed ☞ serving size: 1 cup (8 fl oz) = 263 g; Calories = 373.5; Total Carb (g) = 44.1; Net Carb (g) = 32; Fat (g) = 14; Protein = 20

Soup Bean With Frankfurters Canned Prepared With Equal Volume Water ☞ serving size: 1 cup (8 fl oz) = 250 g; Calories = 187.5; Total Carb (g) = 22; Net Carb (g) = 22; Fat (g) = 7; Protein = 10

Soup Bean With Ham Canned Chunky Ready-To-Serve ☞ serving size: 1 cup (8 fl oz) = 243 g; Calories = 230.9; Total Carb (g) = 27.1; Net Carb (g) = 15.9; Fat (g) = 8.5; Protein = 12.6

Soup Bean With Pork Canned Condensed ☞ serving size: 1/2 cup = 130 g; Calories = 167.7; Total Carb (g) = 22.1; Net Carb (g) = 14.4; Fat (g) = 5.8; Protein = 7.6

Soup Bean With Pork Canned Prepared With Equal Volume Water ☞ serving size: 1 serving 1 cup = 266 g; Calories = 167.6; Total Carb (g) = 22.1; Net Carb (g) = 14.4; Fat (g) = 5.8; Protein = 7.7

Soup Beef And Mushroom Low Sodium Chunk Style ☞ serving size: 1 cup = 251 g; Calories = 173.2; Total Carb (g) = 24.1; Net Carb (g) = 23.5; Fat (g) = 5.8; Protein = 10.8

Soup Beef And Vegetables Canned Ready-To-Serve ☞ serving size: 1 cup = 250 g; Calories = 120; Total Carb (g) = 15.4; Net Carb (g) = 12.4; Fat (g) = 2.9; Protein = 8

Soup Beef And Vegetables Reduced Sodium Canned Ready-To-Serve ☞ serving size: 1 cup = 245 g; Calories = 102.9; Total Carb (g) = 12.2; Net Carb (g) = 10.3; Fat (g) = 2.3; Protein = 8

Soup Beef Barley Ready To Serve ☞ serving size: 1 cup = 208 g; Calories = 108.2; Total Carb (g) = 16.5; Net Carb (g) = 14.6; Fat (g) = 2; Protein = 5.8

Soup Beef Broth Bouillon And Consomme Canned Condensed ☞ serving size: 1/2 cup = 124 g; Calories = 13.6; Total Carb (g) = 0.4; Net Carb (g) = 0.4; Fat (g) = 0; Protein = 3.1

Soup Beef Broth Cubed Dry ☞ serving size: 1 cube = 3.6 g; Calories = 6.1; Total Carb (g) = 0.6; Net Carb (g) = 0.6; Fat (g) = 0.1; Protein = 0.6

Soup Beef Broth Cubed Prepared With Water ☞ serving size: 1 serving 1 cup = 240 g; Calories = 7.2; Total Carb (g) = 0.6; Net Carb (g) = 0.6; Fat (g) = 0.2; Protein = 0.5

Soup Beef Broth Less/reduced Sodium Ready To Serve ☞ serving size: 1 cup = 219 g; Calories = 13.1; Total Carb (g) = 0.4; Net Carb (g) = 0.4; Fat (g) = 0.2; Protein = 2.5

Soup Beef Broth Or Bouillon Canned Ready-To-Serve ☞ serving size: 1 cup = 240 g; Calories = 16.8; Total Carb (g) = 0.1; Net Carb (g) = 0.1; Fat (g) = 0.5; Protein = 2.7

🥣 Soup Beef Broth Or Bouillon Powder Dry ☞ serving size: 1 cube = 3.6 g; Calories = 7.7; Total Carb (g) = 0.6; Net Carb (g) = 0.6; Fat (g) = 0.3; Protein = 0.6

🥣 Soup Beef Broth Or Bouillon Powder Prepared With Water ☞ serving size: 1 serving 1 cup = 240 g; Calories = 7.2; Total Carb (g) = 0.6; Net Carb (g) = 0.6; Fat (g) = 0.2; Protein = 0.5

🥣 Soup Beef Mushroom Canned Condensed ☞ serving size: 1/2 cup (4 fl oz) = 126 g; Calories = 76.9; Total Carb (g) = 6.6; Net Carb (g) = 6.3; Fat (g) = 3; Protein = 5.8

🥣 Soup Beef Mushroom Canned Prepared With Equal Volume Water ☞ serving size: 1 cup (8 fl oz) = 244 g; Calories = 73.2; Total Carb (g) = 6.3; Net Carb (g) = 6.1; Fat (g) = 3; Protein = 5.8

🥣 Soup Beef Noodle Canned Condensed ☞ serving size: 1/2 cup = 125 g; Calories = 83.8; Total Carb (g) = 9; Net Carb (g) = 8.2; Fat (g) = 3.1; Protein = 4.8

🥣 Soup Beef Noodle Canned Prepared With Equal Volume Water ☞ serving size: 1 cup (8 fl oz) = 244 g; Calories = 83; Total Carb (g) = 8.7; Net Carb (g) = 8; Fat (g) = 3; Protein = 4.7

🥣 Soup Beef Stroganoff Canned Chunky Style Ready-To-Serve ☞ serving size: 1 cup = 240 g; Calories = 235.2; Total Carb (g) = 21.6; Net Carb (g) = 20.2; Fat (g) = 11; Protein = 12.2

🥣 Soup Black Bean Canned Condensed ☞ serving size: 1 cup (8 fl oz) = 257 g; Calories = 233.9; Total Carb (g) = 39.6; Net Carb (g) = 22.2; Fat (g) = 3.4; Protein = 12.4

🥣 Soup Bouillon Cubes And Granules Low Sodium Dry ☞ serving size: 1 tsp = 2.6 g; Calories = 11.4; Total Carb (g) = 1.7; Net Carb (g) = 1.7; Fat (g) = 0.4; Protein = 0.4

🥣 Soup Broccoli Cheese Canned Condensed Commercial ☞ serving size: 1 serving 1/2 cup = 121 g; Calories = 105.3; Total Carb (g) = 9.3; Net Carb (g) = 7.1; Fat (g) = 6.4; Protein = 2.5

Soup Cheese Canned Condensed ☞ serving size: 1/2 cup = 124 g; Calories = 101.7; Total Carb (g) = 14; Net Carb (g) = 11.3; Fat (g) = 4.9; Protein = 1

Soup Cheese Canned Prepared With Equal Volume Milk ☞ serving size: 1 cup = 251 g; Calories = 230.9; Total Carb (g) = 16.2; Net Carb (g) = 15.2; Fat (g) = 14.6; Protein = 9.5

Soup Cheese Canned Prepared With Equal Volume Water ☞ serving size: 1 cup (8 fl oz) = 247 g; Calories = 155.6; Total Carb (g) = 10.5; Net Carb (g) = 9.5; Fat (g) = 10.5; Protein = 5.4

Soup Chicken And Vegetable Canned Ready-To-Serve ☞ serving size: 1 cup = 255 g; Calories = 84.2; Total Carb (g) = 11.9; Net Carb (g) = 9.6; Fat (g) = 1.9; Protein = 5

Soup Chicken Broth Canned Condensed ☞ serving size: 1/2 cup (4 fl oz) = 126 g; Calories = 39.1; Total Carb (g) = 1; Net Carb (g) = 1; Fat (g) = 1.3; Protein = 5.6

Soup Chicken Broth Canned Prepared With Equal Volume Water ☞ serving size: 1 cup (8 fl oz) = 244 g; Calories = 39; Total Carb (g) = 0.9; Net Carb (g) = 0.9; Fat (g) = 1.4; Protein = 4.9

Soup Chicken Broth Cubes Dry ☞ serving size: 1 cube = 4.8 g; Calories = 9.5; Total Carb (g) = 1.1; Net Carb (g) = 1.1; Fat (g) = 0.2; Protein = 0.7

Soup Chicken Broth Cubes Dry Prepared With Water ☞ serving size: 1 cup (8 fl oz) = 243 g; Calories = 12.2; Total Carb (g) = 1.5; Net Carb (g) = 1.5; Fat (g) = 0.3; Protein = 1

Soup Chicken Broth Less/reduced Sodium Ready To Serve ☞ serving size: 1 cup = 240 g; Calories = 16.8; Total Carb (g) = 0.9; Net Carb (g) = 0.9; Fat (g) = 0; Protein = 3.3

Soup Chicken Broth Low Sodium Canned ☞ serving size: 1 cup = 240 g; Calories = 38.4; Total Carb (g) = 2.9; Net Carb (g) = 2.9; Fat (g) = 1.4; Protein = 4.8

Soup Chicken Broth Or Bouillon Dry ☞ serving size: 1 cube = 4 g; Calories = 10.7; Total Carb (g) = 0.7; Net Carb (g) = 0.7; Fat (g) = 0.6; Protein = 0.7

Soup Chicken Broth Or Bouillon Dry Prepared With Water ☞ serving size: 1 cup 8 fl oz = 241 g; Calories = 9.6; Total Carb (g) = 0.7; Net Carb (g) = 0.7; Fat (g) = 0.6; Protein = 0.7

Soup Chicken Broth Ready-To-Serve ☞ serving size: 1 cup = 249 g; Calories = 14.9; Total Carb (g) = 1.1; Net Carb (g) = 1.1; Fat (g) = 0.5; Protein = 1.6

Soup Chicken Canned Chunky Ready-To-Serve ☞ serving size: 1 cup = 245 g; Calories = 174; Total Carb (g) = 16.9; Net Carb (g) = 15.4; Fat (g) = 6.5; Protein = 12.4

Soup Chicken Corn Chowder Chunky Ready-To-Serve Single Brand ☞ serving size: 1 serving = 240 g; Calories = 237.6; Total Carb (g) = 18; Net Carb (g) = 15.8; Fat (g) = 15.1; Protein = 7.4

Soup Chicken Gumbo Canned Condensed ☞ serving size: 1/2 cup (4 fl oz) = 126 g; Calories = 56.7; Total Carb (g) = 8.4; Net Carb (g) = 6.4; Fat (g) = 1.4; Protein = 2.7

Soup Chicken Gumbo Canned Prepared With Equal Volume Water ☞ serving size: 1 cup = 244 g; Calories = 56.1; Total Carb (g) = 8.4; Net Carb (g) = 6.4; Fat (g) = 1.4; Protein = 2.6

Soup Chicken Mushroom Canned Condensed ☞ serving size: 1/2 cup = 124 g; Calories = 124; Total Carb (g) = 14.8; Net Carb (g) = 10.9; Fat (g) = 6; Protein = 2

Soup Chicken Mushroom Canned Prepared With Equal Volume Water ☞ serving size: 1 cup (8 fl oz) = 244 g; Calories = 131.8; Total Carb (g) = 9.3; Net Carb (g) = 9; Fat (g) = 9.2; Protein = 4.4

Soup Chicken Noodle Canned Condensed ☞ serving size: 1/2 cup = 124 g; Calories = 59.5; Total Carb (g) = 7.5; Net Carb (g) = 6.4; Fat (g) = 1.9; Protein = 2.9

👄 Soup Chicken Noodle Canned Prepared With Equal Volume Water ☞ serving size: 1 serving 1 cup = 248 g; Calories = 59.5; Total Carb (g) = 7.4; Net Carb (g) = 6.1; Fat (g) = 1.9; Protein = 2.9

👄 Soup Chicken Noodle Dry Mix ☞ serving size: 1 packet = 74 g; Calories = 279; Total Carb (g) = 46.1; Net Carb (g) = 43.8; Fat (g) = 4.8; Protein = 11.4

👄 Soup Chicken Noodle Dry Mix Prepared With Water ☞ serving size: 1 cup = 245 g; Calories = 56.4; Total Carb (g) = 9; Net Carb (g) = 8.8; Fat (g) = 1.4; Protein = 2.1

👄 Soup Chicken Noodle Low Sodium Canned Prepared With Equal Volume Water ☞ serving size: 1 serving 1 cup = 248 g; Calories = 62; Total Carb (g) = 7.3; Net Carb (g) = 6.8; Fat (g) = 2.4; Protein = 3.2

👄 Soup Chicken Noodle Reduced Sodium Canned Ready-To-Serve ☞ serving size: 1 cup = 245 g; Calories = 100.5; Total Carb (g) = 9.4; Net Carb (g) = 7.5; Fat (g) = 3.3; Protein = 8.1

👄 Soup Chicken Rice Canned Chunky Ready-To-Serve ☞ serving size: 1 cup = 240 g; Calories = 127.2; Total Carb (g) = 13; Net Carb (g) = 12; Fat (g) = 3.2; Protein = 12.3

👄 Soup Chicken Vegetable Canned Condensed ☞ serving size: 1/2 cup = 121 g; Calories = 73.8; Total Carb (g) = 8.5; Net Carb (g) = 7.6; Fat (g) = 2.8; Protein = 3.6

👄 Soup Chicken Vegetable With Potato And Cheese Chunky Ready-To-Serve ☞ serving size: 1 cup = 245 g; Calories = 159.3; Total Carb (g) = 12.7; Net Carb (g) = 12; Fat (g) = 10.9; Protein = 2.8

👄 Soup Chicken With Rice Canned Condensed ☞ serving size: 1/2 cup = 126 g; Calories = 85.7; Total Carb (g) = 14.6; Net Carb (g) = 13.4; Fat (g) = 2; Protein = 2.3

👄 Soup Chicken With Rice Canned Prepared With Equal Volume Water ☞ serving size: 1 serving 1 cup = 243 g; Calories =

58.3; Total Carb (g) = 7.1; Net Carb (g) = 6.4; Fat (g) = 1.9; Protein = 3.5

Soup Chili Beef Canned Condensed ☞ serving size: 1 cup (8 fl oz) = 263 g; Calories = 307.7; Total Carb (g) = 49.6; Net Carb (g) = 43; Fat (g) = 6.7; Protein = 13.4

Soup Chili Beef Canned Prepared With Equal Volume Water ☞ serving size: 1 cup = 261 g; Calories = 148.8; Total Carb (g) = 24.1; Net Carb (g) = 21; Fat (g) = 3.2; Protein = 6.5

Soup Chunky Beef Canned Ready-To-Serve ☞ serving size: 1 cup = 245 g; Calories = 161.7; Total Carb (g) = 24.7; Net Carb (g) = 23.2; Fat (g) = 2.7; Protein = 9.7

Soup Chunky Chicken Noodle Canned Ready-To-Serve ☞ serving size: 1 can = 530 g; Calories = 217.3; Total Carb (g) = 23.6; Net Carb (g) = 19.4; Fat (g) = 6.2; Protein = 16.4

Soup Chunky Vegetable Canned Ready-To-Serve ☞ serving size: 1 cup = 230 g; Calories = 89.7; Total Carb (g) = 18.2; Net Carb (g) = 15.6; Fat (g) = 0.8; Protein = 2.6

Soup Chunky Vegetable Reduced Sodium Canned Ready-To-Serve ☞ serving size: 1 cup = 240 g; Calories = 120; Total Carb (g) = 24.7; Net Carb (g) = 22; Fat (g) = 1.2; Protein = 2.8

Soup Clam Chowder Manhattan Canned Condensed ☞ serving size: 1/2 cup (4 fl oz) = 126 g; Calories = 76.9; Total Carb (g) = 12.3; Net Carb (g) = 10.8; Fat (g) = 2.2; Protein = 2.2

Soup Clam Chowder New England Canned Condensed ☞ serving size: 1/2 cup = 126 g; Calories = 90.7; Total Carb (g) = 13; Net Carb (g) = 12.1; Fat (g) = 2.6; Protein = 4

Soup Clam Chowder New England Canned Prepared With Equal Volume Low Fat (2%) Milk ☞ serving size: 1 serving 1 cup = 252 g; Calories = 153.7; Total Carb (g) = 18.8; Net Carb (g) = 18; Fat (g) = 5.1; Protein = 8.2

Soup Clam Chowder New England Canned Ready-To-Serve ☞ serving size: 1 cup = 254 g; Calories = 200.7; Total Carb (g) = 21; Net Carb (g) = 18.5; Fat (g) = 10; Protein = 6.6

Soup Clam Chowder New England Reduced Sodium Canned Ready-To-Serve ☞ serving size: 1 can = 519 g; Calories = 363.3; Total Carb (g) = 29.5; Net Carb (g) = 25.3; Fat (g) = 22; Protein = 12.1

Soup Cream Of Asparagus Canned Condensed ☞ serving size: 1/2 cup (4 fl oz) = 126 g; Calories = 86.9; Total Carb (g) = 10.7; Net Carb (g) = 10.2; Fat (g) = 4.1; Protein = 2.3

Soup Cream Of Asparagus Canned Prepared With Equal Volume Milk ☞ serving size: 1 cup (8 fl oz) = 248 g; Calories = 161.2; Total Carb (g) = 16.4; Net Carb (g) = 15.7; Fat (g) = 8.2; Protein = 6.3

Soup Cream Of Celery Canned Condensed ☞ serving size: 1/2 cup = 126 g; Calories = 90.7; Total Carb (g) = 8.9; Net Carb (g) = 8.1; Fat (g) = 5.6; Protein = 1.7

Soup Cream Of Celery Canned Prepared With Equal Volume Milk ☞ serving size: 1 cup (8 fl oz) = 248 g; Calories = 163.7; Total Carb (g) = 14.5; Net Carb (g) = 13.8; Fat (g) = 9.7; Protein = 5.7

Soup Cream Of Celery Canned Prepared With Equal Volume Water ☞ serving size: 1 cup = 248 g; Calories = 91.8; Total Carb (g) = 9; Net Carb (g) = 8.2; Fat (g) = 5.7; Protein = 1.7

Soup Cream Of Chicken Canned Condensed ☞ serving size: 1/2 cup (4 fl oz) = 126 g; Calories = 113.4; Total Carb (g) = 9; Net Carb (g) = 9; Fat (g) = 7.3; Protein = 3

Soup Cream Of Chicken Canned Condensed Reduced Sodium ☞ serving size: 1/2 cup = 124 g; Calories = 71.9; Total Carb (g) = 11.8; Net Carb (g) = 11.3; Fat (g) = 1.6; Protein = 2.2

Soup Cream Of Chicken Canned Prepared With Equal Volume Milk ☞ serving size: 1 cup (8 fl oz) = 248 g; Calories = 191; Total Carb (g) = 15; Net Carb (g) = 14.7; Fat (g) = 11.5; Protein = 7.5

Soup Cream Of Chicken Dry Mix Prepared With Water ☞ serving size: 1 cup 8 fl oz = 261 g; Calories = 107; Total Carb (g) = 13.3; Net Carb (g) = 13.1; Fat (g) = 5.3; Protein = 1.8

Soup Cream Of Mushroom Canned Condensed ☞ serving size: 1/2 cup = 126 g; Calories = 99.5; Total Carb (g) = 8.6; Net Carb (g) = 7.7; Fat (g) = 6.7; Protein = 1.7

Soup Cream Of Mushroom Canned Condensed Reduced Sodium ☞ serving size: 1 cup = 251 g; Calories = 130.5; Total Carb (g) = 20.3; Net Carb (g) = 18.8; Fat (g) = 4.2; Protein = 3

Soup Cream Of Mushroom Canned Prepared With Equal Volume Low Fat (2%) Milk ☞ serving size: 1 serving 1 cup = 252 g; Calories = 163.8; Total Carb (g) = 14.5; Net Carb (g) = 13.8; Fat (g) = 9; Protein = 6

Soup Cream Of Mushroom Low Sodium Ready-To-Serve Canned ☞ serving size: 1 cup = 244 g; Calories = 129.3; Total Carb (g) = 11.1; Net Carb (g) = 10.6; Fat (g) = 9; Protein = 2.4

Soup Cream Of Nfs ☞ serving size: 1 cup = 244 g; Calories = 141.5; Total Carb (g) = 24.5; Net Carb (g) = 23; Fat (g) = 3; Protein = 5.8

Soup Cream Of Onion Canned Condensed ☞ serving size: 1/2 cup = 126 g; Calories = 110.9; Total Carb (g) = 13.1; Net Carb (g) = 12.6; Fat (g) = 5.3; Protein = 2.8

Soup Cream Of Onion Canned Prepared With Equal Volume Milk ☞ serving size: 1 cup (8 fl oz) = 248 g; Calories = 186; Total Carb (g) = 18.4; Net Carb (g) = 17.6; Fat (g) = 9.4; Protein = 6.8

Soup Cream Of Onion Canned Prepared With Equal Volume Water ☞ serving size: 1 cup (8 fl oz) = 244 g; Calories = 107.4; Total Carb (g) = 12.7; Net Carb (g) = 11.7; Fat (g) = 5.3; Protein = 2.8

Soup Cream Of Potato Canned Condensed ☞ serving size: 1/2 cup = 124 g; Calories = 91.8; Total Carb (g) = 15.9; Net Carb (g) = 14.3; Fat (g) = 2.3; Protein = 1.9

Soup Cream Of Potato Canned Prepared With Equal Volume Milk ☞ serving size: 1 cup (8 fl oz) = 248 g; Calories = 148.8; Total Carb (g) = 17.2; Net Carb (g) = 16.7; Fat (g) = 6.5; Protein = 5.8

Soup Cream Of Potato Canned Prepared With Equal Volume Water ☞ serving size: 1 cup (8 fl oz) = 244 g; Calories = 73.2; Total Carb (g) = 11.5; Net Carb (g) = 11; Fat (g) = 2.4; Protein = 1.8

Soup Cream Of Shrimp Canned Condensed ☞ serving size: 1/2 cup = 126 g; Calories = 90.7; Total Carb (g) = 8.2; Net Carb (g) = 8; Fat (g) = 5.2; Protein = 2.8

Soup Cream Of Shrimp Canned Prepared With Equal Volume Low Fat (2%) Milk ☞ serving size: 1 cup (8 fl oz) = 253 g; Calories = 154.3; Total Carb (g) = 14.3; Net Carb (g) = 14; Fat (g) = 8.2; Protein = 7

Soup Cream Of Shrimp Canned Prepared With Equal Volume Water ☞ serving size: 1 cup = 244 g; Calories = 87.8; Total Carb (g) = 8; Net Carb (g) = 7.7; Fat (g) = 5.1; Protein = 2.7

Soup Cream Of Vegetable Dry Powder ☞ serving size: 1 packet = 18 g; Calories = 80.3; Total Carb (g) = 9.4; Net Carb (g) = 8.8; Fat (g) = 4.3; Protein = 1.4

Soup Egg Drop Chinese Restaurant ☞ serving size: 1 cup = 241 g; Calories = 65.1; Total Carb (g) = 10.3; Net Carb (g) = 9.4; Fat (g) = 1.5; Protein = 2.8

Soup Fruit ☞ serving size: 1 cup = 242 g; Calories = 174.2; Total Carb (g) = 45.5; Net Carb (g) = 43.1; Fat (g) = 0.2; Protein = 1.3

Soup Healthy Choice Chicken And Rice Soup Canned ☞ serving size: 1 serving 1 cup = 240 g; Calories = 88.8; Total Carb (g) = 13.7; Net Carb (g) = 11.8; Fat (g) = 1.3; Protein = 6.1

Soup Healthy Choice Chicken Noodle Soup Canned ☞ serving size: 1 serving 1 cup = 243 g; Calories = 99.6; Total Carb (g) = 12.6; Net Carb (g) = 10.7; Fat (g) = 1.5; Protein = 9

Soup Healthy Choice Garden Vegetable Soup Canned ☞

serving size: 1 serving 1 cup = 246 g; Calories = 125.5; Total Carb (g) = 24.7; Net Carb (g) = 20; Fat (g) = 0.5; Protein = 5.2

🥣 Soup Hot And Sour Chinese Restaurant ☞ serving size: 1 cup = 233 g; Calories = 90.9; Total Carb (g) = 10.1; Net Carb (g) = 9; Fat (g) = 2.8; Protein = 6

🥣 Soup Lentil With Ham Canned Ready-To-Serve ☞ serving size: 1 cup (8 fl oz) = 248 g; Calories = 138.9; Total Carb (g) = 20.2; Net Carb (g) = 20.2; Fat (g) = 2.8; Protein = 9.3

🥣 Soup Minestrone Canned Condensed ☞ serving size: 1/2 cup (4 fl oz) = 123 g; Calories = 83.6; Total Carb (g) = 11.3; Net Carb (g) = 10.3; Fat (g) = 2.5; Protein = 4.3

🥣 Soup Mostly Noodles ☞ serving size: 1 cup = 233 g; Calories = 156.1; Total Carb (g) = 21.4; Net Carb (g) = 20.4; Fat (g) = 6.2; Protein = 3.6

🥣 Soup Mostly Noodles Reduced Sodium ☞ serving size: 1 cup = 233 g; Calories = 123.5; Total Carb (g) = 25.1; Net Carb (g) = 24.2; Fat (g) = 0.9; Protein = 3.9

🥣 Soup Mushroom Barley Canned Condensed ☞ serving size: 1/2 cup (4 fl oz) = 126 g; Calories = 76.9; Total Carb (g) = 12.1; Net Carb (g) = 12.1; Fat (g) = 2.3; Protein = 1.9

🥣 Soup Mushroom With Beef Stock Canned Condensed ☞ serving size: 1/2 cup (4 fl oz) = 126 g; Calories = 85.7; Total Carb (g) = 9.3; Net Carb (g) = 9.2; Fat (g) = 4; Protein = 3.2

🥣 Soup Mushroom With Beef Stock Canned Prepared With Equal Volume Water ☞ serving size: 1 cup (8 fl oz) = 244 g; Calories = 85.4; Total Carb (g) = 9.3; Net Carb (g) = 8.6; Fat (g) = 4; Protein = 3.2

🥣 Soup Nfs ☞ serving size: 1 cup = 241 g; Calories = 57.8; Total Carb (g) = 7.4; Net Carb (g) = 6.2; Fat (g) = 1.9; Protein = 2.9

🥣 Soup Onion Canned Condensed ☞ serving size: 1/2 cup (4 fl oz)

= 123 g; Calories = 56.6; Total Carb (g) = 8.2; Net Carb (g) = 7.4; Fat (g) = 1.8; Protein = 3.8

🥣 Soup Onion Dry Mix ☞ serving size: 1 serving 1 tbsp = 7.5 g; Calories = 22; Total Carb (g) = 4.9; Net Carb (g) = 4.4; Fat (g) = 0; Protein = 0.6

🥣 Soup Onion Dry Mix Prepared With Water ☞ serving size: 1 serving 1 cup = 230 g; Calories = 27.6; Total Carb (g) = 6.4; Net Carb (g) = 5.7; Fat (g) = 0; Protein = 0.7

🥣 Soup Oyster Stew Canned Condensed ☞ serving size: 1/2 cup (4 fl oz) = 123 g; Calories = 59; Total Carb (g) = 4.1; Net Carb (g) = 4.1; Fat (g) = 3.9; Protein = 2.1

🥣 Soup Oyster Stew Canned Prepared With Equal Volume Milk ☞ serving size: 1 cup (8 fl oz) = 245 g; Calories = 134.8; Total Carb (g) = 9.8; Net Carb (g) = 9.8; Fat (g) = 7.9; Protein = 6.2

🥣 Soup Oyster Stew Canned Prepared With Equal Volume Water ☞ serving size: 1 cup (8 fl oz) = 241 g; Calories = 57.8; Total Carb (g) = 4.1; Net Carb (g) = 4.1; Fat (g) = 3.8; Protein = 2.1

🥣 Soup Pea Green Canned Condensed ☞ serving size: 1/2 cup = 128 g; Calories = 160; Total Carb (g) = 25.8; Net Carb (g) = 20.8; Fat (g) = 2.9; Protein = 8.4

🥣 Soup Pea Green Canned Prepared With Equal Volume Milk ☞ serving size: 1 cup (8 fl oz) = 254 g; Calories = 238.8; Total Carb (g) = 32.2; Net Carb (g) = 29.4; Fat (g) = 7; Protein = 12.6

🥣 Soup Pea Green Canned Prepared With Equal Volume Water ☞ serving size: 1 serving 1 cup = 259 g; Calories = 158; Total Carb (g) = 25.6; Net Carb (g) = 20.7; Fat (g) = 2.8; Protein = 8.3

🥣 Soup Pea Low Sodium Prepared With Equal Volume Water ☞ serving size: 1 cup = 259 g; Calories = 160.6; Total Carb (g) = 25.6; Net Carb (g) = 20.7; Fat (g) = 2.8; Protein = 8.3

🥣 Soup Pea Split With Ham Canned Chunky Ready-To-Serve ☞

serving size: 1 cup = 240 g; Calories = 184.8; Total Carb (g) = 26.8; Net Carb (g) = 22.7; Fat (g) = 4; Protein = 11.1

Soup Pea Split With Ham Canned Condensed ☞ serving size: 1/2 cup (4 fl oz) = 135 g; Calories = 190.4; Total Carb (g) = 28.1; Net Carb (g) = 25.8; Fat (g) = 4.4; Protein = 10.4

Soup Pea Split With Ham Canned Prepared With Equal Volume Water ☞ serving size: 1 cup (8 fl oz) = 253 g; Calories = 189.8; Total Carb (g) = 28; Net Carb (g) = 25.7; Fat (g) = 4.4; Protein = 10.3

Soup Ramen Noodle Any Flavor Dry ☞ serving size: 1 package without flavor packet = 81 g; Calories = 356.4; Total Carb (g) = 48.8; Net Carb (g) = 46.5; Fat (g) = 14.3; Protein = 8.2

Soup Ramen Noodle Beef Flavor Dry ☞ serving size: 1 package without flavor packet = 82 g; Calories = 361.6; Total Carb (g) = 49.5; Net Carb (g) = 47; Fat (g) = 14.5; Protein = 8.3

Soup Ramen Noodle Chicken Flavor Dry ☞ serving size: 1 package without flavor packet = 81 g; Calories = 355.6; Total Carb (g) = 48.8; Net Carb (g) = 46.4; Fat (g) = 14.2; Protein = 8.3

Soup Ramen Noodle Dry Any Flavor Reduced Fat Reduced Sodium ☞ serving size: 1 (2/5) oz dry (half noodle block) = 40 g; Calories = 140; Total Carb (g) = 28.4; Net Carb (g) = 27.3; Fat (g) = 1; Protein = 4.4

Soup Shark Fin Restaurant-Prepared ☞ serving size: 1 cup = 216 g; Calories = 99.4; Total Carb (g) = 8.2; Net Carb (g) = 8.2; Fat (g) = 4.3; Protein = 6.9

Soup Swanson Beef Broth Lower Sodium ☞ serving size: 1 cup = 213 g; Calories = 12.8; Total Carb (g) = 0.5; Net Carb (g) = 0.5; Fat (g) = 0.2; Protein = 2.6

Soup Swanson Vegetable Broth ☞ serving size: 1 cup = 220 g; Calories = 13.2; Total Carb (g) = 2.2; Net Carb (g) = 2.2; Fat (g) = 0.2; Protein = 0.5

Soup Tomato Beef With Noodle Canned Condensed ☞ serving size: 1 cup (8 fl oz) = 251 g; Calories = 281.1; Total Carb (g) = 42.3; Net Carb (g) = 39.3; Fat (g) = 8.6; Protein = 8.9

Soup Tomato Beef With Noodle Canned Prepared With Equal Volume Water ☞ serving size: 1 cup = 244 g; Calories = 136.6; Total Carb (g) = 20.6; Net Carb (g) = 19.1; Fat (g) = 4.2; Protein = 4.3

Soup Tomato Bisque Canned Condensed ☞ serving size: 1/2 cup (4 fl oz) = 129 g; Calories = 123.8; Total Carb (g) = 23.8; Net Carb (g) = 22.8; Fat (g) = 2.5; Protein = 2.3

Soup Tomato Bisque Canned Prepared With Equal Volume Milk ☞ serving size: 1 cup (8 fl oz) = 251 g; Calories = 198.3; Total Carb (g) = 29.4; Net Carb (g) = 28.9; Fat (g) = 6.6; Protein = 6.3

Soup Tomato Bisque Canned Prepared With Equal Volume Water ☞ serving size: 1 cup (8 fl oz) = 247 g; Calories = 123.5; Total Carb (g) = 23.7; Net Carb (g) = 23.2; Fat (g) = 2.5; Protein = 2.3

Soup Tomato Canned Condensed ☞ serving size: 1 cup = 148 g; Calories = 97.7; Total Carb (g) = 22.5; Net Carb (g) = 20.9; Fat (g) = 0.7; Protein = 2.2

Soup Tomato Canned Condensed Reduced Sodium ☞ serving size: 1 serving 1/2 cup = 121 g; Calories = 78.7; Total Carb (g) = 16.2; Net Carb (g) = 14.8; Fat (g) = 0.7; Protein = 2

Soup Tomato Canned Prepared With Equal Volume Low Fat (2%) Milk ☞ serving size: 1 serving 1 cup = 252 g; Calories = 138.6; Total Carb (g) = 24.8; Net Carb (g) = 23.5; Fat (g) = 3.1; Protein = 6.1

Soup Tomato Canned Prepared With Equal Volume Water Commercial ☞ serving size: 1 serving 1 cup = 248 g; Calories = 79.4; Total Carb (g) = 18.5; Net Carb (g) = 17.2; Fat (g) = 0.5; Protein = 1.8

Soup Tomato Dry Mix Prepared With Water ☞ serving size: 1 cup 8 fl oz = 265 g; Calories = 100.7; Total Carb (g) = 19; Net Carb (g) = 17.9; Fat (g) = 1.6; Protein = 2.5

Soup Tomato Low Sodium With Water ☞ serving size: 1 serving 1 cup = 248 g; Calories = 74.4; Total Carb (g) = 16.3; Net Carb (g) = 14.8; Fat (g) = 0.7; Protein = 2

Soup Tomato Rice Canned Condensed ☞ serving size: 1/2 cup (4 fl oz) = 129 g; Calories = 120; Total Carb (g) = 22; Net Carb (g) = 20.4; Fat (g) = 2.7; Protein = 2.1

Soup Tomato Rice Canned Prepared With Equal Volume Water ☞ serving size: 1 cup = 247 g; Calories = 116.1; Total Carb (g) = 21.1; Net Carb (g) = 19.4; Fat (g) = 2.6; Protein = 2

Soup Turkey Chunky Canned Ready-To-Serve ☞ serving size: 1 cup (8 fl oz) = 236 g; Calories = 134.5; Total Carb (g) = 14.1; Net Carb (g) = 14.1; Fat (g) = 4.4; Protein = 10.2

Soup Turkey Noodle Canned Prepared With Equal Volume Water ☞ serving size: 1 cup = 244 g; Calories = 68.3; Total Carb (g) = 8.6; Net Carb (g) = 7.9; Fat (g) = 2; Protein = 3.9

Soup Turkey Vegetable Canned Prepared With Equal Volume Water ☞ serving size: 1 cup (8 fl oz) = 241 g; Calories = 72.3; Total Carb (g) = 8.6; Net Carb (g) = 8.2; Fat (g) = 3; Protein = 3.1

Soup Vegetable Beef Canned Condensed ☞ serving size: 1/2 cup = 126 g; Calories = 79.4; Total Carb (g) = 10.2; Net Carb (g) = 8.2; Fat (g) = 1.9; Protein = 5.6

Soup Vegetable Beef Canned Prepared With Equal Volume Water ☞ serving size: 1 cup (8 fl oz) = 244 g; Calories = 75.6; Total Carb (g) = 9.9; Net Carb (g) = 8; Fat (g) = 1.9; Protein = 5.4

Soup Vegetable Beef Microwavable Ready-To-Serve Single Brand ☞ serving size: 1 serving = 292 g; Calories = 128.5; Total Carb (g) = 9.6; Net Carb (g) = 5.3; Fat (g) = 2; Protein = 18.1

Soup Vegetable Canned Low Sodium Condensed ☞ serving size: 1/2 cup = 126 g; Calories = 81.9; Total Carb (g) = 15.3; Net Carb (g) = 12.6; Fat (g) = 1.1; Protein = 2.8

Soup Vegetable Chicken Canned Prepared With Water Low Sodium ☞ serving size: 1 cup = 241 g; Calories = 166.3; Total Carb (g) = 21.1; Net Carb (g) = 20.2; Fat (g) = 4.8; Protein = 12.3

Soup Vegetable Soup Condensed Low Sodium Prepared With Equal Volume Water ☞ serving size: 1 cup = 253 g; Calories = 83.5; Total Carb (g) = 15.3; Net Carb (g) = 12.6; Fat (g) = 1.1; Protein = 2.8

Soup Vegetable With Beef Broth Canned Condensed ☞ serving size: 1/2 cup = 123 g; Calories = 81.2; Total Carb (g) = 13.2; Net Carb (g) = 11.6; Fat (g) = 1.9; Protein = 3

Soup Vegetable With Beef Broth Canned Prepared With Equal Volume Water ☞ serving size: 1 cup (8 fl oz) = 241 g; Calories = 79.5; Total Carb (g) = 12.9; Net Carb (g) = 11.2; Fat (g) = 1.9; Protein = 2.9

Soup Vegetarian Vegetable Canned Condensed ☞ serving size: 1/2 cup = 126 g; Calories = 74.3; Total Carb (g) = 12.3; Net Carb (g) = 11.7; Fat (g) = 2; Protein = 2.2

Soup Wonton Chinese Restaurant ☞ serving size: 1 cup = 223 g; Calories = 71.4; Total Carb (g) = 11.7; Net Carb (g) = 11.3; Fat (g) = 0.6; Protein = 4.6

Soupy Rice Mixture With Chicken And Potatoes Puerto Rican Style ☞ serving size: 1 cup = 240 g; Calories = 268.8; Total Carb (g) = 28.9; Net Carb (g) = 26.8; Fat (g) = 10.4; Protein = 15.2

Soupy Rice With Chicken Puerto Rican Style ☞ serving size: 1 cup, with bone (yield after bone removed) = 215 g; Calories = 324.7; Total Carb (g) = 35.5; Net Carb (g) = 32.4; Fat (g) = 8.6; Protein = 26

Soybean Soup Miso Broth ☞ serving size: 1 cup = 240 g; Calories = 76.8; Total Carb (g) = 5.9; Net Carb (g) = 5; Fat (g) = 3.7; Protein = 5.9

Spaghetti Sauce With Added Vegetables ☞ serving size: 1 cup = 260 g; Calories = 114.4; Total Carb (g) = 17.8; Net Carb (g) = 13.4; Fat (g) = 3.4; Protein = 3.6

Spaghetti Sauce With Meat ☞ serving size: 1 cup = 260 g; Calo-

ries = 231.4; Total Carb (g) = 15.7; Net Carb (g) = 11.8; Fat (g) = 11.6; Protein = 15.4

🍲 Spaghetti Sauce With Meat And Added Vegetables ☞ serving size: 1 cup = 260 g; Calories = 218.4; Total Carb (g) = 14.5; Net Carb (g) = 10.8; Fat (g) = 11; Protein = 15.4

🍲 Spaghetti Sauce With Poultry ☞ serving size: 1 cup = 260 g; Calories = 189.8; Total Carb (g) = 15.7; Net Carb (g) = 11.8; Fat (g) = 6.8; Protein = 16.4

🍲 Spaghetti Sauce With Poultry And Added Vegetables ☞ serving size: 1 cup = 260 g; Calories = 176.8; Total Carb (g) = 14.5; Net Carb (g) = 10.8; Fat (g) = 6.2; Protein = 16.4

🍲 Spaghetti Sauce With Seafood ☞ serving size: 1 cup = 260 g; Calories = 163.8; Total Carb (g) = 17.1; Net Carb (g) = 13.2; Fat (g) = 4.1; Protein = 13.8

🍲 Spaghetti Sauce With Seafood And Added Vegetables ☞ serving size: 1 cup = 260 g; Calories = 150.8; Total Carb (g) = 15.9; Net Carb (g) = 12.3; Fat (g) = 3.5; Protein = 13.8

🍲 Spanish Vegetable Soup Puerto Rican Style ☞ serving size: 1 cup = 250 g; Calories = 260; Total Carb (g) = 13.1; Net Carb (g) = 10.1; Fat (g) = 14.5; Protein = 19.4

🍲 Spinach And Artichoke Dip ☞ serving size: 1 tablespoon = 15 g; Calories = 49.4; Total Carb (g) = 0.7; Net Carb (g) = 0.5; Fat (g) = 5; Protein = 0.6

🍲 Spinach Dip Light ☞ serving size: 1 tablespoon = 15 g; Calories = 24.6; Total Carb (g) = 1.7; Net Carb (g) = 1.7; Fat (g) = 1.9; Protein = 0.3

🍲 Spinach Dip Regular ☞ serving size: 1 tablespoon = 15 g; Calories = 51.8; Total Carb (g) = 0.5; Net Carb (g) = 0.4; Fat (g) = 5.5; Protein = 0.3

🍲 Spinach Dip Yogurt Based ☞ serving size: 1 tablespoon = 15 g;

Calories = 23.7; Total Carb (g) = 0.5; Net Carb (g) = 0.5; Fat (g) = 1.9; Protein = 1.1

Spinach Soup ☞ serving size: 1 cup = 245 g; Calories = 73.5; Total Carb (g) = 7.1; Net Carb (g) = 5.1; Fat (g) = 2.4; Protein = 7.1

Split Pea Soup Canned Reduced Sodium Prepared With Water Or Ready-To Serve ☞ serving size: 1 cup = 253 g; Calories = 179.6; Total Carb (g) = 29.9; Net Carb (g) = 25.1; Fat (g) = 2.3; Protein = 9.7

Split Pea With Ham Soup Canned Reduced Sodium Prepared With Water Or Ready-To-Serve ☞ serving size: 1 cup = 245 g; Calories = 166.6; Total Carb (g) = 27.9; Net Carb (g) = 23.3; Fat (g) = 1.7; Protein = 9.8

Squash Winter Type Soup Home Recipe Canned Or Ready-To-Serve ☞ serving size: 1 cup = 248 g; Calories = 96.7; Total Carb (g) = 10.8; Net Carb (g) = 7.6; Fat (g) = 6.1; Protein = 1.2

Sriracha ☞ serving size: 1 tsp = 6.5 g; Calories = 6; Total Carb (g) = 1.3; Net Carb (g) = 1.1; Fat (g) = 0.1; Protein = 0.1

Sweet And Sour Sauce ☞ serving size: 1 cup = 240 g; Calories = 360; Total Carb (g) = 91.7; Net Carb (g) = 91.5; Fat (g) = 0.1; Protein = 0.7

Sweet And Sour Soup ☞ serving size: 1 cup = 244 g; Calories = 163.5; Total Carb (g) = 11.4; Net Carb (g) = 10.1; Fat (g) = 7.2; Protein = 13.8

Tabasco Sauce ☞ serving size: 1 tsp = 4.7 g; Calories = 0.6; Total Carb (g) = 0; Net Carb (g) = 0; Fat (g) = 0; Protein = 0.1

Teriyaki Sauce ☞ serving size: 2 tbsp = 36 g; Calories = 32; Total Carb (g) = 5.6; Net Carb (g) = 5.6; Fat (g) = 0; Protein = 2.1

Tomato Noodle Soup Canned Prepared With Milk ☞ serving size: 1 cup = 248 g; Calories = 173.6; Total Carb (g) = 30.1; Net Carb (g) = 28.6; Fat (g) = 3.4; Protein = 6.6

Tomato Noodle Soup Canned Prepared With Water Or Ready-To-Serve ☞ serving size: 1 cup = 244 g; Calories = 141.5; Total Carb (g) = 28.8; Net Carb (g) = 27.1; Fat (g) = 1.6; Protein = 4.1

Tomato Relish ☞ serving size: 1 cup = 320 g; Calories = 502.4; Total Carb (g) = 120.4; Net Carb (g) = 112.7; Fat (g) = 1.9; Protein = 7

Tomato Soup Canned Reduced Sodium Prepared With Milk ☞ serving size: 1 cup = 248 g; Calories = 143.8; Total Carb (g) = 22.6; Net Carb (g) = 21.2; Fat (g) = 3.2; Protein = 6.1

Tomato Soup Canned Reduced Sodium Prepared With Water Or Ready-To-Serve ☞ serving size: 1 cup = 244 g; Calories = 80.5; Total Carb (g) = 16.6; Net Carb (g) = 15.1; Fat (g) = 0.7; Protein = 2

Tomato Soup Cream Of Prepared With Milk ☞ serving size: 1 cup = 248 g; Calories = 143.8; Total Carb (g) = 24.9; Net Carb (g) = 23.4; Fat (g) = 3.1; Protein = 5.9

Tomato Soup Nfs ☞ serving size: 1 cup = 244 g; Calories = 80.5; Total Carb (g) = 18.8; Net Carb (g) = 17.4; Fat (g) = 0.5; Protein = 1.8

Tomato Soup Prepared With Water Or Ready-To-Serve ☞ serving size: 1 cup = 244 g; Calories = 80.5; Total Carb (g) = 18.8; Net Carb (g) = 17.4; Fat (g) = 0.5; Protein = 1.8

Tomato Vegetable Soup Prepared With Water ☞ serving size: 1 cup = 241 g; Calories = 79.5; Total Carb (g) = 18.6; Net Carb (g) = 17.2; Fat (g) = 0.5; Protein = 1.8

Turtle And Vegetable Soup ☞ serving size: 1 cup = 244 g; Calories = 102.5; Total Carb (g) = 9.1; Net Carb (g) = 7.4; Fat (g) = 2.3; Protein = 11.6

Tzatziki Dip ☞ serving size: 1 tablespoon = 15 g; Calories = 13.8; Total Carb (g) = 0.6; Net Carb (g) = 0.6; Fat (g) = 1; Protein = 0.8

Vegetable Beef Noodle Soup Prepared With Water ☞ serving size: 1 cup = 244 g; Calories = 78.1; Total Carb (g) = 10.1; Net Carb (g) = 8.1; Fat (g) = 1.9; Protein = 5.5

🍲 Vegetable Beef Soup Canned Prepared With Milk ☞ serving size: 1 cup = 248 g; Calories = 141.4; Total Carb (g) = 16.1; Net Carb (g) = 14.1; Fat (g) = 4.4; Protein = 9.6

🍲 Vegetable Beef Soup Canned Prepared With Water Or Ready-To-Serve ☞ serving size: 1 cup = 244 g; Calories = 78.1; Total Carb (g) = 10; Net Carb (g) = 8.1; Fat (g) = 1.9; Protein = 5.5

🍲 Vegetable Beef Soup Home Recipe ☞ serving size: 1 cup = 241 g; Calories = 132.6; Total Carb (g) = 9.4; Net Carb (g) = 7.5; Fat (g) = 4.4; Protein = 14.1

🍲 Vegetable Beef Soup With Noodles Or Pasta Home Recipe ☞ serving size: 1 cup = 241 g; Calories = 161.5; Total Carb (g) = 13.7; Net Carb (g) = 11.8; Fat (g) = 4.9; Protein = 15.5

🍲 Vegetable Beef Soup With Rice Canned Prepared With Water Or Ready-To-Serve ☞ serving size: 1 cup = 244 g; Calories = 78.1; Total Carb (g) = 10.1; Net Carb (g) = 8.1; Fat (g) = 1.9; Protein = 5.5

🍲 Vegetable Beef Soup With Rice Home Recipe ☞ serving size: 1 cup = 244 g; Calories = 163.5; Total Carb (g) = 15.4; Net Carb (g) = 13.6; Fat (g) = 4.6; Protein = 15.1

🍲 Vegetable Broth ☞ serving size: 1 cup = 221 g; Calories = 11.1; Total Carb (g) = 2.1; Net Carb (g) = 2.1; Fat (g) = 0.2; Protein = 0.5

🍲 Vegetable Dip Light ☞ serving size: 1 tablespoon = 15 g; Calories = 29.6; Total Carb (g) = 2; Net Carb (g) = 2; Fat (g) = 2.3; Protein = 0.3

🍲 Vegetable Dip Regular ☞ serving size: 1 tablespoon = 15 g; Calories = 64.4; Total Carb (g) = 0.5; Net Carb (g) = 0.4; Fat (g) = 6.9; Protein = 0.3

🍲 Vegetable Dip Yogurt Based ☞ serving size: 1 tablespoon = 15 g; Calories = 28.7; Total Carb (g) = 0.6; Net Carb (g) = 0.5; Fat (g) = 2.4; Protein = 1.2

🍲 Vegetable Noodle Soup Canned Prepared With Water Or Ready-

To-Serve ☞ serving size: 1 cup = 241 g; Calories = 72.3; Total Carb (g) = 11.8; Net Carb (g) = 11.1; Fat (g) = 1.9; Protein = 2.1

🥣 Vegetable Noodle Soup Home Recipe ☞ serving size: 1 cup = 241 g; Calories = 113.3; Total Carb (g) = 17.6; Net Carb (g) = 15.2; Fat (g) = 2.8; Protein = 5.3

🥣 Vegetable Soup ☞ serving size: 1 cup = 241 g; Calories = 67.5; Total Carb (g) = 11.8; Net Carb (g) = 11.1; Fat (g) = 1.9; Protein = 2.1

🥣 Vegetable Soup Cream Of Prepared With Milk ☞ serving size: 1 cup = 248 g; Calories = 213.3; Total Carb (g) = 22.4; Net Carb (g) = 21.6; Fat (g) = 9.9; Protein = 9.1

🥣 Vegetable Soup Home Recipe ☞ serving size: 1 cup = 234 g; Calories = 88.9; Total Carb (g) = 14.6; Net Carb (g) = 11.8; Fat (g) = 2; Protein = 4.3

🥣 Vegetable Soup Made From Dry Mix ☞ serving size: 1 cup = 253 g; Calories = 101.2; Total Carb (g) = 11.9; Net Carb (g) = 11.2; Fat (g) = 5.5; Protein = 1.8

🥣 Vegetable Soup Spanish Style Stew Type ☞ serving size: 1 cup = 227 g; Calories = 197.5; Total Carb (g) = 18.2; Net Carb (g) = 14.6; Fat (g) = 7.3; Protein = 15.2

🥣 Vegetable Soup With Chicken Broth Home Recipe Mexican Style ☞ serving size: 1 cup = 232 g; Calories = 141.5; Total Carb (g) = 15.1; Net Carb (g) = 13.7; Fat (g) = 6.9; Protein = 5.7

🥣 Vegetarian Vegetable Soup Prepared With Water ☞ serving size: 1 cup = 241 g; Calories = 72.3; Total Carb (g) = 11.8; Net Carb (g) = 11.1; Fat (g) = 1.9; Protein = 2.1

🥣 Vodka Sauce With Tomatoes And Cream ☞ serving size: 1 cup = 260 g; Calories = 192.4; Total Carb (g) = 8.9; Net Carb (g) = 5.5; Fat (g) = 17.1; Protein = 3.3

🥣 Wasabi ☞ serving size: 1 tablespoon = 20 g; Calories = 58.4; Total Carb (g) = 9.2; Net Carb (g) = 8; Fat (g) = 2.2; Protein = 0.5

Watercress Broth With Shrimp ☞ serving size: 1 cup = 245 g; Calories = 117.6; Total Carb (g) = 3.3; Net Carb (g) = 3; Fat (g) = 4.5; Protein = 15.3

Welsh Rarebit ☞ serving size: 1 tablespoon = 15 g; Calories = 24.5; Total Carb (g) = 1; Net Carb (g) = 1; Fat (g) = 1.8; Protein = 1.1

White Sauce Milk Sauce ☞ serving size: 1 cup = 250 g; Calories = 367.5; Total Carb (g) = 23; Net Carb (g) = 22.5; Fat (g) = 26.9; Protein = 9.3

Worcestershire Sauce ☞ serving size: 1 tbsp = 17 g; Calories = 13.1; Total Carb (g) = 3.3; Net Carb (g) = 3.3; Fat (g) = 0; Protein = 0

Yeast Extract Spread ☞ serving size: 1 tsp = 6 g; Calories = 11.1; Total Carb (g) = 1.2; Net Carb (g) = 0.8; Fat (g) = 0.1; Protein = 1.4

Zucchini Soup Cream Of Prepared With Milk ☞ serving size: 1 cup = 248 g; Calories = 57; Total Carb (g) = 6.8; Net Carb (g) = 5.8; Fat (g) = 2; Protein = 4.2

27

SPICES AND HERBS

🌿 Anise Seeds ☞ serving size: 1 tsp, whole = 2.1 g; Calories = 7.1; Total Carb (g) = 1.1; Net Carb (g) = 0.7; Fat (g) = 0.3; Protein = 0.4

🌿 Apple Cider Vinegar ☞ serving size: 1 tbsp = 14.9 g; Calories = 3.1; Total Carb (g) = 0.1; Net Carb (g) = 0.1; Fat (g) = 0; Protein = 0

🌿 Balsamic Vinegar ☞ serving size: 1 tbsp = 16 g; Calories = 14.1; Total Carb (g) = 2.7; Net Carb (g) = 2.7; Fat (g) = 0; Protein = 0.1

🌿 Basil ☞ serving size: 5 leaves = 2.5 g; Calories = 0.6; Total Carb (g) = 0.1; Net Carb (g) = 0; Fat (g) = 0; Protein = 0.1

🌿 Bay Leaves ☞ serving size: 1 tsp, crumbled = 0.6 g; Calories = 1.9; Total Carb (g) = 0.5; Net Carb (g) = 0.3; Fat (g) = 0.1; Protein = 0.1

🌿 Black Pepper ☞ serving size: 1 tsp, ground = 2.3 g; Calories = 5.8; Total Carb (g) = 1.5; Net Carb (g) = 0.9; Fat (g) = 0.1; Protein = 0.2

🌿 Capers ☞ serving size: 1 tbsp, drained = 8.6 g; Calories = 2; Total Carb (g) = 0.4; Net Carb (g) = 0.2; Fat (g) = 0.1; Protein = 0.2

🌿 Caraway Seed ☞ serving size: 1 tsp = 2.1 g; Calories = 7; Total Carb (g) = 1.1; Net Carb (g) = 0.3; Fat (g) = 0.3; Protein = 0.4

🌿 Cardamom ☞ serving size: 1 tsp, ground = 2 g; Calories = 6.2; Total Carb (g) = 1.4; Net Carb (g) = 0.8; Fat (g) = 0.1; Protein = 0.2

🌿 Cayenne Pepper ☞ serving size: 1 tsp = 1.8 g; Calories = 5.7; Total Carb (g) = 1; Net Carb (g) = 0.5; Fat (g) = 0.3; Protein = 0.2

🌿 Celery Seed ☞ serving size: 1 tsp = 2 g; Calories = 7.8; Total Carb (g) = 0.8; Net Carb (g) = 0.6; Fat (g) = 0.5; Protein = 0.4

🌿 Chili Powder ☞ serving size: 1 tsp = 2.7 g; Calories = 7.6; Total Carb (g) = 1.3; Net Carb (g) = 0.4; Fat (g) = 0.4; Protein = 0.4

🌿 Cinnamon ☞ serving size: 1 tsp = 2.6 g; Calories = 6.4; Total Carb (g) = 2.1; Net Carb (g) = 0.7; Fat (g) = 0; Protein = 0.1

🌿 Coriander Seed ☞ serving size: 1 tsp = 1.8 g; Calories = 5.4; Total Carb (g) = 1; Net Carb (g) = 0.2; Fat (g) = 0.3; Protein = 0.2

🌿 Cumin Seed ☞ serving size: 1 tsp, whole = 2.1 g; Calories = 7.9; Total Carb (g) = 0.9; Net Carb (g) = 0.7; Fat (g) = 0.5; Protein = 0.4

🌿 Curry Powder ☞ serving size: 1 tsp = 2 g; Calories = 6.5; Total Carb (g) = 1.1; Net Carb (g) = 0.1; Fat (g) = 0.3; Protein = 0.3

🌿 Dill ☞ serving size: 5 sprigs = 1 g; Calories = 0.4; Total Carb (g) = 0.1; Net Carb (g) = 0.1; Fat (g) = 0; Protein = 0

🌿 Dill Seed ☞ serving size: 1 tsp = 2.1 g; Calories = 6.4; Total Carb (g) = 1.2; Net Carb (g) = 0.7; Fat (g) = 0.3; Protein = 0.3

🌿 Distilled Vinegar ☞ serving size: 1 tbsp = 14.9 g; Calories = 2.7; Total Carb (g) = 0; Net Carb (g) = 0; Fat (g) = 0; Protein = 0

🌿 Dried Basil ☞ serving size: 1 tsp, leaves = 0.7 g; Calories = 1.6; Total Carb (g) = 0.3; Net Carb (g) = 0.1; Fat (g) = 0; Protein = 0.2

🌿 Dried Chervil ☞ serving size: 1 tsp = 0.6 g; Calories = 1.4; Total Carb (g) = 0.3; Net Carb (g) = 0.2; Fat (g) = 0; Protein = 0.1

🌿 Dried Coriander ☞ serving size: 1 tsp = 0.6 g; Calories = 1.7; Total Carb (g) = 0.3; Net Carb (g) = 0.3; Fat (g) = 0; Protein = 0.1

🌿 Dried Dill Weed ☞ serving size: 1 tsp = 1 g; Calories = 2.5; Total Carb (g) = 0.6; Net Carb (g) = 0.4; Fat (g) = 0; Protein = 0.2

🌿 Dried Marjoram ☞ serving size: 1 tsp = 0.6 g; Calories = 1.6; Total Carb (g) = 0.4; Net Carb (g) = 0.1; Fat (g) = 0; Protein = 0.1

🌿 Dried Oregano ☞ serving size: 1 tsp, leaves = 1 g; Calories = 2.7; Total Carb (g) = 0.7; Net Carb (g) = 0.3; Fat (g) = 0; Protein = 0.1

🌿 Dried Parsley ☞ serving size: 1 tsp = 0.5 g; Calories = 1.5; Total Carb (g) = 0.3; Net Carb (g) = 0.1; Fat (g) = 0; Protein = 0.1

🌿 Dried Rosemary ☞ serving size: 1 tsp = 1.2 g; Calories = 4; Total Carb (g) = 0.8; Net Carb (g) = 0.3; Fat (g) = 0.2; Protein = 0.1

🌿 Dried Spearmint ☞ serving size: 1 tsp = 0.5 g; Calories = 1.4; Total Carb (g) = 0.3; Net Carb (g) = 0.1; Fat (g) = 0; Protein = 0.1

🌿 Dried Tarragon ☞ serving size: 1 tsp, leaves = 0.6 g; Calories = 1.8; Total Carb (g) = 0.3; Net Carb (g) = 0.3; Fat (g) = 0; Protein = 0.1

🌿 Fennel Seed ☞ serving size: 1 tsp, whole = 2 g; Calories = 6.9; Total Carb (g) = 1.1; Net Carb (g) = 0.3; Fat (g) = 0.3; Protein = 0.3

🌿 Fenugreek Seed ☞ serving size: 1 tsp = 3.7 g; Calories = 12; Total Carb (g) = 2.2; Net Carb (g) = 1.3; Fat (g) = 0.2; Protein = 0.9

🌿 Garlic Powder ☞ serving size: 1 tsp = 3.1 g; Calories = 10.3; Total Carb (g) = 2.3; Net Carb (g) = 2; Fat (g) = 0; Protein = 0.5

🌿 Ground Allspice ☞ serving size: 1 tsp = 1.9 g; Calories – 5; Total Carb (g) = 1.4; Net Carb (g) = 1; Fat (g) = 0.2; Protein = 0.1

🌿 Ground Cloves ☞ serving size: 1 tsp = 2.1 g; Calories = 5.8; Total Carb (g) = 1.4; Net Carb (g) = 0.7; Fat (g) = 0.3; Protein = 0.1

🌿 Ground Ginger ☞ serving size: 1 tsp = 1.8 g; Calories = 6; Total Carb (g) = 1.3; Net Carb (g) = 1; Fat (g) = 0.1; Protein = 0.2

🌿 Ground Mace ☞ serving size: 1 tsp = 1.7 g; Calories = 8.1; Total Carb (g) = 0.9; Net Carb (g) = 0.5; Fat (g) = 0.6; Protein = 0.1

🌿 Ground Mustard Seed ☞ serving size: 1 tsp = 2 g; Calories = 10.2; Total Carb (g) = 0.6; Net Carb (g) = 0.3; Fat (g) = 0.7; Protein = 0.5

🌿 Ground Nutmeg ☞ serving size: 1 tsp = 2.2 g; Calories = 11.6; Total Carb (g) = 1.1; Net Carb (g) = 0.6; Fat (g) = 0.8; Protein = 0.1

🌿 Ground Sage ☞ serving size: 1 tsp = 0.7 g; Calories = 2.2; Total Carb (g) = 0.4; Net Carb (g) = 0.1; Fat (g) = 0.1; Protein = 0.1

🌿 Ground Savory ☞ serving size: 1 tsp = 1.4 g; Calories = 3.8; Total Carb (g) = 1; Net Carb (g) = 0.3; Fat (g) = 0.1; Protein = 0.1

🌿 Ground Turmeric ☞ serving size: 1 tsp = 3 g; Calories = 9.4; Total Carb (g) = 2; Net Carb (g) = 1.3; Fat (g) = 0.1; Protein = 0.3

🌿 Horseradish ☞ serving size: 1 tsp = 5 g; Calories = 2.4; Total Carb (g) = 0.6; Net Carb (g) = 0.4; Fat (g) = 0; Protein = 0.1

🌿 Imitation Vanilla Extract ☞ serving size: 1 tsp = 4.2 g; Calories = 10; Total Carb (g) = 0.1; Net Carb (g) = 0.1; Fat (g) = 0; Protein = 0

🌿 Imitation Vanilla Extract (No Alcohol) ☞ serving size: 1 tsp = 4.2 g; Calories = 2.4; Total Carb (g) = 0.6; Net Carb (g) = 0.6; Fat (g) = 0; Protein = 0

🌿 Onion Powder ☞ serving size: 1 tsp = 2.4 g; Calories = 8.2; Total Carb (g) = 1.9; Net Carb (g) = 1.5; Fat (g) = 0; Protein = 0.3

🌿 Paprika ☞ serving size: 1 tsp = 2.3 g; Calories = 6.5; Total Carb (g) = 1.2; Net Carb (g) = 0.4; Fat (g) = 0.3; Protein = 0.3

🌿 Peppermint ☞ serving size: 2 leaves = 0.1 g; Calories = 0.1; Total Carb (g) = 0; Net Carb (g) = 0; Fat (g) = 0; Protein = 0

🌿 Poppy Seeds ☞ serving size: 1 tsp = 2.8 g; Calories = 14.7; Total Carb (g) = 0.8; Net Carb (g) = 0.2; Fat (g) = 1.2; Protein = 0.5

🌿 Poultry Seasoning ☞ serving size: 1 tsp = 1.5 g; Calories = 4.6; Total Carb (g) = 1; Net Carb (g) = 0.8; Fat (g) = 0.1; Protein = 0.1

❧ Pumpkin Pie Spice ☞ serving size: 1 tsp = 1.7 g; Calories = 5.8; Total Carb (g) = 1.2; Net Carb (g) = 0.9; Fat (g) = 0.2; Protein = 0.1

❧ Red Wine Vinegar ☞ serving size: 1 tbsp = 14.9 g; Calories = 2.8; Total Carb (g) = 0; Net Carb (g) = 0; Fat (g) = 0; Protein = 0

❧ Rosemary ☞ serving size: 1 tsp = 0.7 g; Calories = 0.9; Total Carb (g) = 0.1; Net Carb (g) = 0.1; Fat (g) = 0; Protein = 0

❧ Saffron ☞ serving size: 1 tsp = 0.7 g; Calories = 2.2; Total Carb (g) = 0.5; Net Carb (g) = 0.4; Fat (g) = 0; Protein = 0.1

❧ Seasoning Mix Dry Chili Original ☞ serving size: tbsp = 9 g; Calories = 30.2; Total Carb (g) = 5.1; Net Carb (g) = 4.1; Fat (g) = 0.7; Protein = 1

❧ Seasoning Mix Dry Sazon Coriander & Annatto ☞ serving size: 1/4 tsp = 1 g; Calories = 0; Total Carb (g) = 0; Net Carb (g) = 0; Fat (g) = 0; Protein = 0

❧ Seasoning Mix Dry Taco Original ☞ serving size: 2 tsp = 5.7 g; Calories = 18.4; Total Carb (g) = 3.3; Net Carb (g) = 2.6; Fat (g) = 0; Protein = 0.3

❧ Spearmint ☞ serving size: 2 leaves = 0.3 g; Calories = 0.1; Total Carb (g) = 0; Net Carb (g) = 0; Fat (g) = 0; Protein = 0

❧ Spices Thyme Dried ☞ serving size: 1 tsp, leaves = 1 g; Calories = 2.8; Total Carb (g) = 0.6; Net Carb (g) = 0.3; Fat (g) = 0.1; Protein = 0.1

❧ Table Salt ☞ serving size: 1 tsp = 6 g; Calories = 0; Total Carb (g) = 0; Net Carb (g) = 0; Fat (g) = 0; Protein = 0

❧ Thyme (Fresh) ☞ serving size: 1 tsp = 0.8 g; Calories = 0.8; Total Carb (g) = 0.2; Net Carb (g) = 0.1; Fat (g) = 0; Protein = 0

❧ Vanilla Extract ☞ serving size: 1 tsp = 4.2 g; Calories = 12.1; Total Carb (g) = 0.5; Net Carb (g) = 0.5; Fat (g) = 0; Protein = 0

❧ White Pepper ☞ serving size: 1 tsp, ground = 2.4 g; Calories = 7.1; Total Carb (g) = 1.7; Net Carb (g) = 1; Fat (g) = 0.1; Protein = 0.3

🌿 Yellow Mustard ☞ serving size: 1 tsp or 1 packet = 5 g; Calories = 3; Total Carb (g) = 0.3; Net Carb (g) = 0.1; Fat (g) = 0.2; Protein = 0.2

28

VEGETABLES & VEGETABLES PRODUCTS

⬤ Acorn Squash ☞ serving size: 1 cup, cubes = 140 g; Calories = 56; Total Carb (g) = 14.6; Net Carb (g) = 12.5; Fat (g) = 0.1; Protein = 1.1

⬤ Alfalfa Sprouts ☞ serving size: 1 cup = 33 g; Calories = 7.6; Total Carb (g) = 0.7; Net Carb (g) = 0.1; Fat (g) = 0.2; Protein = 1.3

⬤ Amaranth Leaves Raw ☞ serving size: 1 cup = 28 g; Calories = 6.4; Total Carb (g) = 1.1; Net Carb (g) = 1.1; Fat (g) = 0.1; Protein = 0.7

⬤ Arrowhead Raw ☞ serving size: 1 large = 25 g; Calories = 24.8; Total Carb (g) = 5.1; Net Carb (g) = 5.1; Fat (g) = 0.1; Protein = 1.3

⬤ Arrowroot ☞ serving size: 1 cup, sliced = 120 g; Calories = 78; Total Carb (g) = 16.1; Net Carb (g) = 14.5; Fat (g) = 0.2; Protein = 5.1

⬤ Artichoke Cooked From Canned Ns As To Fat Added In Cooking ☞ serving size: 1 small globe = 103 g; Calories = 62.8; Total Carb (g) = 9.2; Net Carb (g) = 4.6; Fat (g) = 2.5; Protein = 3.1

⬤ Artichoke Cooked From Fresh Ns As To Fat Added In Cooking ☞ serving size: 1 small globe = 103 g; Calories = 71.1; Total Carb (g) = 11.9; Net Carb (g) = 6.3; Fat (g) = 2.4; Protein = 2.9

● Artichoke Cooked From Frozen Ns As To Fat Added In Cooking ☞ serving size: 1 cup, hearts = 173 g; Calories = 105.5; Total Carb (g) = 15.4; Net Carb (g) = 7.8; Fat (g) = 4.3; Protein = 5.2

● Artichokes (Globe Or French) ☞ serving size: 1 artichoke, medium = 128 g; Calories = 60.2; Total Carb (g) = 13.5; Net Carb (g) = 6.5; Fat (g) = 0.2; Protein = 4.2

● Arugula ☞ serving size: 1 leaf = 2 g; Calories = 0.5; Total Carb (g) = 0.1; Net Carb (g) = 0; Fat (g) = 0; Protein = 0.1

● Asparagus ☞ serving size: 1 cup = 134 g; Calories = 26.8; Total Carb (g) = 5.2; Net Carb (g) = 2.4; Fat (g) = 0.2; Protein = 3

● Asparagus Cooked Ns As To Form Fat Added In Cooking Ns As To Type Of Fat ☞ serving size: 1 piece = 3 g; Calories = 1; Total Carb (g) = 0.1; Net Carb (g) = 0; Fat (g) = 0.1; Protein = 0.1

● Asparagus Ns As To Form Creamed Or With Cheese Sauce ☞ serving size: 1 cup = 235 g; Calories = 155.1; Total Carb (g) = 8.5; Net Carb (g) = 5.9; Fat (g) = 10.1; Protein = 9.9

● Baby Carrots ☞ serving size: 1 large = 15 g; Calories = 5.3; Total Carb (g) = 1.2; Net Carb (g) = 0.8; Fat (g) = 0; Protein = 0.1

● Baked Acorn Squash ☞ serving size: 1 cup, cubes = 205 g; Calories = 114.8; Total Carb (g) = 29.9; Net Carb (g) = 20.9; Fat (g) = 0.3; Protein = 2.3

● Baked Potato (No Skin) ☞ serving size: 1/2 cup = 61 g; Calories = 56.7; Total Carb (g) = 13.2; Net Carb (g) = 12.2; Fat (g) = 0.1; Protein = 1.2

● Baked Potatoes ☞ serving size: 1 potato large (3 inch to 4-1/4 inch dia) = 299 g; Calories = 275.1; Total Carb (g) = 63; Net Carb (g) = 56.8; Fat (g) = 0.5; Protein = 6.3

● Baked Potatoes (With Skin) ☞ serving size: 1 nlea serving = 148 g; Calories = 137.6; Total Carb (g) = 31.3; Net Carb (g) = 28.1; Fat (g) = 0.2; Protein = 3.7

● Baked Red Potatoes ☞ serving size: 1 potato large (3 inch to 4-1/4 inch dia. = 299 g; Calories = 260.1; Total Carb (g) = 58.6; Net Carb (g) = 53.2; Fat (g) = 0.5; Protein = 6.9

● Baked Russet Potatoes ☞ serving size: 1 potato large (3 inch to 4-1/4 inch dia. = 299 g; Calories = 284.1; Total Carb (g) = 64.1; Net Carb (g) = 57.2; Fat (g) = 0.4; Protein = 7.9

● Balsam-Pear (Bitter Gourd) Leafy Tips Raw ☞ serving size: 1 leaf = 4 g; Calories = 1.2; Total Carb (g) = 0.1; Net Carb (g) = 0.1; Fat (g) = 0; Protein = 0.2

● Bamboo Shoots ☞ serving size: 1 cup (1/2 inch slices) = 151 g; Calories = 40.8; Total Carb (g) = 7.9; Net Carb (g) = 4.5; Fat (g) = 0.5; Protein = 3.9

● Bamboo Shoots (Canned) ☞ serving size: 1 cup (1/8 inch slices) = 131 g; Calories = 24.9; Total Carb (g) = 4.2; Net Carb (g) = 2.4; Fat (g) = 0.5; Protein = 2.3

● Bamboo Shoots (Cooked) ☞ serving size: 1 cup (1/2 inch slices) = 120 g; Calories = 14.4; Total Carb (g) = 2.3; Net Carb (g) = 1.1; Fat (g) = 0.3; Protein = 1.8

● Banana Peppers ☞ serving size: 1 cup = 124 g; Calories = 33.5; Total Carb (g) = 6.6; Net Carb (g) = 2.4; Fat (g) = 0.6; Protein = 2.1

● Bean Sprouts Cooked Ns As To Form Ns As To Fat Added In Cooking ☞ serving size: 1 cup = 129 g; Calories = 103.2; Total Carb (g) = 6.4; Net Carb (g) = 5.4; Fat (g) = 7.5; Protein = 5.9

● Beans Lima Immature Cooked Ns As To Form Fat Added In Cooking Ns As To Type Of Fat ☞ serving size: 1 cup = 185 g; Calories = 216.5; Total Carb (g) = 34.6; Net Carb (g) = 25.2; Fat (g) = 4.2; Protein = 10.9

● Beans Navy Mature Seeds Sprouted Raw ☞ serving size: 1 cup = 104 g; Calories = 69.7; Total Carb (g) = 13.6; Net Carb (g) = 13.6; Fat (g) = 0.7; Protein = 6.4

● Beans Pinto Immature Seeds Frozen Unprepared ☞ serving size: 1/ 3 package (10 oz) = 94 g; Calories = 159.8; Total Carb (g) = 30.6; Net Carb (g) = 25.2; Fat (g) = 0.5; Protein = 9.2

● Beans Shellie Canned Solids And Liquids ☞ serving size: 1 cup = 245 g; Calories = 73.5; Total Carb (g) = 15.2; Net Carb (g) = 6.8; Fat (g) = 0.5; Protein = 4.3

● Beans Snap Green Frozen All Styles Unprepared ☞ serving size: 1 cup = 121 g; Calories = 39.9; Total Carb (g) = 9.1; Net Carb (g) = 6; Fat (g) = 0.3; Protein = 2.2

● Beans Snap Yellow Frozen Cooked Boiled Drained Without Salt ☞ serving size: 1 cup = 135 g; Calories = 37.8; Total Carb (g) = 8.7; Net Carb (g) = 4.7; Fat (g) = 0.2; Protein = 2

● Beans String Cooked From Canned Ns As To Color Fat Added In Cooking Ns As To Type Of Fat ☞ serving size: 1 cup = 140 g; Calories = 56; Total Carb (g) = 5.7; Net Carb (g) = 3.2; Fat (g) = 3.6; Protein = 1.4

● Beet Greens (Raw) ☞ serving size: 1 cup = 38 g; Calories = 8.4; Total Carb (g) = 1.7; Net Carb (g) = 0.2; Fat (g) = 0.1; Protein = 0.8

● Beets (Raw) ☞ serving size: 1 cup = 136 g; Calories = 58.5; Total Carb (g) = 13; Net Carb (g) = 9.2; Fat (g) = 0.2; Protein = 2.2

● Beets Cooked Ns As To Form Ns As To Fat Added In Cooking ☞ serving size: 1 cup, whole = 168 g; Calories = 100.8; Total Carb (g) = 16.2; Net Carb (g) = 13; Fat (g) = 3.6; Protein = 2.8

● Bitter Melon ☞ serving size: 1 cup (1/2 inch pieces) = 93 g; Calories = 15.8; Total Carb (g) = 3.4; Net Carb (g) = 0.8; Fat (g) = 0.2; Protein = 0.9

● Bitter Melon (Cooked) ☞ serving size: 1 cup (1/2 inch pieces) = 124 g; Calories = 23.6; Total Carb (g) = 5.4; Net Carb (g) = 2.9; Fat (g) = 0.2; Protein = 1

● Bok Choy ☞ serving size: 1 cup, shredded = 70 g; Calories = 9.1; Total Carb (g) = 1.5; Net Carb (g) = 0.8; Fat (g) = 0.1; Protein = 1.1

● Borage Raw ☞ serving size: 1 cup (1 inch pieces) = 89 g; Calories = 18.7; Total Carb (g) = 2.7; Net Carb (g) = 2.7; Fat (g) = 0.6; Protein = 1.6

● Breadfruit Cooked Ns As To Fat Added In Cooking ☞ serving size: 1 cup = 257 g; Calories = 336.7; Total Carb (g) = 73.8; Net Carb (g) = 60.5; Fat (g) = 6.9; Protein = 3

● Broadbeans Immature Seeds Raw ☞ serving size: 1 cup = 109 g; Calories = 78.5; Total Carb (g) = 12.8; Net Carb (g) = 8.2; Fat (g) = 0.7; Protein = 6.1

● Broccoflower Cooked Ns As To Fat Added In Cooking ☞ serving size: 1 cup, fresh = 87 g; Calories = 51.3; Total Carb (g) = 5.2; Net Carb (g) = 2.5; Fat (g) = 3.1; Protein = 2.5

● Broccoli ☞ serving size: 1 cup chopped = 91 g; Calories = 30.9; Total Carb (g) = 6; Net Carb (g) = 3.7; Fat (g) = 0.3; Protein = 2.6

● Broccoli (Cooked) ☞ serving size: 1/2 cup, chopped = 78 g; Calories = 27.3; Total Carb (g) = 5.6; Net Carb (g) = 3; Fat (g) = 0.3; Protein = 1.9

● Brussels Sprouts (Cooked) ☞ serving size: 1 sprout = 21 g; Calories = 7.6; Total Carb (g) = 1.5; Net Carb (g) = 1; Fat (g) = 0.1; Protein = 0.5

● Brussels Sprouts (Raw) ☞ serving size: 1 cup = 88 g; Calories = 37.8; Total Carb (g) = 7.9; Net Carb (g) = 4.5; Fat (g) = 0.3; Protein = 3

● Burdock Root Raw ☞ serving size: 1 cup (1 inch pieces) = 118 g; Calories = 85; Total Carb (g) = 20.5; Net Carb (g) = 16.6; Fat (g) = 0.2; Protein = 1.8

● Butterbur (Fuki) Raw ☞ serving size: 1 cup = 94 g; Calories = 13.2; Total Carb (g) = 3.4; Net Carb (g) = 3.4; Fat (g) = 0; Protein = 0.4

Butterhead Lettuce ☞ serving size: 1 cup, shredded or chopped = 55 g; Calories = 7.2; Total Carb (g) = 1.2; Net Carb (g) = 0.6; Fat (g) = 0.1; Protein = 0.7

Butternut Squash ☞ serving size: 1 cup, cubes = 140 g; Calories = 63; Total Carb (g) = 16.4; Net Carb (g) = 13.6; Fat (g) = 0.1; Protein = 1.4

Cabbage ☞ serving size: 1 cup, chopped = 89 g; Calories = 22.3; Total Carb (g) = 5.2; Net Carb (g) = 2.9; Fat (g) = 0.1; Protein = 1.1

Cabbage Chinese (Pak-Choi) Cooked Boiled Drained With Salt ☞ serving size: 1 cup, shredded = 170 g; Calories = 20.4; Total Carb (g) = 3; Net Carb (g) = 1.3; Fat (g) = 0.3; Protein = 2.7

Cabbage Green Cooked Ns As To Fat Added In Cooking ☞ serving size: 1 cup = 155 g; Calories = 65.1; Total Carb (g) = 8.3; Net Carb (g) = 5.5; Fat (g) = 3.5; Protein = 1.9

Cabbage Japanese Style Fresh Pickled ☞ serving size: 1 cup = 150 g; Calories = 45; Total Carb (g) = 8.5; Net Carb (g) = 3.9; Fat (g) = 0.2; Protein = 2.4

Cabbage Mustard Salted ☞ serving size: 1 cup = 128 g; Calories = 35.8; Total Carb (g) = 7.2; Net Carb (g) = 3.2; Fat (g) = 0.1; Protein = 1.4

Cabbage Red Cooked Ns As To Fat Added In Cooking ☞ serving size: 1 cup = 155 g; Calories = 72.9; Total Carb (g) = 10.4; Net Carb (g) = 6.5; Fat (g) = 3.6; Protein = 2.3

Cabbage Savoy Cooked Ns As To Fat Added In Cooking ☞ serving size: 1 cup = 150 g; Calories = 72; Total Carb (g) = 9.2; Net Carb (g) = 4.6; Fat (g) = 3.7; Protein = 3.1

Cactus Cooked Ns As To Fat Added In Cooking ☞ serving size: 1 cup = 154 g; Calories = 52.4; Total Carb (g) = 4.9; Net Carb (g) = 2; Fat (g) = 3.5; Protein = 2

Calabaza Cooked ☞ serving size: 1 cup, cubes = 166 g; Calories = 74.7; Total Carb (g) = 13.1; Net Carb (g) = 8.5; Fat (g) = 2.7; Protein = 1.8

⬤ Canned Asparagus ☞ serving size: 1 cup = 242 g; Calories = 46; Total Carb (g) = 6; Net Carb (g) = 2.1; Fat (g) = 1.6; Protein = 5.2

⬤ Canned Green Beans ☞ serving size: 1 cup = 240 g; Calories = 36; Total Carb (g) = 7.9; Net Carb (g) = 4.3; Fat (g) = 0.4; Protein = 1.7

⬤ Canned Lima Beans ☞ serving size: 1 cup = 248 g; Calories = 176.1; Total Carb (g) = 33.1; Net Carb (g) = 24.1; Fat (g) = 0.7; Protein = 10.1

⬤ Canned Mung Bean Sprouts ☞ serving size: 1 cup = 125 g; Calories = 15; Total Carb (g) = 2.7; Net Carb (g) = 1.7; Fat (g) = 0.1; Protein = 1.8

⬤ Canned Mushrooms ☞ serving size: 1 cup = 156 g; Calories = 39; Total Carb (g) = 7.9; Net Carb (g) = 4.2; Fat (g) = 0.5; Protein = 2.9

⬤ Canned Pimentos ☞ serving size: 1 tbsp = 12 g; Calories = 2.8; Total Carb (g) = 0.6; Net Carb (g) = 0.4; Fat (g) = 0; Protein = 0.1

⬤ Canned Pumpkin ☞ serving size: 1 cup = 245 g; Calories = 83.3; Total Carb (g) = 19.8; Net Carb (g) = 12.7; Fat (g) = 0.7; Protein = 2.7

⬤ Canned Straw Mushrooms ☞ serving size: 1 cup = 182 g; Calories = 58.2; Total Carb (g) = 8.4; Net Carb (g) = 3.9; Fat (g) = 1.2; Protein = 7

⬤ Canned Tomato Paste ☞ serving size: 1/4 cup = 66 g; Calories = 54.1; Total Carb (g) = 12.5; Net Carb (g) = 9.8; Fat (g) = 0.3; Protein = 2.9

⬤ Canned Tomato Puree ☞ serving size: 1 cup = 250 g; Calories = 95; Total Carb (g) = 22.5; Net Carb (g) = 17.7; Fat (g) = 0.5; Protein = 4.1

⬤ Cardoon Raw ☞ serving size: 1 cup, shredded = 178 g; Calories = 30.3; Total Carb (g) = 7.2; Net Carb (g) = 4.4; Fat (g) = 0.2; Protein = 1.3

⬤ Carrot Dehydrated ☞ serving size: 1 cup = 74 g; Calories = 252.3; Total Carb (g) = 58.9; Net Carb (g) = 41.4; Fat (g) = 1.1; Protein = 6

⬤ Carrot Juice Canned ☞ serving size: 1 cup = 236 g; Calories =

94.4; Total Carb (g) = 21.9; Net Carb (g) = 20; Fat (g) = 0.4; Protein = 2.2

● Carrots ☞ serving size: 1 cup chopped = 128 g; Calories = 52.5; Total Carb (g) = 12.3; Net Carb (g) = 8.7; Fat (g) = 0.3; Protein = 1.2

● Carrots Raw Salad ☞ serving size: 1 cup = 175 g; Calories = 364; Total Carb (g) = 30.1; Net Carb (g) = 26; Fat (g) = 27.5; Protein = 2.1

● Carrots Raw Salad With Apples ☞ serving size: 1 cup = 171 g; Calories = 301; Total Carb (g) = 14; Net Carb (g) = 10.4; Fat (g) = 27.3; Protein = 1.4

● Cassava ☞ serving size: 1 cup = 206 g; Calories = 329.6; Total Carb (g) = 78.4; Net Carb (g) = 74.7; Fat (g) = 0.6; Protein = 2.8

● Cauliflower ☞ serving size: 1 cup chopped (1/2 inch pieces) = 107 g; Calories = 26.8; Total Carb (g) = 5.3; Net Carb (g) = 3.2; Fat (g) = 0.3; Protein = 2.1

● Celeriac ☞ serving size: 1 cup = 156 g; Calories = 65.5; Total Carb (g) = 14.4; Net Carb (g) = 11.5; Fat (g) = 0.5; Protein = 2.3

● Celery ☞ serving size: 1 cup chopped = 101 g; Calories = 14.1; Total Carb (g) = 3; Net Carb (g) = 1.4; Fat (g) = 0.2; Protein = 0.7

● Celtuce ☞ serving size: 1 leaf = 8 g; Calories = 1.4; Total Carb (g) = 0.3; Net Carb (g) = 0.2; Fat (g) = 0; Protein = 0.1

● Chamnamul Cooked Ns As To Fat Added In Cooking ☞ serving size: 1 cup = 151 g; Calories = 126.8; Total Carb (g) = 9.2; Net Carb (g) = 6.2; Fat (g) = 9; Protein = 5

● Channa Saag ☞ serving size: 1 cup = 245 g; Calories = 200.9; Total Carb (g) = 22.6; Net Carb (g) = 14.5; Fat (g) = 9.7; Protein = 9.4

● Chantarelle Mushrooms ☞ serving size: 1 cup = 54 g; Calories = 17.3; Total Carb (g) = 3.7; Net Carb (g) = 1.7; Fat (g) = 0.3; Protein = 0.8

● Chard Cooked Ns As To Fat Added In Cooking ☞ serving size: 1

cup, stalk and leaves = 150 g; Calories = 54; Total Carb (g) = 6; Net Carb (g) = 3; Fat (g) = 3; Protein = 2.8

⬤ Chard Swiss Cooked Boiled Drained With Salt ☞ serving size: 1 cup, chopped = 175 g; Calories = 35; Total Carb (g) = 7.2; Net Carb (g) = 3.6; Fat (g) = 0.1; Protein = 3.3

⬤ Chayote Fruit Raw ☞ serving size: 1 cup (1 inch pieces) = 132 g; Calories = 25.1; Total Carb (g) = 6; Net Carb (g) = 3.7; Fat (g) = 0.2; Protein = 1.1

⬤ Chicory Greens ☞ serving size: 1 cup, chopped = 29 g; Calories = 6.7; Total Carb (g) = 1.4; Net Carb (g) = 0.2; Fat (g) = 0.1; Protein = 0.5

⬤ Chicory Roots ☞ serving size: 1 root = 60 g; Calories = 43.2; Total Carb (g) = 10.5; Net Carb (g) = 9.6; Fat (g) = 0.1; Protein = 0.8

⬤ Chives ☞ serving size: 1 tbsp chopped = 3 g; Calories = 0.9; Total Carb (g) = 0.1; Net Carb (g) = 0.1; Fat (g) = 0; Protein = 0.1

⬤ Christophine Cooked Ns As To Fat Added In Cooking ☞ serving size: 1 cup = 165 g; Calories = 69.3; Total Carb (g) = 8.1; Net Carb (g) = 3.7; Fat (g) = 4.2; Protein = 1

⬤ Chrysanthemum ☞ serving size: 1 cup (1 inch pieces) = 25 g; Calories = 6; Total Carb (g) = 0.8; Net Carb (g) = 0; Fat (g) = 0.1; Protein = 0.8

⬤ Chrysanthemum Leaves ☞ serving size: 1 cup, chopped = 51 g; Calories = 12.2; Total Carb (g) = 1.5; Net Carb (g) = 0; Fat (g) = 0.3; Protein = 1.7

⬤ Cilantro ☞ serving size: 1/4 cup = 4 g; Calories = 0.9; Total Carb (g) = 0.2; Net Carb (g) = 0; Fat (g) = 0; Protein = 0.1

⬤ Citronella (Lemon Grass) ☞ serving size: 1 cup = 67 g; Calories = 66.3; Total Carb (g) = 17; Net Carb (g) = 17; Fat (g) = 0.3; Protein = 1.2

⬤ Cobb Salad No Dressing ☞ serving size: 1 cup = 105 g; Calories =

96.6; Total Carb (g) = 2.6; Net Carb (g) = 1.3; Fat (g) = 4.6; Protein = 11.9

⬤ Collards ☞ serving size: 1 cup, chopped = 36 g; Calories = 11.5; Total Carb (g) = 2; Net Carb (g) = 0.5; Fat (g) = 0.2; Protein = 1.1

⬤ Cooked Acorn Squash ☞ serving size: 1 cup, mashed = 245 g; Calories = 83.3; Total Carb (g) = 21.5; Net Carb (g) = 15.2; Fat (g) = 0.2; Protein = 1.6

⬤ Cooked Artichokes (Globe Or French) ☞ serving size: 1 cup = 168 g; Calories = 75.6; Total Carb (g) = 15.4; Net Carb (g) = 7.7; Fat (g) = 0.8; Protein = 5.2

⬤ Cooked Beet Greens ☞ serving size: 1 cup (1 inch pieces) = 144 g; Calories = 38.9; Total Carb (g) = 7.9; Net Carb (g) = 3.7; Fat (g) = 0.3; Protein = 3.7

⬤ Cooked Beets ☞ serving size: 1/2 cup slices = 85 g; Calories = 37.4; Total Carb (g) = 8.5; Net Carb (g) = 6.8; Fat (g) = 0.2; Protein = 1.4

⬤ Cooked Broccoli Raab ☞ serving size: 1 nlea serving = 85 g; Calories = 21.3; Total Carb (g) = 2.7; Net Carb (g) = 0.3; Fat (g) = 0.4; Protein = 3.3

⬤ Cooked Burdock Root ☞ serving size: 1 cup (1 inch pieces) = 125 g; Calories = 110; Total Carb (g) = 26.4; Net Carb (g) = 24.2; Fat (g) = 0.2; Protein = 2.6

⬤ Cooked Butternut Squash ☞ serving size: 1 cup, cubes = 205 g; Calories = 82; Total Carb (g) = 21.5; Net Carb (g) = 14.9; Fat (g) = 0.2; Protein = 1.9

⬤ Cooked Cabbage ☞ serving size: 1/2 cup, shredded = 75 g; Calories = 17.3; Total Carb (g) = 4.1; Net Carb (g) = 2.7; Fat (g) = 0.1; Protein = 1

⬤ Cooked Carrots ☞ serving size: 1 tbsp = 9.7 g; Calories = 3.4; Total Carb (g) = 0.8; Net Carb (g) = 0.5; Fat (g) = 0; Protein = 0.1

● Cooked Cauliflower ☞ serving size: 1/2 cup (1 inch pieces) = 62 g; Calories = 14.3; Total Carb (g) = 2.6; Net Carb (g) = 1.1; Fat (g) = 0.3; Protein = 1.1

● Cooked Celeriac ☞ serving size: 1 cup pieces = 155 g; Calories = 41.9; Total Carb (g) = 9.2; Net Carb (g) = 7.3; Fat (g) = 0.3; Protein = 1.5

● Cooked Celery ☞ serving size: 1 cup, diced = 150 g; Calories = 27; Total Carb (g) = 6; Net Carb (g) = 3.6; Fat (g) = 0.2; Protein = 1.3

● Cooked Chayote ☞ serving size: 1 cup (1 inch pieces) = 160 g; Calories = 38.4; Total Carb (g) = 8.1; Net Carb (g) = 3.7; Fat (g) = 0.8; Protein = 1

● Cooked Chinese Broccoli ☞ serving size: 1 cup = 88 g; Calories = 19.4; Total Carb (g) = 3.4; Net Carb (g) = 1.2; Fat (g) = 0.6; Protein = 1

● Cooked Chrysanthemum ☞ serving size: 1 cup (1 inch pieces) = 100 g; Calories = 20; Total Carb (g) = 4.3; Net Carb (g) = 2; Fat (g) = 0.1; Protein = 1.6

● Cooked Collards ☞ serving size: 1 cup, chopped = 190 g; Calories = 62.7; Total Carb (g) = 10.7; Net Carb (g) = 3.1; Fat (g) = 1.4; Protein = 5.2

● Cooked Crookneck Summer Squash ☞ serving size: 1 cup, sliced = 180 g; Calories = 34.2; Total Carb (g) = 6.8; Net Carb (g) = 4.8; Fat (g) = 0.7; Protein = 1.9

● Cooked Dandelion Greens ☞ serving size: 1 cup, chopped = 105 g; Calories = 34.7; Total Carb (g) = 6.7; Net Carb (g) = 3.7; Fat (g) = 0.6; Protein = 2.1

● Cooked Eggplant ☞ serving size: 1 cup (1 inch cubes) = 99 g; Calories = 34.7; Total Carb (g) = 8.6; Net Carb (g) = 6.2; Fat (g) = 0.2; Protein = 0.8

● Cooked Escarole ☞ serving size: 1 cup = 150 g; Calories = 22.5; Total Carb (g) = 4.6; Net Carb (g) = 0.4; Fat (g) = 0.3; Protein = 1.7

● Cooked Garden Cress ☞ serving size: 1 cup = 135 g; Calories = 31.1; Total Carb (g) = 5.1; Net Carb (g) = 4.2; Fat (g) = 0.8; Protein = 2.6

● Cooked Green Beans (Previously Frozen) ☞ serving size: 1 cup = 135 g; Calories = 37.8; Total Carb (g) = 8.7; Net Carb (g) = 4.7; Fat (g) = 0.2; Protein = 2

● Cooked Green Bell Peppers ☞ serving size: 1 cup, chopped or strips = 135 g; Calories = 37.8; Total Carb (g) = 9.1; Net Carb (g) = 7.4; Fat (g) = 0.3; Protein = 1.2

● Cooked Green Cauliflower ☞ serving size: 1/5 head = 90 g; Calories = 28.8; Total Carb (g) = 5.7; Net Carb (g) = 2.7; Fat (g) = 0.3; Protein = 2.7

● Cooked Green Peas ☞ serving size: 1 cup = 160 g; Calories = 134.4; Total Carb (g) = 25; Net Carb (g) = 16.2; Fat (g) = 0.4; Protein = 8.6

● Cooked Green Peas (Salted) ☞ serving size: 1 cup = 160 g; Calories = 134.4; Total Carb (g) = 25; Net Carb (g) = 16.2; Fat (g) = 0.4; Protein = 8.6

● Cooked Green Snap Beans ☞ serving size: 1 cup = 125 g; Calories = 43.8; Total Carb (g) = 9.9; Net Carb (g) = 5.9; Fat (g) = 0.4; Protein = 2.4

● Cooked Hawaiin Mountain Yam ☞ serving size: 1 cup, cubes = 145 g; Calories = 118.9; Total Carb (g) = 29; Net Carb (g) = 29; Fat (g) = 0.1; Protein = 2.5

● Cooked Hubbard Squash ☞ serving size: 1 cup, cubes = 205 g; Calories = 102.5; Total Carb (g) = 22.2; Net Carb (g) = 12.1; Fat (g) = 1.3; Protein = 5.1

● Cooked Kale ☞ serving size: 1 cup, chopped = 130 g; Calories = 46.8; Total Carb (g) = 6.9; Net Carb (g) = 1.7; Fat (g) = 1.6; Protein = 3.8

● Cooked Kohlrabi ☞ serving size: 1 cup slices = 165 g; Calories = 47.9; Total Carb (g) = 11; Net Carb (g) = 9.2; Fat (g) = 0.2; Protein = 3

● Cooked Leeks ☞ serving size: 1 leek = 124 g; Calories = 38.4; Total Carb (g) = 9.5; Net Carb (g) = 8.2; Fat (g) = 0.3; Protein = 1

#VALUE!

● Cooked Lima Beans ☞ serving size: 1 cup = 170 g; Calories = 209.1; Total Carb (g) = 40.2; Net Carb (g) = 31; Fat (g) = 0.5; Protein = 11.6

● Cooked Lotus Root ☞ serving size: 1/2 cup = 60 g; Calories = 39.6; Total Carb (g) = 9.6; Net Carb (g) = 7.8; Fat (g) = 0; Protein = 1

● Cooked Malabar Spinach ☞ serving size: 1 cup = 44 g; Calories = 10.1; Total Carb (g) = 1.2; Net Carb (g) = 0.3; Fat (g) = 0.3; Protein = 1.3

● Cooked Mustard Greens ☞ serving size: 1 cup, chopped = 140 g; Calories = 36.4; Total Carb (g) = 6.3; Net Carb (g) = 3.5; Fat (g) = 0.7; Protein = 3.6

● Cooked Mustard Spinach ☞ serving size: 1 cup, chopped = 180 g; Calories = 28.8; Total Carb (g) = 5; Net Carb (g) = 1.4; Fat (g) = 0.4; Protein = 3.1

● Cooked Napa Cabbage ☞ serving size: 1 cup = 109 g; Calories = 13.1; Total Carb (g) = 2.4; Net Carb (g) = 2.4; Fat (g) = 0.2; Protein = 1.2

● Cooked New Zealand Spinach ☞ serving size: 1 cup, chopped = 180 g; Calories = 21.6; Total Carb (g) = 3.8; Net Carb (g) = 1.3; Fat (g) = 0.3; Protein = 2.3

● Cooked Nopales ☞ serving size: 1 cup = 149 g; Calories = 22.4; Total Carb (g) = 4.9; Net Carb (g) = 1.9; Fat (g) = 0.1; Protein = 2

● Cooked Okra ☞ serving size: 1/2 cup slices = 80 g; Calories = 17.6; Total Carb (g) = 3.6; Net Carb (g) = 1.6; Fat (g) = 0.2; Protein = 1.5

● Cooked Okra (Previously Frozen) ☞ serving size: 1/2 cup slices = 92 g; Calories = 26.7; Total Carb (g) = 5.9; Net Carb (g) = 4; Fat (g) = 0.2; Protein = 1.5

● Cooked Onions ☞ serving size: 1 cup = 210 g; Calories = 92.4; Total Carb (g) = 21.3; Net Carb (g) = 18.4; Fat (g) = 0.4; Protein = 2.9

● Cooked Oriental Radishes ☞ serving size: 1 cup, sliced = 147 g; Calories = 25; Total Carb (g) = 5; Net Carb (g) = 2.7; Fat (g) = 0.4; Protein = 1

● Cooked Parsnips ☞ serving size: 1/2 cup slices = 78 g; Calories = 55.4; Total Carb (g) = 13.3; Net Carb (g) = 10.5; Fat (g) = 0.2; Protein = 1

● Cooked Podded Peas ☞ serving size: 1 cup = 160 g; Calories = 83.2; Total Carb (g) = 14.4; Net Carb (g) = 9.5; Fat (g) = 0.6; Protein = 5.6

● Cooked Pumpkin ☞ serving size: 1 cup, mashed = 245 g; Calories = 49; Total Carb (g) = 12; Net Carb (g) = 9.3; Fat (g) = 0.2; Protein = 1.8

● Cooked Pumpkin Flowers ☞ serving size: 1 cup = 134 g; Calories = 20.1; Total Carb (g) = 4.4; Net Carb (g) = 3.2; Fat (g) = 0.1; Protein = 1.5

● Cooked Purslane ☞ serving size: 1 cup = 115 g; Calories = 20.7; Total Carb (g) = 4.1; Net Carb (g) = 4.1; Fat (g) = 0.2; Protein = 1.7

● Cooked Red Bell Peppers ☞ serving size: 1 cup, strips = 135 g; Calories = 37.8; Total Carb (g) = 9.1; Net Carb (g) = 7.4; Fat (g) = 0.3; Protein = 1.2

● Cooked Red Cabbage ☞ serving size: 1 leaf = 22 g; Calories = 6.4; Total Carb (g) = 1.5; Net Carb (g) = 1; Fat (g) = 0; Protein = 0.3

● Cooked Rutabagas (Neeps Swedes) ☞ serving size: 1 cup, cubes = 170 g; Calories = 51; Total Carb (g) = 11.6; Net Carb (g) = 8.6; Fat (g) = 0.3; Protein = 1.6

● Cooked Savoy Cabbage ☞ serving size: 1 cup, shredded = 145 g; Calories = 34.8; Total Carb (g) = 7.8; Net Carb (g) = 3.8; Fat (g) = 0.1; Protein = 2.6

● Cooked Scallop Squash ☞ serving size: 1 cup, mashed = 240 g;

Calories = 38.4; Total Carb (g) = 7.9; Net Carb (g) = 3.4; Fat (g) = 0.4; Protein = 2.5

● Cooked Shiitake Mushrooms ☞ serving size: 1 cup pieces = 145 g; Calories = 81.2; Total Carb (g) = 20.9; Net Carb (g) = 17.8; Fat (g) = 0.3; Protein = 2.3

● Cooked Snow Peas ☞ serving size: 1 cup = 160 g; Calories = 67.2; Total Carb (g) = 11.3; Net Carb (g) = 6.8; Fat (g) = 0.4; Protein = 5.2

● Cooked Soybean Sprouts ☞ serving size: 1 cup = 94 g; Calories = 76.1; Total Carb (g) = 6.1; Net Carb (g) = 5.4; Fat (g) = 4.2; Protein = 8

● Cooked Spaghetti Squash ☞ serving size: 1 cup = 155 g; Calories = 41.9; Total Carb (g) = 10; Net Carb (g) = 7.8; Fat (g) = 0.4; Protein = 1

● Cooked Spinach ☞ serving size: 1 cup = 180 g; Calories = 41.4; Total Carb (g) = 6.8; Net Carb (g) = 2.4; Fat (g) = 0.5; Protein = 5.4

● Cooked Summer Squash ☞ serving size: 1 cup, sliced = 180 g; Calories = 36; Total Carb (g) = 7.8; Net Carb (g) = 5.2; Fat (g) = 0.6; Protein = 1.6

● Cooked Swamp Cabbage ☞ serving size: 1 cup, chopped = 98 g; Calories = 19.6; Total Carb (g) = 3.6; Net Carb (g) = 1.8; Fat (g) = 0.2; Protein = 2

● Cooked Sweet Potatoes ☞ serving size: 1 cup = 200 g; Calories = 180; Total Carb (g) = 41.4; Net Carb (g) = 34.8; Fat (g) = 0.3; Protein – 4

● Cooked Sweet White Corn ☞ serving size: 1 ear, small (5-1/2 inch to 6-1/2 inch long) = 89 g; Calories = 86.3; Total Carb (g) = 19.3; Net Carb (g) = 16.9; Fat (g) = 1.3; Protein = 3

● Cooked Swiss Chard ☞ serving size: 1 cup, chopped = 175 g; Calories = 35; Total Carb (g) = 7.2; Net Carb (g) = 3.6; Fat (g) = 0.1; Protein = 3.3

● Cooked Tahitian Taro ☞ serving size: 1 cup slices = 137 g; Calo-

ries = 60.3; Total Carb (g) = 9.4; Net Carb (g) = 9.4; Fat (g) = 0.9; Protein = 5.7

● Cooked Taro ☞ serving size: 1 cup, sliced = 132 g; Calories = 187.4; Total Carb (g) = 45.7; Net Carb (g) = 38.9; Fat (g) = 0.2; Protein = 0.7

● Cooked Tomatoes ☞ serving size: 1 cup = 240 g; Calories = 43.2; Total Carb (g) = 9.6; Net Carb (g) = 7.9; Fat (g) = 0.3; Protein = 2.3

● Cooked Turnip Greens ☞ serving size: 1 cup, chopped = 144 g; Calories = 28.8; Total Carb (g) = 6.3; Net Carb (g) = 1.2; Fat (g) = 0.3; Protein = 1.6

● Cooked Turnips ☞ serving size: 1 cup, cubes = 156 g; Calories = 34.3; Total Carb (g) = 7.9; Net Carb (g) = 4.8; Fat (g) = 0.1; Protein = 1.1

● Cooked White Button Mushrooms ☞ serving size: 1 cup pieces = 156 g; Calories = 43.7; Total Carb (g) = 8.3; Net Carb (g) = 4.8; Fat (g) = 0.7; Protein = 3.4

● Cooked Winter Squash ☞ serving size: 1 cup, cubes = 205 g; Calories = 75.9; Total Carb (g) = 18.1; Net Carb (g) = 12.4; Fat (g) = 0.7; Protein = 1.8

● Cooked Yam ☞ serving size: 1 cup, cubes = 136 g; Calories = 157.8; Total Carb (g) = 37.4; Net Carb (g) = 32.1; Fat (g) = 0.2; Protein = 2

● Cooked Yellow Snap Beans ☞ serving size: 1 cup = 125 g; Calories = 43.8; Total Carb (g) = 9.9; Net Carb (g) = 5.7; Fat (g) = 0.4; Protein = 2.4

● Cooked Yellow Sweet Corn ☞ serving size: 1 ear small (5-1/2 inch to 6-1/2 inch long) = 89 g; Calories = 85.4; Total Carb (g) = 18.7; Net Carb (g) = 16.5; Fat (g) = 1.3; Protein = 3

● Cooked Zucchini ☞ serving size: 1 cup, sliced = 180 g; Calories = 27; Total Carb (g) = 4.8; Net Carb (g) = 3; Fat (g) = 0.7; Protein = 2.1

● Corn Dried Cooked ☞ serving size: 1 oz = 28 g; Calories = 30.5; Total Carb (g) = 4.3; Net Carb (g) = 3.8; Fat (g) = 1.5; Protein = 0.6

● Corn Fritter ☞ serving size: 1 cup = 107 g; Calories = 421.6; Total Carb (g) = 43.7; Net Carb (g) = 41.3; Fat (g) = 24.2; Protein = 8.8

● Corn From Canned Ns As To Color Cream Style ☞ serving size: 1 cup = 256 g; Calories = 184.3; Total Carb (g) = 46.3; Net Carb (g) = 43.3; Fat (g) = 1.1; Protein = 4.5

● Corn Ns As To Form Ns As To Color Cream Style ☞ serving size: 1 cup = 256 g; Calories = 184.3; Total Carb (g) = 46.2; Net Carb (g) = 43.2; Fat (g) = 1.1; Protein = 4.4

● Corn Yellow Whole Kernel Frozen Microwaved ☞ serving size: 1 cup = 141 g; Calories = 159.3; Total Carb (g) = 36.5; Net Carb (g) = 32.8; Fat (g) = 2; Protein = 5.1

● Cornsalad Raw ☞ serving size: 1 cup = 56 g; Calories = 11.8; Total Carb (g) = 2; Net Carb (g) = 2; Fat (g) = 0.2; Protein = 1.1

● Cowpeas (Blackeyes) Immature Seeds Raw ☞ serving size: 1 cup = 145 g; Calories = 130.5; Total Carb (g) = 27.3; Net Carb (g) = 20.1; Fat (g) = 0.5; Protein = 4.3

● Cremini Mushrooms ☞ serving size: 1 cup whole = 87 g; Calories = 19.1; Total Carb (g) = 3.7; Net Carb (g) = 3.2; Fat (g) = 0.1; Protein = 2.2

● Cress Cooked Ns As To Form Ns As To Fat Added In Cooking ☞ serving size: 1 cup = 140 g; Calories = 61.6; Total Carb (g) = 5.1; Net Carb (g) = 4.1; Fat (g) = 4.2; Protein = 2.6

● Cress Garden Cooked Boiled Drained With Salt ☞ serving size: 1 cup = 135 g; Calories = 31.1; Total Carb (g) = 5.1; Net Carb (g) = 4.2; Fat (g) = 0.8; Protein = 2.6

● Crookneck Summer Squash ☞ serving size: 1 cup sliced = 127 g; Calories = 24.1; Total Carb (g) = 4.9; Net Carb (g) = 3.7; Fat (g) = 0.3; Protein = 1.3

● Cucumber ☞ serving size: 1/2 cup slices = 52 g; Calories = 7.8; Total Carb (g) = 1.9; Net Carb (g) = 1.6; Fat (g) = 0.1; Protein = 0.3

● Cucumber Peeled Raw ☞ serving size: 1 cup, pared, chopped = 133 g; Calories = 13.3; Total Carb (g) = 2.9; Net Carb (g) = 1.9; Fat (g) = 0.2; Protein = 0.8

● Dandelion Greens ☞ serving size: 1 cup, chopped = 55 g; Calories = 24.8; Total Carb (g) = 5.1; Net Carb (g) = 3.1; Fat (g) = 0.4; Protein = 1.5

● Dasheen Boiled ☞ serving size: 1 cup, pieces = 142 g; Calories = 200.2; Total Carb (g) = 48.8; Net Carb (g) = 41.6; Fat (g) = 0.2; Protein = 0.7

● Dasheen Fried ☞ serving size: 1 cup, pieces = 123 g; Calories = 311.2; Total Carb (g) = 52.7; Net Carb (g) = 44.9; Fat (g) = 10.9; Protein = 0.8

● Dock Raw ☞ serving size: 1 cup, chopped = 133 g; Calories = 29.3; Total Carb (g) = 4.3; Net Carb (g) = 0.4; Fat (g) = 0.9; Protein = 2.7

● Dried Ancho Peppers ☞ serving size: 1 pepper = 17 g; Calories = 47.8; Total Carb (g) = 8.7; Net Carb (g) = 5.1; Fat (g) = 1.4; Protein = 2

● Dried Chives ☞ serving size: 1 tbsp = 0.2 g; Calories = 0.6; Total Carb (g) = 0.1; Net Carb (g) = 0.1; Fat (g) = 0; Protein = 0

● Dried Fungi Cloud Ears ☞ serving size: 1 cup = 28 g; Calories = 79.5; Total Carb (g) = 20.4; Net Carb (g) = 0.8; Fat (g) = 0.2; Protein = 2.6

● Dried Pasilla Peppers ☞ serving size: 1 pepper = 7 g; Calories = 24.2; Total Carb (g) = 3.6; Net Carb (g) = 1.7; Fat (g) = 1.1; Protein = 0.9

● Dried Shiitake Mushrooms ☞ serving size: 1 mushroom = 3.6 g; Calories = 10.7; Total Carb (g) = 2.7; Net Carb (g) = 2.3; Fat (g) = 0; Protein = 0.3

● Dried Spirulina Seaweed ☞ serving size: 1 cup = 112 g; Calories = 324.8; Total Carb (g) = 26.8; Net Carb (g) = 22.7; Fat (g) = 8.7; Protein = 64.4

● Drumstick Pods Raw ☞ serving size: 1 cup slices = 100 g; Calories = 37; Total Carb (g) = 8.5; Net Carb (g) = 5.3; Fat (g) = 0.2; Protein = 2.1

● Edamame Frozen Unprepared ☞ serving size: 1 cup = 118 g; Calories = 128.6; Total Carb (g) = 9; Net Carb (g) = 3.3; Fat (g) = 5.6; Protein = 13.2

● Egg Curry ☞ serving size: 1 cup = 236 g; Calories = 184.1; Total Carb (g) = 16.7; Net Carb (g) = 12.7; Fat (g) = 10.2; Protein = 7.9

● Eggplant ☞ serving size: 1 cup, cubes = 82 g; Calories = 20.5; Total Carb (g) = 4.8; Net Carb (g) = 2.4; Fat (g) = 0.2; Protein = 0.8

● Endive ☞ serving size: 1/2 cup, chopped = 25 g; Calories = 4.3; Total Carb (g) = 0.8; Net Carb (g) = 0.1; Fat (g) = 0.1; Protein = 0.3

● Enoki Mushrooms ☞ serving size: 1 large = 5 g; Calories = 1.9; Total Carb (g) = 0.4; Net Carb (g) = 0.3; Fat (g) = 0; Protein = 0.1

● Epazote Raw ☞ serving size: 1 tbsp = 0.8 g; Calories = 0.3; Total Carb (g) = 0.1; Net Carb (g) = 0; Fat (g) = 0; Protein = 0

● Eppaw Raw ☞ serving size: 1 cup = 100 g; Calories = 150; Total Carb (g) = 31.7; Net Carb (g) = 31.7; Fat (g) = 1.8; Protein = 4.6

● Escarole Cooked Ns As To Fat Added In Cooking ☞ serving size: 1 cup = 135 g; Calories = 63.5; Total Carb (g) = 4; Net Carb (g) = 0.3; Fat (g) = 4.6; Protein = 1.5

● Fennel ☞ serving size: 1 cup, sliced = 87 g; Calories = 27; Total Carb (g) = 6.4; Net Carb (g) = 3.7; Fat (g) = 0.2; Protein = 1.1

● Fireweed Leaves Raw ☞ serving size: 1 cup, chopped = 23 g; Calories = 23.7; Total Carb (g) = 4.4; Net Carb (g) = 2; Fat (g) = 0.6; Protein = 1.1

● Flowers Or Blossoms Of Sesbania Squash Or Lily Ns As To Fat Added In Cooking ☞ serving size: 1 cup = 109 g; Calories = 39.2; Total Carb (g) = 3.5; Net Carb (g) = 2.5; Fat (g) = 2.8; Protein = 1.2

● Freeze-Dried Parsley ☞ serving size: 1 tbsp = 0.4 g; Calories = 1.1; Total Carb (g) = 0.2; Net Carb (g) = 0; Fat (g) = 0; Protein = 0.1

● Garden Cress ☞ serving size: 1 cup = 50 g; Calories = 16; Total Carb (g) = 2.8; Net Carb (g) = 2.2; Fat (g) = 0.4; Protein = 1.3

● Garlic ☞ serving size: 1 cup = 136 g; Calories = 202.6; Total Carb (g) = 45; Net Carb (g) = 42.1; Fat (g) = 0.7; Protein = 8.7

● Ginger ☞ serving size: 1 tsp = 2 g; Calories = 1.6; Total Carb (g) = 0.4; Net Carb (g) = 0.3; Fat (g) = 0; Protein = 0

● Ginger Root Pickled Canned With Artificial Sweetener ☞ serving size: 2 tablespoon = 25 g; Calories = 5; Total Carb (g) = 1.2; Net Carb (g) = 0.6; Fat (g) = 0; Protein = 0.1

● Gourd Dishcloth (Towelgourd) Raw ☞ serving size: 1 cup (1 inch pieces) = 95 g; Calories = 19; Total Carb (g) = 4.1; Net Carb (g) = 3.1; Fat (g) = 0.2; Protein = 1.1

● Gourd White-Flowered (Calabash) Raw ☞ serving size: 1/2 cup (1 inch pieces) = 58 g; Calories = 8.1; Total Carb (g) = 2; Net Carb (g) = 1.7; Fat (g) = 0; Protein = 0.4

● Grape Leaves Canned ☞ serving size: 1 leaf = 4 g; Calories = 2.8; Total Carb (g) = 0.5; Net Carb (g) = 0.1; Fat (g) = 0.1; Protein = 0.2

● Grape Leaves Raw ☞ serving size: 1 cup = 14 g; Calories = 13; Total Carb (g) = 2.4; Net Carb (g) = 0.9; Fat (g) = 0.3; Protein = 0.8

● Green Banana Cooked In Salt Water ☞ serving size: 1 small = 54 g; Calories = 47.5; Total Carb (g) = 12.3; Net Carb (g) = 10.9; Fat (g) = 0.2; Protein = 0.6

● Green Banana Fried ☞ serving size: 1 slice = 23 g; Calories = 33.8; Total Carb (g) = 5.5; Net Carb (g) = 4.9; Fat (g) = 1.5; Protein = 0.3

● Green Bell Peppers ☞ serving size: 1 cup, chopped = 149 g; Calories = 29.8; Total Carb (g) = 6.9; Net Carb (g) = 4.4; Fat (g) = 0.3; Protein = 1.3

● Green Cauliflower ☞ serving size: 1 cup = 64 g; Calories = 19.8; Total Carb (g) = 3.9; Net Carb (g) = 1.9; Fat (g) = 0.2; Protein = 1.9

● Green Chili Peppers ☞ serving size: 1 cup = 139 g; Calories = 29.2; Total Carb (g) = 6.4; Net Carb (g) = 4; Fat (g) = 0.4; Protein = 1

● Green Leaf Lettuce ☞ serving size: 1 cup shredded = 36 g; Calories = 5.4; Total Carb (g) = 1; Net Carb (g) = 0.6; Fat (g) = 0.1; Protein = 0.5

● Green Plantains Boiled ☞ serving size: 1 slice = 27 g; Calories = 31.3; Total Carb (g) = 8.4; Net Carb (g) = 7.8; Fat (g) = 0.1; Protein = 0.2

● Green Snap Beans (Raw) ☞ serving size: 1 cup 1/2 inch pieces = 100 g; Calories = 31; Total Carb (g) = 7; Net Carb (g) = 4.3; Fat (g) = 0.2; Protein = 1.8

● Green Tomatoes ☞ serving size: 1 cup = 180 g; Calories = 41.4; Total Carb (g) = 9.2; Net Carb (g) = 7.2; Fat (g) = 0.4; Protein = 2.2

● Greens Cooked Ns As To Form Ns As To Fat Added In Cooking ☞ serving size: 1 cup = 151 g; Calories = 69.5; Total Carb (g) = 7.7; Net Carb (g) = 2.8; Fat (g) = 3.9; Protein = 2.9

● Homemade Mashed Potatoes With Milk And Butter ☞ serving size: 1 cup = 210 g; Calories = 237.3; Total Carb (g) = 35.3; Net Carb (g) = 32.2; Fat (g) = 8.9; Protein = 3.9

● Hot Green Chili Peppers ☞ serving size: 1 pepper = 45 g; Calories = 18; Total Carb (g) = 4.3; Net Carb (g) = 3.6; Fat (g) = 0.1; Protein = 0.9

● Hubbard Squash ☞ serving size: 1 cup, cubes = 116 g; Calories = 46.4; Total Carb (g) = 10.1; Net Carb (g) = 5.6; Fat (g) = 0.6; Protein = 2.3

● Hungarian Peppers ☞ serving size: 1 pepper = 27 g; Calories = 7.8; Total Carb (g) = 1.8; Net Carb (g) = 1.5; Fat (g) = 0.1; Protein = 0.2

● Hyacinth-Beans Immature Seeds Raw ☞ serving size: 1 cup = 80

g; Calories = 36.8; Total Carb (g) = 7.4; Net Carb (g) = 4.7; Fat (g) = 0.2; Protein = 1.7

● Iceberg Lettuce ☞ serving size: 1 cup shredded = 72 g; Calories = 10.1; Total Carb (g) = 2.1; Net Carb (g) = 1.3; Fat (g) = 0.1; Protein = 0.7

● Irishmoss Seaweed ☞ serving size: 2 tbsp (1/8 cup) = 10 g; Calories = 4.9; Total Carb (g) = 1.2; Net Carb (g) = 1.1; Fat (g) = 0; Protein = 0.2

● Jai Monk's Food ☞ serving size: 1 cup = 188 g; Calories = 167.3; Total Carb (g) = 28.9; Net Carb (g) = 24.2; Fat (g) = 3.7; Protein = 9.6

● Jalapeno Peppers ☞ serving size: 1 cup, sliced = 90 g; Calories = 26.1; Total Carb (g) = 5.9; Net Carb (g) = 3.3; Fat (g) = 0.3; Protein = 0.8

● Jerusalem-Artichokes Raw ☞ serving size: 1 cup slices = 150 g; Calories = 109.5; Total Carb (g) = 26.2; Net Carb (g) = 23.8; Fat (g) = 0; Protein = 3

● Jews Ear ☞ serving size: 1 cup slices = 99 g; Calories = 24.8; Total Carb (g) = 6.7; Net Carb (g) = 6.7; Fat (g) = 0; Protein = 0.5

● Jute Potherb Raw ☞ serving size: 1 cup = 28 g; Calories = 9.5; Total Carb (g) = 1.6; Net Carb (g) = 1.6; Fat (g) = 0.1; Protein = 1.3

● Kale ☞ serving size: 1 cup 1 inch pieces, loosely packed = 16 g; Calories = 5.6; Total Carb (g) = 0.7; Net Carb (g) = 0.1; Fat (g) = 0.2; Protein = 0.5

● Kale Frozen Unprepared ☞ serving size: 1/3 package (10 oz) = 94 g; Calories = 26.3; Total Carb (g) = 4.6; Net Carb (g) = 2.7; Fat (g) = 0.4; Protein = 2.5

● Kanpyo ☞ serving size: 1 strip = 6.3 g; Calories = 16.3; Total Carb (g) = 4.1; Net Carb (g) = 3.5; Fat (g) = 0; Protein = 0.5

● Kelp Seaweed ☞ serving size: 2 tbsp (1/8 cup) = 10 g; Calories = 4.3; Total Carb (g) = 1; Net Carb (g) = 0.8; Fat (g) = 0.1; Protein = 0.2

⬤ Ketchup ☞ serving size: 1 tbsp = 17 g; Calories = 17.2; Total Carb (g) = 4.7; Net Carb (g) = 4.6; Fat (g) = 0; Protein = 0.2

⬤ Kidney Bean Sprouts ☞ serving size: 1 cup = 184 g; Calories = 53.4; Total Carb (g) = 7.5; Net Carb (g) = 7.5; Fat (g) = 0.9; Protein = 7.7

⬤ Kimchi ☞ serving size: 1 cup = 150 g; Calories = 22.5; Total Carb (g) = 3.6; Net Carb (g) = 1.2; Fat (g) = 0.8; Protein = 1.7

⬤ Kohlrabi ☞ serving size: 1 cup = 135 g; Calories = 36.5; Total Carb (g) = 8.4; Net Carb (g) = 3.5; Fat (g) = 0.1; Protein = 2.3

⬤ Lambsquarters Cooked Boiled Drained Without Salt ☞ serving size: 1 cup, chopped = 180 g; Calories = 57.6; Total Carb (g) = 9; Net Carb (g) = 5.2; Fat (g) = 1.3; Protein = 5.8

#VALUE!

⬤ Laver Seaweed ☞ serving size: 10 sheets = 26 g; Calories = 9.1; Total Carb (g) = 1.3; Net Carb (g) = 1.3; Fat (g) = 0.1; Protein = 1.5

⬤ Leek Cooked Ns As To Fat Added In Cooking ☞ serving size: 1 leek (about 6-3/4" long, 1" dia) = 84 g; Calories = 69.7; Total Carb (g) = 12.1; Net Carb (g) = 10.6; Fat (g) = 2.2; Protein = 1.3

⬤ Leeks ☞ serving size: 1 cup = 89 g; Calories = 54.3; Total Carb (g) = 12.6; Net Carb (g) = 11; Fat (g) = 0.3; Protein = 1.3

⬤ Lentil Sprouts ☞ serving size: 1 cup = 77 g; Calories = 81.6; Total Carb (g) = 17.1; Net Carb (g) = 17.1; Fat (g) = 0.4; Protein = 6.9

⬤ Lettuce Cooked Ns As To Fat Added In Cooking ☞ serving size: 1 cup = 86 g; Calories = 43; Total Carb (g) = 3.7; Net Carb (g) = 2.2; Fat (g) = 3; Protein = 1.1

⬤ Lima Beans Immature Seeds Raw ☞ serving size: 1 cup = 156 g; Calories = 176.3; Total Carb (g) = 31.5; Net Carb (g) = 23.8; Fat (g) = 1.3; Protein = 10.7

⬤ Lotus Root ☞ serving size: 10 slices (2-1/2 inch dia) = 81 g; Calories = 59.9; Total Carb (g) = 14; Net Carb (g) = 10; Fat (g) = 0.1; Protein = 2.1

● Low Sodium Ketchup ☞ serving size: 1 tbsp = 17 g; Calories = 17.2; Total Carb (g) = 4.7; Net Carb (g) = 4.6; Fat (g) = 0; Protein = 0.2

● Low Sodium Sour Pickles ☞ serving size: 1 cup, chopped or diced = 143 g; Calories = 15.7; Total Carb (g) = 3.2; Net Carb (g) = 1.5; Fat (g) = 0.3; Protein = 0.5

● Low Sodium Sweet Pickles ☞ serving size: 1 slice = 6 g; Calories = 7.3; Total Carb (g) = 2; Net Carb (g) = 2; Fat (g) = 0; Protein = 0

● Luffa Cooked Ns As To Fat Added In Cooking ☞ serving size: 1 cup = 183 g; Calories = 84.2; Total Carb (g) = 8; Net Carb (g) = 3.6; Fat (g) = 5.4; Protein = 3.3

● Maitake Mushrooms ☞ serving size: 1 cup diced = 70 g; Calories = 21.7; Total Carb (g) = 4.9; Net Carb (g) = 3; Fat (g) = 0.1; Protein = 1.4

● Mashed Sweet Potatoes ☞ serving size: 1 cup = 255 g; Calories = 257.6; Total Carb (g) = 59.1; Net Carb (g) = 54.8; Fat (g) = 0.5; Protein = 5.1

● Mixed Vegetables Cooked Ns As To Form Fat Added In Cooking Ns As To Type Of Fat ☞ serving size: 1 cup = 187 g; Calories = 147.7; Total Carb (g) = 23.8; Net Carb (g) = 15.7; Fat (g) = 3.7; Protein = 5.2

● Mixed Vegetables Cooked Ns As To Form Fat Not Added In Cooking ☞ serving size: 1 cup = 182 g; Calories = 118.3; Total Carb (g) = 23.7; Net Carb (g) = 15.7; Fat (g) = 0.3; Protein = 5.2

● Mixed Vegetables Cooked Ns As To Form Made With Butter ☞ serving size: 1 cup = 187 g; Calories = 151.5; Total Carb (g) = 23.7; Net Carb (g) = 15.7; Fat (g) = 4.1; Protein = 5.2

● Mixed Vegetables Cooked Ns As To Form Made With Margarine ☞ serving size: 1 cup = 187 g; Calories = 144; Total Carb (g) = 23.8; Net Carb (g) = 15.7; Fat (g) = 3.1; Protein = 5.2

● Mixed Vegetables Cooked Ns As To Form Made With Oil ☞ serving size: 1 cup = 187 g; Calories = 159; Total Carb (g) = 23.8; Net Carb (g) = 15.7; Fat (g) = 4.8; Protein = 5.2

● Mixed Vegetables Cooked Ns As To Form Ns As To Fat Added In Cooking ☞ serving size: 1 cup = 187 g; Calories = 147.7; Total Carb (g) = 23.8; Net Carb (g) = 15.7; Fat (g) = 3.7; Protein = 5.2

● Morel Mushrooms ☞ serving size: 1 cup = 66 g; Calories = 20.5; Total Carb (g) = 3.4; Net Carb (g) = 1.5; Fat (g) = 0.4; Protein = 2.1

● Mountain Yam Hawaii Raw ☞ serving size: 1/2 cup, cubes = 68 g; Calories = 45.6; Total Carb (g) = 11.1; Net Carb (g) = 9.4; Fat (g) = 0.1; Protein = 0.9

● Mung Bean Sprouts ☞ serving size: 1 cup = 104 g; Calories = 31.2; Total Carb (g) = 6.2; Net Carb (g) = 4.3; Fat (g) = 0.2; Protein = 3.2

● Mushroom Asian Cooked From Dried ☞ serving size: 1 cup = 145 g; Calories = 81.2; Total Carb (g) = 20.7; Net Carb (g) = 17.7; Fat (g) = 0.3; Protein = 2.3

● Mushrooms Portobellos Grilled ☞ serving size: 1 cup sliced = 121 g; Calories = 35.1; Total Carb (g) = 5.4; Net Carb (g) = 2.7; Fat (g) = 0.7; Protein = 4

● Mushrooms Shiitake Cooked With Salt ☞ serving size: 1 cup pieces = 145 g; Calories = 81.2; Total Carb (g) = 20.9; Net Carb (g) = 17.8; Fat (g) = 0.3; Protein = 2.3

● Mushrooms Shiitake Stir-Fried ☞ serving size: 1 cup whole = 89 g; Calories = 34.7; Total Carb (g) = 6.8; Net Carb (g) = 3.6; Fat (g) = 0.3; Protein = 3.1

● Mushrooms Stuffed ☞ serving size: 1 stuffed cap = 24 g; Calories = 67.2; Total Carb (g) = 6.5; Net Carb (g) = 6; Fat (g) = 3.6; Protein = 2.6

● Mushrooms White Cooked Boiled Drained With Salt ☞ serving size: 1 cup pieces = 156 g; Calories = 43.7; Total Carb (g) = 8.3; Net Carb (g) = 4.8; Fat (g) = 0.7; Protein = 3.4

● Mustard Cabbage Cooked Ns As To Fat Added In Cooking ☞ serving size: 1 cup = 175 g; Calories = 50.8; Total Carb (g) = 3; Net Carb (g) = 1.3; Fat (g) = 3.7; Protein = 2.7

● Mustard Greens ☞ serving size: 1 cup, chopped = 56 g; Calories = 15.1; Total Carb (g) = 2.6; Net Carb (g) = 0.8; Fat (g) = 0.2; Protein = 1.6

● Mustard Greens Frozen Unprepared ☞ serving size: 1 cup, chopped = 146 g; Calories = 29.2; Total Carb (g) = 5; Net Carb (g) = 0.2; Fat (g) = 0.4; Protein = 3.6

● Mustard Spinach ☞ serving size: 1 cup, chopped = 150 g; Calories = 33; Total Carb (g) = 5.9; Net Carb (g) = 1.7; Fat (g) = 0.5; Protein = 3.3

● Nopales ☞ serving size: 1 cup, sliced = 86 g; Calories = 13.8; Total Carb (g) = 2.9; Net Carb (g) = 1; Fat (g) = 0.1; Protein = 1.1

● Okra ☞ serving size: 1 cup = 100 g; Calories = 33; Total Carb (g) = 7.5; Net Carb (g) = 4.3; Fat (g) = 0.2; Protein = 1.9

● Okra Cooked Ns As To Form Ns As To Fat Added In Cooking ☞ serving size: 1 cup = 189 g; Calories = 83.2; Total Carb (g) = 11.8; Net Carb (g) = 8; Fat (g) = 3.9; Protein = 3

● Onion Rings Breaded Par Fried Frozen Unprepared ☞ serving size: 6 rings = 85 g; Calories = 219.3; Total Carb (g) = 26; Net Carb (g) = 24.4; Fat (g) = 12; Protein = 2.7

● Onion Rings From Fresh Batter-Dipped Baked Or Fried ☞ serving size: 10 small rings (1" - 2" dia) = 48 g; Calories = 157.4; Total Carb (g) = 15.2; Net Carb (g) = 14.4; Fat (g) = 9.3; Protein = 3.3

● Onions ☞ serving size: 1 cup, chopped = 160 g; Calories = 64; Total Carb (g) = 14.9; Net Carb (g) = 12.2; Fat (g) = 0.2; Protein = 1.8

● Onions Canned Solids And Liquids ☞ serving size: 1 onion = 63 g; Calories = 12; Total Carb (g) = 2.5; Net Carb (g) = 1.8; Fat (g) = 0.1; Protein = 0.5

● Onions Cooked Ns As To Form Ns As To Fat Added In Cooking
☞ serving size: 1 cup = 215 g; Calories = 86; Total Carb (g) = 13.9; Net
Carb (g) = 10; Fat (g) = 3.2; Protein = 1.6

● Onions Dehydrated Flakes ☞ serving size: 1 tbsp = 5 g; Calories
= 17.5; Total Carb (g) = 4.2; Net Carb (g) = 3.7; Fat (g) = 0; Protein = 0.5

● Onions Pearl Cooked Ns As To Form ☞ serving size: 1 cup = 185
g; Calories = 51.8; Total Carb (g) = 12.3; Net Carb (g) = 9.8; Fat (g) =
0.1; Protein = 1.3

#VALUE!

● Oriental Radishes ☞ serving size: 1 cup slices = 116 g; Calories =
20.9; Total Carb (g) = 4.8; Net Carb (g) = 2.9; Fat (g) = 0.1; Protein =
0.7

● Oyster Mushrooms ☞ serving size: 1 large = 148 g; Calories =
48.8; Total Carb (g) = 9; Net Carb (g) = 5.6; Fat (g) = 0.6; Protein = 4.9

● Palm Hearts (Canned) ☞ serving size: 1 cup = 146 g; Calories =
40.9; Total Carb (g) = 6.8; Net Carb (g) = 3.2; Fat (g) = 0.9; Protein =
3.7

● Palm Hearts Cooked Assume Fat Not Added In Cooking ☞
serving size: 1 cup = 146 g; Calories = 166.4; Total Carb (g) = 37.2; Net
Carb (g) = 35; Fat (g) = 0.3; Protein = 3.9

● Parsley ☞ serving size: 1 cup chopped = 60 g; Calories = 21.6;
Total Carb (g) = 3.8; Net Carb (g) = 1.8; Fat (g) = 0.5; Protein = 1.8

● Parsnips ☞ serving size: 1 cup slices = 133 g; Calories = 99.8; Total
Carb (g) = 23.9; Net Carb (g) = 17.4; Fat (g) = 0.4; Protein = 1.6

● Pea Sprouts ☞ serving size: 1 cup = 120 g; Calories = 148.8; Total
Carb (g) = 32.5; Net Carb (g) = 32.5; Fat (g) = 0.8; Protein = 10.6

● Peas ☞ serving size: 1 cup = 145 g; Calories = 117.5; Total Carb (g)
= 21; Net Carb (g) = 12.7; Fat (g) = 0.6; Protein = 7.9

● Peas Ns As To Form Creamed ☞ serving size: 1 cup = 244 g;

Calories = 263.5; Total Carb (g) = 29.3; Net Carb (g) = 23; Fat (g) = 11.7; Protein = 11.2

● Pepeao Dried ☞ serving size: 1 cup = 24 g; Calories = 71.5; Total Carb (g) = 19.5; Net Carb (g) = 19.5; Fat (g) = 0.1; Protein = 1.2

● Pepper Raw Nfs ☞ serving size: 1 piece = 10 g; Calories = 2.4; Total Carb (g) = 0.5; Net Carb (g) = 0.3; Fat (g) = 0; Protein = 0.1

● Pepper Sweet Red Raw ☞ serving size: 1 piece = 10 g; Calories = 3.1; Total Carb (g) = 0.6; Net Carb (g) = 0.4; Fat (g) = 0; Protein = 0.1

● Peppers Green Cooked Fat Added In Cooking Ns As To Type Of Fat ☞ serving size: 1 piece = 6 g; Calories = 2.9; Total Carb (g) = 0.4; Net Carb (g) = 0.3; Fat (g) = 0.2; Protein = 0.1

● Peppers Sweet Red Cooked Boiled Drained With Salt ☞ serving size: 1 tbsp = 12 g; Calories = 3.1; Total Carb (g) = 0.7; Net Carb (g) = 0.6; Fat (g) = 0; Protein = 0.1

● Pickled Beets ☞ serving size: 1 cup slices = 227 g; Calories = 147.6; Total Carb (g) = 37; Net Carb (g) = 35.1; Fat (g) = 0.2; Protein = 1.8

● Pickles Chowchow With Cauliflower Onion Mustard Sweet ☞ serving size: 1 cup = 245 g; Calories = 296.5; Total Carb (g) = 65.3; Net Carb (g) = 61.6; Fat (g) = 2.2; Protein = 3.7

● Pigeonpeas Immature Seeds Raw ☞ serving size: 1 cup = 154 g; Calories = 209.4; Total Carb (g) = 36.8; Net Carb (g) = 28.9; Fat (g) = 2.5; Protein = 11.1

● Pinacbet ☞ serving size: 1 cup = 214 g; Calories = 96.3; Total Carb (g) = 11.3; Net Carb (g) = 8.8; Fat (g) = 5.4; Protein = 2.3

● Plantain Boiled Ns As To Green Or Ripe ☞ serving size: 1 slice = 27 g; Calories = 31.3; Total Carb (g) = 8.4; Net Carb (g) = 7.8; Fat (g) = 0.1; Protein = 0.2

● Plantain Fried Ns As To Green Or Ripe ☞ serving size: 1 slice =

27 g; Calories = 65.1; Total Carb (g) = 11; Net Carb (g) = 10.2; Fat (g) = 2.7; Protein = 0.5

⬤ Plantain Ripe Rolled In Flour Fried ☞ serving size: 1 piece (2-1/2" long) = 45 g; Calories = 110.3; Total Carb (g) = 16.4; Net Carb (g) = 15.3; Fat (g) = 5.4; Protein = 0.9

⬤ Poi ☞ serving size: 1 cup = 240 g; Calories = 268.8; Total Carb (g) = 65.4; Net Carb (g) = 64.4; Fat (g) = 0.3; Protein = 0.9

⬤ Potato Boiled Nfs ☞ serving size: 1 baby potato = 60 g; Calories = 75; Total Carb (g) = 12.3; Net Carb (g) = 11.4; Fat (g) = 2.5; Protein = 1.1

⬤ Potato Boiled Ready-To-Heat ☞ serving size: 1 baby potato = 60 g; Calories = 75; Total Carb (g) = 12.3; Net Carb (g) = 11.4; Fat (g) = 2.5; Protein = 1.1

⬤ Potato Flour ☞ serving size: 1 cup = 160 g; Calories = 571.2; Total Carb (g) = 133; Net Carb (g) = 123.5; Fat (g) = 0.5; Protein = 11

⬤ Potato Nfs ☞ serving size: 1 baby potato = 60 g; Calories = 75; Total Carb (g) = 12.3; Net Carb (g) = 11.4; Fat (g) = 2.5; Protein = 1.1

⬤ Pumpkin Cooked Ns As To Form Ns As To Fat Added In Cooking ☞ serving size: 1 cup, mashed = 250 g; Calories = 80; Total Carb (g) = 12; Net Carb (g) = 9.3; Fat (g) = 3.6; Protein = 1.8

⬤ Pumpkin Flowers ☞ serving size: 1 cup = 33 g; Calories = 5; Total Carb (g) = 1.1; Net Carb (g) = 1.1; Fat (g) = 0; Protein = 0.3

⬤ Pumpkin Leaves Cooked Boiled Drained With Salt ☞ serving size: 1 cup = 71 g; Calories = 14.9; Total Carb (g) = 2.4; Net Carb (g) = 0.5; Fat (g) = 0.2; Protein = 1.9

⬤ Pumpkin Raw ☞ serving size: 1 cup (1 inch cubes) = 116 g; Calories = 30.2; Total Carb (g) = 7.5; Net Carb (g) = 7; Fat (g) = 0.1; Protein = 1.2

⬤ Purslane ☞ serving size: 1 cup = 43 g; Calories = 8.6; Total Carb (g) = 1.5; Net Carb (g) = 1.5; Fat (g) = 0.2; Protein = 0.9

● Radicchio ☞ serving size: 1 cup, shredded = 40 g; Calories = 9.2; Total Carb (g) = 1.8; Net Carb (g) = 1.4; Fat (g) = 0.1; Protein = 0.6

● Radish Daikon Cooked Ns As To Fat Added In Cooking ☞ serving size: 1 cup = 153 g; Calories = 65.8; Total Carb (g) = 5.1; Net Carb (g) = 2.8; Fat (g) = 4.9; Protein = 1

● Radish Sprouts ☞ serving size: 1 cup = 38 g; Calories = 16.3; Total Carb (g) = 1.4; Net Carb (g) = 1.4; Fat (g) = 1; Protein = 1.5

● Radishes ☞ serving size: 1 cup slices = 116 g; Calories = 18.6; Total Carb (g) = 3.9; Net Carb (g) = 2.1; Fat (g) = 0.1; Protein = 0.8

● Radishes Hawaiian Style Pickled ☞ serving size: 1 cup = 150 g; Calories = 42; Total Carb (g) = 7.8; Net Carb (g) = 4.5; Fat (g) = 0.5; Protein = 1.7

● Radishes Oriental Cooked Boiled Drained With Salt ☞ serving size: 1 cup slices = 147 g; Calories = 25; Total Carb (g) = 5; Net Carb (g) = 2.7; Fat (g) = 0.4; Protein = 1

● Radishes Oriental Dried ☞ serving size: 1 cup = 116 g; Calories = 314.4; Total Carb (g) = 73.5; Net Carb (g) = 45.8; Fat (g) = 0.8; Protein = 9.2

● Ratatouille ☞ serving size: 1 cup = 214 g; Calories = 139.1; Total Carb (g) = 12.8; Net Carb (g) = 9.4; Fat (g) = 9.8; Protein = 2.1

● Rutabaga Cooked Ns As To Fat Added In Cooking ☞ serving size: 1 cup, pieces = 175 g; Calories = 80.5; Total Carb (g) = 11.6; Net Carb (g) = 8.6; Fat (g) = 3.7; Protein = 1.6

● Rutabagas (Neeps Swedes) ☞ serving size: 1 cup, cubes = 140 g; Calories = 51.8; Total Carb (g) = 12.1; Net Carb (g) = 8.9; Fat (g) = 0.2; Protein = 1.5

● Rutabagas Cooked Boiled Drained With Salt ☞ serving size: 1/2 cup, mashed = 120 g; Calories = 36; Total Carb (g) = 8.2; Net Carb (g) = 6.1; Fat (g) = 0.2; Protein = 1.1

● Salsify (Vegetable Oyster) Raw ☞ serving size: 1 cup slices = 133 g; Calories = 109.1; Total Carb (g) = 24.7; Net Carb (g) = 20.4; Fat (g) = 0.3; Protein = 4.4

● Sambar Vegetable Stew ☞ serving size: 1 cup = 248 g; Calories = 208.3; Total Carb (g) = 28.8; Net Carb (g) = 19.1; Fat (g) = 6.6; Protein = 10.7

● Sauerkraut ☞ serving size: 1 cup = 142 g; Calories = 27; Total Carb (g) = 6.1; Net Carb (g) = 2; Fat (g) = 0.2; Protein = 1.3

● Sauteed Green Bell Peppers ☞ serving size: 1 cup chopped = 115 g; Calories = 133.4; Total Carb (g) = 4.9; Net Carb (g) = 2.8; Fat (g) = 13.6; Protein = 0.9

● Savoy Cabbage ☞ serving size: 1 cup, shredded = 70 g; Calories = 18.9; Total Carb (g) = 4.3; Net Carb (g) = 2.1; Fat (g) = 0.1; Protein = 1.4

● Scallop Squash ☞ serving size: 1 cup slices = 130 g; Calories = 23.4; Total Carb (g) = 5; Net Carb (g) = 3.4; Fat (g) = 0.3; Protein = 1.6

● Seaweed Agar Raw ☞ serving size: 2 tbsp (1/8 cup) = 10 g; Calories = 2.6; Total Carb (g) = 0.7; Net Carb (g) = 0.6; Fat (g) = 0; Protein = 0.1

● Seaweed Canadian Cultivated Emi-Tsunomata Dry ☞ serving size: 1/4 cup = 5 g; Calories = 13; Total Carb (g) = 2.3; Net Carb (g) = 0.5; Fat (g) = 0.1; Protein = 0.8

● Seaweed Canadian Cultivated Emi-Tsunomata Rehydrated ☞ serving size: 1/4 cup = 25 g; Calories = 7.8; Total Carb (g) = 1.4; Net Carb (g) = 0.3; Fat (g) = 0; Protein = 0.5

● Seaweed Cooked Fat Added In Cooking Ns As To Type Of Fat ☞ serving size: 1 cup = 96 g; Calories = 58.6; Total Carb (g) = 4.7; Net Carb (g) = 4.4; Fat (g) = 3.2; Protein = 5.4

● Seaweed Cooked Made With Butter ☞ serving size: 1 cup = 96 g; Calories = 53.8; Total Carb (g) = 4.7; Net Carb (g) = 4.4; Fat (g) = 2.7; Protein = 5.4

● Seaweed Cooked Made With Oil ☞ serving size: 1 cup = 96 g; Calories = 58.6; Total Carb (g) = 4.7; Net Carb (g) = 4.4; Fat (g) = 3.2; Protein = 5.4

● Seaweed Cooked Ns As To Fat Added In Cooking ☞ serving size: 1 cup = 96 g; Calories = 58.6; Total Carb (g) = 4.7; Net Carb (g) = 4.4; Fat (g) = 3.2; Protein = 5.4

● Seaweed Raw ☞ serving size: 1 cup = 80 g; Calories = 30.4; Total Carb (g) = 6.7; Net Carb (g) = 6.1; Fat (g) = 0.2; Protein = 1.9

● Serrano Peppers ☞ serving size: 1 cup, chopped = 105 g; Calories = 33.6; Total Carb (g) = 7; Net Carb (g) = 3.2; Fat (g) = 0.5; Protein = 1.8

● Sesbania Flower Cooked Steamed With Salt ☞ serving size: 1 cup = 104 g; Calories = 21.8; Total Carb (g) = 5.3; Net Carb (g) = 5.3; Fat (g) = 0.1; Protein = 1.2

● Sesbania Flower Cooked Steamed Without Salt ☞ serving size: 1 cup = 104 g; Calories = 22.9; Total Carb (g) = 5.4; Net Carb (g) = 5.4; Fat (g) = 0.1; Protein = 1.2

● Sesbania Flower Raw ☞ serving size: 1 flower = 3 g; Calories = 0.8; Total Carb (g) = 0.2; Net Carb (g) = 0.2; Fat (g) = 0; Protein = 0

● Seven-Layer Salad Lettuce Salad Made With A Combination Of Onion Celery Green Pepper Peas Mayonnaise Cheese Eggs And/or Bacon ☞ serving size: 1 cup = 119 g; Calories = 270.1; Total Carb (g) = 6.7; Net Carb (g) = 5.1; Fat (g) = 24.6; Protein = 5.7

● Shallots ☞ serving size: 1 tbsp chopped = 10 g; Calories = 7.2; Total Carb (g) = 1.7; Net Carb (g) = 1.4; Fat (g) = 0; Protein = 0.3

● Shallots Freeze-Dried ☞ serving size: 1 tbsp = 0.9 g; Calories = 3.1; Total Carb (g) = 0.7; Net Carb (g) = 0.6; Fat (g) = 0; Protein = 0.1

● Shiitake Mushrooms ☞ serving size: 1 piece whole = 19 g; Calories = 6.5; Total Carb (g) = 1.3; Net Carb (g) = 0.8; Fat (g) = 0.1; Protein = 0.4

● Snow Peas ☞ serving size: 1 cup, chopped = 98 g; Calories = 41.2; Total Carb (g) = 7.4; Net Carb (g) = 4.9; Fat (g) = 0.2; Protein = 2.7

● Sour Pickled Cucumber ☞ serving size: 1 cup = 155 g; Calories = 17.1; Total Carb (g) = 3.5; Net Carb (g) = 1.6; Fat (g) = 0.3; Protein = 0.5

● Soybean Sprouts ☞ serving size: 1/2 cup = 35 g; Calories = 42.7; Total Carb (g) = 3.4; Net Carb (g) = 3; Fat (g) = 2.4; Protein = 4.6

● Spaghetti Squash ☞ serving size: 1 cup, cubes = 101 g; Calories = 31.3; Total Carb (g) = 7; Net Carb (g) = 5.5; Fat (g) = 0.6; Protein = 0.7

● Spinach ☞ serving size: 1 cup = 30 g; Calories = 6.9; Total Carb (g) = 1.1; Net Carb (g) = 0.4; Fat (g) = 0.1; Protein = 0.9

● Spring Onions ☞ serving size: 1 cup, chopped = 100 g; Calories = 32; Total Carb (g) = 7.3; Net Carb (g) = 4.7; Fat (g) = 0.2; Protein = 1.8

● Squash Fritter Or Cake ☞ serving size: 1 fritter = 24 g; Calories = 86.2; Total Carb (g) = 8.6; Net Carb (g) = 7.9; Fat (g) = 5.1; Protein = 1.7

● Squash Spaghetti Cooked Ns As To Fat Added In Cooking ☞ serving size: 1 cup, cooked = 160 g; Calories = 72; Total Carb (g) = 10; Net Carb (g) = 7.8; Fat (g) = 3.8; Protein = 1.1

● Squash Summer All Varieties Cooked Boiled Drained With Salt ☞ serving size: 1 cup slices = 180 g; Calories = 36; Total Carb (g) = 7.8; Net Carb (g) = 5.2; Fat (g) = 0.6; Protein = 1.6

● Summer Squash ☞ serving size: 1 cup, sliced = 113 g; Calories = 18.1; Total Carb (g) = 3.8; Net Carb (g) = 2.5; Fat (g) = 0.2; Protein = 1.4

● Sun-Dried Hot Chile Peppers ☞ serving size: 1 cup = 37 g; Calories = 119.9; Total Carb (g) = 25.9; Net Carb (g) = 15.2; Fat (g) = 2.2; Protein = 3.9

● Sun-Dried Tomatoes ☞ serving size: 1 cup = 54 g; Calories = 139.3; Total Carb (g) = 30.1; Net Carb (g) = 23.5; Fat (g) = 1.6; Protein = 7.6

● Swamp Cabbage ☞ serving size: 1 cup, chopped = 56 g; Calories

= 10.6; Total Carb (g) = 1.8; Net Carb (g) = 0.6; Fat (g) = 0.1; Protein = 1.5

● Swamp Cabbage (Skunk Cabbage) Cooked Boiled Drained With Salt ☞ serving size: 1 cup, chopped = 98 g; Calories = 19.6; Total Carb (g) = 3.6; Net Carb (g) = 1.8; Fat (g) = 0.2; Protein = 2

● Sweet Onions ☞ serving size: 1 nlea serving = 148 g; Calories = 47.4; Total Carb (g) = 11.2; Net Carb (g) = 9.8; Fat (g) = 0.1; Protein = 1.2

● Sweet Pickled Cucumbers ☞ serving size: 1 cup, chopped = 160 g; Calories = 145.6; Total Carb (g) = 33.8; Net Carb (g) = 32.2; Fat (g) = 0.7; Protein = 0.9

● Sweet Pickled Relish ☞ serving size: 1 tbsp = 15 g; Calories = 19.5; Total Carb (g) = 5.3; Net Carb (g) = 5.1; Fat (g) = 0.1; Protein = 0.1

● Sweet Potato And Pumpkin Casserole Puerto Rican Style ☞ serving size: 1 cup = 266 g; Calories = 601.2; Total Carb (g) = 106.2; Net Carb (g) = 100.3; Fat (g) = 18.5; Protein = 8

● Sweet Potato Baked Peel Eaten Fat Added In Cooking Ns As To Type Of Fat ☞ serving size: 1 small = 80 g; Calories = 100; Total Carb (g) = 16.7; Net Carb (g) = 14; Fat (g) = 3.2; Protein = 1.6

● Sweet Potato Boiled Ns As To Fat Added In Cooking ☞ serving size: 1 small = 80 g; Calories = 86.4; Total Carb (g) = 13.5; Net Carb (g) = 11.5; Fat (g) = 3.4; Protein = 1.1

● Sweet Potato Candied ☞ serving size: 1 piece = 45 g; Calories = 80.1; Total Carb (g) = 16.9; Net Carb (g) = 16.1; Fat (g) = 1.4; Protein = 0.5

● Sweet Potatoes ☞ serving size: 1 cup, cubes = 133 g; Calories = 114.4; Total Carb (g) = 26.8; Net Carb (g) = 22.8; Fat (g) = 0.1; Protein = 2.1

● Sweet Red Bell Peppers ☞ serving size: 1 cup, chopped = 149 g; Calories = 38.7; Total Carb (g) = 9; Net Carb (g) = 5.9; Fat (g) = 0.5; Protein = 1.5

● Sweet White Corn ☞ serving size: 1 ear, small (5-1/2 inch to 6-1/2 inch long) = 73 g; Calories = 62.8; Total Carb (g) = 13.9; Net Carb (g) = 11.9; Fat (g) = 0.9; Protein = 2.4

● Sweet Yellow Peppers ☞ serving size: 1 pepper, large (3-3/4 inch long, 3 inch dia) = 186 g; Calories = 50.2; Total Carb (g) = 11.8; Net Carb (g) = 10.1; Fat (g) = 0.4; Protein = 1.9

● Swiss Chard ☞ serving size: 1 cup = 36 g; Calories = 6.8; Total Carb (g) = 1.4; Net Carb (g) = 0.8; Fat (g) = 0.1; Protein = 0.7

● Tahitian Taro ☞ serving size: 1 cup slices = 125 g; Calories = 55; Total Carb (g) = 8.6; Net Carb (g) = 8.6; Fat (g) = 1.2; Protein = 3.5

● Tannier Cooked ☞ serving size: 1 cup = 190 g; Calories = 290.7; Total Carb (g) = 68.7; Net Carb (g) = 58.1; Fat (g) = 0.5; Protein = 3.9

● Tannier Fritters Puerto Rican Style ☞ serving size: 1 fritter (2-1/2" x 1-1/2"x 1/2") = 20 g; Calories = 46.8; Total Carb (g) = 5.5; Net Carb (g) = 4.7; Fat (g) = 2.2; Protein = 1.3

● Taro ☞ serving size: 1 cup, sliced = 104 g; Calories = 116.5; Total Carb (g) = 27.5; Net Carb (g) = 23.3; Fat (g) = 0.2; Protein = 1.6

● Thistle Leaves Cooked Ns As To Fat Added In Cooking ☞ serving size: 1 cup = 185 g; Calories = 81.4; Total Carb (g) = 6.8; Net Carb (g) = 5.5; Fat (g) = 5.6; Protein = 3.4

● Tomatillos ☞ serving size: 1 medium = 34 g; Calories = 10.9; Total Carb (g) = 2; Net Carb (g) = 1.3; Fat (g) = 0.4; Protein = 0.3

● Tomato And Onion Cooked Ns As To Fat Added In Cooking ☞ serving size: 1 cup = 242 g; Calories = 87.1; Total Carb (g) = 12.8; Net Carb (g) = 10.8; Fat (g) = 3.8; Protein = 2.5

● Tomato And Vegetable Juice Low Sodium ☞ serving size: 1 cup = 242 g; Calories = 53.2; Total Carb (g) = 11.1; Net Carb (g) = 9.2; Fat (g) = 0.2; Protein = 1.5

● Tomato Aspic ☞ serving size: 1 cup = 227 g; Calories = 63.6; Total Carb (g) = 10.7; Net Carb (g) = 10; Fat (g) = 0.6; Protein = 5.8

● Tomato Juice Canned With Salt Added ☞ serving size: 1 cup = 243 g; Calories = 41.3; Total Carb (g) = 8.6; Net Carb (g) = 7.6; Fat (g) = 0.7; Protein = 2.1

● Tomato Juice Canned Without Salt Added ☞ serving size: 1 cup = 243 g; Calories = 41.3; Total Carb (g) = 8.6; Net Carb (g) = 7.6; Fat (g) = 0.7; Protein = 2.1

● Tomato Products Canned Puree With Salt Added ☞ serving size: 1 cup = 250 g; Calories = 95; Total Carb (g) = 22.5; Net Carb (g) = 17.7; Fat (g) = 0.5; Protein = 4.1

● Tomato Products Canned Sauce ☞ serving size: 1 cup = 245 g; Calories = 58.8; Total Carb (g) = 13; Net Carb (g) = 9.3; Fat (g) = 0.7; Protein = 2.9

● Tomatoes ☞ serving size: 1 cup cherry tomatoes = 149 g; Calories = 26.8; Total Carb (g) = 5.8; Net Carb (g) = 4; Fat (g) = 0.3; Protein = 1.3

● Tomatoes Cooked From Fresh Ns As To Method ☞ serving size: 1 cup = 240 g; Calories = 43.2; Total Carb (g) = 9.6; Net Carb (g) = 7.9; Fat (g) = 0.3; Protein = 2.3

● Tomatoes Cooked Ns As To Form Ns As To Method ☞ serving size: 1 small = 82 g; Calories = 14.8; Total Carb (g) = 3.3; Net Carb (g) = 2.7; Fat (g) = 0.1; Protein = 0.8

● Tomatoes Sun-Dried Packed In Oil Drained ☞ serving size: 1 cup = 110 g; Calories = 234.3; Total Carb (g) = 25.7; Net Carb (g) = 19.3; Fat (g) = 15.5; Protein = 5.6

● Turnip Cooked Ns As To Form Ns As To Fat Added In Cooking ☞ serving size: 1 cup, pieces = 160 g; Calories = 65.6; Total Carb (g) = 6.7; Net Carb (g) = 3.7; Fat (g) = 3.8; Protein = 2.4

● Turnip Greens ☞ serving size: 1 cup, chopped = 55 g; Calories = 17.6; Total Carb (g) = 3.9; Net Carb (g) = 2.2; Fat (g) = 0.2; Protein = 0.8

● Vegetable Juice Bolthouse Farms Daily Greens ☞ serving size: 1 cup = 269 g; Calories = 83.4; Total Carb (g) = 21.9; Net Carb (g) = 16.8; Fat (g) = 0.1; Protein = 1.3

● Vegetable Juice Cocktail Canned ☞ serving size: 1 cup = 253 g; Calories = 55.7; Total Carb (g) = 9.8; Net Carb (g) = 8.5; Fat (g) = 0.8; Protein = 2.4

● Vegetable Juice Cocktail Low Sodium Canned ☞ serving size: 1 cup = 254 g; Calories = 48.3; Total Carb (g) = 9.7; Net Carb (g) = 8.5; Fat (g) = 0.8; Protein = 2.3

● Vegetable Stew Without Meat ☞ serving size: 1 cup = 239 g; Calories = 133.8; Total Carb (g) = 23; Net Carb (g) = 18.7; Fat (g) = 2.3; Protein = 6.4

● Vegetable Tempura ☞ serving size: 1 cup = 63 g; Calories = 147.4; Total Carb (g) = 12.8; Net Carb (g) = 11.8; Fat (g) = 9.9; Protein = 2.3

● Wakame ☞ serving size: 2 tbsp (1/8 cup) = 10 g; Calories = 4.5; Total Carb (g) = 0.9; Net Carb (g) = 0.9; Fat (g) = 0.1; Protein = 0.3

● Wasabi Root ☞ serving size: 1 cup, sliced = 130 g; Calories = 141.7; Total Carb (g) = 30.6; Net Carb (g) = 20.5; Fat (g) = 0.8; Protein = 6.2

● Water Chestnut ☞ serving size: 1 cup = 158 g; Calories = 123.2; Total Carb (g) = 30.4; Net Carb (g) = 24.2; Fat (g) = 0.1; Protein = 2.2

● Waterchestnuts Chinese (Matai) Raw ☞ serving size: 1/2 cup slices = 62 g; Calories = 60.1; Total Carb (g) = 14.8; Net Carb (g) = 13; Fat (g) = 0.1; Protein = 0.9

● Waterchestnuts Chinese Canned Solids And Liquids ☞ serving size: 1/2 cup slices = 70 g; Calories = 35; Total Carb (g) = 8.6; Net Carb (g) = 6.9; Fat (g) = 0; Protein = 0.6

● Watercress ☞ serving size: 1 cup, chopped = 34 g; Calories = 3.7; Total Carb (g) = 0.4; Net Carb (g) = 0.3; Fat (g) = 0; Protein = 0.8

● Waxgourd (Chinese Preserving Melon) Raw ☞ serving size: 1

cup, cubes = 132 g; Calories = 17.2; Total Carb (g) = 4; Net Carb (g) = 0.1; Fat (g) = 0.3; Protein = 0.5

● White Button Mushrooms ☞ serving size: 1 cup, pieces or slices = 70 g; Calories = 15.4; Total Carb (g) = 2.3; Net Carb (g) = 1.6; Fat (g) = 0.2; Protein = 2.2

● White Button Mushrooms (Stir-Fried) ☞ serving size: 1 cup sliced = 108 g; Calories = 28.1; Total Carb (g) = 4.4; Net Carb (g) = 2.4; Fat (g) = 0.4; Protein = 3.9

● White Icicle Radishes (Daikon) ☞ serving size: 1/2 cup slices = 50 g; Calories = 7; Total Carb (g) = 1.3; Net Carb (g) = 0.6; Fat (g) = 0.1; Protein = 0.6

● Winged Beans Immature Seeds Raw ☞ serving size: 1 cup slices = 44 g; Calories = 21.6; Total Carb (g) = 1.9; Net Carb (g) = 1.9; Fat (g) = 0.4; Protein = 3.1

● Winter Melon Cooked ☞ serving size: 1 cup = 175 g; Calories = 24.5; Total Carb (g) = 5.3; Net Carb (g) = 3.5; Fat (g) = 0.4; Protein = 0.7

● Winter Squash ☞ serving size: 1 cup, cubes = 116 g; Calories = 39.4; Total Carb (g) = 10; Net Carb (g) = 8.2; Fat (g) = 0.2; Protein = 1.1

● Witloof Chicory ☞ serving size: 1 head = 53 g; Calories = 9; Total Carb (g) = 2.1; Net Carb (g) = 0.5; Fat (g) = 0.1; Protein = 0.5

● Yam ☞ serving size: 1 cup, cubes = 150 g; Calories = 177; Total Carb (g) = 41.8; Net Carb (g) = 35.7; Fat (g) = 0.3; Protein = 2.3

● Yambean (Jicama) Raw ☞ serving size: 1 cup slices = 120 g; Calories = 45.6; Total Carb (g) = 10.6; Net Carb (g) = 4.7; Fat (g) = 0.1; Protein = 0.9

● Yardlong Bean Raw ☞ serving size: 1 cup slices = 91 g; Calories = 42.8; Total Carb (g) = 7.6; Net Carb (g) = 7.6; Fat (g) = 0.4; Protein = 2.6

● Yautia ☞ serving size: 1 cup, sliced = 135 g; Calories = 132.3; Total Carb (g) = 31.9; Net Carb (g) = 29.9; Fat (g) = 0.5; Protein = 2

● Yellow Onions ☞ serving size: 1 cup chopped = 87 g; Calories = 107; Total Carb (g) = 6.8; Net Carb (g) = 5.4; Fat (g) = 9.4; Protein = 0.8

● Yellow Snap Beans ☞ serving size: 1 cup 1/2 inch pieces = 100 g; Calories = 31; Total Carb (g) = 7.1; Net Carb (g) = 3.7; Fat (g) = 0.1; Protein = 1.8

● Yellow Sweet Corn ☞ serving size: 1 cup = 145 g; Calories = 124.7; Total Carb (g) = 27.1; Net Carb (g) = 24.2; Fat (g) = 2; Protein = 4.7

● Yellow Tomatoes ☞ serving size: 1 cup, chopped = 139 g; Calories = 20.9; Total Carb (g) = 4.1; Net Carb (g) = 3.2; Fat (g) = 0.4; Protein = 1.4

● Yuca Fries ☞ serving size: 1 cup = 140 g; Calories = 373.8; Total Carb (g) = 48.6; Net Carb (g) = 46.4; Fat (g) = 19.5; Protein = 1.7

● Zucchini ☞ serving size: 1 cup, chopped = 124 g; Calories = 21.1; Total Carb (g) = 3.9; Net Carb (g) = 2.6; Fat (g) = 0.4; Protein = 1.5

HEALTH AND NUTRITION WEBSITES

American Diabetes Association

(www.diabetes.org)

American Heart Association

(www.americanheart.org)

Centers for Disease Control and Prevention

(www.cdc.gov/healthyweight)

Cooking Light

(www.cookinglight.com)

Eating Well

(www.eatingwell.com)

eMedicine Health

(www.emedicinehealth.com)

Fruits and Vegetables Matter

(www.fruitsandveggiesmatter.gov)

Health

(www.health.com)

Hormone Foundation

(www.hormone.org)

National Heart, Lung, Blood Institute

(www.nhlbi.nih.gov)

National Institute on Aging

(www.nia.nih.gov)

National Institutes of Health

(http://health.nih.gov)

Nutrition.gov (www.nutrition.gov)

Prevention (www.prevention.com)

Made in United States
Orlando, FL
04 December 2022

25516926R10430